PEDIATRICS:
A Competency-Based Companion

PEDIATRICS:
A Competency-Based Companion

Maureen C. McMahon MD

Assistant Professor of Pediatrics
Jefferson Medical College
Thomas Jefferson University
Philadelphia, Pennsylvania
General Pediatrician
Nemours/Alfred I. duPont Hospital for Children
Wilmington, Delaware
Lankenau Medical Center, Main Line Health System
Wynnewood, Pennsylvania

Glenn R. Stryjewski MD, MPH

Associate Professor
Department of Pediatrics
Jefferson Medical College
Thomas Jefferson University
Philadelphia, Pennsylvania
Pediatric Intensivist
Nemours/Alfred I. duPont Hospital for Children
Wilmington, Delaware

Series Editor: Barry D. Mann MD, FACS

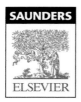

SAUNDERS

ELSEVIER

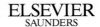

1600 John F. Kennedy Blvd.
Ste 1800
Philadelphia, PA 19103-2899

Notices

Knowledge and best practice in this field are constantly changing. As new research and
experience broaden our understanding, changes in research methods, professional
practices, or medical treatment may become necessary.

Practitioners and researchers must always rely on their own experience and
knowledge in evaluating and using any information, methods, compounds, or
experiments described herein. In using such information or methods, they should be
mindful of their own safety and the safety of others, including parties for whom they
have a professional responsibility.

With respect to any drug or pharmaceutical products identified, readers are advised
to check the most current information provided (i) on procedures featured or (ii) by the
manufacturer of each product to be administered to verify the recommended dose or
formula, the method and duration of administration, and contraindications. It is the
responsibility of practitioners, relying on their own experience and knowledge of their
patients, to make diagnoses, to determine dosages and the best treatment for each
individual patient, and to take all appropriate safety precautions.

To the fullest extent of the law, neither the Publisher nor the authors, contributors,
or editors, assume any liability for any injury and/or damage to persons or property as
a matter of products liability, negligence or otherwise, or from any use or operation of
any methods, products, instructions, or ideas contained in the material herein.

Library of Congress Cataloging-in-Publication Data
Pediatrics : a competency-based companion / [edited by] Maureen McMahon,
Glenn Stryjewski.
      p. ; cm.—(Competency-based companion)
    Includes bibliographical references and index.
    ISBN 978-1-4160-5350-7 (pbk. : alk. paper)
    1. Pediatrics.   2. Clinical competence.   3. Patients—Care.   4. Physician and patient.
I. McMahon, Maureen (Maureen C.)   II. Stryjewski, Glenn.   III. Series: Competency-based
companion.
    [DNLM: 1. Pediatrics.   2. Clinical Competence.   3. Patient Care.   4. Physician—
Patient Relations. WS 21]
    RJ45.P3976 2011
    618.92—dc22

                                                                2011005356

Acquisitions Editor: James Merritt
Developmental Editor: Christine Abshire
Publishing Services Manager: Anne Altepeter
Senior Project Manager: Beth Hayes
Project Manager: Louise King
Design Direction: Louis Forgione

Working together to grow
libraries in developing countries
www.elsevier.com | www.bookaid.org | www.sabre.org

ELSEVIER   BOOK AID International   Sabre Foundation

Printed in China

Last digit is the print number: 9   8   7   6   5   4   3   2   1

Educator's Foreword

Medical education has changed dramatically in recent years. The ultimate goal, to develop a pediatrician who can practice "competently and independently," remains the same. However, the route to this end has been altered. It is no longer adequate to assume that trainees will learn how to care for patients appropriately and gain the necessary medical knowledge for pediatrics just by "showing up" and participating in the daily routine of medical school rotations and residency training. Medical educators must now prove that they have included all of the key components of medical training (the six core competencies) in their programs. They must have evaluation tools to show that their trainees have grasped these concepts. Likewise, one can no longer assume that medical students and pediatric residents will communicate well with patients and families or that they will act professionally in their daily work. Educators must now demonstrate that they have taught and assessed the interpersonal and communication skills and professionalism of their graduates. Furthermore, trainees must now learn to function effectively as part of a larger health-care system and use resources effectively. They must evaluate their own patient care and practice evidence-based medicine.

Changing the culture of medical education is not easy. Medical educators are obligated to change the way students and residents *think*. The six core competencies must be incorporated into the daily lives of trainees so they approach each patient and each challenge in medicine with them in mind.

Pediatrics: A Competency-Based Companion will play a vital role in our changing educational culture. This is not just another traditional textbook. It is instead a unique guide that effectively helps readers to tackle pediatric problems in a systematic manner, with the core competencies in the foreground. The distinctive format encourages trainees to think differently and logically. Whereas many "old" textbooks supply an arsenal of medical information, this comprehensive text covers much more. Practical concepts learned from experience are combined with evidence from scientific studies. Early chapters teach how to succeed as a medical student or a pediatric resident in clinical settings and independent study. Other contributions advise trainees to function as part of a medical team, on inpatient wards and outpatient clinics. Later sections show how to approach an ill child with a specific complaint or medical problem. Each chapter emphasizes what to do first and how to develop a differential diagnosis when confronted with a simple or puzzling case. All chapters remind the reader to treat patients, families, and colleagues with respect and compassion. Authors stress the importance of including the family in medical decisions. The authors and editors are skillful clinicians and talented teachers. They have a wealth of knowledge and experience to share.

This important new book will undoubtedly have a great impact on medical education. I congratulate the authors and editors for having the courage to change our approach to pediatrics. I applaud their effort to modify traditional readings and develop a new thought process, with an eye toward competence in all areas. This book is exceptional and exciting. Our medical students and pediatric residents will be better for it.

Steven M. Selbst MD
Pediatric Residency Program Director
Jefferson Medical College/Nemours/Alfred I. duPont Hospital for Children

Pediatrician's Foreword

In September 1999 the board of the Accreditation Council for Graduate Medical Education (ACGME) approved the Outcome Project. In the decade that has followed there have been significant changes in graduate and undergraduate medical education stimulated by the project. The Outcome Project is a long-term initiative by which the ACGME intended to increase emphasis on educational outcomes. In its role as the accreditation agency for graduate medical education programs, the ACGME wanted to shift from looking at the structure and process of education, which are assessments of potential, to the measurement of outcomes and actual accomplishments. The project defined the six areas of competence: patient care, medical knowledge, professionalism, systems-based practice, practice-based learning and improvement, and interpersonal and communication skills. Clearly, these are not unique and fully distinct areas of competence, but they do define the breadth and depth of what a trainee must know to practice in the twenty-first century. Since the launch of the project there have been many years of moving from concept to program requirements and ultimately to an understanding of what these terms mean and how to use them for enhanced learning and improved clinical practice.

From a pediatrician's point of view, *Pediatrics: A Competency-Based Companion* takes the aforementioned training paradigm and moves it into the reality of clinical practice. Using the competency framework, the authors and editors provide the pediatrician with a concise set of information points that will help guide practice. The chapters each start with a clinical scenario, and that is the vantage point of a practitioner. It is not a starting point of a theory or a topical matter but the setting of a commonly seen patient in a clinical context. Next the reader is provided medical knowledge—not an expansive amount of knowledge, but a quantum the practitioner needs to know for clinical thinking, history, physical examination, and laboratory testing considerations. Where this text breaks new ground is in the consideration of interpersonal communication, professionalism, practice-based learning, and systems-based practice. These topics place the book uniquely in the twenty-first century and adjust the practitioner's thinking and action in important new directions. Beyond the chapters on all the key well child and ill child conditions, the chapters on giving bad news, difficult encounters, teamwork, and patient safety are unique and very important. Introductory chapters on each of the competencies and on how to be successful in the student and resident roles are also unique.

The authors have taken the Outcome Project framework and applied it to a new and innovative learning tool useful to all of us who are providing care. I applaud these efforts and look forward to putting the book to work in my own practice. It is indeed a welcome companion.

Stephen Ludwig MD
Philadelphia, Pennsylvania

Preface of the Series Editor

At the turn of this millennium, when the Accreditation Council for Graduate Medical Education (ACGME) brought forth the idea of competency categories, it was left to the discretion of individual program directors to define and develop competency content and then to teach and to evaluate according to it. Elsevier's *Competency-Based Companion Series* is the first publisher's attempt to demonstrate that the ACGME competencies are indeed the real components of what makes the art and science of doctoring a multidimensional profession.

Surgery: A Competency-Based Companion, the first volume of the series, was the initial effort to define the specifics of what we mean by each competency. When editing the surgery volume, I personally called upon more than 100 surgical educators to offer specific examples of how they defined behaviors in the six ACGME competency categories. Early in the process it became clear that authors had different understandings of what might be meant by each of the competencies. Hence, defining this six-pronged curriculum as it pertained specifically to surgery was not a simple task, but it did prove to be an enriching educational journey.

Even as *Surgery: A Competency-Based Companion* was being compiled, a poignant question asked was, "Why crowd a book addressed to students and residents, who are hungry for *clinical science,* with the 'fluffy' issues of Interpersonal and Communication Skills, Professionalism, or how to make one's practice System-Based?" Dr. Michael Belden's *Obstetrics and Gynecology: A Competency-Based Companion,* the second book of the series, demonstrated quite clearly that these hard-to-measure "fluffy" competencies are actually quite *integral* to the clinical science of a women's health curriculum and should not be separated from it.

Similarly, in *Pediatrics: A Competency-Based Companion,* Drs. Maureen McMahon and Glenn Stryjewski have demonstrated that studying Interpersonal Skills, Professionalism and how to make the System work for children and for their families is a vital part of learning to be a successful pediatrician. To my read, their journey into delineation of the competencies has lead to the discovery that the tenets of Professionalism appear to remain constant, hardly differing from our discoveries in the Surgery and Obstetrics/Gynecology volumes. On the other hand, they have demonstrated that Interpersonal and Communication Skills in pediatrics is a triangulation: physician, child, family. There are specific sets of skills required for communication with the child, but always a need to communicate with parents and families;

and occasionally, additional skills are required to bring child and family in sync. Whereas the previous volumes highlight the ever-present need to make the **System** work for our patients, in pediatrics there are moral mandates for the physician to make the System work specifically for the less fortunate: the indigent, children hampered by congenital problems, those challenged by disabilities, and those whose chronic illnesses require significant system support. I congratulate Dr. McMahon and Dr. Stryjewski for their excellent work, and I salute Elsevier for the courage and persistence to believe that this series will ultimately have an impact on the quality of medical education.

Barry D. Mann MD

Preface

Pediatrics: A Competency-Based Companion is modeled after the template designed by Barry Mann in *Surgery: A Competency-Based Companion.* Our goal is simple and timely: to illustrate application of the six Accreditation Council for Graduate Medical Education competencies across clinical settings where pediatric care is provided, including the newborn nursery, the outpatient office well child and episodic care, the hospital inpatient setting, the neonatal intensive care unit, the pediatric intensive care unit, and the emergency department.

Section I contains chapters that outline the essential components and implementation of each competency. In addition, practical topics on successful performance in the pediatric clerkship, junior resident performance in continuity clinic and the inpatient setting, history taking and physical examination, and note writing and oral presentations provide valuable guidance to the reader. Online features include chapters on competency-based career planning, organization and time management, and nonclinical activities.

Each clinical chapter contains a specific case or topic in the context of the six competencies: medical knowledge, patient care, interpersonal and communication skills, professionalism, practice-based learning and improvement, and systems-based practice. Medical knowledge and patient care are expanded and referenced to the pertinent sections of *Nelson Essentials of Pediatrics,* sixth edition. Vertical reads have been created for interpersonal and communication skills, professionalism, and systems-based practice by abstracting the respective components of these competencies from each chapter to form a mini-curriculum in each of the three topics available in the online version. Most chapters contain a reference to an article that provides either an excellent overview of the subject or has historical significance related to the topic to facilitate the readers' practice-based learning and improvement. Our target audiences are medical students in the pediatric clerkship and junior pediatric residents. When providing education to this audience, we hope faculty will find this to be an innovative and useful educational tool.

In the process of dissecting each competency, our own awareness was raised regarding what comes naturally as we provide care. Excellent care can be delivered when all the competencies are considered and applied. Perhaps this is a novel way of thinking, as we have focused on the value of medical knowledge and patient care for so many years. By breaking down the components of truly comprehensive care, this book aims to facilitate a practical working sense of the competencies and how they can be integrated in our daily practice. This will hopefully promote a reshaping of our thought process regarding how we approach clinical care and raise the standard of care we provide.

We have strived to avoid redundancy where there is potential for significant overlap, i.e., between interpersonal/communication skills and professionalism. This book leans heavily toward the clinical, with a cross-sectional demonstration of the six competencies in common clinical scenarios. It is not a comprehensive resource on each topic; the collation to *Nelson Essentials of Pediatrics,* suggested websites, and a practice-based learning and improvement article in most chapters all expand on what is offered here. The overarching goal is to provide a road map for learners to navigate implementation of the six competencies in patient care.

Maureen C. McMahon and Glenn R. Stryjewski

Acknowledgments

Glenn and I have many to thank for their roles in each phase of this project. Jim Merritt, senior acquisitions editor at Elsevier, was instrumental along with Dr. Mann in designing the series, and has been an overarching support for Glenn and me throughout the project. Christine Abshire, developmental editor at Elsevier, has been a tremendous guide, providing expertise and experience to help us navigate the process, and as such, has been our steadfast anchor and contact through the entire process. We are truly grateful for her unwavering assistance that has added quality to our work. Beth Hayes, senior project manager, has piloted us through the final stages in review of copy edits and page proofs. She, too, has been a tremendous resource for guidance, support, and keeping us on a timeline to bring the project to completion. Thank you to Tilda Mann for her artistic expertise in sketching for Teaching Visual: Examination of the Middle Ear.

Thank you to all of our section editors: Jennifer Miller, David Rappaport, Helen Towers, Sharon Calaman, Magdy Attia, and Cynthia McIntosh. Without you, our focus would have been lost. The Competency editors, Lindsey Lane in Professionalism, Marsha Anderson in Interpersonal and Communication Skills, and Nik Tchopev in Systems-Based Practice, deserve special thanks for their input on each of the clinical chapters. And to our authors: We thank you and express huge gratitude to you for sticking with it, and bringing the project to completion. We have been truly impressed with the quality of writing and clinical experience brought to the table. The world of pediatric education is blessed to have all of you among its ranks.

A very special thank you to Dr. Barry Mann for recruiting us, and for bringing his wisdom, mentoring, and clinical writing expertise to support us at every step. It has been an honor and a privilege for us to be a part of this project.

Maureen C. McMahon and Glenn R. Stryjewski

I would like to thank my wife, Alison, and my children, Sophia and Isabella, to whom I dedicate my contributions to this book. I sit and type this as you patiently wait for me to be with you. This is an experience I know you are far too familiar with. As the family of a pediatric critical care specialist, you know the meaning of an absent husband and father; however, you still seem to relish every minute we spend together. I hope you always understand that these interruptions in our lives are spent to better the world around us. I know that you see the value of this endeavor and are willing to selflessly accept my absence, even at such a young age. And especially to my wife, who shoulders this burden as I disappear in the night or fail to reappear the next day as expected. Thank you for all that you are.

Glenn R. Stryjewski

I would like to acknowledge the tremendous input of Barry Mann, and thank him for the mentoring and quality editing that has added so much to this volume. Barry was one of my instructors in surgery in the third-year clerkship and a fourth-year elective in general surgery at the Medical College of Pennsylvania, and he truly stands out as an excellent clinician, a wonderful teacher and mentor, and a friend. I am honored to have been a part of this project and thank him for all his support.

I also thank my entire family for their support and understanding, most especially my parents, Kathleen and Joseph McMahon, to whom I dedicate my contributions here.

Maureen C. McMahon

Contributors

Elizabeth E. Adams DO
Associate Professor, Division of General Pediatrics, Pennsylvania State Children's Hospital, Hershey, Pennsylvania

R. Jason Adams MD
Assistant Professor of Pediatrics, Department of Emergency Medicine, Children's Hospital of Pittsburgh, Pittsburgh, Pennsylvania

Marilee C. Allen MD
Professor of Pediatrics, Neonatology and Neurodevelopmental Disabilities, The Johns Hopkins School of Medicine, Baltimore, Maryland

Benjamin Alouf MD
Attending Physician, Nemours/Alfred I. duPont Hospital for Children, Wilmington, Delaware; Assistant Professor of Pediatrics, Jefferson Medical College, Philadelphia, Pennsylvania

Gina Amoroso DO
Assistant Clinical Professor, Department of Pediatrics, Jefferson Medical College, Thomas Jefferson University, Philadelphia, Pennsylvania; General Pediatrician, Department of Pediatrics, Nemours/Alfred I. duPont Hospital for Children, Wilmington, Delaware

Tara Andersen DO
Clinical Assistant Professor, Department of Pediatrics, Des Moines University; Pediatric Hospitalist, Mercy Children's Center, Mercy Medical Center, Des Moines, Iowa

Marsha S. Anderson MD
Associate Professor of Pediatrics, Assistant Dean for Longitudinal Curriculum, Department of Pediatrics, University of Colorado School of Medicine; Associate Pediatric Residency Program Director, Department of Pediatrics, The Children's Hospital, Denver, Colorado

Magdy W. Attia MD
Professor of Pediatrics, Jefferson Medical College, Philadelphia, Pennsylvania; Academic Chief, Division of Pediatric Emergency Medicine, Department of Pediatrics, Associate Director, Emergency Services, Director, Pediatric Emergency Medicine Fellowship Program, Nemours/Alfred I. duPont Hospital for Children, Wilmington, Delaware

Jacquelyn M. Aveta MD, FAAP
Attending Physician, Department of Pediatrics, The Children's Hospital of Philadelphia; Clinical Assistant Professor of Pediatrics, School of Medicine, University of Pennsylvania, Philadelphia, Pennsylvania

Louis E. Bartoshesky MD, MPH
Professor of Pediatrics, Medical Genetics, Jefferson Medical College; Chair, Pediatrics, Christiana Care Health System; Attending Geneticist, Nemours/Alfred I. duPont Hospital for Children, Wilmington, Delaware

Sara L. Beers MD
Assistant Professor of Pediatrics, Emergency Medicine, University of Texas Southwestern Medical School; Attending Physician, Pediatric Emergency Medicine, Children's Medical Center, Dallas, Texas

Amanda E. Bennett MD, MPH
Attending Physician, Developmental-Behavioral Pediatrics, University of Pennsylvania; Pediatrics, The Children's Hospital of Philadelphia, Philadelphia, Pennsylvania

Faizah N. Bhatti MD, MS
Assistant Professor of Pediatrics, Section on Neonatal-Perinatal Medicine, The University of Oklahoma Health Sciences Center, Oklahoma City, Oklahoma

Nathan J. Blum MD
Professor of Pediatrics, University of Pennsylvania School of Medicine; Attending, Department of Developmental-Behavioral Pediatrics, The Children's Hospital of Philadelphia, Philadelphia, Pennsylvania

Christopher P. Bonafide MD
Instructor in Pediatrics, Division of General Pediatrics, University of Pennsylvania School of Medicine; Attending Physician, Division of General Pediatrics, The Children's Hospital of Philadelphia, Philadelphia, Pennsylvania

Robert L. Bonner Jr. MD
Assistant Professor of Pediatrics, Department of General Pediatrics, Drexel University College of Medicine; Medical Director, General Pediatrics Outpatient Services, St. Christopher's Hospital for Children, Philadelphia, Pennsylvania

Denise Bratcher DO
Professor of Pediatrics, Department of Pediatrics, Section of Infectious Diseases, University of Missouri–Kansas City School of Medicine; Director, Pediatrics Residency Program, Children's Mercy Hospital, Kansas City, Missouri

Hal C. Byck MD
Clinical Associate Professor, Department of General Pediatrics, Jefferson Medical College, Thomas Jefferson University, Philadelphia, Pennsylvania; General Pediatrician, Department of Pediatrics, Nemours/Alfred I. duPont Hospital for Children, Wilmington, Delaware

Sharon Calaman MD
Assistant Professor of Pediatrics, Pediatrics, Section of Critical Care,
Drexel University College of Medicine; Pediatric Intensivist,
St. Christopher's Hospital for Children, Philadelphia, Pennsylvania

Rosemary Casey MD
Associate Professor of Pediatrics, Department of General Pediatrics,
Jefferson Medical College, Thomas Jefferson University, Philadelphia,
Pennsylvania; General Pediatrician, Pediatrics, Main Line Health System,
Lankenau Hospital, Wynnewood, Pennsylvania

Lindsay Chase MD
Assistant Professor of Pediatrics, Pediatric Hospital Medicine, Baylor
College of Medicine, Texas Children's Hospital, Houston, Texas

Aaron S. Chidekel MD
Associate Professor of Pediatrics, Department of Pediatrics, Jefferson
Medical College, Thomas Jefferson University, Philadelphia, Pennsylvania;
Chief, Division of Pediatric Pulmonology, Nemours/Alfred I. duPont
Hospital for Children, Wilmington, Delaware

Arun Chopra MD
Assistant Professor of Pediatrics, Drexel University College of Medicine;
Attending Physician, Pediatrics, Division of Critical Care, Saint Christopher's
Hospital for Children, Philadelphia, Pennsylvania

Edelveis R. M. Clapp DO
Assistant Professor of Pediatrics, Division of General Pediatrics, Pennsylvania
State Medical College; General Pediatrician, Department of Pediatrics,
Pennsylvania State Hershey Medical Center, Hershey, Pennsylvania

Deborah M. Consolini MD
Assistant Professor of Pediatrics, Department of Pediatrics, Jefferson
Medical College, Thomas Jefferson University, Philadelphia, Pennsylvania;
General Pediatrician, Department of Pediatrics, Diagnostic Referral
Division, Nemours/Alfred I. duPont Hospital for Children, Wilmington,
Delaware

Kathryn Rausch Crowell MD
Assistant Professor of Pediatrics, Department of Pediatrics, Pennsylvania
State University School of Medicine; General Pediatrician, Department of
Pediatrics, Pennsylvania State University Children's Hospital, Hershey,
Pennsylvania

Mario Cruz MD
Assistant Professor of Pediatrics, Pediatrics, Drexel University College of
Medicine; Attending Physician, General Pediatrics, St. Christopher's
Hospital for Children, Philadelphia, Pennsylvania

Ashley Daly MD, FAAP
Assistant Professor of Pediatrics, University of Missouri–Kansas City School
of Medicine; Medical Director, Pediatric Hospital Medicine Services,
Kansas City, Missouri

Reza J. Daugherty MD
Assistant Professor of Pediatrics, Department of Pediatrics, Thomas Jefferson University, Philadelphia, Pennsylvania; Attending Physician, Pediatric Emergency Medicine, Nemours/Alfred I. duPont Hospital for Children, Wilmington, Delaware

Cynthia DeLago MD, MPH
Associate Professor of Pediatrics, Department of Pediatrics, Jefferson Medical College, Thomas Jefferson University; Medical Director, Pediatrics and Adolescent Ambulatory Center, Department of Pediatrics, Albert Einstein Medical Center, Philadelphia, Pennsylvania

Craig C. DeWolfe MD, MEd
Assistant Professor of Pediatrics, Department of Pediatrics, George Washington University School of Medicine; Pediatric Hospitalist, Children's National Medical Center, Washington, DC

Rachel A. B. Dodge MD, MPH
Assistant Professor of Pediatrics, Division of General Pediatrics and Adolescent Medicine, Johns Hopkins University; Medical Director, Foster Care, The MATCH Program, Baltimore City Department of Social Services, Baltimore HealthCare Access, Inc., Baltimore, Maryland

Cara B. Doughty MD, MEd
Assistant Professor of Pediatrics, Pediatric Emergency Medicine, Baylor College of Medicine, Texas Children's Hospital, Houston, Texas

Maria C. Dycoco MD, FAAP
Associate Director of Medical Student Education, Section of General Pediatrics, Children's Mercy Hospital and Clinics; Assistant Professor of Pediatrics, University of Missouri–Kansas City, Kansas City, Missouri

Stephen C. Eppes MD
Professor of Pediatrics, Jefferson Medical College, Thomas Jefferson University, Philadelphia, Pennsylvania; Chief, Division of Infectious Diseases, Nemours/Alfred I. duPont Hospital for Children, Wilmington, Delaware

Christiana R. Farkouh MD, MPH
Assistant Clinical Professor of Pediatrics, Division of Neonatology, Columbia University School of Physicians and Surgeons; Attending Neonatologist, Morgan Stanley Children's Hospital of New York–Presbyterian, New York, New York

Gerald M. Fendrick MD
Clinical Professor of Pediatrics, Jefferson Medical College, Thomas Jefferson University Hospital; Chief of Pediatrics, Our Lady of Lourdes Medical Center, Camden, New Jersey

Gary Frank MD, MS
Clinical Assistant Professor, General Pediatrics, Emory University School of Medicine; Medical Director for Quality and Medical Management, Children's Healthcare of Atlanta, Atlanta, Georgia

Meg A. Frizzola DO
Critical Care Fellow, Critical Care and Anesthesia, Thomas Jefferson University, Philadelphia, Pennsylvania; Critical Care Fellow, Critical Care and Anesthesia, Nemours/Alfred I. duPont Hospital for Children, Wilmington, Delaware

Kate L. Fronheiser MD
Clinical Assistant Professor of Pediatrics, Department of General Pediatrics, Jefferson Medical College, Thomas Jefferson University, Philadelphia, Pennsylvania; Hospitalist, Department of Pediatrics, Nemours/Alfred I. duPont Hospital for Children, Wilmington, Delaware

Cara Garofalo MD
Assistant Professor, Department of Pediatrics, Drexel University College of Medicine; Attending Cardiologist, St. Christopher's Hospital for Children, Philadelphia, Pennsylvania

John Carlton Gartner Jr. MD
Professor of Pediatrics, Vice Chair, Department of Pediatrics, Jefferson Medical College, Thomas Jefferson University, Philadelphia, Pennsylvania; Pediatrician-in-Chief, General Pediatrics/Diagnostic Referral Division, Nemours/Alfred I. duPont Hospital for Children, Wilmington, Delaware

Cynthia Gibson MD, FAAP
Medical Director, Pediatric Hospitalists, Pediatric Critical Care Physician, Assistant Professor of Pediatrics, Virginia Commonwealth University School of Medicine; Department of Pediatrics, INOVA Fairfax Hospital for Children, Falls Church, Virginia

Nilufer R. Goyal MD, FAAP
Consultant Pediatrician, General Pediatrics, Fresno, California

Nicole A. Green MD
Fellow in Pediatric Emergency Medicine, Emergency Medicine, Nemours/Alfred I. duPont Hospital for Children, Wilmington, Delaware

Christopher J. Haines DO, FAAP, FACEP
Assistant Professor of Emergency Medicine and Pediatrics, Drexel University College of Medicine; Director, Department of Emergency Medicine, Medical Director, Critical Care Transport Team, St. Christopher's Hospital for Children, Philadelphia, Pennsylvania

Sandra Gibson Hassink MD, FAAP
Assistant Professor of Pediatrics, Jefferson Medical College, Thomas Jefferson University, Philadelphia, Pennsylvania; Director, Nemours Obesity Initiative, Nemours/Alfred I. duPont Hospital for Children, Wilmington, Delaware

Theresa Hetzler MD
Associate Professor of Clinical Pediatrics, New York Medical College; Academic General Pediatrician, Maria Fareri Children's Hospital, Westchester Medical Center, Valhalla, New York

John M. Howard DO
Pediatric Emergency Medicine Fellow, Thomas Jefferson University, Philadelphia, Pennsylvania; Pediatric Emergency Medicine Fellow, Nemours/Alfred I. duPont Hospital for Children, Wilmington, Delaware

Deborah Hsu MD, MEd
Associate Professor of Pediatrics, Pediatric Emergency Medicine, Baylor College of Medicine, Texas Children's Hospital, Houston, Texas

Lisa Humphrey MD
Medical Director, Palliative Care Program, Assistant Professor of Pediatrics, Case Western Reserve University, Cleveland, Ohio

Matthew J. Kapklein MD, MPH
Assistant Professor, Department of Pediatrics, New York Medical College; Director, Pediatric Residency Program, Attending Physician, Pediatric Intensive Care Unit, Pediatric Emergency Department, Maria Fareri Children's Hospital, Westchester Medical Center, Valhalla, New York

Aaron D. Kessel MD
Assistant Professor of Pediatrics, Hofstra North Shore–Long Island Jewish School of Medicine, Hofstra University, Hempstead, New York; Pediatric Critical Care Medicine, Cohen Children's Medical Center of New York, New Hyde Park, New York

James S. Killinger MD
Assistant Professor of Pediatrics, Department of Pediatrics, Albert Einstein College of Medicine of Yeshiva University, Bronx, New York; Attending Physician, Pediatric Critical Care Medicine, The Children's Hospital at Montefiore, Bronx, New York

Jane F. Knapp MD
Professor of Pediatrics, Associate Dean, University of Missouri–Kansas City School of Medicine; Associate Chair for Pediatrics, Chair, Department of Medical Education, Children's Mercy Hospitals and Clinics, Kansas City, Missouri

Ganga Krishnamurthy MD
Garrett Isaac Neubauer Assistant Professor of Pediatrics, Director of Neonatal Cardiac Care, Morgan Stanley Children's Hospital of New York–Presbyterian; Attending, Columbia University Medical Center, New York, New York

Patrice Kruszewski DO
Department of Pediatrics, Nemours/Alfred I. duPont Hospital for Children, Wilmington, Delaware

Dennis Z. Kuo MD, MHS
Assistant Professor of Pediatrics, Center for Applied Research and Evaluation, Department of Pediatrics, University of Arkansas for Medical Sciences; General Pediatrician, Arkansas Children's Hospital, Little Rock, Arkansas

J. Lindsey Lane MD
*Vice Chair for Education, The Children's Hospital, University of Colorado–
Denver, Aurora, Colorado*

Robert LaTerra MD
*Graduate Medical Student, Jefferson Medical College, Thomas Jefferson
University, Philadelphia, Pennsylvania*

Jane S. Lee MD, MPH
*Assistant Professor of Pediatrics, Division of Neonatology, Department of
Pediatrics, Columbia University School of Physicians and Surgeons;
Neonatologist, Director of Neonatal Follow-Up Program, Division of
Neonatology, Morgan Stanley Children's Hospital of New York–Presbyterian,
New York, New York*

Jannet Lee-Jayaram MD
*Assistant Professor of Pediatrics, Department of Pediatrics, John A. Burns
School of Medicine, University of Hawaii–Mānoa, Honolulu, Hawaii*

Kelly R. Leite DO
*Associate Professor of Pediatrics, General Pediatrics, Pennsylvania State
College of Medicine; Director, Pediatric Residency Program, Pennsylvania
State Children's Hospital, Hershey, Pennsylvania*

John M. Loiselle MD
*Associate Professor of Pediatrics, Jefferson Medical College, Thomas
Jefferson University, Philadelphia, Pennsylvania; Chief, Division of
Emergency Medicine, Department of Pediatrics, Nemours/Alfred I. duPont
Hospital for Children, Wilmington, Delaware*

Justin F. Lynn MD, MPH
*Clinical Assistant Professor of Pediatrics, Department of General Pediatrics,
Temple University School of Medicine, Philadelphia, Pennsylvania; Pediatric
Hospitalist, Pediatrics, Crozer-Chester Medical Center, Chester, Pennsylvania*

Barry D. Mann MD, FACS
*Chief Academic Officer, Main Line Health System; Executive Director, the
Walter and Leonore Annenberg Conference Center for Medical Education,
Wynnewood, Pennsylvania; Professor of Surgery, Jefferson Medical College,
Thomas Jefferson University, Philadelphia, Pennsylvania*

Keith J. Mann MD
*Assistant Professor of Pediatrics, University of Missouri–Kansas City School
of Medicine; Medical Director, Quality and Safety, Children's Mercy
Hospitals and Clinics, Kansas City, Missouri*

Ruth D. Mayforth MD, PhD
Consultant Pediatric Surgeon, Kijabe, Kenya

Jennifer L. McCullough MD
*Assistant Professor of Pediatrics, Children's Mercy Hospitals and Clinics;
Pediatric Gastroenterologist, Department of Pediatrics, Gastroenterology
Section, University of Missouri–Kansas City, Kansas City, Missouri*

Cynthia McIntosh MD
Assistant Clinical Professor of Pediatrics, Thomas Jefferson School of Medicine, Philadelphia, Pennsylvania; Courtesy Staff, General Pediatrics, Nemours/Alfred I. duPont Hospital for Children, Wilmington, Delaware

Maureen C. McMahon MD
Assistant Professor of Pediatrics, Jefferson Medical College, Thomas Jefferson University, Philadelphia, Pennsylvania; General Pediatrician, Nemours/Alfred I. duPont Hospital for Children, Wilmington, Delaware; Lankenau Medical Center, Main Line Health System, Wynnewood, Pennsylvania

Anne M. Meduri MD
Developmental Pediatrician, Division of Developmental Medicine, Nemours/ Alfred I. duPont Hospital for Children, Wilmington, Delaware

Suzanne Swanson Mendez MD
Clinical Instructor of Pediatrics, Pediatrics, Stanford University, Palo Alto, California; Pediatric Hospitalist, Medical Director of Pediatric Unit, Pediatrics, Santa Clara Valley Medical Center, San Jose, California

Carolyn Milana MD
Assistant Professor of Pediatrics, Department of Pediatrics, State University of New York–Stony Brook, Stony Brook, New York

Jennifer R. Miller MD
Assistant Professor, Associate Director, Pediatric Residency Program, Division of General Pediatrics, Pennsylvania State Hershey Children's Hospital, Hershey, Pennsylvania

Marilyn C. Morris MD, MPH
Assistant Professor of Clinical Pediatrics, Department of Pediatrics, Columbia University, The Children's Hospital of New York, New York, New York

Jason Newland MD
Department of Pediatrics, Children's Mercy Hospitals and Clinics, University of Missouri–Kansas City School of Medicine, Kansas City, Missouri

Kathleen B. O'Brien MD
Pediatric Sports Medicine, Department of Orthopedics, Nemours/Alfred I. duPont Hospital for Children, Wilmington, Delaware

Robert Palermo DO
Pediatric Resident, Department of Pediatrics, Jefferson Medical College, Thomas Jefferson University, Philadelphia, Pennsylvania; Pediatric Resident, Pediatrics, Nemours/Alfred I. duPont Hospital for Children, Wilmington, Delaware

Christopher P. Raab MD
Clinical Instructor, Jefferson Medical College, Thomas Jefferson University, Philadelphia, Pennsylvania; Pediatrician, Division of Diagnostic Referral, Division of Solid Organ Transplant, Nemours/Alfred I. duPont Hospital for Children, Wilmington, Delaware

Tara M. Randis MD
Assistant Professor of Pediatrics, Division of Neonatology, Department of Pediatrics, Columbia University Medical Center, New York, New York

David I. Rappaport MD
Clinical Assistant Professor of Pediatrics, Department of General Pediatrics, Jefferson Medical College, Thomas Jefferson University, Philadelphia, Pennsylvania; Hospitalist, General Pediatrics, Nemours/Alfred I. duPont Hospital for Children, Wilmington, Delaware

Veniamin Ratner MD
Assistant Professor of Pediatrics, Department of Pediatrics, Physicians and Surgeons College, Columbia University, New York, New York

Deena K. Roemer
Volunteer, the Walter and Leonore Annenberg Conference Center for Medical Education, Lankenau Medical Center, Main Line Health System, Wynnewood, Pennsylvania

Carolyn M. Rosen MD
Assistant Professor of Pediatrics, Department of Pediatrics, Mount Sinai Medical Center, New York, New York

Jennifer R. Rosenthal MD
Pediatrician, Rady Children's Hospital–San Diego, San Diego, California

Jody Ross MD
Department of Pediatrics, University Physicians Group, Pennsylvania State Hershey Medical Center, Hershey, Pennsylvania

Sara L. P. Ross MD
Assistant Professor of Pediatrics, Pediatric Critical Care Medicine, Albert Einstein College of Medicine; Pediatric Critical Care Medicine, Fellowship Program Director, Children's Hospital at Montefiore, Bronx, New York

Linda M. Sacks MD
Associate Clinical Professor, Department of Pediatrics, Mercer University School of Medicine, Savannah Campus; Co-Director, Nurseries, Memorial University Medical Center, Savannah, Georgia

David J. Sas DO, MPH
Assistant Professor of Pediatrics, Division of Pediatric Nephrology, Medical University of South Carolina Children's Hospital, Charleston, South Carolina

Marilyn Scharbach MD
Department of Pediatrics, New York Medical College, Valhalla, New York

Christine M. Schlichting MD
Associate Professor of Anesthesiology, Drexel University College of Medicine; Attending, Section of Critical Care Medicine, Department of Pediatrics, St. Christopher's Hospital for Children, Philadelphia, Pennsylvania

Steven M. Selbst MD
Professor of Pediatrics, Vice-Chair for Education, Pediatric Residency Program Director, Department of Pediatrics, Jefferson Medical College, Thomas Jefferson University, Philadelphia, Pennsylvania; Attending Physician, Division of Emergency Medicine, Nemours/Alfred I. duPont Hospital for Children, Wilmington, Delaware

Kathleen Senn MD
Assistant Professor of Pediatrics, Department of Pediatrics, University of Missouri–Kansas City; General Pediatrician, Pediatrics, The Children's Mercy Hospitals and Clinics, Kansas City, Missouri

Venkat R. Shankar MD, MBA
Associate Professor, Department of Pediatrics, Drexel University College of Medicine; Chief, Section of Critical Care, Department of Pediatrics, St. Christopher's Hospital for Children, Philadelphia, Pennsylvania

Paul M. Shore MD, MS
Assistant Professor of Pediatrics, Department of Pediatrics, Drexel University College of Medicine; Attending Physician, Section of Pediatric Critical Care Medicine, St. Christopher's Hospital for Children, Philadelphia, Pennsylvania

Lewis P. Singer MD, FCCM
Professor of Clinical Pediatrics, Department of Pediatrics, Albert Einstein College of Medicine; Chief, Division of Pediatric Critical Care Medicine, The Children's Hospital at Montefiore, Bronx, New York

Sabina B. Singh MD
Assistant Professor of Pediatrics and Emergency Medicine, St. Christopher's Hospital for Children, Philadelphia, Pennsylvania

Maria Stephan MD
Associate Professor, Department of Pediatrics, University of Texas Southwestern Medical School; Attending Physician, Division of Emergency Medicine, Children's Medical Center of Dallas, Dallas, Texas

Glenn R. Stryjewski MD, MPH
Associate Professor, Department of Pediatrics, Jefferson Medical College, Thomas Jefferson University, Philadelphia, Pennsylvania; Pediatric Intensivist, Nemours/Alfred I. duPont Hospital for Children, Wilmington, Delaware

Todd Sweberg MD
Assistant Professor of Pediatrics, Hofstra North Shore–Long Island Jewish School of Medicine, Hofstra University, Hempstead, New York;, Pediatric Critical Care Medicine, Cohen Children's Medical Center of New York, New Hyde Park, New York

Danna Tauber MD, MPH
Assistant Professor, Department of Pediatrics, Drexel University College of Medicine; Attending, Section of Pulmonology, St. Christopher's Hospital for Children, Philadelphia, Pennsylvania

Nik Tchopev MD, MBA
Medical Director, Johns Hopkins Healthcare, Glen Burnie, Maryland; Instructor in Medicine, Department of Medicine–Division of General Internal Medicine, Instructor in Pediatrics, Department of Pediatrics– Division of General Pediatrics and Adolescent Medicine, Johns Hopkins University School of Medicine; Active Staff, The Johns Hopkins Hospital, Baltimore, Maryland

Rebecca Tenney-Soeiro MD
Clinical Assistant Professor of Pediatrics, General Pediatrics, University of Pennsylvania School of Medicine; Attending Physician, General Pediatrics Inpatient Service and Integrated Care Service, Pediatrics, Children's Hospital of Philadelphia, Philadelphia, Pennsylvania

Helen M. Towers MD
Associate Clinical Professor of Pediatrics, Department of Pediatrics, Columbia University Medical Center, New York, New York

Judith A. Turow MD
Clinical Associate Professor of Pediatrics, Division of Pediatrics, Jefferson Medical College, Thomas Jefferson University Hospital, Philadelphia, Pennsylvania

Daniel Walmsley DO
Assistant Professor of Pediatrics, Department of General Pediatrics, Jefferson Medical College, Thomas Jefferson University; General Pediatrician and Hospitalist, Department of Pediatrics, Nemours Pediatrics at Philadelphia, Thomas Jefferson University Hospital, Philadelphia, Pennsylvania

Kristi Williams MD
Assistant Professor of Pediatrics, General Pediatrics, University of Missouri– Kansas City School of Medicine; General Pediatrician, Department of Pediatrics, Section of General Pediatrics, Children's Mercy Hospitals and Clinics, Kansas City, Missouri

English Willis MD
Director, Clinical Risk Management and Safety Surveillance, Merck & Co., Whitehouse Station, New Jersey

Rachel Wohlberg Friedberg MD
Pediatric Hospitalist, Scottish Rite Pediatric and Adolescent Consultants, Children's Healthcare of Atlanta at Scottish Rite, Atlanta, Georgia

Paul K. Woolf MD
Department of Pediatrics, New York Medical College, Valhalla, New York

Marcy E. Yonker MD, FAHS
Director, Pediatric Headache Program, Division of Neurology, Phoenix Children's Hospital, Phoenix, Arizona; Clinical Associate Professor of Pediatrics, University of Arizona, Tucson, Arizona

Matthew Zinn DO
Third Year Pediatric Resident, Department of Pediatrics, Jefferson Medical College, Thomas Jefferson University, Philadelphia, Pennsylvania; Nemours/ Alfred I. duPont Hospital for Children, Wilmington, Delaware

Arezoo Zomorrodi MD
Attending Physician, Division of Emergency Medicine, Nemours/Alfred I. duPont Hospital for Children, Wilmington, Delaware; Department of Pediatrics, Jefferson Medical College, Thomas Jefferson University, Philadelphia, Pennsylvania

Contents

Section I
INTRODUCTION TO THE COMPETENCIES

Section Editor

Glenn R. Stryjewski MD, MPH

Section Contents

Online Appendices are accessible at www.studentconsult.com.

Chapter 1
How to Study This Book

Maureen C. McMahon MD,
Glenn R. Stryjewski MD, MPH,
and Barry D. Mann MD, FACS

How does one define a good pediatrician? Is it a physician with an extensive fund of knowledge, or one who can deliver care compassionately? Perhaps it is one who can communicate well with patients and their families, or one who can lead a medical team to the correct diagnosis and treatment plan? Perhaps the best pediatrician is one who masters all of these skills? Students and residents in pediatrics are confronted with the task of acquiring large amounts of medical knowledge in the limited time of a clerkship or a rotation, a daunting task unto itself. However, how does one acquire those "other" attributes, such as professionalism and the ability to communicate? The purpose of this book is to provide the learner an efficient method of learning these attributes simultaneously with and in the context of the necessary medical knowledge. This book is by no means an exhaustive compendium of all pediatric knowledge. Rather, this book sets out to help the student acquire knowledge of the processes that define a good pediatrician. To help the reader accomplish this, the remainder of this chapter outlines the structure of this book and provides a few suggestions for prioritizing reading and study of the concepts presented.

STRUCTURE OF THE BOOK

This book contains three basic types of chapters. The first type comprises 56 case-based chapters based on common chief complaints found typically in specific practice sites within pediatrics:

The outpatient office
The inpatient ward
The newborn nursery
The neonatal intensive care unit (NICU)
The pediatric intensive care unit (PICU)
The emergency department

Embedded within these sections and two additional sections (Section I: Introduction to the Competencies and Section VIII: Applications and Challenges) are 47 non–case-based chapters that deal with unique aspects of pediatrics such as survival tools for the resident and teamwork skills.

Finally, there are five Teaching Visuals chapters. These chapters are meant to reinforce the concept that in order to teach a subject the student must have mastery of the material. These chapters provide not only useful review of key material, but also tips on how to educate patients and their families.

ORGANIZING STRUCTURE

At the turn of this millennium, the Accreditation Council for Graduate Medical Education (ACGME) introduced the six competencies into the language of medical instruction. Medical educators must now verify that trainees are competent in Patient Care, Medical Knowledge, Practice-Based Learning and Improvement, Interpersonal and Communication Skills, Professionalism, and Systems-Based Practice.[1] Each of these competencies is explained and expanded in the next several introductory sections. In each case-based chapter, the six ACGME competencies are color coded for easy identification:

Patient Care
Medical Knowledge
Practice-Based Learning and Improvement
Interpersonal and Communication Skills
Professionalism
Systems-Based Practice

Competency definitions according to the ACGME are provided in Appendix 1.

CHAPTER ELEMENTS

A paragraph entitled **Speaking Intelligently** sums up the "big picture" in language that you might use with a colleague. **Clinical Thinking, History, Physical Examination, Tests for Consideration,** and **Imaging Considerations** constitute the most important aspects of the evaluation process.

The Clinical Entities boxes outline the entities considered in the differential diagnoses. The diagnoses listed for each case emphasize the most common diagnoses and are therefore typically fewer in number. Low-frequency diagnoses are described in the **Zebra Zone.**

Each case includes issues and solutions about Practice-Based Learning and Improvement, **Interpersonal and Communication Skills, Professionalism,** and the **Systems-Based Practice** competencies.

SUGGESTIONS FOR READING

Begin by making a reading schedule based on your rotation assignment (e.g., if you start on the "Newborn Nursery," read the Newborn Nursery section first). If your rotation provides you no obvious cue for where to start, read the outpatient section first.

Knowledge of the common differential diagnoses will orient you to educational conversation on rounds, because the underlying issue in patient-related discussions is the differentiation of one diagnostic possibility from another. If you do not know the differential diagnosis of wheezing, it is difficult to participate in a discussion about its evaluation or treatment.

If you do not have time to read a complete chapter or section, read the Differential Diagnosis and the corresponding Clinical Entities boxes. Then use **Clinical Thinking, History, Physical Examination, Tests for Consideration,** and **Imaging Considerations** to understand the basic differentiation of one clinical entity from another. Note that many Clinical Entities entries are referenced to a chapter in *Nelson Essentials of Pediatrics,* 6th edition. Look for **"Nelson Essentials"** and the chapter number. **To access the information in Nelson Essentials, go to the Elsevier Student Consult website (http://www.studentconsult.com) and register using the PIN code in the front cover of this book.**

TEACHING AND LEARNING ACTIVITIES

Teaching a peer is often a great way to reinforce your own knowledge, and diagramming for a patient can add substantially to the physician-patient relationship. Five Teaching Visuals, such as drawing and/or diagramming various entities, have been included throughout the book.

THE COMPETENCIES AND VERTICAL READS

The pediatricians who contributed to this book incorporated aspects of **Patient Care, Medical Knowledge, Practice-Based Learning and Improvement, Interpersonal and Communication Skills, Professionalism,** and **Systems-Based Practice** in the context of their cases. This book is organized to allow for a "vertical read," whereby readers may focus their study on each specific competency. Vertical reads of the **Interpersonal and Communication Skills, Professionalism,** and **Systems-Based Practice** are available online at http://www.studentconsult.com and can be accessed as noted above.

A NOTE ABOUT PRACTICE-BASED LEARNING AND IMPROVEMENT

Evidence-based information has been abstracted and provided to demonstrate how problems can be solved by examining best evidence. At times the Evidence-Based material included in Practice-Based Learning and Improvement represents the most up-to-date review of a topic. At times, an evidence-based study has been abstracted that remains of some historical importance.

Performing routine and accurate self-assessment is an important part of effective practice. A *Competency Self-Assessment Form* is in Appendix 2 at the end of Section I and available online at http://www.studentconsult.com. This form was designed to provide you with an opportunity to assess your performance regarding patients in whose care you have participated.

We hope that the features and organization of this volume will facilitate a productive and enjoyable learning process.

Reference

1. Accreditation Council for Graduate Medical Education: *General Competencies*. Available at http://www.acgme.org/outcome/comp/compFull.asp.

Chapter 2
Medical Knowledge

Ashley Daly MD, FAAP *and Keith J. Mann* MD

INTRODUCTION

At face value, medical knowledge seems like the most straightforward of the competencies to teach and assess. However, we practice medicine in a time of rapid change with exposure to an overwhelming amount of information. Estimates suggest that the volume of medical knowledge doubles every 6 to 8 years. Physicians must first acquire a basic foundation of medical knowledge through formal education. The assessment of this basic knowledge is accomplished by a series of certifying examinations culminating in a specialties professional board certifying examination. Physicians must also learn, however, to constantly review this expanse of medical literature in an effort to stay up to date with the latest research and technology. While doing this, physicians must learn clinical reasoning and critical thinking skills that allow them not only to remember and understand the knowledge they acquire, but also to apply that knowledge to different clinical situations.

DEFINITION AND IMPORTANCE OF MEDICAL KNOWLEDGE

Medical knowledge is the clinical information a physician must have to practice medicine competently. But medical knowledge encompasses far more than the basic sciences and the memorization of clinical information. The Accreditation Council for Graduate Medical Education (ACGME) further defines medical knowledge as it relates to residents: "Residents must demonstrate knowledge about established and evolving biomedical, clinical, and cognate sciences and the application of this knowledge to patient care. Residents are expected to: (1) Demonstrate an investigatory and analytic thinking approach to clinical situations and (2) Know and apply the basic and clinically supportive sciences which are appropriate to their discipline."[1] Thus medical knowledge, in addition to the factual information obtained in study, includes the assessment and evidence-based application of that knowledge through critical thinking skills and clinical reasoning.

There are two main components of medical knowledge described by Rider in *A Practical Guide to Teaching and Assessing the ACGME Core Competencies* that help in understanding the complex nature of this competency. These are "public knowledge" and "personal knowledge." Physicians attend medical school courses, read textbooks, take tests and quizzes, participate in didactic lectures, and read journal articles, which all relate to our public knowledge. This public knowledge is, in short, information the medical community has access to. Our personal knowledge is essentially the knowledge that allows a physician to make clinical judgments based on clinical reasoning.[2] This type of knowledge incorporates both the tangible and intangible information we have accumulated through training. It is the personal charts, note cards, and study material we have from our medical school classes. It is the diagnoses and cases in which we have been intimately involved, whether during core rotations, during residency, or during postresidency clinical practice.

Our professional knowledge, the combination of both public and personal knowledge, is constantly changing, and the process of acquiring and maintaining this knowledge can be overwhelming. We must continue to develop this professional knowledge as we make clinical decisions, as we practice, as we attend continuing medical education opportunities, and as we read and interpret the medical literature.

SPECIFIC STRATEGIES FOR TEACHING AND ASSESSING MEDICAL KNOWLEDGE

An individual's personal medical knowledge is dynamic, and there are both objective and subjective tools for teaching and assessing a medical student's or resident's acquisition of level-appropriate medical knowledge. Because several tools both teach and simultaneously assess this competency, the two will be discussed together.

Institutions that support medical education are challenged to invest financial, technologic, and personnel resources to ensure that a high level of medical knowledge is taught and assessed. The personnel are frequently attending-level physicians and university faculty who must be the leaders in training a new generation of learners. The idea of physician educators with adult students (medical students and residents) is not new; thus there is much experience to rely on. In fact, much has been studied about how adults learn and how to maximize the educational process for the adult learner. One can refer to a hierarchy of competence and skills as the learner becomes more experienced and knowledgeable.

This original taxonomy for adult education was described by Benjamin Bloom in 1956.[3] Physicians have adapted his model to explain how one learns in the clinical arena and have used the concepts for optimal knowledge attainment.[4] The initial component is knowledge, which is the factual information that underlies the basic and clinical sciences. Factual medical information is often taught through didactic conferences and encouraged through self-directed learning. The second step is comprehension, in which the learner attaches meaning to that factual information and can, in his/her own mind, begin to execute a task associated with this knowledge. Next the learner applies this oral and/or written information by actually executing a skill. In medicine, this is often done through the completion of a history, physical examination, and diagnostic evaluation. The fourth step allows the learning physician to analyze various signs and symptoms to decide which are pertinent and to form a differential diagnosis based on this information. The final two components of adult learning as described by Bloom are synthesis and evaluation. Learners who achieve this advanced level of learning can put information into a functional whole, make decisions on that synthesized information, and evaluate the decisions that they make in a systematic fashion. The revised Bloom's taxonomy may be even more applicable to medical education. The steps include remembering, understanding, applying, analyzing, evaluating, and creating.[5]

From the above taxonomy it becomes clear why medical knowledge, a seemingly straightforward competency, can be so difficult to teach and assess. Knowledge as we often see it is simply the first rung on the ladder of a complex learning process. As one progresses through training, the emphasis on cognitive and diagnostic reasoning, the latter stages of the learning hierarchy, becomes more important. Thus, in addition to didactic education associated with the acquisition of factual knowledge, programs must provide educational strategies to promote clinical reasoning that allows for growth. Academic faculty within these programs must also have the skills to promote graded and gradually autonomous critical thinking. A senior resident should be able to analyze a clinical situation more readily and efficiently than a medical student just as a senior faculty member should be capable of higher clinical synthesis than junior faculty. The key elements in progressing through the stages of higher-level learning combine basic medical knowledge, the context of the clinical situation, and personal experience and practice.[6]

Many medical schools and residencies use problem-based learning as another strategy to teach clinical reasoning and simulate experiential learning. This mode of gathering information uses a team approach to teach the individual learner where to find answers to clinical questions and to afford the opportunity for the group to raise clinical questions and teaching opportunities. At the same time, the individual learner also has a self-directed responsibility within the group to search for unanswerable questions in the group setting and present these findings to the group.

Medical knowledge, clinical decision making, and critical thinking must also be taught simultaneously with the skills needed to acquire and interpret the growing body of medical literature. Residency programs address this through the systematic teaching of evidence-based practice. Residents must be able to ask clinical questions, search the literature for answers, and appraise the articles that answer their questions. Residency programs can address this through specific rotations geared toward evidence-based medicine, through regular journal clubs, and through the judicious use of clinical practice guidelines in the care of patients. Programs that encourage best practice, such as antimicrobial stewardship programs, also are a way to promote quality care and teach evidence-based practice.

SUMMARY

In conclusion, medical knowledge is the one competency we have been teaching and assessing for years. In pediatrics, the American Board of Pediatrics requires pediatricians to pass a knowledge-based examination to become board certified. However, recognition that medical knowledge is so much more than factual recall is critical to the success of medical students and residents. Promoting clinical reasoning and critical thinking through various teaching strategies can accomplish this task while also providing a method of assessment built into the educational process.

References

1. Joyce B: *An introduction to competency-based residency education: Facilitator's guide to the ACGME.* Available at http://www.acgme.org.
2. Rider EA: *A practical guide to teaching and assessing the ACGME Core Competencies,* Marblehead, MA, 2007, HCPro, pp 85-86.
3. Bloom BS, Engelhart MD, Hill HH, et al: The taxonomy and illustrative materials. In Bloom BS, editor: *Taxonomy of educational objectives, the classification of educational goals, handbook 1: Cognitive domain,* New York, 1956, David McKay, pp 62-197.
4. Nkanginieme K: Clinical diagnosis as a dynamic cognitive process: Application of Bloom's taxonomy for educational objective in the cognitive domain. *Med Educ Online* 2:1, 1997.
5. Anderson LW, Krathwohl DR, editors: *A taxonomy for learning, teaching and assessing: A revision of Bloom's taxonomy of educational objectives: Complete edition,* New York, 2001, Longman.
6. Bowen J: Education strategies to promote clinical diagnostic reasoning. *N Engl J Med* 355:2217-2225, 2006.

Chapter 3
Patient Care

Jennifer L. McCullough MD
and Jason Newland MD

INTRODUCTION

Patient care is at the foundation of becoming an effective clinician and is truly at the center of all of the Accreditation Council for Graduate Medical Education (ACGME) core competencies. Effective patient care encompasses excellent communication, professional behavior, a solid knowledge base, self-reflection skills, principles of lifelong learning, and an understanding of the health-care system. For most students and residents, caring for patients was the initial stimulus for entering medical school and the basis for pursuing a residency program; however, the all-encompassing nature of patient care is often not realized early in training. For educators, teaching and assessing this competency and providing effective feedback are thus critical to resident education and development.

DEFINITIONS OF PATIENT CARE

The ACGME expects "residents to provide patient care that is compassionate, appropriate, and effective for the treatment of health problems and the promotion of health."[1] The American Board of Pediatrics (ABP) has developed general guidelines for the pediatric competencies and states that for patient care "residents must be able to provide family centered patient care that is developmentally and age appropriate, compassionate, and effective for the treatment of health problems and the promotion of health."[2] The ABP pediatric-specific components of patient care competency include:

- Gather essential and accurate information about the patient using medical interviewing, physical examination, diagnostic studies, and developmental assessment.
- Make informed diagnostic and therapeutic decisions based on patient information, current scientific evidence, and clinical judgment: use effective and appropriate clinical problem-solving skills, understand the limits of one's knowledge and expertise, use consultants and referrals appropriately.

- Develop and carry out patient care management plans.
- Prescribe and perform competently all medical procedures considered essential for the scope of practice.
- Counsel patients and families: to take measures needed to enhance or maintain health and function and prevent disease and injury; by encouraging them to participate actively in their care by providing information necessary to understand illness and treatment, share decisions, and obtain informed consent; by providing comfort and allaying fear.
- Provide effective health-care services and anticipatory guidance.
- Use information technology to optimize patient care.

STRATEGIES FOR LEARNING PATIENT CARE

The ACGME outlines the content that should be taught under the patient care competency. This includes specialty-specific skills that address key skill sets, specialty-specific procedural knowledge, and knowledge about information technology. Learning can take place in the following settings: clinical teaching, lectures/seminars/conferences, role modeling, workshops, simulations, and self-directed learning through case-based modules. Teaching methods should include didactic conferences, clinical teaching, case-based teaching, role modeling, journal club, mentoring, morbidity and mortality (M&M) conferences, simulation, self-directed learning modules, individual or group projects, research projects, and chart audit. Simulation is defined as recreating a medical situation that contains the visual, auditory, and tactile information that might be experienced in an actual clinical encounter. Importantly, simulation takes place in a safe environment that does not pose risk to a patient and can provide learners with experiences that they might not encounter during their clinical duties.

Passive methods of instruction, including case conferences, didactics, and M&M conference, are also important in educating residents on patient care. Through M&M and case conferences, trainees are able to critically appraise a patient's case and subsequent care, to develop their own thoughts on how things may have been done differently or how the disease process works more thoroughly. This takes the trainee away from the bedside to review a case in detail from an outsider's view and to learn from other specialties' viewpoints. Didactic conferences enhance patient care by providing the fundamentals of medical knowledge and current guidelines for treatment strategies.

ASSESSING PATIENT CARE

Important to all competencies are the assessment tools that are in place to ensure successful accomplishment. Many methods exist for assessing competencies for patient care. In many situations the teaching methods instituted will dictate the type of assessment tool that is used. Assessment tools for evaluating patient care include:

■ Attending evaluation
■ Peer evaluation
■ Global rating of live/recorded performance
■ Checklist evaluation of live/recorded performance
■ Standardized patients/parents
■ Objective structured clinical examination
■ Oral examination
■ Procedural skills documentation
■ Pediatric Advanced Life Support/Neonatal Resuscitation Program
■ Mock codes
■ Portfolio

Although most programs use an attending evaluation, the most comprehensive method for evaluating the patient care competency is the 360-degree global evaluation. This tool incorporates the evaluations of all members of the health-care team—attending physician, nursing staff, allied health professionals, and resident colleagues—and/or the patient and his/her family. Reliable and valid multidisciplinary evaluation instruments have been developed to use with patients and the health-care team.[3]

Competency in patient care encompasses both medical and procedural skills. Although evaluations can aid in overall performance, more specific assessments must be made on specific medical and procedural skills. The checklist evaluation of live performance requires the resident to perform the skill in the presence of an evaluator. A checklist is often completed as the resident performs the task (e.g., history and physical examination, lumbar puncture, and family counseling).

Another method of assessing the patient care competency is through the use of objective structured clinical examinations (OSCEs). Specific aspects of the patient care competencies can be tested using OSCEs, various skills are observed and feedback is provided, and improvement and growth in patient care can be elicited. Standardizing the OSCE is essential to ensuring that it evaluates the intended part of the competency. Standardization can be attained through the use of standardized patients and families. Thoroughly reviewed case scenarios that simulate real clinical scenarios are imperative for the success of this evaluation tool. OSCEs have been demonstrated to be both valid and reliable in assessing neonatal-perinatal trainees.[4]

As discussed above, simulators are an exciting new advancement increasingly being used in medical education. Simulators provide an excellent way to assess the competency of certain procedural skills before actual interactions with a patient. In addition, simulators provide instant feedback and allow for a skill to be practiced numerous times in one setting.

A procedure logbook is another method of helping assess procedural competency. Although logs do not specifically demonstrate competency, they can be used as a threshold that must be performed before a more formal evaluation by a faculty member. These logs can also be used in clinical skills laboratories in which simulators are used.

The final type of evaluation method is the use of a portfolio. A portfolio encompasses all of the competencies and provides a place where the resident can maintain his/her accomplishments, evaluations, presentations, and patient and procedural logbooks. A portfolio is an excellent place to encourage the resident to critically reflect about the management or treatment of specific patients. The review of these portfolios allows the faculty to observe and document the progress a resident is making in fulfilling all of the competencies, including patient care.

CONCLUSION

Being competent in patient care is crucial to a resident's role as a physician. Patient care encompasses a wide variety of skills and is taught in a diversity of ways. Although no more important than any of the other core competencies, patient care includes elements from all and is often what defines us as physicians.

References

1. Accreditation Council for Graduate Medical Education: *ACGME outcome project.* Available at http://www.acgme.org/outcome/.
2. Pediatric General Competencies. Available at https://www.abp.org/ABPWebSite/resident/gencomp.pdf.
3. Violato C, Lockyer JM, Fidler H: Assessment of pediatricians by a regulatory authority. *Pediatrics* 117:796-802, 2005.
4. Jefferies A, Simmons B, Tabak D, et al: Using an objective structured clinical examination (OSCE) to assess multiple physician competencies in postgraduate training. *Med Teacher* 29:183-191, 2007.

Chapter 4
Professionalism

Maria C. Dycoco MD, FAAP

The test of the morality of a society is what it does for its children.
Dietrich Bonhoeffer

There is an unwritten contract between patients and physicians based on the mutual understanding that professionalism is an expected characteristic of the competent physician. This contract includes mutual respect, honesty, and trust, and within this contract, the patient's welfare and safety must be the physician's primary concerns. In the ever-changing world of medicine with challenges such as climbing costs of health care, increasing cultural diversity, the heightened awareness of medical errors, the threat of malpractice suits, and the influence of managed care on medical decisions, this contract is continually tested. The resulting challenge to the physician is to develop and maintain the trust that is so integral to the successful ongoing care of the patient. In order to accomplish this, communication skills and professional behavior become paramount to those practicing medicine.

DEFINITIONS OF PROFESSIONALISM

Professionalism is defined by the Accreditation Council for Graduate Medical Education (ACGME) as follows:

Residents must demonstrate a commitment to carrying out professional responsibilities and an adherence to ethical principles. Residents are expected to demonstrate[1]:

- Compassion, integrity, and respect for others
- Responsiveness to patient needs that supersedes self-interest
- Respect for patient privacy and autonomy
- Accountability to patients, society and the profession
- Sensitivity and responsiveness to a diverse patient population, including but not limited to diversity in gender, age, culture, race, religion, disabilities, and sexual orientation

The American Medical Association's proposed definition of professional competence is "the habitual and judicious use of communication, knowledge, technical skills, clinical reasoning, emotions, values, and reflection in daily practice for the benefit of the individual and community being served."[2] Organizations in multiple fields of medicine have developed their own definitions for professionalism, but overall most of the descriptions have been similar in their ideals and framework. Pediatrics differs from other fields in that a pediatrician has the responsibility to effectively interact with the child as the patient and the child's parents/family as the decision maker, while also communicating appropriately with other supporting staff and fellow colleagues. This creates unique circumstances that must be considered when defining professionalism in pediatrics.

The American Board of Pediatrics (ABP) published *Foundations for Evaluating the Competency of Pediatricians* in 1974.[3] This publication was the Board's initial attempt to define the skills that would be expected of the pediatrician, including interpersonal skills, technical skills, clinical judgment, knowledge, and attitudes. Residencies were asked over the next several years to evaluate the these skills and to assess their trainees in the performance of these skills and professionalism.

More recently, the ABP has worked on defining professionalism as it pertains to pediatrics in the *Program Director's Guide to the ABP: Resident Evaluation, Tracking & Certification* published in 2003.[4] Professionalism was defined to include, but not be limited to, the principles set as guidelines that should be used in the training and evaluation of this competency. The eight principles are described below[4,5]:

- **Honesty and integrity:** Physicians should be honest and fair in all communications and interactions with their patients.
- **Reliability and responsibility:** Physicians should be accountable to their patients and their families, fellow colleagues, and the community, which includes recognizing errors made and discussing the consequences of their actions with possible alternatives or solutions.
- **Respect for others:** Physicians should treat all patients with respect and sensitivity in regard to gender, race, and cultural differences and also maintain patient confidentiality when appropriate.
- **Compassion/sympathy:** Physicians should attempt to recognize the pain, discomfort, and anxiety of the patients and their families and respond appropriately to help relieve pain and deal with these emotions.
- **Self-improvement:** Physicians should strive to improve by participating in educational activities, reading current literature, learning from past errors, reflecting on past actions through self-evaluation, and accepting feedback from other colleagues and patients.
- **Self-awareness/knowledge of limits:** Physicians should acknowledge the limitations of their own experience and recognize situations in which further guidance from consultants is needed.
- **Communication and collaboration:** Physicians should communicate effectively with their patients, their families, and the medical team in order to provide comprehensive care and meet the goals of the team and the patients. The pediatrician must take into consideration the ability of the pediatric patient to understand the situation and include him/her in the development of the goals in care when appropriate.
- **Altruism and advocacy:** Physicians should put the best interest of the patient above all others, including themselves.

IMPORTANCE OF PROFESSIONALISM

Health-care providers frequently face challenges to their professionalism. Communication with patients who speak a different language, the lack of medical knowledge on a given topic, the bevy of false information available on the Internet, the challenge of an angry parent, and the second-guessing of a peer all provide unique challenges and test professional competence. These obstacles pose a unique but important challenge to medical schools, residency programs, and the practicing physician undergoing maintenance of certification. Many recent studies have supported the necessity to instill the principles of professionalism early in the training of future physicians. Patients are more likely to adhere to treatment recommendations when they feel they truly trust their caregiver.[6] Patients are also more likely to continue care with and recommend a doctor to others if they believe the caregiver practices in a professional manner.[7] It has been shown that disciplinary action against a practicing physician by a medical board is strongly associated with past unprofessional behavior in medical school,[8] and that patients are more likely to take legal action against physicians if the caregiver's behavior was perceived as unprofessional.[9] These emphasize the importance of teaching this competency early in training, because physicians will be faced with difficult situations and affected by their choices and actions throughout their careers.

STRATEGIES FOR LEARNING AND ASSESSING PROFESSIONALISM

As previously mentioned, the development of tools for learning and assessing professionalism has been challenging. As a student transitions from medical school through residency and eventually to being a practicing physician, he/she gradually develops clinical and professional skills. Similar to the acquisition of medical knowledge and development of clinical skills, tools for teaching professionalism should proceed along this continuum and must be appropriate for the environment and level of training of the learner. Some researchers have proposed plans to promote institutional change and educational activities in professionalism. For example, Inui wrote a paper, *A Flag in the Wind: Educating for Professionalism in Medicine,*[10] which describes an agenda for institutional change to promote the education of professionalism at all levels of an organization, from the CEOs to the residents and students. Faculty role modeling is a vital mode of learning professionalism because the understanding of professionalism by medical students and residents is affected much more by what they observe during their clinical experiences than by what may be included in a formal curriculum.

Several methods of evaluation have been developed in attempts to assess the professionalism of a caregiver, including self-assessment, direct observation, 360-degree evaluations, objective structured clinical examinations, peer assessments, physician portfolios, educational vignettes on ethical issues, and patient/parent surveys. Numerous studies have evaluated some of these assessment tools in the area of competency in professionalism. The consensus of the studies suggests that a multisource evaluation that includes self-evaluation along with input from the patient and/or parent, the supervising faculty, and other members of the health-care team is a valid and effective mode of assessing professional competence and positively affects communication skills and the professional behavior of physicians during their training.[2] Adequate mentoring, feedback, and remediation systems have also been found to be key components[2] in a successful program for teaching and assessing professionalism, and these cannot be accomplished without adequate faculty development in these areas.

CONCLUSION

The pediatrician has the unique opportunity to touch the lives of his/her patients as their health-care provider, confidante, teacher, child advocate, counselor, and friend. The obligation to protect the welfare of young patients and their families should not be compromised by the barriers and influences that exist in today's world of medicine. Pediatricians who successfully accomplish this task while also upholding the responsibilities to the rest of the health-care team, the community, and the profession of medicine demonstrate the values that exemplify professionalism in pediatrics. Training programs, hospitals, and governing medical boards should ensure that doctors are taught to

Table 4-1 Professionalism Definitions		
Accreditation Council for Graduate Medical Education	**American Board of Pediatrics**	**Cases**
Compassion, integrity, and respect for others	**Honesty and integrity**	5, 27, 28, 33
Responsiveness to patient needs that supersedes self-interest	**Reliability and responsibility**	2, 3, 9, 17, 21, 22, 25, 29, 30, 37
Respect for patient privacy and autonomy	**Respect for others**	1, 20, 32, 39, 42, 47, 54
Sensitivity and responsiveness to a diverse patient population	**Compassion/ sympathy**	4, 7, 19, 24, 35, 49
	Self-improvement	13, 15, 16, 31, 40
	Self-awareness/ knowledge of limits	8, 10, 18, 38, 41, 48, 56
	Communication and collaboration	6, 11, 26, 33, 36, 44, 47, 51, 52, 55
Accountability to patients, society, and the profession	**Altruism and advocacy**	4, 12, 14, 23, 34, 43, 45, 46, 50, 53

maintain these standards, because all physicians have a duty to be true to their profession and provide the comprehensive, quality, and professional care that every patient deserves. Table 4-1 lists the definitions of professionalism covered above and the cases in the book in which those definitions are discussed.

References

1. Common Program Requirements: General Competencies. ACGME Outcome Project. February 13, 2007. ACGME. 11 Oct. 2010. Available at http://www.acgme.org/outcome/comp/GeneralCompetenciesStandards21307.pdf.
2. Epstein RM, Hundert EM: Defining and assessing professional competence. *JAMA* 287(2):226-235, 2002.
3. American Board of Pediatrics: *Foundations for evaluating the competency of pediatricians*, Chapel Hill, NC, 1974, American Board of Pediatrics.
4. American Board of Pediatrics: Appendix F: Professionalism. In *Program director's guide to the ABP: Resident evaluation, tracking and certification*, Chapel Hill, NC, 2003, American Board of Pediatrics.
5. Fallat ME, Glover J, Committee on Bioethics: Professionalism in pediatrics. *Pediatrics* 120(4):1123-1133, 2007.
6. Hall MA, Zheng B, Dugan E, et al: Measuring patients' trust in their primary care providers. *Med Care Res Rev* 59:293-318, 2002.
7. Hauck FR, Zyzanski SJ, Alemango SA, Medalie JH: Patient perceptions of humanism in physicians: Effects on positive health behaviors. *Fam Med* 22:447-452, 1990.
8. Papadakis MA, Teherani A, Banach MA, et al: Disciplinary action by medical boards and prior behavior in medical school. *N Engl J Med* 353:2673-2682, 2005.
9. Hickson GB, Federspiel CF, Pichert JW, et al: Patient complaints and malpractice risk. *JAMA* 287:2951-2957, 2002.
10. Inui TS: *A flag in the wind: Educating for professionalism in medicine*, Washington, DC, 2003, Association of American Medical Colleges. Available at http://www.regenstrief.org/Members/tiunui/bio/

Chapter 5
Interpersonal and Communication Skills

Kathleen Senn MD

The intimate and very human relationship that a doctor and patient share may be the greatest privilege awarded a physician. To be a part of another's most joyful and sorrowful moments, and entrusted with another's health, places the physician in a unique role. This role is extraordinary in pediatrics because parents entrust the health and well-being of their children to the pediatrician. Good interpersonal and effective communication skills are paramount for these doctor-patient and doctor-family relationships to succeed. The Accreditation Council for Graduate Medical Education (ACGME) has acknowledged this by including these skills in their set of core competencies. The objective of this chapter is to define the interpersonal and communication skills competency, discuss its importance, and review strategies for teaching and assessing this competency.

DEFINITIONS OF INTERPERSONAL AND COMMUNICATION SKILLS

The ACGME has set forth three main elements of the communication and interpersonal skills competency that postgraduate residents should demonstrate.[1] Also, a consensus statement known as the Kalamazoo statement and the Kalamazoo report was developed by leaders in medical education.[2] Although these documents were designed to apply generally across all medical specialties, the focus of this chapter will be the application to pediatrics.

There are three elements of the ACGME Interpersonal and Communication Skills competency that physicians should master, and each will be discussed in depth.

1. "Create and sustain a therapeutic and ethically sound relationship with patients and their families."[1] There are several concrete behaviors that help develop therapeutic and ethical relationships. First, it is important to always focus your complete attention on the patient and family (being "in the moment") during conversations. Second, it is essential to explore and understand the patient or parent's ideas, concerns, values, and feelings, even if they are negative or unpleasant, because this demonstrates respect for the autonomy of the patient. Third, the relationship is strengthened when there are openness and honesty that allow for the admission and repair of mistakes and the expression of authentic sorrow.[1,2] Finally, an approach that recognizes and honors diversity is another skill that allows a physician to foster a therapeutic relationship. By the year 2020, 44.5% of American children 0 to 19 years of age will belong to a racial or ethnic minority group.[4] Given these changing demographics, cultural competence is vital for developing successful relationships with families. The pediatrician must be aware of the many potential barriers to quality health care that a racial or ethnic minority family may confront, not only to understand how these may affect patients' care, but also to advocate for them. These barriers may include poverty; geographic factors; racism and other forms of prejudice; nonnative languages, including cultural variations in verbal and nonverbal communication; low-literacy; and culturally based beliefs surrounding illness, health, and death.[4]

The relationship with the pediatric patient is unique because it involves connecting not only with the child but also with the immediate family, other caregivers, and/or extended family. This situation brings its own challenges and rewards. The relationship with a family is often dynamic as family members enter or leave the family circle. It may also involve the challenging task of working with members of the family who are in conflict with one another or working with a family in crisis. On a positive note, it can be very rewarding to help a family engage their strengths or overcome their weaknesses in support of their child (e.g., ceasing tobacco use in a family that includes a child with asthma).

2. "Use effective listening skills to facilitate the relationship. Elicit and provide information using effective non-verbal, explanatory, questioning, and writing skills. Respond promptly to patient's queries and requests."[1] This competency element may be, in part, accomplished using the model of child- and parent-centered interviewing. This model allows the patient/parent to lead the discussion to the concerns that are most important in his/her eyes. Rather than following the doctor's agenda, it allows the patient to tell his/her own story. The parent is acknowledged as being the expert on his/her own child. The pediatrician is charged with finding an appropriate balance between centering the interview on the child or the parent, depending on the child's level of development and ability to participate. This style requires several key skills. Active listening involves hearing the patient's words in such a way that the patient feels understood. This may be accomplished by nonverbal cues and positive body language such as good eye contact, nodding, and leaning forward. Verbal skills include reflecting a patient's words back to him/her, paraphrasing back to the patient in your own words what you think has been said, and therapeutic pauses. Other verbal skills that facilitate the dialogue include using open-ended and closed-ended questions appropriately, asking for clarification when needed, and avoiding interrupting the speaker.[1]

Understanding the perspective of the family is also an important skill. Identify in a nonjudgmental way the emotions and feeling that you hear conveyed by the words, tone, or body language of the parent/child, and acknowledge this verbally to the speaker. For example, "You sound frustrated" (sad, angry, etc). Often bringing highly charged emotions out in the open both validates the speaker and subsequently diffuses the negativity of the situation so that you may move forward with the interview more productively.

The importance of effective communication of information back to the family cannot be overlooked. A correct diagnosis is in vain if the family is unable or unwilling to follow the treatment plan. Ensure that an agreement with the family is reached. The pediatrician should use language that is understandable, ask the parent to repeat what he/she heard, and ask for questions. Finally, the pediatrician should provide support in the form of appropriate follow-up care.[1-3]

3. "Work effectively with others as a member or leader of the healthcare team or other professional group. In all areas of communication and interaction show respect and empathy toward colleagues and learners."[1] Excellent patient care depends on the cooperation and clear communication of the entire health-care team. Elements of a highly effective team include respect, honesty, and integrity. Respectful treatment includes being truthful and responsible, following through on commitments, honoring the expertise of other health-care professionals, being open to learning from others, and being collaborative in patient care.

Acknowledge and respect the unique contributions that each professional makes to the health-care team. In interactions with colleagues, the pediatrician should be proactive in communication and take full responsibility for being understood by others. Resolve conflicts quickly and directly by discussing the issue with the relevant parties, instead of with other staff or parents. Advocate for a consensus treatment plan that takes into account all subspecialists, ancillary health-care providers, or support personnel involved. Parents who get the same message from all of their providers view their child's care as coming from a coordinated team, as opposed to receiving care piecemeal from a variety of individuals. Give and be open to receiving honest, constructive feedback from other health-care providers,[1] and agree to make adjustments to a plan with the team to provide the best and most integrated care possible.

WHY ARE INTERPERSONAL AND COMMUNICATION SKILLS IMPORTANT?

It is important to actively emphasize communication and interpersonal skills during medical training because they can be easily forgotten in the effort to master medical knowledge. Good communication skills have been found to lead to better patient outcomes, more efficient care, increased patient satisfaction, and physician satisfaction.[1] In addition, mastering these competencies is required by various medical organizations and regulatory bodies such as the United States Medical Licensing Examination Clinical Skills Exam, American Association of Medical Colleges, the Accreditation Council for Graduate Medical Education, and the American Board of Medical Specialties.

It is well documented that good interpersonal and communication skills result in a more effective doctor-patient relationship and better health outcomes. Effective communication is correlated with improved patient adherence, fewer medication errors, better management of chronic conditions, fewer malpractice claims, and a reduction in diagnostic testing and referrals.

Good interpersonal and communication skills are also correlated with increased patient satisfaction. Patient and family satisfaction is improved when physicians can express emotion nonverbally and are sensitive to nonverbal cues.[5] One study showed that parental perception of physician's qualities such as caring, openness to communication, and apparent level of concern were key factors in the parent's decision to continue the relationship with the provider.[6]

Good interpersonal and communication skills can provide the physician with a sense of satisfaction. Skillful interaction with a parent or child typically gives immediate positive feedback and builds confidence. When a physician truly values the whole patient, he/she in turn is reaffirming the worth of his/her work, thus reducing burnout and dissatisfaction.

Finally, care from an empathetic, respectful physician is important because it is what we would wish for ourselves, our friends, and our family.

LEARNING STRATEGIES

Good interpersonal and communication skills may not be automatically acquired in the course of medical training. As with other clinical skills, these skills are in part a set of tools that can be learned and taught.[1]

An international group of medical education leaders has developed a consensus of teaching strategies for interpersonal and communication competencies. These strategies are applicable for undergraduate, graduate, and postgraduate medical education across all specialties.[1] One method is physician self-awareness and self-reflection. Physician attitudes about various issues such as death and dying, gender, race, anger, and bad news influence how the provider interacts with patients. A lack of self-awareness of our own biases surrounding these issues may lead to behaviors that interfere with the doctor-patient relationship, and thus the physician's ability to discuss sensitive topics, to be supportive and empathetic, to obtain necessary data, and to reach an agreement with the patient.[1] The consensus statement suggests several strategies for learning self-awareness. These include individual work such as journaling or reading, one-on-one sessions with a mentor, and small group discussions. Other strategies for learning effective listening and communication skills include role modeling at the bedside, observation in real time with feedback, working with a standardized patient, role-playing, videotape review, and workshops.

The assessment of competency in interpersonal skills and communication can take several forms. The assessment tools most highly recommended by the ACGME include rating of direct or video observation of interactions with real or simulated patients, patient ratings by real or simulated patients, and 360-degree evaluations by patients, family, nursing, faculty, peers, and self.[7] The objective structured clinical examination (OSCE) with a real or simulated patient is a reliable method used by many medical schools and postgraduate training programs to

Table 5-1 Interpersonal and Communication Skills	
Skill	**Cases**
Create and sustain a therapeutic and ethically sound relationship with patients and their families.[1]	1, 2, 4, 16, 29, 32, 43, 44, 46, 49, 51, 52, 54
Use effective listening skills to facilitate the relationship.[1]	34, 49
Elicit and provide information using effective nonverbal, explanatory, questioning, and writing skills.[1]	3, 6, 7, 8, 9, 10, 12, 15, 18, 19, 21, 22, 25, 27, 28, 30, 32, 35, 36, 37, 38, 41, 42, 45, 47, 51, 55
Respond promptly to patient's queries and requests.[1]	35
Work effectively with others as a member or leader of the health-care team or other professional group. In all areas of communication and interaction show respect and empathy toward colleagues and learners.[1]	5, 11, 13, 14, 17, 20, 23, 24, 26, 30, 31, 33, 39, 40, 48, 50, 53, 56

assess multiple physician competencies, including communication and interpersonal skills.[8-10] In this model, the examinee moves through various standardized stations and is observed completing isolated portions of an encounter and then is rated by the examiner, and possibly the patient. The mini-clinical evaluation exercise (mini-CEX) is another popular evaluation method used to assess multiple competencies in interactions with actual patients. Through the use of standardized or real patients, observable behaviors can be evaluated and feedback provided in real time.

CONCLUSION

Mastery of the interpersonal and communication skills competency is essential for a successful, effective, and satisfying career in pediatrics. It will allow you to create and sustain deep and meaningful relationships with children and their families, to communicate skillfully during patient interactions, and to be a vital part of a health-care team, providing care to children and their families.

Table 5-1 lists each skill discussed above and the cases in the book in which those skills are applied to the practice of pediatrics.

References

1. Rider E: Competency 1: Interpersonal and communication skills. In *A practical guide to teaching and assessing the ACGME core competencies*, Marblehead, MA, 2007, HCPro, Inc.

2. All Participants in the Bayer-Fetzer Conference on Physician-Patient Communication in Medical Education: Essential elements of communication in medical encounter: The Kalamazoo consensus statement. *Acad Med* 76(4):390-393, 2001.

3. Committee on Hospital Care: Family-centered care and the pediatrician's role. *Pediatrics* 112(3):691-696, 2003.

4. Committee on Pediatric Workforce: Ensuring culturally effective pediatric care: Implications for education and health policy. *Pediatrics* 114(6):1677-1685, 2004.

5. DiMatteo MR, Taranta A, Friedman HS, Prince LM: Predicting patient satisfaction from physicians' nonverbal communication skills. *Med Care* 18:376-387, 1980.

6. Young PC, Wasserman RC, McAullife T, et al: Why families change pediatricians. *Am J Dis Child* 139(7):683-686, 1985.

7. Accreditation Council for Graduate Medical Education: *Toolbox of assessment methods, version 1.1,* 2001. Available at http://www.acgme.org/outcome/assess/toolbox.asp.

8. Jefferies A, Simmons B, Tabak D, et al: Using an objective structured clinical examination (OSCE) to assess multiple physician competencies in postgraduate training. *Med Teach* 29(2-3):183-191, 2007.

9. Bergus GR, Kreiter CD: The reliability of summative judgments based on objective structured clinical examination cases distributed across the clinical year. *Med Educ* 41(7):661-666, 2007.

10. Rider EA, Hinrichs MM, Lown BA: A model for communication skills assessment across the undergraduate curriculum. *Med Teach* 28(5):e127-e134, 2006.

Chapter 6
Practice-Based Learning and Improvement

Kristi Williams MD and Jane F. Knapp MD

INTRODUCTION

The Accreditation Council for Graduate Medical Education (ACGME) core competency of Practice-Based Learning and Improvement (PBLI) best summarizes the knowledge that caring for patients is a powerful way to learn.[1] In addition, it helps us to understand that this learning experience is most beneficial when we measure our processes of care and spend time in self-reflection. Finally, attaining competency in PBLI provides the physician with skills that will be useful over the course of his/her career.

The objectives of this chapter are to define the competency of PBLI and provide strategies for teaching PBLI during a pediatric residency training program.

DEFINITION

PBLI encompasses evaluation of patient care practices, appraisal and assimilation of scientific evidence, and subsequent improvement in patient care. The ACGME delineates six aspects of PBLI that provide a stepwise approach for physicians to successfully incorporate PBLI into daily practice. Table 6-1 lists the six aspects of PBLI.

THE IMPORTANCE OF SKILLS IN PBLI

The competency of PBLI is important because it teaches pediatricians how to monitor the quality of their work, improve their care of children, and keep up with new developments in pediatric medicine. As the American Board of Pediatrics adopts and implements Maintenance of Certification, understanding the core principles of PBLI becomes critical for the practicing pediatrician in order to maintain board certification. The four-step Maintenance of Certification process will entail assessment of the following:

- Professional standing
- Knowledge assessment
- Cognitive expertise
- Performance in practice

This last criterion will require comprehension and documentation of an approach to PBLI.

Table 6-1 The ACGME Six Aspects of PBLI

- Analyze practice experience and perform practice-based improvement activities using a systematic methodology
- Locate, appraise, and assimilate evidence from scientific studies related to their patients' health problems
- Obtain and use information about their own population of patients and the larger population from which their patients are drawn
- Apply knowledge of study designs and statistical methods to the appraisal of clinical studies and other information on diagnostic and therapeutic effectiveness
- Use information technology to manage information, access on-line medical information, and support their own education
- Facilitate the learning of students and other health care-professionals

STRATEGIES FOR LEARNING PBLI

Individualized Learning Plans

Individualized learning plans (ILPs) place the learner in control and at the center of learning.[1] Several steps go into preparing an ILP. These include reflection on career goals, determining learning needs for each goal, and forming enabling strategies to attain the goals. After creating the ILP, physicians periodically reflect on the learning goals to determine if they have been met. As each goal is met, the physician sets new learning goals for achievement. The choice of goal, methodology to achieve the goal, and the time frame set for each goal are specific to the physician's individual learning style, exemplifying the basic principles of self-directed learning. Challenges to ILPs include not knowing what to set as reasonable goals, not having time to focus on goals, and difficulty evaluating progress toward goals. Despite these challenges, residents found that ILPs helped them to concentrate on specific areas in which to gain knowledge and experience.[2]

Small-Group Learning Programs

Small-group learning programs provide a forum for physicians to meet and discuss specific clinical problems. Together, they can reflect on and share their experiences as well as review current information applicable to the clinical situations presented. One residency program established a pediatric digital library and learning collaboratory that residents and attending physicians use in multiple practice settings to broaden their pediatric knowledge.[3] Each clinical case begins with a question that serves to stimulate and direct discussion. A brief discussion of the topic, highlighted learning points, and further questions to consider follow the clinical vignette. Lastly, an accompanying list states the competencies that were met through the discussion of the clinical case. The database of clinical cases serves as a bank from which physicians can choose cases (based on disease, symptom, specialty, age, or posted date) as a means for self-study and review.

Evidence-Based Medicine

The ability to identify gaps in knowledge, formulate clinical questions, conduct literature searches, and apply the newly gained knowledge to clinical situations defines evidence-based medicine (EBM). Many residency programs have developed an EBM curriculum through which residents learn how to efficiently search the literature, critically appraise study results, and implement changes in patient care practices based on what they have learned. Journal clubs may be an adjunct to the EBM curriculum, allowing residents to gain more experience critically appraising the medical literature. Implementing EBM skills into daily practice improves patient care by increasing the likelihood that therapies provided are the current standard of care.

Periodic Chart Reviews and Morbidity and Mortality Conferences

A method to evaluate if patient care practices reflect the standard of care includes periodic chart reviews. A more structured venue for chart review occurs with preparation and presentation of Morbidity and Mortality (M&M) conferences. Both methods require reflection on cases to evaluate areas for improvement in patient care. Chart reviews may reveal system-wide issues that need improvement; improvement projects provide a means to address these issues.[6]

Quality Improvement Projects

Ideas for quality improvement projects may spring from clinical questions that arise in the course of patient care or after chart reviews. Following the processes outlined in various continuous quality improvement curricula, residents can implement aspects of PBLI. In this process, residents gain the tools to critically evaluate practices and systems and integrate the information to develop and carry out projects that would improve their individual practices and the larger systems within which they work.[5]

CONCLUSION

Practice-based learning and improvement, when incorporated into daily patient care practices, provide physicians with the skills to evaluate their work, to identify gaps in knowledge and skills, and to implement improvements in their practices to improve their care of patients. Residency programs, including pediatric programs, have begun incorporating strategies to teach and assess the skills of PBLI. The ability to use the skills of PBLI to improve the care of children and their families is unique to pediatrics and thus important to the training of pediatric residents.

References

1. Challis M: AMEE medical education guide no. 19: Personal learning plans. *Med Teach* 22(3):225-236, 2000.
2. Stuart E, Sectish TC, Huffman LC: Are residents ready for self-directed learning? A pilot program of individualized learning plans in continuity clinic. *Ambul Pediatr* 5:298-301, 2005.
3. The Pediatric Digital Library and Learning Collaboratory: Available at http://www.pediatriceducation.org.

4. Kravet SJ, Howell E, Wright SM: Morbidity and Mortality conference, grand rounds, and the ACGME's core competencies. *J Gen Intern Med* 21:1192-1194, 2006.
5. Weingart SN, Tess A, Driver J, et al: Creating a quality improvement elective for medical house officers. *J Gen Intern Med* 19:861-967, 2004.

Chapter 7
Systems-Based Practice

Tara Andersen DO and Denise Bratcher DO

Very few doctors understand what is happening to the health care system in which they practice, why the system is changing so rapidly, and what they can do about it.[1]

Systems-based practice is widely regarded as one of the most challenging competencies to understand and implement. The Accreditation Council for Graduate Medical Education (ACGME) requires that all residents demonstrate an "awareness of and responsiveness to the larger context and system of health care and the ability to effectively call on system resources to provide care that is of optimal value."[2] To better understand this concept, we must ask the following question: How can we best provide safe, effective, efficient, equitable, and patient-centered care? Within the answer to this question lies the essence of systems-based practice.

DEFINITIONS OF SYSTEMS-BASED PRACTICE

Systems-based practice is formally defined by the ACGME as "the use of health-care services for patient care, and how the costs of providing those services can affect the delivery of care."[3] This competency, stated simply, concerns the *business* of health care. Effective and efficient patient care is at the root of systems-based practice. Physicians can best provide optimal care by understanding the *structure, process, economics,* and *politics* of the health-care industry.

IMPORTANCE OF SYSTEMS-BASED PRACTICE

Physicians must understand how their actions affect others within their profession, health-care organization, and society as a whole to recognize the importance of and truly understand the *structure* of the health-care industry. Through this critical self-evaluation they begin to realize the impact of their actions on others. It is also critical for physicians to observe and understand the interconnectedness of the entire health-care system and how a system failure in one area can have a deleterious downstream effect on patient care. Structure and process drive behavior; thus flaws within structure and process can lead to medical errors. Within this understanding lies the critical role of both root cause analysis and systematic quality improvement. When flaws in structure or process are observed, a systematic approach to problem identification and subsequent quality improvement provides a vehicle for both education and change.

Physicians also need to demonstrate understanding of the *economics* of health care. More specifically, residents must understand methods that different health-care systems use to control costs and allocate resources. This will assist physicians in learning to provide high-quality patient care that is cost-effective and use resources to the patients' optimal benefit.

Finally, physicians need to understand the *politics* of medicine. Students and residents must learn to be advocates for their patients; they need to be equipped with the tools to ensure that their patients receive high-quality care at all times. They must be able to help their patients navigate complex health-care systems with ease.

STRATEGIES FOR LEARNING SYSTEMS-BASED PRACTICE

Many areas encompassed within this competency, such as understanding the broad health-care system and how to bill and code effectively, have traditionally been learned as a function of experience. The challenge posed to educational programs is to discern how to replace the slow process of gradual exposure to the various aspects of the health-care system with an effective, comprehensive educational curriculum.

Many different teaching tactics have been attempted with varying degrees of success. This section will highlight four categories of strategies: patient care review projects, simulation, web-based modules, and formal didactic learning.

Patient Care Review Projects

Patient safety is the driving force for much of the systems-based practice competency. Assessment of patient care delivery and its impact on patient safety can aid in the learning of systems-based practice.

Tomolo and colleagues[4] developed an educational tool, named the Outcomes Card, to assist residents in this process. Residents were asked to identify cases in which patient safety was at risk and to track several important factors (type of case, type of event, error type, systems involved, and system failures). The use of outcomes cards can help demonstrate the complexities of the systems involved and the impact the health-care system has on patient care delivery.

Allen and colleagues also suggest that independent learning projects are effective in teaching systems-based practice.[5] Residents in their internal medicine program independently identified a health-care system or delivery issue. They used seminars to initially educate residents about health-care systems, followed by reinforcement via active learning through their own projects, called the Health Systems Independent Study Project (HSISP). Participating residents found that these projects help them relate systems-based practice with their own clinical practice and gain a focused understanding of their health-care system.

Students and residents can also gain exposure to systems-based problems associated with errors through involvement with hospital-wide Morbidity and Mortality (M&M) committees/conferences as well as quality improvement (QI) committees/projects.[3,6] At Children's Mercy Hospital, we have implemented a systems-based approach to evaluating cases submitted for M&M conference. A multidisciplinary committee, involving nursing staff and physicians with various specialties, ranging from QI to evidence-based medicine, evaluates all cases in a systematic fashion to identify where within our system we may best be able to institute further "checks and balances" to ensure high-quality patient care.

Simulation

Another method of active learning that may be used in the teaching of systems-based practice involves simulation of actual patient care. Zenni and co-workers[7] used scenario-based learning to give pediatric residents first-hand experience with the difficulties of being a parent to a child requiring complex medical care. Emphasis was placed on identifying and accessing community resources to solve problems. This project ultimately helped residents to develop empathy and compassion as well as an improved understanding of barriers that families face to obtaining adequate medical care.

Matter and colleagues[8] used a slightly different program to help their internal medicine residents understand what challenges their patients face after hospital discharge. They found that by having their residents perform home visits on patients, the residents gained a greater understanding of difficulties their patients encounter at home with applying and adhering to discharge plans as well as an increased awareness of home needs of various patients.

Many hospitals are beginning to form family advisory boards, which can be a great resource to pediatric residents in providing a parent's perspective of medical care. Opportunities for residents to shadow patients and families can provide a unique, first-hand view of the patient's perspective.

Web-Based Knowledge

Web-based modules are also being used successfully by many residency programs as teaching aids. Kerfoot and co-workers[9] performed a large

Table 7-1 Health-Care Systems	
Systems	**Cases**
Medical management	
Care management	21, 24, 26, 27, 28, 29, 32, 54, 55
Disease management	10
Case management	10, 22
Prescription drug benefits and formulary	47
Hospital clinical pathways	30, 33, 43
Health-care technology	
Benchmarking	16
Place of service and level of care	
Office-based care	9, 40
Emergency department and urgent care	12, 49
Acute care hospital	42, 44
Home health care	14, 18, 19
Hospice and end-of-life care	
Health law	1, 53, 56
Informed consent and The Patient Care Partnership (formerly known as The Patient Bill of Rights)	3, 15, 48
Medical malpractice and liability insurance	13, 51, 52
Fraud and abuse	
Health-care economics	
Claims, coding, and billing	20, 46
Cost of health care	5, 6, 8, 25, 31, 38, 39, 45
Managed care	
Medicare, Medicaid, Tricare, HMOs, PPOs Providers	50
Member benefits	11, 23
Services requiring authorization	11, 23
Quality improvement	4, 7, 17, 35, 36, 37
NCQA/HEDIS, TJC	2, 41
IOM, AHRQ	34

AHRQ, Agency for Healthcare Research and Quality; *HEDIS,* Healthcare Effectiveness Data and Information Set; *HMO,* heath maintenance organization; *IOM,* Institute of Medicine; *NCQA,* National Committee for Quality Assurance; *PPO,* preferred provider organization; *TJC,* The Joint Commission.

study across multiple medical specialties and found that web-based education on patient safety and the U.S. health-care system resulted in statistically significant increases in knowledge for participants.

Formal Didactic Education

In addition to the previously discussed innovative learning approaches, it appears that traditional didactic learning remains effective in teaching many areas of systems-based practice. Kravet and colleagues describe an interdisciplinary case-based conference developed to improve understanding of resource management in their internal medicine residents.[10] Each conference begins with a case presentation followed by discussion of follow-up information, review of itemized hospital bill and coding issues, and discussion of hospital reimbursement.

CONCLUSION

The importance of understanding and implementing of systems-based practice can be widely generalized; this set of concepts is not just important to physicians. In fact, anyone who works within any sort of organization or industry must master these skills to become truly effective. The nebulous nature of these new ACGME expectations may make this competency seem superfluous to the practice of medicine and education of residents on how to be a "good doctor." However, although systems-based practice may initially seem to be the most daunting of the competencies to integrate into an educational program, it becomes evident with more understanding of the breadth of this topic how truly important each component is to the foundation of a solid, well-rounded pediatrician.

Table 7-1 lists the health-care systems and the cases in the book in which those parts are discussed in context of the practice of pediatrics.

References

1. Relman AS: Education to defend professional values in the new corporate age. *Acad Med* 73:1229-1233, 1998.
2. Available at. http://www.acgme.org/outcome/comp/compMin.asp.
3. Rider EA, Nawotniak RH, Smith G: *A practical guide to teaching and assessing the ACGME core competencies*, Marblehead, MA, 2007, HCPro, Inc.
4. Tomolo A, Caron A, Perz ML, et al: The outcomes card: Development of a systems-based practice educational tool. *J Gen Intern Med* 20:769-771, 2005.
5. Allen E, Zerzan J, Choo C, et al: Teaching systems-based practice to residents by using independent study projects. *Acad Med* 80:125-128, 2005.
6. Kravet SJ, Howell E, Wright SM: Morbidity and mortality conference, grand rounds, and the ACGME's core competencies. *J Gen Intern Med* 21:1192-1194, 2006.

7. Zenni EA, Ravago L, Ewart C, et al: A walk in the patients' shoes: A step toward competency development in systems-based practice. *Ambul Pediatr* 6:54-57, 2006.
8. Matter CA, Speice JA, McCann R, et al: Hospital to home: Improving internal medicine residents' understanding of the needs of older persons after a hospital stay. *Acad Med* 78:793-797, 2003.
9. Kerfoot BP, Conlin PR, Travison T, McMahon GT: Web-based education in systems-based practice: A randomized trial. *Arch Intern Med* 167:361-366, 2007.
10. Kravet SJ, Wright SM, Carrese JA: Teaching resource and information management using an innovative case-based conference. *J Gen Intern Med* 16:399-403, 2001.

Chapter 8
How to Succeed in the Pediatric Clerkship

J. Lindsey Lane MD

INTRODUCTION

How does one define success on the pediatric clerkship? Getting a high grade and performing well on the examination are important. However, it is equally important to focus on personal growth and strive to become a reflective practitioner who is skilled and engaged in continuous learning and self-improvement. This is the ultimate measure of success.

GENERAL OVERVIEW OF APPROACH TO THE CLERKSHIP

The six competencies (patient care, medical knowledge, practice-based learning and improvement, interpersonal and communication skills, professionalism, systems-based practice) introduced by the Accreditation Council for Graduate Medical Education (ACGME) describe core areas in medical practice and the skills within each area in general terms. The challenge for students is to focus on the specific competencies, skills, and learning goals that match their learning level within the pediatric clinical training experience. The pediatric clerkship director is responsible for defining, based on national standards,[1] the expectations for what is to be learned; transmitting this information to students and teachers; and providing appropriate learning opportunities. However, the learning process and eventual outcomes will depend on the student's approach.[2]

Most students will have a variety of experiences on the pediatric clerkship. The newborn nursery, inpatient service, outpatient, and subspecialty offices and community sites are all common training areas. Students will have to adapt to new clinical expectations and different team structure and work systems several times within a short time period. This can be especially difficult for students who take time to adapt and feel comfortable in new situations. An orientation given at each training site will decrease "newcomer anxiety"; however, it is very important for students to ask about the specific expectations at a new training locale if orientation is inadequate. Asking recent students is helpful; however, interns, residents, and attending physicians may all have different expectations, and a student may have to ask each of these members of the team to clearly transmit his/her expectations.

It is essential for students to present themselves well and to have a good attitude. Studies show that about half of a student's grade is based on assessment of their nonverbal behaviors[3]; therefore always be aware of how others might perceive your behavior. The shy, quiet student may be perceived as disinterested and should be sure to behave in ways that dispel this erroneous impression—for example, offering to do research about a patient problem or staying late to help with patient care. Being pushy, very solicitous, and trying too hard to impress are at the other end of the spectrum and are equally undesirable. Aim to be neither underconfident nor overconfident. Try to find and fit into the rhythm of work of your preceptor or team and intellectually, physically, and emotionally help them care for patients. Students who do this not only gain greater personal satisfaction, but also receive more teaching and more clinical opportunities.

It is imperative for students to monitor their progress and ask their teachers to observe them and give them feedback. Without feedback, students evaluate their performance and progress on self-assessment—which is inaccurate at best. Ideally, observation and feedback should be built into the program. If it is not, the student should suggest to the clerkship director that this part of the teaching program be developed.

Now let's consider the individual competencies and how a student's approach to learning within these areas will ensure success. Each competency is listed as follows with elements gleaned from the definitions. See Appendix 1 ACGME General Competencies for a complete listing of the competencies and their definitions from the ACGME.

MEDICAL KNOWLEDGE

Elements

- Investigatory and analytic thinking
- Knowledge and application of basic sciences

One model of learning[4] describes learning in the following terms: "deep," "strategic," and "surface." Deep learning is based on three motivational factors (intrinsic motivation, vocational interest, and personal understanding) and three learning processes (making links across material, searching for a deeper understanding of the material, and looking for general principles). Strategic learning is motivated by a desire to be successful and leads to patchy and variable understanding. Surface learning is motivated by fear of failure and a desire to complete a course, with students tending to rely on learning by rote and focusing on particular tasks.

Studies show that, of all the learning approaches, medical students who are strategic learners score highest on examinations. Deep learners, however, perform well in clinical situations when working with faculty and residents evaluating and managing patients. Therefore a combination of strategic and deep learning is ideal. Always think rigorously and share your knowledge and insights, but do not be afraid to say "I don't know" or "I do not understand."

PATIENT CARE

Elements

- Caring and respectful behaviors
- Interviewing
- Informed decision making
- Developing and carrying out patient management plans
- Counseling and educating patients and families
- Performance of procedures
- Routine physical examination
- Medical procedures
- Preventive health services
- Working within a team

Because pediatrics spans a wide age range, students often find it challenging to adapt to the different developmental stages of the patients. There are differences in what must be included in a history, different elements in the physical examination, and different approaches to adopt for successful data gathering that vary with the age of the patient. Technical procedures are also more difficult and challenging, and students will be invited to do only the most straightforward and on cooperative patients. However, if you are not invited, you should ask to be involved in procedures because students who show an interest are more likely to be allowed to attempt procedures. Rounds offer opportunities for students to present in front of patients and share information. This can be intimidating at first, but by carefully watching how attendings and residents approach this task—and as always asking for guidance and feedback—it is possible to become relatively comfortable fairly quickly.

One important tip: Always know everything about your patients—you will learn from them and remember them forever.

INTERPERSONAL AND COMMUNICATION SKILLS

Elements

- Creation of therapeutic relationships with patients
- Listening skills

Excellent interpersonal and communication skills improve patient adherence (compliance) and improve your relationship with peers, colleagues, and other members of the medical team.[5] There is always more to learn, and you should watch the master clinician communicators and emulate them. Also, observe closely and never adopt the habits of individuals with inferior skills or the demeanor of those around you if it is anything less than excellent, compassionate, and caring.

PROFESSIONALISM

Elements

- Respect, altruism
- Ethically sound practice
- Sensitivity to cultural, age, gender, disability issues

Many studies show a worsening of professional behavior as training progresses.[6] Medicine is stressful; being a medical student is *very* stressful, and you must be aware that the process of training may erode your empathy and inclination to care. Always put yourself in the shoes of the patient and family members to understand what they are experiencing and how they are responding. Talking with peers and seeking out forums in the medical school where you can discuss the daily challenges to professionalism is useful for helping you stay "on course."[7]

PRACTICE-BASED LEARNING AND IMPROVEMENT

Elements

- Analyzing own practice for needed improvements
- Use of evidence from scientific studies
- Application of research and statistical methods
- Use of information technology
- Facilitating learning of others

During the clerkship you will probably be asked to research and give short presentations on topics pertaining to your patients. Make a habit of formulating "well-built" clinical questions[8] about diagnosis, therapy, prognosis, prevention, and education. Try to synthesize the clinical information and evidence and format it to answer the relevant clinical questions that you have generated. Make a habit of asking "why?"—not to the point of being annoying—to trigger exploration of clinical problems and critical review of the literature. This is the deep learning process that is the hallmark of growth as a physician. You are also most likely to be the person on the team closest to your basic science education. You should capitalize on this and try to incorporate basic science information into your presentations for the members of your team who have forgotten it!

SYSTEMS-BASED PRACTICE

Elements

- Understanding interaction of own practice with the larger system
- Knowledge of practice and delivery systems
- Practicing cost-effective care
- Advocating for patients within the health-care system

Students will get glimpses of the four elements of systems-based practice during their clinical work. Paying close attention to the functioning of the health-care system and thinking about cost-effectiveness when engaged in patient care are important. Advocacy is an area in which students can make great contributions.[9] Seeking out opportunities to advocate for their patients and learn about the broader scope of advocacy is important for professional growth and development as a reflective practitioner.

CONCLUSION

The bottom line for success: keep a sense of humor, keep a sense of perspective, and remember that it is all about the patients.

References

1. Council on Medical Student Education in Pediatrics Curriculum: Available at http://www.comsep.org/.
2. Kolb DA: *Learning-Style Inventory*, Boston, MA, 1976, McBer & Co.
3. Rosenblum ND, Wetzel M, Platt O, et al: Predicting medical student success in a clinical clerkship by rating students' nonverbal behavior. *Arch Pediatr Adolesc Med* 148:213-219, 1994.
4. Cassidy S, Eachus P: Learning style, academic belief systems, self-report student proficiency and academic achievement in higher education. *Educ Psychol* 20:307-322, 2000.
5. Novack DH: Clinical review: Therapeutic aspects of the clinical encounter. *J Gen Intern Med* 2:346-355, 1987.
6. Hojat M, Mangione S, Nasca TJ, et al: An empirical study of decline in empathy in medical school. *Med Educ* 38:934–941, 2004.

7. Inui TS: *A flag in the wind: Education for professionalism in medicine*. Association of American Medical Colleges, 2003, pp 1-37. Available at http://www.regenstrief.org/Members/tinui/bio/flaginthewind.
8. Richardson WS, Wilson MC, Nishikawa J, Hayward RSA: The well-built clinical question: A key to evidence-based decisions. *ACP Journal Club* 123:A12, 1995 Nov-Dec.
9. Shon DA: *The reflective practitioner*. New York, NY, 1983, Basic Books.

Chapter 9
How to Succeed as a Junior Resident: Continuity Clinic and Inpatient Wards

Theresa Hetzler MD *and*
Matthew J. Kapklein MD, MPH

CONTINUITY CLINIC

Introduction

Continuity clinic provides a longitudinal educational experience spanning the 3 years of pediatric residency. Although continuity clinics vary from program to program, all afford a learning experience quite different from the inpatient ward or intensive care unit. It is an ideal site to work on all of the core competencies.

MEDICAL KNOWLEDGE

There is a core fund of knowledge you will need to succeed. A thorough understanding of the well child examination and how to approach it is imperative. At each examination you must know the normal developmental and behavioral milestones, appropriate diet, and age-appropriate essential components of the physical examination, screening tools, anticipatory guidance, and immunization schedule. Although the immunization schedule may vary over time, risks and benefits of vaccine components are relatively constant. Likewise, age-appropriate developmental milestones and injury prevention can be committed to memory. Knowing these by heart will save you time during the visit.

You should be familiar with resources available at your continuity site to aid you in the encounter, as well as online resources.

PATIENT CARE

The continuity clinic is the optimal setting for developing and assessing longitudinal therapeutic relationships with patients and families. You will learn the generalist's approach to common ambulatory pediatric problems, as well as the specific skills needed to provide anticipatory guidance, developmental and behavioral screening, immunizations, preventive care, and coordination of care. The beauty of continuity clinic is that you will be able to observe your skills in these areas evolve over time.

Your role as primary care provider allows you to provide services aimed at maintaining wellness and preventing health problems. Following your patients over time, you have the opportunity to give them the tools necessary to become healthy adults. At routine well-child visits, you will give patients and their families age-appropriate anticipatory guidance to assist them between visits (see Chapters 16, and 18 to 24).

Here are some tips that will aid in mastering these skills. From the beginning, identify yourself as the child's doctor, even though you are still in training. Give the family a business card with your name, the office or clinic number, and the off-hours emergency number. This will help establish continuity and help you gain the family's trust. Assisting the family in scheduling follow-up appointments specifically with you will help establish an ongoing relationship. Maintaining your continuity log (specific procedures will differ by program) from day 1 will help you track your patient panel throughout your training.

INTERPERSONAL AND COMMUNICATION SKILLS

Communication is key in working not only with your patients and their families but also within the health-care team. Effective communication requires use of appropriate language based on the educational, socioeconomic, and cultural backgrounds of your patients and their families. These will be unique to each continuity site and each patient encounter. For a successful visit, you must start on an appropriate playing field with your patient and family. By inquiring into the family situation and engaging in a brief conversation with the family, you can get a feel for the level of education and understanding of English. Based on these, the patient's history should be elicited with questions aimed at an appropriate level of understanding. An interpreter should participate in any encounter in which you are not fluent in the language the historian speaks. Know your patients: Learn about the cultures seen in your practice setting, and do not hesitate to ask for help in understanding them.

In addition to communicating effectively with your patients, you will need to master skills to communicate effectively with the health-care team. In the continuity setting, this means nurses, receptionists, and schedulers as well as consultants, agencies, and other physicians (residents and faculty) on your team. Of equal or greater importance are your written communication skills. The medical record will be your connection to other practitioners and staff on days you are not present at the continuity site. Maintaining clear, legible, comprehensive notes will help make you an effective communicator (see Chapters 11, Note Writing, and 12, Oral Presentations).

PROFESSIONALISM

An important first step in professional behavior is demonstrating appropriate respect for the setting, your patients, and yourself. Regardless of where it is, your continuity site is your office, and you should look like a doctor while you are there. Grooming is important, as well as attire. Your program will let you know what is acceptable at each site. Your dress is a sign of respect for the relationship you have with your patient. Your verbal and nonverbal behaviors will also be a measure of your respect for that relationship.

During the encounter, listening attentively and responding compassionately and honestly are evidence of professionalism. Be honest with families when you do not know an answer, and seek help appropriately. Remember that these are **your** patients; acknowledge this ownership by demonstrating your reliability and accountability to your patients and responsibility for your decisions.

Maintaining confidentiality of patient information is especially important. Whenever you exchange information with other practitioners, make sure to have permission to do so from the patient or family. Be conscious of where you are discussing this information. Are you in a room set aside for patient discussions with your preceptor, or in a hallway outside the waiting room, where others may hear?

Many medical students and pediatric residents come from different socioeconomic and cultural backgrounds than the patients served by their continuity clinics. "Cultural competency" means being sensitive to patients' cultures and recognizing the role of those cultures in all spheres, including the perceived need for health care and treatment compliance. It is important to become culturally competent in the populations for whom you frequently provide care.

PRACTICE-BASED LEARNING AND IMPROVEMENT

Residents develop longitudinal relationships not only with their patients, but with their continuity preceptors. This relationship is unique in residency because of its longevity and consistent contact. Most residents find it safe and comfortable, and often a mentoring relationship. Why is this important? Many residents struggle with soliciting feedback from supervisors and critically reviewing their own practice. The preceptor is in a unique position to give you ongoing feedback. Use your preceptor as a resource by asking relevant questions regarding diagnoses, therapies, management, and clinical practice.

Other resources at your continuity site include online resources, texts, and clinical guidelines. You should become familiar with resources at your disposal at your site. Texts available through the American Academy of Pediatrics (AAP), such as the *Report of the Committee on Infectious Diseases* (the *Red Book*) and *Bright Futures: Guidelines for Health Supervision of Infants, Children, and Adolescents,* are valuable resources and should be available at your site. The *Red Book* provides you with current AAP recommendations for diagnosing, treating, and preventing infectious disease. *Bright Futures* provides comprehensive health supervision guidelines, including recommendations on immunizations, routine health screening, and anticipatory guidance. Access to current literature and the ability to interpret it will permit you to give your patients up-to-date, appropriate care.

To best serve your patients you must understand the community in which they live. Learn about the community you serve. Familiarize yourself with the health risks and needs of your population, and put them in the context of available resources. For many people, residency training also means moving to a new city or community. If you are unfamiliar with the community, take a field trip through the neighborhoods you are serving, learn about the specific ethnic groups or other subpopulations, and speak to long-time staff members at your continuity site familiar with the population and the available resources.

SYSTEMS-BASED PRACTICE

There are hospital-based clinics, community-based clinics, and private practices in which residents receive their continuity experience. Each site has its own unique characteristics regarding payer types, insurance carriers, billing practices, and available resources. Providing the best care for your patients not only depends on your medical knowledge, but also on your applying it with attention to outcome, cost-effectiveness, risk benefit, and patient/family preference. You will acquire cost-consciousness skills during your continuity experience.

Here are some ways you can incorporate the tenets of cost-conscious medicine into your training:

- **Think before you act.** Listen closely to your patient before ordering sophisticated tests. A careful history may provide you with more infor- mation than an expensive test. Beware of the costs of diagnostic tests and medications, and consider generic medications when appropriate.
- **Choose diagnostic tests carefully.** Learn the most common diagnoses based on history and physical presentation, then consider studies that will confirm or reject them. Always ask yourself what

information you will get from a test that will change the patient's management.

- **Talk to patients/families about medications.** Explain the price difference between generic and brand-name medications. Consider which medications are covered by specific insurance plans, and select effective medications that will require as little out-of-pocket expense from your patients as possible.
- **Get help from online formularies and other practice software.** Use resources at your site to compare prices and take cost into consideration when making prescribing decisions.
- **Follow accepted practice guidelines.** Practice guidelines help control practice variation and often take into account cost-effectiveness.
- **Use your preceptor as a resource.** Learn from your attendings who have had experience negotiating the health-care system and understanding your patient population.
- **Do not underutilize tests, procedures, or referrals simply to cut costs.** Remember, your primary concern is to be cost-effective without compromising care.

You will play the role of coordinator of the health-care team. This is of particular importance for children with complex diagnoses and medical needs. For these patients in particular, you should become familiar with the other physicians and professionals involved with their care. Identify local resources such as early intervention, child welfare services, support groups, and early childhood care and educational services. Understanding obstacles families may encounter and learning to navigate the system will improve your ability to advocate for your patients.

THE INPATIENT WARDS

Introduction

Students and residents spend a large portion of their training working on inpatient wards. Lessons learned in this setting often influence the way physicians practice for the rest of their careers. Hospital wards can also be daunting places, filled with new and potentially frightening experiences. Learning how to navigate the wards can help one become more facile in all competency areas.

MEDICAL KNOWLEDGE

Patient interactions give young doctors first-hand experience with disease processes and problems that may have seemed more abstract up to that point. Each interaction can advance one's medical knowledge. Pathology encountered on inpatient wards leads to questions about disease processes, methods of treatment, and controversies regarding treatment options. The successful student or resident uses these cases as opportunities to learn more by turning to "the literature" for answers. Do not be afraid to use textbooks during the early phases of your training—you need to know the basics before you start asking about the current controversies. Once you have a knowledge foundation, up-to-date, peer-reviewed journals should be your principal sources of information about common disease processes and their management.

PATIENT CARE

If one were to ask pediatric residents to rank the six core competencies by the amount of time and energy devoted to them, most would put patient care at the top. To succeed, we must ensure that our patients receive safe and timely care, which often requires careful planning and coordination of services by the medical team.

It is important to remember that the tasks that seem most important to you may be less so to patients and their families. For example, in pediatrics, every needlestick counts. If a patient requires an IV placement and has a timed blood draw, care should be taken to accomplish these tasks at the same time, thereby saving the patient an extra needlestick. This type of consideration allows for optimal patient care and comfort and is appreciated by families. Every hour without food also counts. If a patient requires procedural sedation, the expert house officer schedules carefully so as to avoid extra days in the hospital or unnecessary hours on an empty stomach.

The workload on inpatient wards can sometimes seem overwhelming. Patients and families (who are dealing with the stresses of hospitalized children) do not care how busy or overworked you are, nor is "I'm busy" ever an acceptable response to a concern raised by a parent, patient, or staff member. Our job is to make sure that we address our patients' needs, and if we're too busy to do so, to get help.

INTERPERSONAL AND COMMUNICATION SKILLS

Life on the wards basically consists of moving from one interaction to the next. Each conversation with an inpatient's family is designed to serve a function and must be handled with thought and planning. Some conversations elicit information from the patient or family; others deliver news, be it good, bad, or neither; still others are used to comfort, empathize, or even just chat. Each interaction requires preparation with regard to location, word choice, and those present. All must be undertaken with respect for the patient, acknowledgment of level of understanding, and empathy.

Learning to approach and address patients appropriately based on developmental level and situation is a skill. Attention should be paid to how a patient likes to be addressed, whom the patient would like present for interactions, and so on. Patients do not like to feel they are being rushed—so even if you are pressed for time, try to avoid letting families feel that way. Give opportunities to ask questions and a way to contact you if they have more. Physicians who take the time to explain plans, give reasonable time frames with respect to test results, and allow patients to voice concerns establish easier working relationships with families. A good motto on the inpatient wards is, "Underpromise and overdeliver"—nothing disappoints a family more than when physicians create an expectation (for when a test result will be available, for example) then fail to meet it; better to give families a pleasant surprise by getting something done faster than you said you would.

One of the most crucial communications on the inpatient wards is when residents transfer care of patients to one another, often called "handoff" or "signout." Physicians must learn to sign out accurately, including medically relevant facts and discarding all nonpertinent information. Likewise, notes in medical records must be accurate and factual and allow other caregivers to comprehend patients' current status and reason for treatment plans. Any unexpected or important events, findings, or laboratory values should be documented similarly—dated, legible, and signed.

PROFESSIONALISM

Being a professional begins with looking the part. Patients and their families expect a certain level of dress and grooming from physicians. Most hospitals have dress codes for employees—this usually means business-casual attire. Professional attire also means clean scrubs and laboratory coats. Patients do not need to see that their physician has been busy taking care of other patients by examining the stains on his/her clothing. Each hospital and residency program will have its own rules and culture regarding when and where scrub attire is acceptable.

Timing is an important aspect of success on the wards. Arriving at work on time shows that you respect not only your patients, but your colleagues as well. A typical day on the inpatient wards is tightly structured, with lectures and meetings between rounds and patient care. Punctuality allows these events to start on time, thereby not delaying other important tasks for you and your colleagues.

Timing also means getting work done in an appropriate time frame. On the inpatient wards, there are multiple tasks to complete for any given patient. Calling consults, speaking to referring physicians, arranging for studies, and performing timed blood draws all will have specific times by which they need to be accomplished. Successful students and residents devise methods to track these time-sensitive assignments.

Nowhere will your ability to maintain respectful communication be tested more than on the inpatient wards. This means being courteous even when others do not reciprocate. It means speaking to patients and staff calmly and politely, regardless of how they address you. If you are tempted to argue and escalate a tense situation, politely stepping away from the situation is usually the more professional course. Patients and their families are not required to behave professionally; other health-care personnel are, but sometimes do not. Unprofessional behavior in others is not a justification for responding in kind. The true test of our professionalism is how we behave when it is challenged.

PRACTICE-BASED LEARNING AND IMPROVEMENT

The amount of information to absorb and apply on the inpatient wards can seem endless. The student or novice house officer may feel that he/she lacks the basics, let alone the advanced knowledge required to answer current controversies about common problems. There are those rare diagnoses or presentations that arise that deserve reading time. A good study guide is as follows: Read **something** (starting with book chapters, working up to review articles and original research publications) about every patient you admit. This will quickly allow you to become expert in common inpatient conditions while giving you a background on rarer conditions. Once acquired, medical knowledge should be communicated to others. Information obtained to answer a query raised on inpatient rounds should be brought back to the group and shared among colleagues, allowing everyone to benefit from each other's labors.

With so many skills to learn, it is common to feel overwhelmed and to wonder how your performance compares with that of your peers. Both of these feelings are normal, and the latter should be encouraged. Part of success on the wards is the ability to self-reflect. Ask yourself questions like, "Is my patient care as good as it should be?" and "Am I learning and studying enough?" These questions should prompt requests for feedback from those with whom you interact regularly and encourage you to explore ways to improve.

SYSTEMS-BASED PRACTICE

The system of a hospital can be overwhelming to families, who often must navigate this complicated structure without guidance. A physician on the inpatient wards is in a key position to help coordinate care and make things run as smoothly as possible. As a patient advocate, the physician contacts the appropriate consultants—including noncaregivers like social workers and case managers—to provide needed services. Prompt and proper completion of paperwork and prescriptions ensures that patients receive the care they require. By providing a smooth transition between hospital and home care, one can make families' experience of the inpatient ward less stressful.

Chapter 10
History and Physical Examination

Matthew J. Kapklein MD, MPH

INTRODUCTION

A chapter on history and physical examination (H&P) in a medical text is
a bit like a chapter on gravity and Newtonian physics in a book on
aviation: they are the foundation on which the entire field is built.
Everything we do as professionals, we do for a reason—or at least we
should. The skilled technician knows what to do; the reflective
practitioner knows why to do it. Good strategic planning is an important
component of any endeavor and requires a mission statement as well as
goals and objectives for achieving it. What follows is an attempt to place
the pediatric H&P in this context, using the framework of the American
Academy of Pediatrics' (AAP's) mission statement, goals gleaned from
the Accreditation Council for Graduate Medical Education's (ACGME's)
component skills in the six core competencies, and one author's
objectives. See Appendix 1 ACGME General Competencies for a complete
listing of the competencies and their definitions from the ACGME.

PROFESSION: PEDIATRICIAN

Mission: Attain optimal physical, mental, and social health and
   well-being for all infants, children, adolescents, and young adults.
Activity: History and physical examination (H&P).

PATIENT CARE

Goal 1: Gather essential and accurate information about patients.
Objectives: Most think of this as the primary goal of the H&P,
   with historical information obtained first (via interviewing) and
   examination findings later (via "laying hands"). In fact, history
   taking starts before the interview begins and continues after it
   ends. Likewise, the physical examination begins the moment you
   hear or see the patient and ends only when he/she is out of reach
   of your senses.
   Before medical school, we live for decades during which we
   develop skills in reading people. You are allowed, even encouraged,
   to use those skills in addition to the ones you paid to learn.
   Indeed, these may tell you whether the time is even appropriate

for information gathering or for immediate intervention, or both in tandem. An experienced pediatrician can, on entering a room and from several feet away, perform a large portion of a child's examination without touching the child or entering his/her personal space. This is fortunate, because many of our patients do not like it when we touch them, or even get close.

Goal 2: Communicate effectively, and demonstrate caring and respectful behaviors with patients and their families.

Objectives: The key word here is *demonstrate*. You may respect or care a great deal about a patient and family, but if they cannot discern it, then as far as they are concerned you do not. Likewise, there may be times when, for a variety of reasons, we do **not** highly respect a particular family. At these times demonstrating that we **do** becomes even more important. It is easy to act our best when we feel good; the challenge is doing so when we do not.

"You never get a second chance to make a first impression," which becomes harder to change as time goes on. Eye contact, posture, vocal tone, facial expression—these behaviors form others' major impressions of you. Maya Angelou said, "I've learned that people will forget what you said, people will forget what you did, but people will never forget how you made them feel." For many, any trip to a physician is anxiety provoking; the stress of a sick child compounds this anxiety exponentially. Feeling someone cares about them goes a long way toward making people feel better— which is, after all, what we are trying to do.

Goal 3: Make informed decisions about interventions based on patient information and preferences.

Objectives: Although most "decisions" made during this initial interaction are about navigating the interaction itself, it is also when you learn about the aforementioned "preferences." You may be told outright what those preferences are; other times you must infer. The relationship between behavior and preferences may not be obvious. For example, if a family comes to you by ambulance, it could be because of perceived or actual degree of illness, lack of alternate transportation or ability to afford it, lack of consideration of alternatives, or any combination thereof. Each possibility reveals different familial concerns.

Goal 4: Perform a competent physical examination.

Objectives: Notice that this is separate from the goal of information gathering. Notice also that a "competent" examination is not necessarily the same as a "complete" one. The common rookie mistake is to do a comprehensive examination in every situation, irritating patients and delaying care. Examination is as much a matter of knowing what not to include as what to include. We must limit our violation of patients' privacy without sacrificing their health. Even for the routine, screening well child visit, the "complete" examination is in context of what you are screening for. A note stating, "Soft, active bowel sounds, no rebound tenderness, no guarding" for the abdominal examination of a healthy child is largely irrelevant, because abnormalities in these areas matter more for acute problems (e.g., pain, vomiting). A screening examination concerns itself more with occult problems, with a note stating "no masses or organomegaly," for example. masses or organomegaly, for example. Just as when you order laboratory tests, your examination should not be a "fishing expedition"—you should fish for something in particular.

MEDICAL KNOWLEDGE

Goal 5: Know and apply the basic and clinically supportive sciences that are appropriate.

Objectives: The reason physicians—not laypeople or robots—do H&Ps is that we have knowledge uniquely suited to guiding the encounter. Many questions we ask could be asked by someone without medical expertise. Even components of the physical are noted by caregivers as the reason they bring children to medical attention: breathing fast, listlessness, color change, and so on. But knowing what children's problems **could be** is what allows us to ask pointed questions and do a directed examination, to figure out what the problems **are.**

Goal 6: Demonstrate an investigative and analytic thinking approach to clinical situations.

Objectives: "The will to doubt" is one of our most important assets as clinicians. H&Ps require constant hypothesis-testing, weighing data to separate signal from noise. Every complaint plants a differential diagnosis in your mind. Investigating and analyzing mean constantly clarifying, challenging, and reprioritizing that differential, **while** interacting with the patient. Although the case presentation usually follows a ritualized order, in the interview it is often necessary to "skip ahead" or "backtrack" if new information opens a previously unconsidered line of questioning. Indeed, a caregiver's response to a question may seem to contradict a previous answer and demand that you retrace your steps. Likewise, physical findings may bring to mind new questions, or a historical element may require clarification by "prematurely" performing a portion of the examination.

PRACTICE-BASED LEARNING AND IMPROVEMENT

Goal 7: Assimilate evidence from scientific studies related to patients' health problems.

Objectives: How can one assimilate evidence from studies before even formulating a plan? First, formulating the plan begins with the first scrap of information about the patient, even just a chief complaint. Second, studies on the predictive value of historical and physical findings themselves allow us to optimize our own practice by performing evidence-based H&P examination.

Goal 8: Obtain and use information about one's own patient population and the larger population from which one's patients are drawn.
Objectives: Everything we and our patients do is a function of genetics and environment. Physicians rarely perform comprehensive, statistically rigorous analyses of the communities they serve, but stick to the tried-and-true method of getting to know a community by getting to know its people, one family at a time. The H&P is often a first step in that process.

Goal 9: Facilitate the learning of students and other health-care professionals.
Objectives: By the end of the first month of residency, pediatricians-in-training have probably interviewed and examined nearly as many children as they had through the entirety of medical school. By explicitly acting as a **role model** for good interviewing and examination techniques and using well-timed, tactful opportunities to answer questions for your students, you impart knowledge while you acquire it.

Goal 10: Analyze practice experience, and perform practice-based improvement activities using a systematic methodology.
Objectives: Among the many types of information you receive from your H&P is ongoing feedback on the interaction itself. Your phrases, movements, and expressions all elicit responses from patients and families; your job is to note what works and what does not. Use this information systematically to make sure each interaction is better than the ones before. In many residency programs, H&Ps are periodically observed and evaluated by faculty: these are valuable tools for improving technique, often identifying behaviors or deficiencies of which we are unaware.

INTERPERSONAL AND COMMUNICATION SKILLS

Goal 11: Use effective listening skills, and elicit information using effective nonverbal, explanatory, questioning, and writing skills.
Objectives: Much of our training in interviewing focuses on what to say and when to say it. Equally important is knowing what **not** to say and when **not** to say it. Nodding, smiling responsively, maintaining eye contact, leaning forward, making "reinforcing sounds" ("yes," "I see," and so on) all maximize the useful data obtained from the encounter. Of equal or greater importance is

providing historians with gentle, appropriate redirection—many details have little if any medical significance. As you gain in experience and confidence, you will learn which lines of questioning and conversation are "dead ends" and how to steer an interview back on course.

Goal 12: Create and sustain a therapeutic and ethically sound relationship with patients.

Objectives: This means more than just demonstrating caring and respect. It may also mean letting one's guard down: showing vulnerability and uncertainty in addition to the humility we should always show. Imagine you are in a foreign country, incapable of being understood by anyone other than your family. You are also sick—making you frightened and upset, impairing your family's ability to comfort you. Finally, the people in this country are 12 times your size and frequently touch you in unfamiliar ways, sometimes even hurt you. This is a sick toddler's experience of a physician visit. You want to establish trust with patients; on the other hand, they probably should not trust you if you are about to hurt them. Maintaining your eye level at theirs and a nonthreatening distance when you can, modulating facial expression and vocal tone in developmentally appropriate ways— these can help young patients understand that you want to help.

PROFESSIONALISM

Goal 13: Demonstrate respect, compassion, and integrity; a responsiveness to the needs of patients that supersedes self-interest; accountability to patients; and a commitment to excellence and ongoing professional development.

Objectives: Once again the key word: *demonstrate.* This demonstration can be as simple as a validation of the family's experience or a considerate gesture, like a tissue to a crying parent or a basin to a vomiting child. The medical analogue of "Never let them see you sweat" is "Never let them hear you complain." Families come to you for your help and empathy, and you should not request or expect it from them. Families may express empathy for the tired-looking house officer, which should be accepted graciously. But **do not** state that you are overwhelmed, performing inadequately, or, worst of all, not enjoying your job. (If you **are** overwhelmed or performing inadequately, you should be seeking help. If you do not enjoy your job, you should be looking for a new one.)

Goal 14: Demonstrate a commitment to ethical principles pertaining to confidentiality of patient information and informed consent.

Objectives: Establishing patients' trust requires that they know that the information they reveal to you will be used only to help them and be shared only with others for the same purpose. Some enter the relationship knowing this; for others, like a suspicious adolescent, you may need to state so explicitly. It helps to acknowledge (in words, tone, and posture) that the information you are discussing is sensitive and private. We need informed consent for everything we do (including H&Ps), because everything we do—including obtaining personal information—has risks.

Goal 15: Demonstrate sensitivity and responsiveness to patients' culture, gender, and disabilities.

Objectives: We all have prejudices, whether we admit them or not. These do not always take the form of mistrust, fear, or hatred, nor are they necessarily directed at racial, ethnic, or cultural groups. There may be behaviors that, when anyone exhibits them, push our buttons and make us feel or act in ways we do not like. Your feelings about such things must remain invisible during patient interactions. We want families to be comfortable sharing information, but we may also believe some children are being raised to hold unhealthy views or values. In other words, our mission may yield conflicting goals. Our society has decided that parents are those best qualified to make health decisions for their children. It simply **does not matter** how families' decisions make you feel—as long as they are not acting illegally, your job is not only to tolerate, but to support and encourage them. They need to see you do this.

SYSTEMS-BASED PRACTICE

Goal 16: Practice cost-effective health care and resource allocation that do not compromise quality of care.

Objectives: Nothing saves the health-care system money like a good H&P. Every time you successfully diagnose someone without the aid of laboratory tests, you save the cost of those tests. There's something satisfying about knowing that you yourself have all the tools you need to take care of people—it is a bit like knowing you can run a marathon, even though you have a driver's license.

Goal 17: Understand how patient care affects the health-care organization and the larger society, and how these elements affect practice.

Objectives: This skill is difficult to define practically. Everything we do exists in multiple contexts. When we enter a room to take an H&P, we must focus not only on the patient, but on the room, the building the room occupies, the companies that pay to operate it, the legal structure that allows those payments, and so on. We may not like to think so, but when we interact with patients we represent not only ourselves, but our employers, our profession, and "the system."

CONCLUSION

Every professional activity we undertake requires that we understand why we are doing it and what we are trying to accomplish. The more we maintain awareness of these goals, the better able we are to fulfill them.

Chapter 11
Note Writing

Matthew J. Kapklein MD, MPH

Medical records serve many purposes in day-to-day medical practice. They are chronologic logs of events during a hospital stay or series of office visits. They document medical thought process. They serve as a conduit of communication from one provider to another. They also often are examined by nonproviders for determining payment for services, gathering information for litigation, aiding in quality improvement, and myriad other reasons.

MEDICAL KNOWLEDGE

For most medical documentation, not much medical knowledge is required. A notable exception is in the writing of assessments (including differential diagnoses) and plans. Clearly, differential diagnoses for any given problem require the ability to fit a set of data points into a recognizable pattern. A well-written differential diagnosis is prioritized in order of likelihood, specific to that patient and follows logically from the data you have presented.

PATIENT CARE

The medical record serves as an aid to patient care by facilitating interprovider transfer of information. When you are writing your notes, it is useful to maintain the following mindset: "What information would another physician need to take care of this patient if I was unavailable?" The role of event notes, procedure notes, and course summaries in this approach is obvious. But in no area is this mindset more important than in writing the routine progress note.

Two formats for progress notes have gained popularity: SOAP and RICHMeN or systems-based. The SOAP format is familiar to most of us:

Subjective: A narrative description of any relevant events since the last entry, as well as any communications or concerns on the part of the patient

Objective: A listing of physical findings, laboratory values, and other measurable data

Assessment/**P**lan: A listing of the patient's active problems (using the information listed above) and the plan for managing them

In the systems-based format, laboratory values, medications, and other data are categorized by organ system. It often follows this order:

Respiratory
Infectious/Immunologic
Cardiovascular
Hematologic
Metabolic/Nutritional
Neurologic

In this format, subjective material (recent events, patient complaints) and physical findings can go either before the "systems" or within them. After the systems are reviewed, an assessment and plan should follow. This format has the disadvantage that items may appropriately go in several systems, and some data do not seem to fit into any system. In addition, a rigid order of presentation may bury the most important information at the end. Finally, pieces of data must often be drawn from several "systems" in order to synthesize an assessment.

Despite its drawbacks, the systems-based format assists the note writer in remembering all relevant information to be transmitted in the note.

INTERPERSONAL AND COMMUNICATION SKILLS

Notes in patients' medical records are written on many occasions. These include:

Admission history and physical: Initial data obtained at time of admission, including medical thought process and plan

Procedure note: Documents the relevant events of an operative or other procedure

Event note: Updates the reader about a specific (usually urgent) event or set of events (e.g., multidisciplinary meeting, acute clinical change, unanticipated event, death)

Consultation note: Provides input on aspects of a patient's care, often specifically used to communicate thought processes or recommendations

Off-service or transfer note: A summary of a patient's course up to that point, designed to assist in transferring care

Progress note: Periodic "update" for the reader on events and other changes since the last entry

In general, notes should be written with the presumption that the reader has read (or at least has access to) all other notes that came before. Any repetition of previously documented information should be done with this in mind and for the purpose of summarizing or documenting the writer's awareness of that information. For example, a patient transferred within an institution from a medical ward to an intensive care unit usually is accompanied by a summary of the patient's course in the transfer note. Your note need not be a complete repetition of the transfer note. Rather, your acceptance note may include documentation of having read the transfer note ("Transfer note read and appreciated."), understood it (a brief summary of the important events and problems), examined the data yourself (any differences between the transferring physician's history and examination findings/impressions and your own), but most importantly, should include **your** assessment and plan.

Regardless of the occasion on which they are written, medical notes should all have some things in common:

- Date and time
- Legibility
- Accepted language and terminology
  - Professional tone
  - Use of only accepted abbreviations
- Signature with name printed and method of contacting signer (e.g., pager number)

PROFESSIONALISM

Patients have access to their medical records, and all notes should be written as if the patient may read them. Keeping patients' rights to access their medical records in mind is a good way to make sure chart communication maintains a professional tone.

A few things to remember:

- Avoid colloquialisms and slang.
- Do not carry on arguments in the chart.
- Do not express frustration in the chart.
- Keep language objective and descriptive.
- Do not simply copy others' material and claim it as your own.

Medical note writing is a skill that is acquired over time. Maintaining perspective on the many purposes and uses of medical documentation will help you as you develop it.

PRACTICE-BASED LEARNING AND IMPROVEMENT

Early in medical training—during medical school and into residency—medical record notes require cosignature from supervising physicians. A good cosigner reads the note carefully, amends it as necessary at the bottom, and gives verbal feedback. A good trainee takes the extra step to solicit feedback on notes if it is not offered.

SYSTEMS-BASED PRACTICE

It is important to remember that non–health-care personnel may read your notes as well.

Insurance companies and other payers use medical documentation to determine whether they agree with the services for which hospitals and physicians charge. In addition, medical services are often billed by the level of complexity they involve. To justify that a patient's care is "highly complex," there must be written proof of that complexity or the patient's insurance company may refuse to pay the charge or state that a lower fee is indicated. Indeed, if medical documentation does not clearly state a reason for the service (including, for example, admission to a hospital), payment for that entire service may be denied.

Medical records are also carefully scrutinized as evidence in malpractice litigation. The phrase "Not documented, not done" has been popularized by plaintiffs' attorneys in an effort to portray medical records as encyclopedically comprehensive and to state that the absence of documentation of an action constitutes "proof" that it was not performed. This premise, of course, is not true. It is impossible to document every action and microevent in a patient's care without videotaping every moment, perhaps not even then. This said, all important events should be documented—even though it is not always possible to know what events are important at the time they are happening. It is difficult to recall specific details when questioned about events months or years after they happen.

Medical records are legal documents and may be examined by attorneys or law enforcement officials; it is important that corrections to statements made in the record are done appropriately. Erasure and blacking- or whiting-out entries are forbidden, as is backdating or "back-timing." If a statement needs correction, it should have a simple horizontal line drawn through it and the initials of the writer placed next to it, with an explanation written below the entry. If a statement needs to be added, a dated and timed amendment should be written. **Never** change a note after it has been signed and placed in the chart.

Chapter 12
Oral Presentations

Matthew J. Kapklein MD, MPH

Oral presentations take a myriad of forms and occur in multiple settings. What follows is a sample of presentation types and the settings in which they may be encountered:

Formal, complete presentations: Case conferences
Summary presentations: Attending rounds
Focused presentations: Consultation requests
Systems-based presentations: Work rounds on complex patients
Problem-based presentations: Transfers of care between residents
Bullet updates: Transfers of care on mutually known patients

Each has its own unique skill set, but some principles apply to all.
Oral presentations follow different structures. Most medical students are taught the classic, complete, formal presentation format, which is rarely used in daily medical practice. For example, birth history, feeding history, growth/development, immunizations, family history, social history, and review of systems are not included in most presentations pediatricians make to each other. Far more important are an assessment and proposed plan, which should be parts of *every* presentation.

INTERPERSONAL AND COMMUNICATION SKILLS

As in all communication, presentations should be approached with advance knowledge of the **goals** and **frame of reference** of speaker and listeners, as well as the **context** in which the exchange is taking place. Let's take an example of an infant who presents to an emergency department (ED) with evidence of congestive heart failure (CHF) (failure to thrive, dyspnea with feeding, a murmur on auscultation, and cardiomegaly on chest radiograph). As the resident caring for the child, you may present this case several times:

Listener	Presentation Type	Your Goals
ED attending	Summary	Summarize history/examination/ assessment, develop plan
Hospitalist	Summary	Acceptance for hospital admission
Cardiologist	Focused	Request echocardiogram
Ward resident	Problem-based	Transfer care, summarize course and current plans
Department chair	Formal	Education on diagnosis/ management of CHF

The amount of detail you provide for each presentation will also differ depending on the context.

People think in terms of narrative, and patients/caregivers tend to tell their medical histories in the forms of stories. However, many details of these narratives add little, if anything, to the medical history. Compare the following:

> XZ is a 6-month-old boy who presents with a 2-month history of failing to gain weight. He was a full-term baby. He was growing well up to age 4 months, when he was noted to have gained only 4 ounces in the previous month. At that time he was being fed with Enfamil. His mother brought him to her pediatrician, who recommended changing his formula to Similac, which she did. Two weeks later he returned for a weight check, which showed that his weight had gone up 2 ounces, but the mother recalls that this was measured on a different scale than the previous visit. His mother says he did not seem to like the Similac because he cried and fussed while eating. He returned to his pediatrician another 2 weeks later and this time was remeasured on the same scale as the first visit, and was found to have not gained weight since the 4-month visit. Because of the fussing with feeds, the pediatrician changed the formula to Nutramigen, which the mother says he also does not like.

With this:

> XZ is a 6-month-old former full-term boy who presents with a 2-month history of failure to thrive. He cries and fusses with feeding, and his formula has been changed several times.

There is no meaningful difference between these two presentations. However, the listener will stop paying attention during the first presentation and probably miss important information that comes later. One of our difficult tasks is to **edit** the information we transmit, trusting ourselves to decide which details are important and trusting our audiences to ask the questions left unanswered.

There are a few rules of thumb that are useful in optimizing presentation quality:

1. KISS ("**K**eep **I**t **S**hort and **S**imple"). Presentations should rarely be longer than 3 minutes. House officers who fear "missing something" and wish to be perceived as "attentive to detail" may not trust themselves to identify those data points that are meaningless, so they include all of them, hoping listeners will edit out the unimportant ones themselves. You must trust yourself to decide which details need not be stated.
2. Trust your memory. Nothing shortens an audience's attention span more than a speaker who does not make eye contact, and by simply reading your admission note from a piece of paper you will be unable to engage your audience.

3. Everything you say should follow logically from something you've already said. As soon as you utter an age and presenting complaint, a set of questions and diagnoses begins to form in your listeners' minds. Every item in the history should answer a question raised by the presenting complaint, every item in the physical by something in the history. This is what differentiates pertinent negatives from unimportant ones—pertinent negatives are those a listener would logically want to know based on the history. For example, a case presentation about a patient with a headache should mention the absence of papilledema, but not the absence of an umbilical hernia.

4. Beware of the "surprise ending." Although a key element may not have become evident until sometime after the initial history was obtained, important information should not be withheld to build up the suspense. Let's say you admitted a child with pallor and jaundice, worked him up for hemolytic anemia, found he had G6PD deficiency, then went back and determined he had eaten fava beans. The fava beans belong in the **opening sentences** of the presentation.

5. Avoid the temptation to tell a story. Patients generally give details of the history in chronologic order, but these elements can be compressed and rearranged as you see fit. If you find yourself using the phrase "and then," you are probably not summarizing enough. Likewise, it is unlikely that any person other than the patient needs to be mentioned; if you are mentioning things parents or other physicians did, said, or thought, you're probably leaving too much in.

PATIENT CARE

We transmit information to other caregivers in order to allow ourselves, our listener(s), or both to take better care of patients. Always consider presentations in context: What am I trying to accomplish by presenting this case? If I am asking for advice, what information does the listener need in order to make a recommendation? If I have a specific patient-care goal in mind, what are the important pieces of data that **support** that goal? If I am transferring care to another physician, what information does that person need in order to take care of this patient for the next hour? Fifteen hours? Forever?

Your differential diagnosis is the differential diagnosis for **that patient,** *not* for that patient's complaint. The differential diagnosis of abdominal pain in children could easily fill two single-spaced pages in a textbook. Your job is to generate a differential diagnosis for your patient based on that child's particular history and physical findings, as well as your knowledge of epidemiology. Your differential diagnosis should include *only* items that you are seriously considering, not just ones you saw on a list. If your history and physical have already ruled out a diagnosis, *do not* include it in your differential.

MEDICAL KNOWLEDGE

The only way you will be able to present a coherent assessment and differential diagnosis is if you have sufficient knowledge to compare the information you have presented with recognizable patterns. The only way you will know what information to present is if you know what patterns are suggested by the presenting complaint. The only way you will be able to obtain the history and physical in the first place is if you have an idea of what you are looking for.

Maintaining an investigatory and analytic approach to clinical situations means being willing to retrace your steps. If, as you put together the information you obtained, a previously unconsidered diagnosis occurs to you, go back and ask the relevant questions. If, as you read about one of the items in your differential, you realize that a pertinent physical finding (positive or negative) was not adequately investigated, go back and reexamine. If a laboratory result suggests diagnostic possibilities that hadn't been on your list before, reconsider your thought process.

PROFESSIONALISM

We can demonstrate professional behavior in many ways as we present cases:

1. Choose language that demonstrates compassion and respect for our patients. There is a difference between neutral abbreviations (e.g., "MR/CP" for "mental retardation and cerebral palsy") and disrespectful ones (e.g., "gork"). Relating family concerns during a presentation should be done in a way that demonstrates respect for those concerns, regardless of whether you share them.
2. Choose communication styles that demonstrate respect for your colleagues. Eye rolling, sarcasm, and dismissiveness do nothing to add to your stature and do not make you appear smart or funny—they do the opposite.
3. Include families in the discussion. There are very few elements of presentations that parents are not fully entitled to hear. In fact, they can often clarify details and provide important feedback. In the rare instance of a parent hindering the flow of a presentation, a skilled supervising physician can usually redirect the conversation appropriately.
4. Be inclusive of input and opinion. If someone asks a question, answer it straightforwardly, even if you believe you already have. If someone disagrees with your assessment, he/she is entitled to do so, and you are entitled to rebut—both must be done respectfully.
5. Be aware of your surroundings. Although we are often pressed for time and must take advantage of available opportunities for transmission of information, be aware that your audience may

include unintended members. Patients are entitled to privacy and confidentiality of medical information—make sure that the only people listening to the presentation are people who should be.

PRACTICE-BASED LEARNING AND IMPROVEMENT

Good presentation skills do not develop overnight. Solicit feedback through the entire process: from your supervising resident as you obtain your data and prepare your presentation, from your supervising physician after rounds, from your colleagues during and after transferring care. The only way to improve will be for you to identify how you are and are not meeting your audience's needs.

There is no such thing as a case with nothing to be learned from it. The evidence-based practitioner thinks about the elements of each case that make it both similar to and different from others. It is these elements that guide further reading: What are the characteristics of this patient that make diagnosis/management challenging? Do the similarities between this case and others I have seen justify my treating them in the same way? These questions, arising at the bedside and focusing on clinical, answerable matters, are the seeds of meaningful literature searches and useful information.

SYSTEMS-BASED PRACTICE

Oral presentations done in the context of transferring care (also called "handoff" or "sign-out") deserve special mention, because these transactions are particularly risky and can be the source of medical errors. Handoffs have been the subject of much scrutiny and study, and various methods have been advocated for improving their accuracy and efficiency, with the goal of improving patient safety. Several institutions have implemented specific formats and policies regarding this type of communication. Handoffs now often occur using specific verbal formats, paper forms, even computer programs. "Closed-loop communication" refers to repeating back information at the end of an interaction and is helpful in ensuring accurate care plans.

Appendix 1
ACGME General Competencies

ACGME GENERAL COMPETENCIES
VERSION 1.3 (9.28.99)

The residency program must require its residents to develop the competencies in the six areas below to the level expected of a new practitioner. Toward this end, programs must define the specific knowledge, skills, and attitudes required and provide educational experiences as needed in order for their residents to demonstrate the competencies.

Patient Care

Residents must be able to provide patient care that is compassionate, appropriate, and effective for the treatment of health problems and the promotion of health. Residents are expected to:

- communicate effectively and demonstrate caring and respectful behaviors when interacting with patients and their families
- gather essential and accurate information about their patients
- make informed decisions about diagnostic and therapeutic interventions based on patient information and preferences, up-to-date scientific evidence, and clinical judgment
- develop and carry out patient management plans
- counsel and educate patients and their families
- use information technology to support patient care decisions and patient education
- perform competently all medical and invasive procedures considered essential for the area of practice
- provide health-care services aimed at preventing health problems or maintaining health
- work with health-care professionals, including those from other disciplines, to provide patient-focused care

Medical Knowledge

Residents must demonstrate knowledge about established and evolving biomedical, clinical, and cognate (e.g., epidemiologic and social-behavioral) sciences and the application of this knowledge to patient care. Residents are expected to:

- demonstrate an investigatory and analytic thinking approach to clinical situations
- know and apply the basic and clinically supportive sciences that are appropriate to their discipline

Practice-Based Learning and Improvement

Residents must be able to investigate and evaluate their patient care practices, appraise and assimilate scientific evidence, and improve their patient care practices. Residents are expected to:

- analyze practice experience and perform practice-based improvement activities using a systematic methodology
- locate, appraise, and assimilate evidence from scientific studies related to their patients' health problems
- obtain and use information about their own population of patients and the larger population from which their patients are drawn
- apply knowledge of study designs and statistical methods to the appraisal of clinical studies and other information on diagnostic and therapeutic effectiveness
- use information technology to manage information, access on-line medical information, and support their own education
- facilitate the learning of students and other health-care professionals

Interpersonal and Communication Skills

Residents must be able to demonstrate interpersonal and communication skills that result in effective information exchange and teaming with patients, their patients' families, and professional associates. Residents are expected to:

- create and sustain a therapeutic and ethically sound relationship with patients
- use effective listening skills and elicit and provide information using effective nonverbal, explanatory, questioning, and writing skills
- work effectively with others as a member or leader of a health-care team or other professional group

Professionalism

Residents must demonstrate a commitment to carrying out professional responsibilities, adherence to ethical principles, and sensitivity to a diverse patient population. Residents are expected to:

- demonstrate respect, compassion, and integrity; a responsiveness to the needs of patients and society that supersedes self-interest; accountability to patients, society, and the profession; and a commitment to excellence and ongoing professional development
- demonstrate a commitment to ethical principles pertaining to provision or withholding of clinical care, confidentiality of patient information, informed consent, and business practices
- demonstrate sensitivity and responsiveness to patients' culture, age, gender, and disabilities

Systems-Based Practice

Residents must demonstrate an awareness of and responsiveness to the larger context and system of health care and the ability to effectively call on system resources to provide care that is of optimal value. Residents are expected to:

- understand how their patient care and other professional practices affect other health-care professionals, the health-care organization, and the larger society and how these elements of the system affect their own practice
- know how types of medical practice and delivery systems differ from one another, including methods of controlling health-care costs and allocating resources
- practice cost-effective health care and resource allocation that does not compromise quality of care
- advocate for quality patient care and assist patients in dealing with system complexities
- know how to partner with health-care managers and health-care providers to assess, coordinate, and improve health care and know how these activities can affect system performance

From ACGME Competency definitions: Used with permission of Accreditation Council for Graduate Medical Education © ACGME 2011. Please see the ACGME website: www.acgme.org for the most current version.

Appendix 2
Competency Self-Assessment Form: Pediatrics

Competency Self-Assessment Form: Pediatrics

Patient Summary:

Dx:

Patient Care

Was I complete in my history and physical examination? Was my clinical reasoning appropriate and sound?

Medical Knowledge

Do I understand the basics of the patient's most likely disease processes?

Practice-Based Learning and Improvement

Did I use evidence-based medicine? Did I increase my fund of knowledge regarding pediatrics?

Interpersonal and Communication Skills

Did I work well with the team providing care? Was I respectful and compassionate in my interactions with the patient and his/her family?

Professionalism

Did I function at the highest possible level? What can I do to improve my medical professionalism?

Systems-Based Practice

Did the medical system work at its best for the welfare of the patient? How can I facilitate improvements?

Section II
THE OUTPATIENT OFFICE

Section Editor

Maureen C. McMahon MD

EPISODIC CARE

Subsection Editor

Cynthia McIntosh MD

Section Contents

Chapter 13
Essentials of the Pediatric Well Child Visit

Maureen C. McMahon MD

There are multiple components of the pediatric well child visit that provide an overall snapshot of the child's well-being and an opportunity to identify concerns. *Bright Futures: Guidelines for Health Supervision of Infants, Children, and Adolescents,* published by the American Academy of Pediatrics (AAP) describes four activities in the health supervision visit: disease detection, disease prevention, health promotion, and anticipatory guidance. The Bright Futures model is centered on a strength-based approach whose goal is to identify and build on the strengths in each family. It is important for the pediatrician to realize that often everything cannot be addressed in a single encounter. The allotted time for the visit is about 20 minutes. A key to effectiveness is to assess the family situation, know your patient, and target what will be most useful to them. The frequency of well visits in the first 2 years of life provides an opportunity to assess and address nonemergent issues over time. Parental concerns should be elicited and addressed, and the parental-child interaction should be observed at each visit. Other priorities will be specific to the child's age and expected developmental milestones. With older children, school performance should be discussed.

During each well visit encounter growth, development, and sensory functions (hearing and vision) are assessed, and immunizations are administered according to the AAP recommended schedule. A complete physical examination is recommended. Growth charts and the 2011 recommended immunization schedule are included at the end of this chapter (Figures 13-1 to 13-9). When assessing development, it is important to understand there is a range of normal for attainment of each milestone. Development may occur in spurts separated by plateaus, rather than follow a smooth trajectory. Also, the rate of development in an otherwise normal child can sometimes be impacted and slowed significantly by a major acute illness, a chronic health condition, or major surgery.

Our chief purpose here is to demonstrate application of the six Accreditation Council for Graduate Medical Education (ACGME) competencies in well child care. To that effect, there are eight well visit chapters, and each provides an introduction to the well visit with specific examples of how each competency can be applied in well child care. Additional details for each age-group can be found in *Bright Futures*. Chapter 14 provides an overview of developmental surveillance and screening, and Chapter 15 provides an overview of anticipatory guidance using *Bright Futures* as a framework. (*Bright Futures: Guidelines for health supervision of infants, children and adolescents,* ed 3, Elk Grove, IL, 2008, American Academy of Pediatricians.)

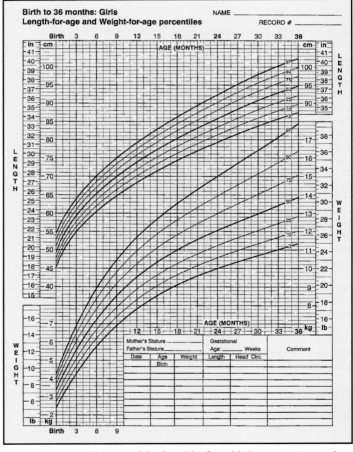

Figure 13-1 Length and weight for girls, from birth to age 36 months.

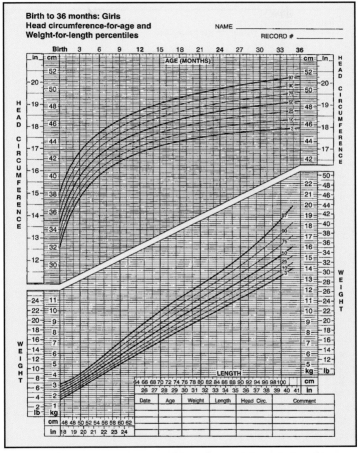

Figure 13-2 Head circumference and length-to-weight ratio for girls, from birth to age 36 months.

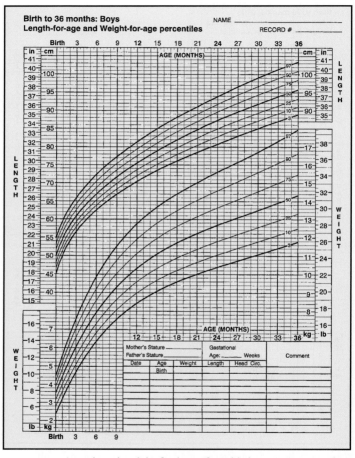

Figure 13-3 Length and weight for boys, from birth to age 36 months.

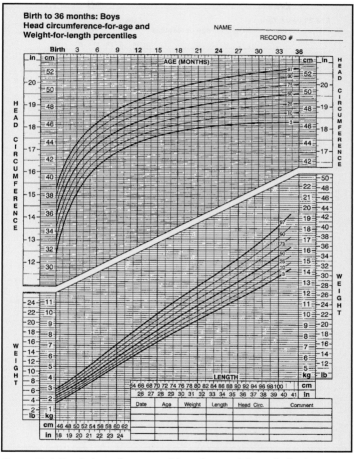

Figure 13-4 Head circumference and length-to-weight ratio for boys, from birth to age 36 months.

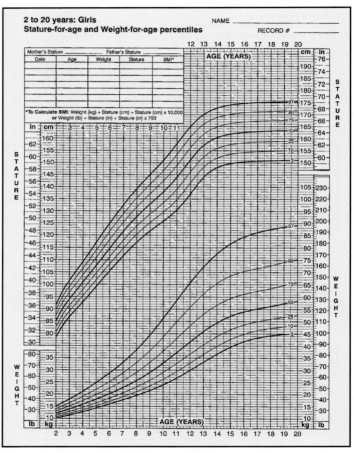

Figure 13-5 Stature and weight for girls ages 2 to 20 years.

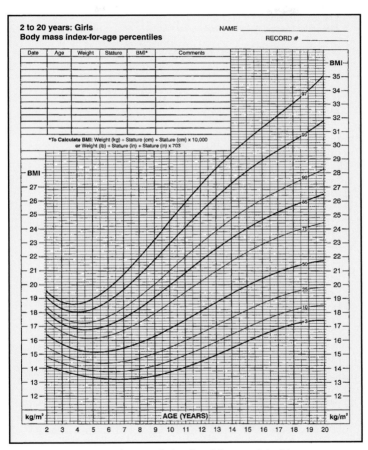

Figure 13-6 Body mass index for girls ages 2 to 20 years.

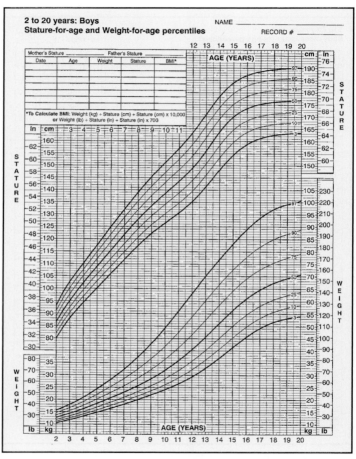

Figure 13-7 Stature and weight for boys ages 2 to 20 years.

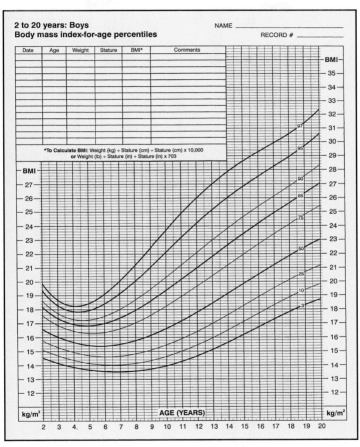

Figure 13-8 Body mass index for boys ages 2 to 20 years.

Vaccine ▼ Age ▶	Birth	1 month	2 months	4 months	6 months	12 months	15 months	18 months	19–23 months	2–3 years	4–6 years
Hepatitis B[1]	HepB	HepB				HepB					
Rotavirus[2]			RV	RV	RV[2]						
Diphtheria, Tetanus, Pertussis[3]			DTaP	DTaP	DTaP	*see footnote[3]*	DTaP				DTaP
Haemophilus influenzae type b[4]			Hib	Hib	Hib[4]	Hib					
Pneumococcal[5]			PCV	PCV	PCV	PCV				PPSV	
Inactivated Poliovirus[6]			IPV	IPV		IPV					IPV
Influenza[7]						Influenza (Yearly)					
Measles, Mumps, Rubella[8]						MMR		*see footnote[8]*			MMR
Varicella[9]						Varicella		*see footnote[9]*			Varicella
Hepatitis A[10]						HepA (2 doses)				HepA Series	
Meningococcal[11]										MCV4	

Range of recommended ages for all children

Range of recommended ages for certain high-risk groups

Figure 13-9A Recommended immunization schedule for infants and children, from birth through age 6 years. This schedule includes recommendations in effect as of December 21, 2010. Any dose not administered at the recommended age should be administered at a subsequent visit, when indicated and feasible. For those who fall behind or start late, see the catch-up schedule at http://www.cdc.gov. The use of a combination vaccine generally is preferred over separate injections of its equivalent component vaccines. Considerations should include provider assessment, patient preference, and the potential for adverse events. Providers should consult the relevant Advisory Committee on Immunization Practices statement for detailed recommendations: http://www.cdc.gov/vaccines/pubs/acip-list.htm. Clinically significant adverse events that follow immunization should be reported to the Vaccine Adverse Event Reporting System (VAERS) at http://www.vaers.hhs.gov or by telephone, 800-822-7967.

1. Hepatitis B vaccine (HepB). (Minimum age: birth)

At birth:
- Administer monovalent HepB to all newborns before hospital discharge.
- If mother is hepatitis B surface antigen (HBsAg)-positive, administer HepB and 0.5 mL of hepatitis B immune globulin (HBIG) within 12 hours of birth.
- If mother's HBsAg status is unknown, administer HepB within 12 hours of birth. Determine mother's HBsAg status as soon as possible and, if HBsAg-positive, administer HBIG (no later than age 1 week).

Doses following the birth dose:
- The second dose should be administered at age 1 or 2 months. Monovalent HepB should be used for doses administered before age 6 weeks.
- Infants born to HBsAg-positive mothers should be tested for HBsAg and antibody to HBsAg 1 to 2 months after completion of at least 3 doses of the HepB series, at age 9 through 18 months (generally at the next well-child visit).
- Administration of 4 doses of HepB to infants is permissible when a combination vaccine containing HepB is administered after the birth dose.
- Infants who did not receive a birth dose should receive 3 doses of monovalent HepB on a schedule of 0, 1, and 6 months.
- The final (3rd or 4th) dose in the HepB series should be administered no earlier than age 24 weeks.

2. Rotavirus vaccine (RV). (Minimum age: 6 weeks)
- Administer the first dose at age 6 through 14 weeks (maximum age: 14 weeks 6 days). Vaccination should not be initiated for infants aged 15 weeks 0 days or older.
- The maximum age for the final dose in the series is 8 months 0 days.
- If Rotarix is administered at ages 2 and 4 months, a dose at 6 months is not indicated.

3. Diphtheria and tetanus toxoids and acellular pertussis vaccine (DTaP). (Minimum age: 6 weeks)
- The fourth dose may be administered as early as age 12 months, provided at least 6 months have elapsed since the third dose.

4. Haemophilus influenzae type b conjugate vaccine (Hib). (Minimum age: 6 weeks)
- If PRP-OMP (PedvaxHIB or Comvax [HepB-Hib]) is administered at ages 2 and 4 months, a dose at age 6 months is not indicated.
- Hiberix should not be used for doses at ages 2, 4, or 6 months for the primary series but can be used as the final dose in children aged 12 months through 4 years.

5. Pneumococcal vaccine. (Minimum age: 6 weeks for pneumococcal conjugate vaccine [PCV]; 2 years for pneumococcal polysaccharide vaccine [PPSV])
- PCV is recommended for all children aged younger than 5 years. Administer 1 dose of PCV to all healthy children aged 24 months through 59 months who are not completely vaccinated for their age.
- A PCV series begun with 7-valent PCV (PCV7) should be completed with 13-valent PCV (PCV13).
- A single supplemental dose of PCV13 is recommended for all children aged 14 through 59 months who have received an age-appropriate series of PCV7.
- A single supplemental dose of PCV13 is recommended for all children aged 60 through 71 months with underlying medical conditions who have received an age-appropriate series of PCV7.
- The supplemental dose of PCV13 should be administered at least 8 weeks after the previous dose of PCV7. See *MMWR* 2010;59(No. RR-11).

- Administer PPSV at least 8 weeks after last dose of PCV to children aged 2 years or older with certain underlying medical conditions, including a cochlear implant.

6. Inactivated poliovirus vaccine (IPV). (Minimum age: 6 weeks)
- If 4 or more doses are administered prior to age 4 years an additional dose should be administered at age 4 through 6 years.
- The final dose in the series should be administered on or after the fourth birthday and at least 6 months following the previous dose.

7. Influenza vaccine (seasonal). (Minimum age: 6 months for trivalent inactivated influenza vaccine [TIV]; 2 years for live, attenuated influenza vaccine [LAIV])
- For healthy children aged 2 years and older (i.e., those who do not have underlying medical conditions that predispose them to influenza complications), either LAIV or TIV may be used, except LAIV should not be given to children aged 2 through 4 years who have had wheezing in the past 12 months.
- Administer 2 doses (separated by at least 4 weeks) to children aged 6 months through 8 years who are receiving seasonal influenza vaccine for the first time or who were vaccinated for the first time during the previous influenza season but only received 1 dose.
- Children aged 6 months through 8 years who received no doses of monovalent 2009 H1N1 vaccine should receive 2 doses of 2010-2011 seasonal influenza vaccine. See *MMWR* 2010;59(No. RR-8):33–34.

8. Measles, mumps, and rubella vaccine (MMR). (Minimum age: 12 months)
- The second dose may be administered before age 4 years, provided at least 4 weeks have elapsed since the first dose.

9. Varicella vaccine. (Minimum age: 12 months)
- The second dose may be administered before age 4 years, provided at least 3 months have elapsed since the first dose.
- For children aged 12 months through 12 years the recommended minimum interval between doses is 3 months. However, if the second dose was administered at least 4 weeks after the first dose, it can be accepted as valid.

10. Hepatitis A vaccine (HepA). (Minimum age: 12 months)
- Administer 2 doses at least 6 months apart.
- HepA is recommended for children aged older than 23 months who live in areas where vaccination programs target older children, who are at increased risk for infection, or for whom immunity against hepatitis A is desired.

11. Meningococcal conjugate vaccine, quadrivalent (MCV4). (Minimum age: 2 years)
- Administer 2 doses of MCV4 at least 8 weeks apart to children aged 2 through 10 years with persistent complement component deficiency and anatomic or functional asplenia, and 1 dose every 5 years thereafter.
- Persons with human immunodeficiency virus (HIV) infection who are vaccinated with MCV4 should receive 2 doses at least 8 weeks apart.
- Administer 1 dose of MCV4 to children aged 2 through 10 years who travel to countries with highly endemic or epidemic disease and during outbreaks caused by a vaccine serogroup.
- Administer MCV4 to children at continued risk for meningococcal disease who were previously vaccinated with MCV4 or meningococcal polysaccharide vaccine after 3 years if the first dose was administered at age 2 through 6 years.

Continued

The Recommended Immunization Schedules for Persons Aged 0 Through 18 years are approved by the Advisory Committee on Immunization Practices (**http://www.cdc.gov/vaccines/recs/acip/**), the American Academy of Pediatrics (**http://www.aap.org**), and the American Academy of Family Physicians (**http:www.aafp.org**).
Department of Health and Human Services • Centers for Disease Controld and Prevention

Figure 13-9A, cont'd.

A

Vaccine ▼ Age ▶	7–10 years	11–12 years	13–18 years
Tetanus, Diphtheria, Pertussis[1]		Tdap	Tdap
Human Papillomavirus[2]	see footnote[2]	HPV (3 doses)(females)	HPV series
Meningococcal[3]	MCV4	MCV4	MCV4
Influenza[4]		Influenza (Yearly)	
Pneumococcal[5]		Pneumococcal	
Hepatitis A[6]		HepA Series	
Hepatitis B[7]		Hep B Series	
Inactivated Poliovirus[8]		IPV Series	
Measles, Mumps, Rubella[9]		MMR Series	
Varicella[10]		Varicella Series	

Legend:
- Range of recommended ages for all children
- Range of recommended ages for catch-up immunization
- Range of recommended ages for certain high-risk groups

Figure 13-9B Recommended immunization schedule for children, ages 7 to 18 years. This schedule includes recommendations in effect as of December 21, 2010. Any dose not administered at the recommended age should be administered at a subsequent visit, when indicated and feasible. For those who fall behind or start late, see this schedule and the catch-up schedule at http://www. cdc.gov. The use of a combination vaccine generally is preferred over separate injections of its equivalent component vaccines. Considerations should include provider assessment, patient preference, and the potential for adverse events. Providers should consult the relevant Advisory Committee on Immunization Practices statement for detailed recommendations: http://www.cdc.gov/ vaccines/pubs/acip-list.htm. Clinically significant adverse events that follow immunization should be reported to the Vaccine Adverse Event Reporting System (VAERS) at http://www.vaers.hhs.gov or by telephone, 800-822-7967.

1. **Tetanus and diphtheria toxoids and acellular pertussis vaccine (Tdap).**
(Minimum age: 10 years for Boostrix and 11 years for Adacel)
   - Persons aged 11 through 18 years who have not received Tdap should receive a dose followed by Td booster doses every 10 years thereafter.
   - Persons aged 7 through 10 years who are not fully immunized against pertussis (including those never vaccinated or with unknown pertussis vaccination status) should receive a single dose of Tdap. Refer to the catch-up schedule if additional doses of tetanus and diphtheria toxoid–containing vaccine are needed.
   - Tdap can be administered regardless of the interval since the last tetanus and diphtheria toxoid–containing vaccine.

2. **Human papillomavirus vaccine (HPV).** (Minimum age: 9 years)
   - Quadrivalent HPV vaccine (HPV4) or bivalent HPV vaccine (HPV2) is recommended for the prevention of cervical precancers and cancers in females.
   - HPV4 is recommended for prevention of cervical precancers, cancers, and genital warts in females.
   - HPV4 may be administered in a 3-dose series to males aged 9 through 18 years to reduce their likelihood of genital warts.
   - Administer the second dose 1 to 2 months after the first dose and the third dose 6 months after the first dose (at least 24 weeks after the first dose).

3. **Meningococcal conjugate vaccine, quadrivalent (MCV4).** (Minimum age: 2 years)
   - Administer MCV4 at age 11 through 12 years with a booster dose at age 16 years.
   - Administer 1 dose at age 13 through 18 years if not previously vaccinated.
   - Persons who received their first dose at age 13 through 15 years should receive a booster dose at age 16 through 18 years.
   - Administer 1 dose to previously unvaccinated college freshmen living in a dormitory.
   - Administer 2 doses at least 8 weeks apart to children aged 2 through 10 years with persistent complement component deficiency and anatomic or functional asplenia, and 1 dose every 5 years thereafter.
   - Persons with HIV infection who are vaccinated with MCV4 should receive 2 doses at least 8 weeks apart.
   - Administer 1 dose of MCV4 to children aged 2 through 10 years who travel to countries with highly endemic or epidemic disease and during outbreaks caused by a vaccine serogroup.
   - Administer MCV4 to children at continued risk for meningococcal disease who were previously vaccinated with MCV4 or meningococcal polysaccharide vaccine after 3 years (if first dose administered at age 2 through 6 years) or after 5 years (if first dose administered at age 7 years or older).

4. **Influenza vaccine (seasonal).**
   - For healthy nonpregnant persons aged 7 through 18 years (i.e., those who do not have underlying medical conditions that predispose them to influenza complications), either LAIV or TIV may be used.
   - Administer 2 doses (separated by at least 4 weeks) to children aged 6 months through 8 years who are receiving seasonal influenza vaccine for the first time or who were vaccinated for the first time during the previous influenza season but only received 1 dose.
   - Children 6 months through 8 years of age who received no doses of monovalent 2009 H1N1 vaccine should receive 2 doses of 2010–2011 seasonal influenza vaccine. See *MMWR* 2010;59(No. RR-8):33–34.

5. **Pneumococcal vaccines.**
   - A single dose of 13-valent pneumococcal conjugate vaccine (PCV13) may be administered to children aged 6 through 18 years who have functional or anatomic asplenia, HIV infection or other immunocompromising condition, cochlear implant or CSF leak. See *MMWR* 2010;59(No. RR-11).
   - The dose of PCV13 should be administered at least 8 weeks after the previous dose of PCV7.
   - Administer pneumococcal polysaccharide vaccine at least 8 weeks after the last dose of PCV to children aged 2 years or older with certain underlying medical conditions, including a cochlear implant. A single revaccination should be administered after 5 years to children with functional or anatomic asplenia or an immunocompromising condition.

6. **Hepatitis A vaccine (HepA).**
   - Administer 2 doses at least 6 months apart.
   - HepA is recommended for children older than 23 months who live in areas where vaccination programs target older children, or who are at increased risk for infection, or for whom immunity against hepatitis A is desired.

7. **Hepatitis B vaccine (HepB).**
   - Administer the 3-dose series to those not previously vaccinated. For those with incomplete vaccination, follow the catch-up schedule.
   - A 2-dose series (separated at least 4 months) of adult formulation Recombivax HB is licensed for children aged 11 through 15 years.

8. **Inactivated poliovirus vaccine (IPV).**
   - The final dose in the series should be administered on or after the fourth birthday and at least 6 months following the previous dose.
   - If both OPV and IPV were administered as part of a series, a total of 4 doses should be administered, regardless of the child's current age.

9. **Measles, mumps, and rubella vaccine (MMR).**
   - The minimum interval between the 2 doses of MMR is 4 weeks.

10. **Varicella vaccine.**
   - For persons aged 7 through 18 years without evidence of immunity (see *MMWR* 2007;56[No. RR-4]), administer 2 doses if not previously vaccinated or the second dose if only 1 dose has been administered.
   - For persons aged 7 through 12 years, the recommended minimum interval between doses is 3 months. However, if the second dose was administered at least 4 weeks after the first dose, it can be accepted as valid.
   - For persons aged 13 years and older, the minimum interval between doses is 4 weeks.

The Recommended Immunization Schedules for Persons Aged 0 Through 18 Years are approved by the Advisory Committee on Immunization Practices (http://www.cdc.gov/vaccines/recs/acip), the American Academy of Pediatrics (http://www.aap.org), and the American Academy of Family Physicians (http:www.aafp.org).
Department of Health and Human Services • Centers for Disease Controls and Prevention

Figure 13-9B, cont'd.

B

Chapter 14
Developmental Screening and Surveillance

Carolyn M. Rosen MD

Medical Knowledge and Patient Care

One of the more important tasks of the primary care physician is early detection of children with developmental disabilities. It is estimated that approximately 16% to 18% of all children have developmental disabilities and only 20% to 30% of these children are detected before school entrance.[1] Earlier detection of a potential problem may lead to earlier referrals to appropriate services such as Early Intervention and improvement in outcomes.

Developmental Screening

The importance of developmental screening in the primary care setting was emphasized in the recent American Academy of Pediatrics (AAP) Policy Statement "Identifying Infants and Young Children with Developmental Disorders in the Medical Home: An Algorithm for Developmental Surveillance and Screening" published in *Pediatrics* in July 2006. The policy statement recommends that developmental surveillance be done at every well child preventive visit. If surveillance identifies a developmental concern, a standardized developmental screening tool should be used. In addition, in order to detect delays in children at low risk, screening tools should be used at the 9-month, 18-month, and 24- or 30-month well child visits.[2]

The **developmental domains** that need to be assessed **cover four main areas: (1) motor, which includes gross motor and fine motor development; (2) communication, which includes speech and expressive and receptive language; (3) cognition, which includes language as well as visual-motor coordination and problem solving; and (4) social-emotional, which includes temperament and behavioral responses to people and the surrounding environment.** Specific details on age-specific milestones for each of these categories can be found in the chapters describing the age-specific well child visits.

Developmental Surveillance

It is important to understand the difference between developmental surveillance and developmental screening. Surveillance is the ongoing process that is longitudinal and cumulative and helps primary care providers identify children who *may be* at risk for developmental delay. Surveillance includes eliciting and attending to parents' concerns about their child's development; documenting and maintaining a developmental history; making accurate observations of the child; identifying risk and protective factors, which include the child's environment, genetic, social, and demographic factors; and maintaining an accurate record and documenting the process and findings.[2]

Developmental screening refers to the administration of a brief standardized validated instrument that is both sensitive and specific for detecting developmental delays. The screen will hopefully identify children with subtle delays who would have otherwise been missed. **If surveillance points to possible risks or this is a 9-month, 18-month, or 24- to 30-month visit, a development screen should be performed. In addition, the AAP** in collaboration with Bright Futures also **recommends that a specific autism screen be performed at the 18- and 24-month visits.**[3] (See the age-specific well child visit chapters for more details.) It is important to note that these tests are only screens; therefore children may be identified as not meeting certain developmental milestones who are actually within the range of normal. All results must be interpreted within the context of the primary care provider's knowledge of the child's medical history and environment, social, and historical risks.

Choosing the correct instrument to use can also be somewhat complicated. Factors that play into this decision include the screen's reliability, validity, sensitivity, and specificity. In addition, different screens rely on obtaining information from either the parent or the child or both. Depending on the format of the screen, ease of use, time for administration, and parental literacy level may also play a role in the primary care provider's decision regarding various screening tools. A list of several screening tools can be found in both *Nelson Textbook of Pediatrics,* 18th edition (Chapter 15, Developmental Screening and Surveillance) and the AAP's policy statement regarding developmental surveillance and screening.[2]

When Developmental Delay is Identified

Once a possible developmental delay has been identified, it is important for the primary care physician to make the appropriate referrals. This includes a referral for a more comprehensive developmental assessment by a specialist such as a developmental or neurodevelopmental pediatrician. In addition, referrals for interventional services should be made. Even if a child does not yet have a diagnosis, services such as speech therapy, occupational therapy, or physical therapy can be started. If a child is younger than 3 years old, this is usually done through Early Intervention. Once a child is 3 years of age, services may be obtained either through the county intermediate unit, or the local school district or board of education, according to custom in the specific location. See Chapter 25, The Special Needs Child.

Assessing a child's development is a continual process performed by the primary care physician throughout the course of childhood. Although much focus is placed on younger children, it is important to remember that school-age children and adolescent children require ongoing surveillance too. School success and peer interactions become more important as the child ages. As the child ages, learning disabilities, attention issues, such as attention-deficit/hyperactivity disorder, and behavioral problems may become apparent. The primary care pediatrician must continue to screen for these disorders, make appropriate referrals and remain a resource and advocate for the family.

Practice-Based Learning and Improvement

Title
The Denver Developmental Screening Test

Authors
Frankenburg WK, Dodds JB

Reference
Pediatr 71:181-191, 1967

Historical significance/comments
A description of an early development screening tool for use in the primary care setting

Interpersonal and Communication Skills

Discuss Abnormal Screening Results: Share Information Using Language the Family Can Understand

Discussion of abnormal screening results can be very frightening for families. Parents who have raised concerns themselves may be more amenable to discussing abnormal results than a parent who has noted no abnormalities. It is important to emphasize that there is a range of normal and that further testing may show that there is no problem requiring intervention. Explaining the results of the screening tests needs to be done in understandable terms for the family (this includes both normal and abnormal findings). Some suggestions of easy-to-understand terms describing developmental delays include "behind other children" or "having difficulties with . . ."

Professionalism

Communication and Collaboration: Build a Partnership With Parents

Some parents may be in denial when a possible delay is found (for example, "I didn't start talking until I was over 2 years old, and I am just fine"). It is very important to continue to work with such parents and maintain an ongoing open relationship so a future plan of action can be developed in partnership with the parent.

Be available to the parent as questions come up during the evaluation process.

Encourage parents to be aware of the importance of development in their child, and suggest ways for them to help their child (such as reading to their child from a young age).

Systems-Based Practice

Government-Mandated Support Services for Children

Pediatricians need to be aware of and comfortable using various local and state services and resources available for supporting children with developmental delay. Some examples include the Early Intervention and Head Start programs.

The **Early Intervention** program (Part C of Individuals with Disabilities Education Act [IDEA] of 2004) is a federal grant program that assists states in operating a comprehensive, coordinated, multidisciplinary, interagency system of early intervention services for infants and toddlers with disabilities from birth to age 3 and their families (http://www.medicalhomeinfo.org/health/ei.html).

The **Head Start** program provides grants to local public and private nonprofit and for-profit agencies to provide comprehensive child development services to economically disadvantaged children and families, with a special focus on helping preschoolers develop the early reading and math skills they need to be successful in school. Head Start programs promote school readiness by enhancing the social and cognitive development of children through the provision of educational, health, nutritional, social, and other services to enrolled children and families. They engage parents in their children's learning and help them in making progress toward their educational, literacy, and employment goals. Significant emphasis is placed on the involvement of parents in the administration of local Head Start programs (http://www.acf.hhs.gov/programs/ohs/).

In addition, physicians should be able assist parents of older children in applying for evaluations/services through the local school district or board of education by writing letters on their behalf and providing relevant information.

Other Resources
Promoting child development. In Hagan JF, Shaw JS, Duncan PM (eds): *Bright Futures: Guidelines for health supervision of infants, children, and adolescents,* 3rd ed. Elk Grove Village, IL, American Academy of Pediatrics, 2008, pp 39-75.

References

1. Glascoe FP, Shapiro HL: *Introduction to developmental and behavioral screening.* Available at section on learning, http://www.dbpeds.org
2. Identifying infants and young children with developmental disorders in the medical home: An algorithm for developmental surveillance and screening. *Pediatrics* 118:405-420, 2006.
3. Recommendations for preventive pediatric health care. *Pediatrics* 120:1376, 2007.

Chapter 15
Anticipatory Guidance

English Willis MD

Medical Knowledge and Patient Care

Anticipatory guidance (AG) is age and developmentally appropriate health advice focused on improving the health, safety, and physical and emotional well-being of children and adolescents. This preventive advice, valued by parents, guardians, and patients, is dedicated to helping families understand what to expect during their child's or adolescent's current and approaching stage of development.[1] The continuity relationship between the physician and family makes this the ideal setting for AG discussions, because many of the topics are discussed longitudinally. To be effective, the AG should be patient specific and culturally relevant.[2]

The health education provided by pediatricians is intended to increase parent and patient knowledge, and hopefully it has a positive impact on behaviors that promote health and well-being and prevent disease and injury. The number of potential topics and their content are extensive. Although there are no mandatory issues to be covered, there are standard topics for consideration. These include:

- Healthy eating
- Prevention of illness and injury
- Environmental health

- Child development
- Promotion of literacy
- Media use
- Nutrition
- Oral health
- Sexual health
- Substance abuse
- Social development
- Family relationships
- Parental health
- Community interactions
- Self-responsibility
- School/vocational achievement

Most pediatricians recognize the importance of providing health advice but are challenged on how to cover the topics effectively and efficiently.[3,4] The best advice is given and received by the family when there is a strong doctor–patient–child relationship. To create a patient-focused visit, families find it helpful to receive personalized advice with a discussion reflecting their child's age and developmental level, along with cultural traditions of the family. This avoids "running the list" and allows time to prioritize and focus the discussion on topics that are both interesting and relevant to the patient and family.

Environmental, cultural, and economic shifts have made AG more important than ever. For many, the support provided by extended family members is less available, and the demands of working outside the home have resulted in less parental time and less energy to learn independently about these topics. Parents want, need, and expect their pediatrician to provide them with child-rearing information and preventive advice. To enhance the parental response to AG it is important to learn what families already know and are currently doing to promote health and then select topics to clarify misconceptions, reinforce healthy family practices, and introduce new information.[1]

Physicians report that limited time and lack of confidence in counseling techniques and benefits are barriers to effective provision of guidance.[4] Ideally, counseling moments are discussed naturally and seamlessly during the visit. Counseling should be woven into all interactions with the family to include your direct observations during the visit, as well as questions during the history and physical examination. Make the history interactive by not only asking questions but also providing timely information. For example, when taking the dietary history, use this as an opportunity to recommend healthy foods and eating habits not mentioned by the parent, or discuss alternative foods and physical activities to reduce the risk for obesity. Advise teenagers about weight and healthy eating habits while exploring their perception of body image. When assessing the developmental status, use this opportunity to educate the parents regarding anticipated milestones, recommendations for skills improvement such as reading, recommendations for television viewing, and personal and environmental measures for injury prevention. The physical examination provides many opportunities for focused health education. Discuss proper oral health care during the dental examination. If bruises or lacerations are observed, this is an ideal time to discuss safety and injury prevention. Direct observations of infant/toddler temperament or parent-child interactions can be made during the office visit. These observations may provide insight into the parent-child dynamics and lead to discussions about normal behavior and temperament.

Practice-Based Learning and Improvement

Become familiar with resources that provide health and safety topics for age-appropriate AG. **Bright Futures, third edition,** provides a comprehensive list of topics to cover at each of the standard well child/adolescent care visits. Stay current with the published literature on AG to include new information on issues of health promotion, illness and injury prevention, and reducing environmental risks. Know the environmental and injury risk statistics for your practice community, and use these to effect change or to educate your parents and patients.

Interpersonal and Communication Skills

Share Useful and Specific Information

Advice should be given respectfully without a dogmatic or judgmental tone, and should be culturally relevant and age and developmentally appropriate. Take time to explore cultural beliefs and practices of the family and their views and concerns regarding any recommendations. Incorporating cultural or family beliefs in your counseling will strengthen the doctor-parent relationship. It may also expand the pediatrician's knowledge and empathy and overall confidence with counseling.

Parents and patients are part of the health-care team; whenever possible try to incorporate their thoughts and ideas into your agreed plan. Try to avoid lecturing. Engage parents and patients in a discussion, and provide reasons for recommending a preventive measure or counseling them on a behavior change.

- Use a medically trained translator or a language translation telephone service whenever caring for parents or children with limited English proficiency. Never use the children as your translator to communicate with parents or guardians.
- Use language-appropriate printed handouts to supplement verbal discussions on AG.
- Document all topics discussed with parents and patients.

Professionalism

Demonstrate Respect for Others

When giving anticipatory guidance it is important to be flexible and accommodate the personal style or preference of the parents and their family and cultural traditions. When an issue is of minor importance and does not affect the health, safety, and well-being of the child, the family should be supported in their approach even if it differs from the approach the physician normally recommends. If an issue does affect the health, safety, and well-being of the child, it must be addressed directly, but with sensitivity and with sufficient time for an open discussion with the parents.

- Read, ask questions, and become familiar with cultural practices that may involve nontraditional methods of child rearing, nutrition, or health-care beliefs.
- To ensure the best possible health care for the child, maintain open communication and a collaborative relationship with families who choose to use or explore alternative care or complementary medical treatments.
- Commit to lifelong learning, and explore new methods to supplement your verbal recommendations for AG. These may include preselected websites or computer kiosks designed to provide health promotion information. Be aware of health-promoting community resources.

Systems-Based Practice

Clinical Practice Guidelines: Address Anticipatory Guidance and Preventive Health

Recommendations and clinical practice guidelines (CPGs) addressing anticipatory guidance and preventive health are derived from several sources: *Bright Futures: Guidelines for Health Supervision of Infants, Children, and Adolescents*[2]; the U.S. Preventive Services Task Force[5]; and the policy statements of the AAP.[6,7] *Bright Futures* (http://mchb. hrsa.gov) is *"a set of principles, strategies, and tools that are theory based, evidence driven, and systems oriented that can be used to improve the health and well-being of all children through culturally appropriate interventions that address the current and emerging health promotion needs at the family, clinical practice, community, health system, and policy levels."* The Bright Futures project was sponsored by the Maternal and Child Health Bureau of the U.S. Public Health Service and the Medicaid Bureau of the Health Care Financing Administration (now the Centers for Medicare and Medicaid Services). It promotes identification of family strengths and family empowerment. **There are six core concepts: partnership,**

communication, health promotion and illness prevention, time management, education, and advocacy. In addition to health supervision visit guidelines, there are multiple **health promotion themes, such as child development, mental health, healthy weight, healthy sexual development and sexuality, and safety and injury prevention.**

Bright Futures, third edition, has replaced all other guidelines such as Guidelines for Adolescent Preventive Services (GAPS) published by the American Medical Association and the American Academy of Pediatrics Guidelines for Health Supervision.

Many of Bright Future's health promotion topics reflect the Healthy People 2010 national disease prevention and health promotion objectives.[8] Healthy People 2010 has two overarching goals: (1) to increase quality and years of healthy life and (2) to eliminate health disparities. To achieve these goals, 10 health indicators for the nation have been targeted: physical activity, overweight and obesity, tobacco use, substance abuse, responsible sexual behavior, mental health, injury prevention, environmental quality, immunizations, and access to care.

Pediatricians often cite lack of time and inadequately developed office systems as barriers that negatively impact delivery of AG.[4] Advocate within your institution and with insurance carriers and public and political agencies for changes to improve the promotion of health and the prevention of disease and injury in your practice community.

References

1. Green M, Palfrey JS, editors: *Bright Futures Guidelines for health supervision of infants, children, and adolescents*, ed 2, Arlington, VA, National Center for Education in Maternal and Child Health, 2002.
2. Hagan JF, Shaw JS, Duncan PM, editors: *Bright Futures Guidelines for health supervision of infants, children, and adolescents*, ed 3, Elk Grove Village, IL, American Academy of Pediatrics, 2008.
3. Schuster MA, Duan N, Regalado M, Klein DJ: Anticipatory guidance: What information do parents receive? What information do they want? *Arch Pediatr Adolesc Med* 154:1191-1198, 2000.
4. Rosenthal MS, Lannon CM, et al: A randomized trial of practice-based education to improve delivery systems for anticipatory guidance. *Arch Pediatr Adolesc Med* 159:456-463, 2005.
5. U.S. Preventive Services Task Force, Agency for Healthcare Research and Quality. Available at http://www.ahrq.gov/clinic/prevenix.htm
6. American Academy of Pediatrics: *Pediatric clinical practice guidelines and policy*, ed 5, Elk Grove, IL, American Academy of Pediatrics, 2005.
7. Belamarich PF, Gandica R, Stein REK, Racine AD: Drowning in a sea of advice: Pediatricians and American Academy of Pediatrics policy statements. *Pediatrics* 2006;118:e964-e978.
8. U.S. Department of Health and Human Services: *Healthy People 2010: Understanding and improving health*, 2nd ed. Washington, DC, Government Printing Office, 2000.

Chapter 16
The Newborn Well Child Visit

Jacquelyn M. Aveta MD, FAAP

Speaking Intelligently

The first newborn visit ideally occurs within a few days after hospital discharge.[1] I first congratulate the parents and then elicit their questions and concerns. The infant is carefully evaluated for jaundice. If the infant is breastfeeding, determine if the mother's milk is in and if the baby is feeding well and gaining weight. Establishment of successful feeding and weight gain is marked by return to birth weight by 10 to 14 days of age for breastfed and formula-fed infants. All prenatal data, including ultrasounds, are reviewed, and any needed follow-up is arranged.

Medical Knowledge and Patient Care

History

The first newborn office visit is comprehensive and may require more time and organization than subsequent infant well visits.[1] Ask the parents, especially first-time parents, how they are adjusting to caring for their newborn. Asking if they have questions or concerns will guide the visit.

- **Prenatal.** The prenatal history and testing, as well as newborn nursery data, should be reviewed with the parents. Were there any complications, such as gestational diabetes or hypertension? Review maternal laboratory results: gonorrhea, chlamydia, syphilis, hepatitis B, group B streptococcus, and human immunodeficiency virus (HIV). Is there a maternal history of genital herpes? Review time of diagnosis and treatment. Were prenatal tests done, such as chorionic villus sampling (CVS), amniocentesis, or fetal ultrasound? Inquire about drug and alcohol use, cigarette smoking, and use of over-the-counter, prescription, or herbal medications.
- **Birth History.** Review the birth history, including duration of labor, method of delivery, and any signs of fetal distress (e.g., meconium-stained amniotic fluid, low scalp pH). Review the Apgar scores. Was any resuscitation performed? Was the infant in the term nursery or the neonatal intensive care unit? Review the birth and discharge weights, length, and head circumference. Note percentiles, and compare with present measurements. Has the

infant gained weight since discharge? It is not unusual for a neonate to lose up to 10% of birth weight in the first 2 to 3 days, after which a gain of 20 to 30 g per day is expected. Obtain the newborn screen results. Most states have a mandatory newborn hearing screening program (see Chapter 58, Newborn Hearing Screen). All infants should be assessed for jaundice before discharge. Some infants may have transcutaneous or serum bilirubin assessment, along with prompt outpatient follow-up for ongoing surveillance and management (see Chapter 60, Jaundice). Check if the first hepatitis B vaccine was administered.

- **Family History.** Obtain a thorough family history. Note any hereditary conditions (e.g., sickle cell disease, metabolic defects), birth anomalies, any infant death, and mental health disorders. Social history should include the educational level and occupation of the parents, who lives in the household with the baby, and who will be the primary care provider(s). Ask about environmental tobacco smoke exposure.

- **Nutrition.** Next, obtain information specific to the newborn. Starting with nutrition, is the baby breastfed or bottle fed? If breastfed, there is colostrum for the first few days before the milk comes in.[1] Breastfeeding every 1 to 3 hours for 15 to 30 minutes on one or both breasts is not unusual (see Chapter 56, Infant Feeding) Remind the new mother that the amount of breast milk produced depends on how often the baby feeds—more feeding yields more subsequent milk production—that is, production matches demand. A lactation consultant can be quite helpful if there is difficulty establishing successful feeding. The newborn will require careful monitoring of weight and possible supplementation with infant formula to prevent excessive weight loss and dehydration. Breast milk contains little vitamin D, and hence daily supplementation is recommended. Check any maternal medication for compatibility with breastfeeding. There are multiple options for the formula-fed infant, with milk- and soy-based formulas most common. These are available in powder, concentrate, and ready to feed forms. Review the type of formula and method of preparation, ensuring that the correct amount of water is used. Note that neither the water nor bottles require sterilization. Formula-fed babies usually feed every 3 to 4 hours, initially taking $\frac{1}{2}$ ounce per feeding and gradually increasing to about 4 to 6 ounces every 3 to 4 hours by 2 months of age. The newborn should not be given any plain water or food.

- **Voiding and Stooling.** Assess the voiding and stooling patterns. In the first few days, there may be little urine. After that a well neonate will typically have about eight wet diapers per day. Early on, there may be an orange or red discoloration, sometimes called "brick dust urine," which is typically due to passage of urate crystals. Although benign, it is considered a sign of dehydration, and formula supplementation may be indicated in a breastfed neonate. The first bowel movement usually occurs within the first 24 hours of life, with all normal newborns having passed meconium by 48 hours. By the end of the first week, meconium is replaced by a softer, lighter stool. The passage of stool varies, with some newborns having anywhere from 12 stools per day to 1 stool per week. It can vary from soft and more formed to wet, yellow, and seedy. It should not contain blood or be hard. Also note that the stool pattern may vary in an individual newborn on a day-to-day basis.

- **Sleep.** All newborns should be placed to sleep on their back in their own sleep space (bassinette, crib, or cradle). This decreases the risk for sudden infant death syndrome (SIDS). There should be no pillows, toys, or excessive blankets. Sleep positioning devices are not recommended by the American Academy of Pediatrics (AAP). Newborns usually sleep 14 to 16 hours per day. Nearly all do not sleep through the night.

Physical Examination

Perform a complete physical examination and developmental surveillance (see Chapter 54, The Newborn Examination). Does the baby gaze at faces and track to midline? Do the eyes close on transition from a dark to well-lit room? Does the baby cry? Is there a startle response to sound? When placed prone, does the baby attempt to raise his/her head? Perform the physical examination in full view of the caregivers, so significant findings can be discussed and reassurance provided where appropriate. Most will examine the chest first in a quiet infant. Auscultate for a murmur or heart rate irregularity. Peripheral pulmonic stenosis is a benign systolic ejection murmur heard best at both upper sternal borders with radiation to the axillae and back. It results from turbulent flow in small branch pulmonary arteries. Weak or absent femoral pulses require prompt evaluation for coarctation of the aorta (see Chapter 65, The Newborn With a Murmur). Count the respiratory rate for 1 full minute. The lungs should be clear, but nasal stuffiness and sneezing are not uncommon. Inspect and palpate the abdomen for masses. In a crying infant, palpation is easier during inspiration. Other key features of the neonatal examination include assessment of fontanelles, presence of cephalohematoma, bilateral red reflexes, hip examination including symmetry of skin folds, muscle tone, and checking the umbilical stump and circumcision healing. Note symmetry of movement—the healthy newborn assumes a flexed posture and moves all extremities equally. Primitive reflexes such as the startle, fencing, stepping, and grasp should be identical on the right and left sides. Ear malformations may be a clue to an underlying renal anomaly. Inspect the skin throughout the examination. Normal findings are bluish hands and feet (acrocyanosis), peeling dry skin, and the classic markings of capillary nevi on the eyelids, forehead, and nape of neck. Mongolian spots, blue or purple-gray flat spots, occur on the back and buttocks of dark-skinned babies (Figure 16-1). Milia are simple inclusion cysts that appear as discrete white bumps, usually on the

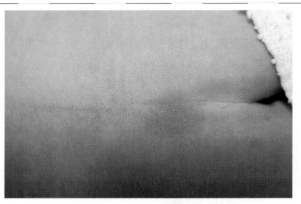

Figure 16-1 Mongolian spots.

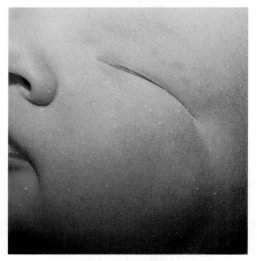

Figure 16-2 Milia.

nose (Figure 16-2). The benign rash of erythema toxicum neonatorum appears as 1- to 3-mm papules on an erythematous base in a diffuse pattern, by the second to third day of life (Figure 16-3). A baby with neonatal pustular melanosis will have 2- to 4-mm nonerythematous vesicles and/or pigmented macules with a collarette of flaking in previous area of vesicles (Figure 16-4). These benign lesions usually disappear by 3 months of age. If there is any question of herpes simplex or staphylococcal skin infection, further evaluation is urgently needed.

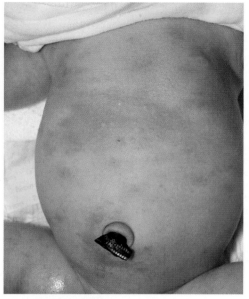

Figure 16-3 Erythema toxicum neonatorum.

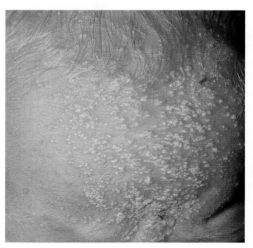

Figure 16-4 Neonatal pustular melanosis.

Interpersonal and Communication Skills

Look for Postpartum Depression: Gather Information Using Active Listening and Verbal Techniques

It is recommended that pediatricians routinely screen for postpartum depression. Unrecognized maternal depression can adversely affect maternal–child attachment and impact the child's emotional development as well as quality of care.[2] Use active listening technique, making eye contact and speaking words of encouragement as needed to facilitate a dialogue with the mother. The opportunity to observe a seasoned clinician in this setting can be invaluable. The U.S. Public Health two-question screen for depression is quick and simple to administer. (1) Have you been feeling down, depressed, or hopeless? (2) Have you had little interest or pleasure in doing things? If there are positive answers, elicit if there is any history of depression and any prior treatment for mental health disorders. Explore the family situation, and identify available family and social supports. If there is concern about depression, explore whether the mother has thoughts of harming herself or her infant, because suicidal ideation or thoughts of harming the baby would require urgent psychiatric referral. In some patients, prompt referral to a mental health professional may be indicated, or perhaps close follow-up by telephone or another office visit in a few days will suffice. (See Chapter 61, Feeding Difficulty in the Newborn.)

Professionalism

Use Compassion and Empathy When Dealing With a New Mother

The immediate postpartum period may be difficult for a new mother for many reasons: anxiety about the health of the infant; pain, especially after a cesarean section or difficult vaginal delivery; sleepiness and confusion related to narcotics given for pain; and frustration when there are difficulties initiating breastfeeding are a few examples. All these issues may be magnified for a first-time mother. It is important for the physician to recognize how these factors can affect a new mother and understand the need to repeat information and provide ongoing assurance and support.

Practice-Based Learning and Improvement: Screening for Developmental Dysplasia of the Hip

Title
Clinical practice guideline: Early detection of developmental dysplasia of the hip

Author
American Academy of Pediatrics, Committee on Quality Improvement, Subcommittee on Developmental Dysplasia of the Hip

Reference
Pediatrics 105(4):896-905, 2000

Problem
Developmental dysplasia of the hip (DDH) is relatively uncommon but important to detect and treat to promote healthy development and function of the hips and avoid development of avascular necrosis and premature osteoarthritis. In addition, a missed diagnosis of DDH can result in a malpractice claim.

Historical significance/comments
The guideline provides a paradigm for screening and referral and reviews the spectrum of DDH. Because this can be an evolving process, screening is recommended through the first 12 months of life. See Chapter 17, Teaching Visual: Examination of the Infant Hip.

Systems-Based Practice

Understand Procedures and Terminology for Claims, Coding, and Billing of the First Newborn Well Visit

Depending on the clinical circumstances and work performed, the first office visit for a newborn may be coded either as a new or established well child visit (CPT code 99381 or 99391), or as a new or problem-oriented patient visit (99202-99205 or 99212-99215). CPT stands for the American Medical Association's Current Procedural Terminology—the most widely accepted medical nomenclature used to report medical procedures and services under public and private health insurance programs. It is important for the physician to recognize that both the CPT Manual and Centers for Medicare and Medicaid Services Documentation Guidelines for Evaluation and Management Services define a new patient as "one who has not received any professional services from the physician or another physician of the same specialty who belongs to the same group practice within 3 years." If the newborn was cared for in the hospital by the same primary care physician or another group member who will provide office care, the first well visit is billed as an established patient well visit. Similarly, a first newborn office visit for a feeding problem is billed as a new patient visit if the infant received in-hospital care from another pediatric group.

References

1. Hagan JF, Shaw JS, Duncan PM, editors: *Bright Futures: Guidelines for health supervision of infants, children, and adolescents*, ed 3, Elk Grove Village, IL, American Academy of Pediatrics, 2008.
2. Chaudron LH, Szilagyi PG, Campbell AT: Legal and ethical considerations: Risks and benefits of post partum depression screening at well-child visits. *Pediatrics* 119:123-128, 2007.

Chapter 17
Teaching Visual: Examination of the Infant Hip

Maureen C. McMahon MD

Objectives

- Describe the abnormalities in developmental dysplasia of the hip (DDH).
- Explain that DDH may be present at birth or evolve in the postnatal period.
- Demonstrate and describe performance of the Ortolani and Barlow maneuvers.
- Explain the significance of positive Ortolani and Barlow maneuvers.

Medical Knowledge

Because the hip contains a high percentage of cartilage at birth, regular examinations are performed during the first year of life to detect abnormalities as the hip grows and undergoes ossification. The goals are to detect developing dysplasia, to prevent or successfully treat hip dislocation, and to avoid development of avascular necrosis (AVN) of the femoral head. DDH may include underdevelopment or dysplasia of the acetabulum, or the femoral head may be abnormally positioned within the acetabulum, which may lead to frank dislocation (luxation), partial dislocation (subluxation), or instability, whereby the femoral head slides in and out of the acetabulum.[1] Risk factors for DDH include female gender, firstborn child, breech presentation, or a family history of DDH.[2]

The Ortolani and Barlow maneuvers are performed on infants from birth through 12 weeks of age. **The Barlow maneuver is a gentle attempt to sublux or dislocate the femoral head from an unstable hip. The Ortolani maneuver is an attempt to relocate a dislocated hip.** If either the Ortolani or Barlow is elicited, it is a positive examination for DDH. After 12 weeks of age, these maneuvers become increasingly less reliable.[1,2] Limitation of abduction is the most reliable sign of DDH after 3 months of age. Normal abduction is symmetric and nearly complete; that is, the knees should come close to touching the examination table[3]. Asymmetry of thigh and gluteal folds or suspected leg length discrepancy raises suspicion for DDH, but is not diagnostic.[1] In the neonate, soft tissue "clicks" are common and are usually due to ligamentous laxity caused by maternal hormones and do not indicate DDH. It is important to distinguish a soft tissue "click" from the rarely felt "clunk" of frank femoral head dislocation.

The infant is ideally examined in a quiet state lying supine. With the diaper open, first observe for symmetry of the anterior thigh creases (Figure 17-1).

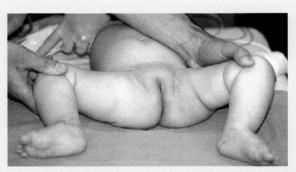

Figure 17-1 Note asymmetric anterior thigh creases in an infant with developmental dysplasia of the hip.

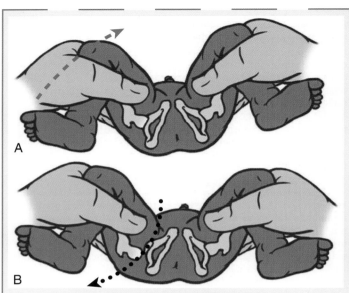

Figure 17-2 The Barlow provocative test.

Next the knees and hips are flexed while the feet are held flat on the table. Note if the height of the knees is equal. With a posteriorly dislocated hip, the leg on the affected side will appear shorter (a positive Galeazzi sign).

Method of Hip Assessment

The hip is assessed by examining one side at a time. To examine the right hip, flex the infant's knees and hips to 90 degrees. The left hip is held stable with the examiner's right hand, and the examiner's left thumb is placed on the infant's right knee as the second and third fingers gently grasp the posterolateral thigh.

The **Barlow maneuver** is performed by **adducting the hip while simultaneously applying gentle posterior pressure to the thigh** (Figure 17-2, *A*). If the femoral head dislocates, a "clunk" is felt as it exits the acetabulum (Figure 17-2, *B*).

Next perform the **Ortolani maneuver** on the right hip by positioning the left thumb on the right medial thigh and the second and third digits on the right greater trochanter. *The thigh is gently lifted anteriorly while simultaneously abducting from midline.* A "clunk" will be appreciated when a dislocated femoral head is relocated in the acetabulum. These maneuvers are then performed on the left hip. (See Figure 17-3.)

The baby is then turned prone. While the examiner holds and gently extends both legs together, the gluteal and posterior thigh folds are checked for symmetry. **See Nelson Essentials 199.**

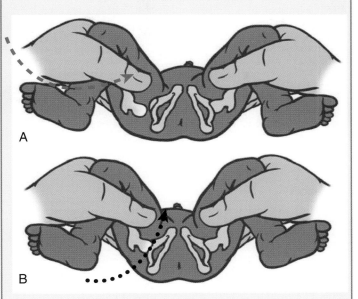

Figure 17-3 The Ortolani test.

See Nelson Essentials 39.

Interpersonal and Communication Skills

Communicate With Parents Using Understandable Language

Explain to the parents that you will examine their baby's hips at every well visit until the first birthday as the hip joint grows and develops around the femur. Explain that we examine using two specific maneuvers to check for joint stability. Early detection of abnormalities is important because treatment almost always results in normal hip formation. I explain that well-formed hips are essential to successful development of walking and prevention of arthritis and other degenerative changes in adulthood.

Explain that many infants cry while the hips are manipulated, but the maneuvers are not straining the joint or inducing pain.

Parents will often become anxious if I note an abnormality. A true "clunk" with a positive Ortolani or Barlow maneuver will require timely evaluation by a pediatric orthopedist (within a few days if possible), and timely counseling of parents. Parents usually have many questions and are often very concerned about having to wait before seeing the orthopedist. I explain that a few days' lag before initiating treatment is generally safe. Initial treatment is usually a Pavlik harness to position the legs in abduction to promote hip relocation. In some cases, casting is required, and still rarer, some infants require open surgery for full correction. Progress in hip growth is followed with ultrasound in the young infant, and after several months plain x-ray is used to monitor new bone formation.

References

1. Committee on Quality Improvement, Subcommittee on Developmental Dysplasia of the Hip: American Academy of Pediatrics clinical practice guideline: Early detection of developmental dysplasia of the hip. *Pediatrics* 105(4):896-905, 2000.
2. Kliegman RM, Behrman RE, Jenson HB, Stanton BF: *Nelson textbook of pediatrics*, ed 18, Philadelphia, 2007, Saunders.
3. Algranati PS: *The pediatric patient: An approach to history and physical examination*, Baltimore, MD, 1992, Williams & Wilkins.

Chapter 18
The 1-, 2-, and 4-Month Well Child Visits

Dennis Z. Kuo MD, MHS

Speaking Intelligently

Early infancy is a time of rapid growth and change as the infant develops increasing awareness of the environment and motor skills begin to emerge. Key elements of these visits include eliciting parental concerns, monitoring growth percentiles, developmental surveillance, administering immunizations, and providing individualized anticipatory guidance. Many infants transition to a group day care setting when the mother resumes employment outside the home. Parents have usually become comfortable caring for their baby. It is important to acknowledge this and provide reassurance that the infant is growing and developing as expected.

Medical Knowledge and Patient Care

In early infancy the excitement of a new baby settles down into a routine. Parents become attuned to responding to their child's needs and wants, and the child begins to smile, coo, and laugh. Many parents simply want to know "Is my child healthy and normal?" Almost all infants you will see are, in fact, healthy, normal, and growing well. Time should be devoted to reassurance and giving parents a vote of confidence in their parenting skills.

- **Nutrition.** The child grows quickly at this age. Typical weight gain is 20 to 30 g/day. Length typically increases 3.5 cm/month and head circumference 2 cm/month. The child should be fed with either breast milk or iron-fortified formula. If the mother is breastfeeding, the milk supply and the feeding routine are generally well established at this age. Encourage the breastfeeding mother to exclusively breastfeed through 6 months of age. Solid foods such as iron-fortified baby cereals can be introduced to formula-fed infants at 4 to 6 months of age. Starting solids earlier is discouraged because oral motor skills are not adequately developed, nutrition may be adversely affected, and there may be an increased incidence of allergies. Solids are introduced to allow the baby to try new textures and flavors, but breast milk or formula remains the principal source of nutrition until 6 months of age.

- **Development.** As the infant grows, he/she acquires new motor, language, and social skills in a predictable sequence. These skills, called developmental milestones, are important for assessing the developmental trajectory. At the 1-month visit, the child may be smiling and holding his/her head up briefly. At 2 months, the child will be smiling socially, visually tracking across the midline, and holding his/her head up steadily. By the 4-month visit, the child will be cooing, starting to babble and laugh, reaching for an object, pushing up on his/her arms, and visually tracking around the room.
- **Teaching parents to recognize a sick child.** Although infants may get common colds, they are also susceptible to more serious invasive illnesses such as bacteremia or urinary tract infections. Teach parents how to recognize a sick child. Under 3 months of age, a child who feels warm, is fussy, or is feeding poorly should have a rectal temperature taken. If the temperature is above 100.4° F, the family should call the physician immediately so the infant can be evaluated for infection. Over the age of 3 months, the family should call for fussiness, labored breathing, poor feeding, or high fever.
- **Immunizations.** Immunizations are important to protect against childhood diseases. The 2-month-old can receive up to eight vaccines: diphtheria, tetanus, pertussis, *Haemophilus influenzae* type b, pneumococcus, hepatitis B, polio, and rotavirus. Several vaccines are combined to reduce the number of shots. Parents should be counseled about the benefits and risks of each vaccine, but discuss that the risk of each vaccine is exceedingly low compared with the actual disease.
- **Common questions at the young infant checkup include:**
  - *Is my baby eating enough?* Too much? Infants usually self-regulate how much to feed. Hunger cues (rooting, sucking on a hand, then finally crying) and satiety cues (sleepy, not interested in feeding) are important to recognize. A consistent growth curve reassures parents. It is difficult to overfeed an infant at this age, but counsel parents that crying infants may simply want to be held and not fed.
  - *Why is my baby congested all the time?* Young infants frequently sound congested because they are obligate nose breathers and have small nasal passages. Residual estrogen from pregnancy and reflux can also exacerbate congestion. The congestion rarely bothers infants, and as long as the infant is feeding well, little more than reassurance is needed. Congestion typically resolves by 6 months. Over-the-counter cough and cold medicines are never indicated in this age-group.

- *Why is my baby fussy?* Crying and fussiness tend to increase over the first several months and peak around 4 months of age. Although a definition of colic exists (3 hours of crying a day, 3 days a week), the official definition matters little if the parents are stressed.[1] Find out how easy feeds are, whether there is any blood in the stool, and how the parents are coping with the crying. Reassurance and empathy are important to manage this difficult time. Parents can be given permission to put the child down in a safe place and take a brief break when they feel overwhelmed.

Elements of Patient Care

- **General:** Establish the visit tone in a positive, enthusiastic manner. Greet the parents and the baby by name and correct gender, and introduce yourself if it is your first time meeting the family. Take note of where the child and the family are sitting and how they are interacting. Is the baby being held by the parent? Does the parent appear happy, sad, fearful, or angry?
- **History:** Begin with open-ended questions, and let the parent set the agenda. Appropriate open-ended questions include "How is she doing?" or "Do you have any questions about her?" Once the parents have answered, you may ask more specific questions. Ask about temperament, sleep position and location, and bowel and bladder habits. Ask about milestones the child has reached. For breastfed babies, ask how long the child is breastfeeding and whether there are problems with latch, milk supply, or nipple soreness. For formula-fed babies, ask how many ounces per feed and how often. Finally, be sure to ask how the family is doing. Maternal depression affects 14% of new mothers, and you may be the first health professional to discover it and intervene[2] (see Chapter 16, The Newborn Well Child Visit and Chapter 61, Feeding Difficulty in the Newborn).
- **Physical Examination:** Begin by observing the child without touching him/her. Notice the child's tone and body position. Is the child moving his/her arms and legs freely? Know the developmental stage of the child—the 1-month-old should focus on your face briefly, but the 4-month-old should be able to track your face in all directions. Do not forget to adjust expectations for gestational age. The child should be fully undressed for the examination, save for the diaper initially. A complete physical examination is important. Begin with the lungs and the heart, because the infant may start crying when you press on the abdomen or look in the ears. Pay particular attention to heart murmurs, abdominal masses, hip stability, and whether both testes are down in males. Check the infant's tone, because head lag should disappear by 4 months.
- **Anticipatory Guidance:** Common topics to discuss include development, safety, and diet.[3] Discuss when to call the office and how to call. Infants should be placed on their backs to sleep to

decrease the risk for sudden infant death syndrome (SIDS). The child must be in an appropriate car seat when in a moving vehicle. Advise parents to never leave a child unattended on an elevated surface or in a bathtub, even for a second. Discuss plans for child care. Finally, emphasize that babies cannot be spoiled by too much holding or attention. Encourage tummy time while awake to prevent positional plagiocephaly.

Practice-Based Learning and Improvement

Title
American Academy of Pediatrics Policy Statement. Breastfeeding and the Use of Human Milk

Reference
Pediatrics 115(2):496-506, 2005

Historical significance/comments:
This policy statement summarizes the benefits of exclusive breastfeeding and lists recommendations for pediatricians and other health-care professionals to assist in initiation and maintenance of breastfeeding. In addition, contraindications to breastfeeding are reviewed. According to the National Immunization Survey, 43% of children born in 2007 were breastfeeding at 6 months, below the Health People 2010 goal of 50%. In addition, many of these infants receive formula supplementation and hence are not exclusively breastfed.

Interpersonal and Communication Skills

Gather Information Using Nonverbal and Verbal Techniques

The pediatrician can be a tremendous resource for information and support. During the young infant visits, the parents are getting to know *you*. Take time to develop rapport with the family, empowering the parents to feel comfortable taking care of their child, and educating parents on how to best work with you. Reassurance, empathy, and support are paramount to the successful well child visit at this age. Engage in active listening by nodding, using "uh-huh," and repeating what you have heard. Be sure to allow parents enough opportunity to describe their questions, and avoid interrupting. Discuss concerns with a soothing and reassuring tone, but convey that you will address them as quickly as possible. If you are asked a question for which you do not know the answer, it is okay to say, "I do not know, but I will find out for you." Explain any findings in clear, everyday language. Check periodically for parental understanding. End by asking parents what additional questions they have, and tell them when the next well visit is due.

Professionalism

Communication and Collaboration: Respect Nontraditional Arrangements

Physicians should work with the family to meet the individual needs of the child and family, while respecting personal preferences, cultural differences, and experiences the family may have had.[3] Some health and care recommendations should be negotiated. Many parents will look to their physician as a source of information and guidance, but they may have very strong ideas about some issues. Be sensitive to family and community preferences. Know, understand, and respect the family and caregiver arrangements, especially for nontraditional families.

Systems-Based Practice

Patient-Centered Care

Patient-centered care is one of the six domains of quality outlined by the Institute of Medicine. This model is based on convenience and accessibility for patients and families.[4] It requires offering same-day service, open access or flexible scheduling, and expanded office hours. Patients would be provided access to their medical information and partner with the physician in making health-care decisions. Institutions with electronic medical record systems may allow patients limited access to the record, such as immunizations, growth charts, medication lists, and select laboratory results. In addition, there may be e-mail access to office staff requesting routine appointments and prescription renewal. Care should be comprehensive and coordinated. These tenets, which have been adopted to varying degrees across the United States, are ingredients of the medical home concept advocated by the American Academy of Pediatrics (see Chapter 25, The Special Needs Child).

References

1. Reijneveld SA, Brugman E, Hirasing RA: Excessive infant crying: The impact of varying definitions. *Pediatrics* 108:893-897, 2001.
2. Chaudron LH, Szilagyi PG, Campbell AT, et al: Legal and ethical considerations: Risks and benefits of postpartum depression screening at well-child visits. *Pediatrics* 119:123-128, 2007.
3. Hagan JF, Shaw JS, Duncan PM, editors: *Bright Futures: Guidelines for health supervision of infants, children, and adolescents*, ed 3, Elk Grove Village, IL, 2008, American Academy of Pediatrics. Available at http://www.brightfutures. org.
4. Davis K: A 2020 vision of patient-centered primary care. *J Gen Int Med* 20(10):953-957, 2005.

Chapter 19
The 6-Month Well Child Visit

Kelly R. Leite DO

Speaking Intelligently

The 6-month-old has developed into a curious and social infant who most enjoys interacting with his/her parents. Reciprocal smiles and vocalizations create strong emotional attachment and enjoyment. The infant is beginning to distinguish strangers and will often prefer familiar people. Sitting balance and early mobility are emerging. In addition to visual cues, the curious infant now learns through oral exploration of his/her environment. The parents are now well accustomed to the well visit format and vaccination schedule. Discussion of environmental safety and "babyproofing" the home to facilitate safe exploration and infant development is a high priority for this visit. By 6 months of age, complementary solid foods are required for optimal growth and prevention of iron deficiency.

Medical Knowledge and Patient Care

The 6-month-old shows continued developmental gains and increasing interaction with others, while exhibiting a strong attachment to his/her parents. While sitting in his/her parent's lap the infant will often be happy and responsive, but may quickly cry when approached by others. The infant may now resist when a nurse attempts to obtain vital signs, weight, and measurements or examine him/her. These early signs of stranger awareness and strong attachment to parents are a direct result of the infant's increased recognition of others. The infant may now display some resistance with familiar friends or routine babysitters. Parents may report that he/she has difficulty separating from them at day care or with a familiar caregiver. Offer reassurance that this behavior is normal. Infants develop a sense that their parents exist when not in sight before they develop object permanence, though many at this age will look for objects out of sight and show interest in simple interactive games such as hide-and-seek.

History

- **Growth Assessment.** Assess growth by reviewing the growth curves for weight, length, head circumference, and weight to length ratio. If the infant is maintaining similar percentiles as compared with previous visits, the velocity of growth is intact. Channeling to a lower percentile may occur during the first year of life as a normal trend, but this is a gradual change influenced by genetic potential. If there is an upward trend in weight percentile, an accurate history will determine if the infant is overfed. Acute changes in growth parameters warrant a detailed history and focused physical examination and possible imaging or laboratory testing.

- **Nutrition.** To assess nutritional status, begin by inquiring how often the infant breastfeeds and the length of feeds. For formula-fed infants, ask how many ounces are consumed per feed and how many bottles per day. Caloric needs are around 90 to 100 kcal/kg/day. Many infants have started complementary solid foods before 6 months. Most infants between 4 and 6 months have developed appropriate head and neck control, can sit well with support, and have effective oral motor abilities. If solids have already been started, inquire about specific foods and amount and if there have been any adverse reactions. Solids are necessary at this age due to an increased iron requirement, and this should be explained if solid food has not been initiated. Single-grain infant cereals such as rice, barley, and oatmeal are the recommended initial food given their iron fortification, easy digestibility, and relatively low potential for allergic reaction. Additional foods, once the infant is easily taking cereal for a few weeks, include pureed or soft fruits, vegetables, and meat to offer a balanced diet. Review the importance of feeding solids twice a day, placing the infant in a high chair or infant seat, and offering pureed food with a spoon. Remind the parents that it often takes several attempts before the infant accepts spoon feeding and initial intake is often just a few spoonfuls. New foods should be introduced every 5 to 7 days to ensure time to watch for adverse reactions. Avoid adding spices, salt, and sugar. Juice is not a necessary part of the diet. Review the foods to avoid because of high allergic potential and choke hazard: peanut products, shellfish, eggs, popcorn, whole grapes, hot dogs, and dry foods that do not easily break apart.[1] Honey should be discouraged until age 2 years because of the increased risk for infant botulism. Infants should always be supervised at mealtimes. Continue supplemental vitamin D (400 international units daily) for breastfeeding babies, especially if they are dark skinned or have limited exposure to sunlight.[2]

   Fluoride supplementation is started in breastfed infants and those who receive formula prepared with water that is low or deficient in fluoride (<0.3 ppm).[2] Initial tooth eruption may begin at any time between 6 and 12 months. Lower central incisors often erupt first. Oral health risk assessments should occur routinely with the first tooth eruption. Encourage parents to gently brush or wipe teeth with a soft cloth daily. Discourage supine bottle drinking and bottle propping because of the strong evidence of increased dental caries and otitis media.[3,4]

- **Development.** The infant's ability to eat finger foods provides information about **fine motor skills.** The addition of soft finger foods cut into small pieces is appropriate at this time. Because infants at this stage use a raking motion to pick up objects, it is important to limit the amount of finger foods offered at one time. For other fine motor skills, ask if the infant helps to hold the bottle or has started to drink from a cup. Observe if the infant transfers an object from one hand to another.

    For **gross motor development,** observe if the infant is sitting with good head control with or without support. Some will be able to sit without support. Observe the infant prone. Is the infant able to push his/her body up on his/her hands? Do the parents report the infant has rolled over from prone to supine and supine to prone? When held standing, the infant should bear full weight and may "bounce" up and down. If some but not all of these skills are being observed and reported, reassure the parent that progress will continue in an infant with normal muscle tone. Some minor delay in gross motor development may be due to inadequate tummy time. Encourage increased tummy time while the infant is awake to increase muscle strength and coordination. An interim follow-up visit can be scheduled for surveillance of motor development if there is concern for an evolving delay.[5]

    Parents typically note **increasing vocalization.** Infants who were laughing and imitating vowel sounds at the last visit are now starting to combine syllables and may say "da-da" nonspecifically. Receptive language assessment is somewhat limited: does the infant turn to the parent's voice and perhaps turn when his/her name is called? Let parents know that reading books, singing, and talking to their infant will provide important stimulation for language and social development.

- **Sleep.** A bedtime routine will help establish **good sleep hygiene.** Infants should be put in the crib awake for naps and bedtime, allowing them to learn to fall asleep. Review the importance of putting the infant to sleep on his/her back, but it is now okay for him to roll over to sleep in the side or prone position. Most 6-month-olds require two naps a day.

Physical Examination

The physical examination should be complete with clothing removed. Begin with the infant on the parent's lap, where he/she will feel secure. Auscultate the heart and lungs, assess the fontanelle, elicit red reflexes, and perform the ear examination in the parent's lap. The infant should visually fix on an object and be able to follow it 180 degrees. Transfer to the examination table for the remainder of the examination with the parent next to the baby. Other essential components of the examination include checking the abdomen for masses, the hips for symmetric abduction and muscle tone, and the skin examination for birthmarks and rashes.

Practice-Based Learning and Improvement

Title
Policy statement: Eye examination in infants, children, and young adults by pediatricians

Authors
American Academy of Pediatrics, Committee on Practice and Ambulatory Medicine and Section on Ophthalmology, American Association of Certified Orthoptists, American Association for Pediatric Ophthalmology and Strabismus, and American Academy of Ophthalmology

Reference
Pediatrics 111(4):902-907, 2003

Historical significance/comments
Eye examinations should be performed at all well visits, beginning with the newborn visit. This policy statement addresses risk assessment and age-appropriate vision screening. It is critically important to detect and treat any condition interfering with visual pathway development. For infants and children up to 3 years, determine if parents have any concerns about the child's vision, strabismus, or drooping eyelids. Inquire if there is a high-risk condition such as prematurity, cataract, or developmental delay. Check red reflexes, lid position, ocular motility, and pupillary reflex. Any concern warrants a referral to ophthalmology. From birth to age 3 years, the primary care ocular evaluation includes ocular history, vision assessment (age-appropriate ability to fix and follow), external inspection of the eyes and lids, pupil examination, and red reflex examination.

Interpersonal and Communication Skills

Establish Rapport by Encouraging Partnership Between the Physician and the Family

Anticipatory guidance is a major component of each health supervision visit (see Chapter 15, Anticipatory Guidance). Being able to provide effective anticipatory guidance to families requires well-developed interpersonal skills. After 6 months, the pediatrician has usually had time to get to know the family and form a partnership in which meaningful advice can be provided. The goal is to anticipate needs for the next phase of development so that a brief meaningful dialogue can occur without providing an overload of information. Share the information using language the family can understand, and be receptive to questions. Teaching with a nonjudgmental attitude can increase parental willingness to learn new child care–related skills and view the pediatrician as a useful mentor.

For the 6-month-old the biggest developmental change is gaining the ability to move about. Infants between 6 and 9 months of age will learn to crawl and scoot around to inspect their surroundings. In addition, they will be able to pick up small items with a primitive pincer grasp. Specifically, ask the parents to crawl around at home to inspect for potential hazards such as: electric sockets, dangling cords, drawers easily opened and small objects on the floor. Hot liquids and hot appliances should be kept out of reach. Discourage the use of infant walkers because of the significant risk for injury.[8] An infant should never be left unattended on a bed or changing table or in a tub or other body of water. All medications and household cleaning agents should be locked in an out-of-reach cabinet. Other topics may include use of a rear-facing car seat, risk of environmental tobacco smoke exposure, and storage of guns in the home. The amount of guidance provided is individualized for each family.[7]

Professionalism

Reliability and Responsibility: Acknowledge and Discuss Errors

The recommended immunization schedule and vaccine types are complex, frequently updated, and include multiple new combination vaccines. Because of this it takes time and focus to review a child's records accurately and decide if immunizations should be administered. Another challenge is to figure out which immunizations are due for children who for various reasons are "behind on their shots." These factors make the ordering and administration of vaccines error prone. Should an error in administration occur, the physician must determine at which point in the process the error occurred and implement a review and education process with the office care delivery team (physician, nursing, and administrative). This process must be done in a positive manner without assigning blame. The team must review the systems and procedures related to vaccine ordering and administration and, if necessary, make modifications to prevent future errors. When an error occurs, the parents must be notified with full disclosure and the conversation documented in the chart. An incident or variance report should be completed and remain separate from the patient's chart.

Systems-Based Practice

Managed Care Providers

Managed care organizations (MCOs) are required to maintain provider networks with adequate numbers of primary care physicians, specialists, and tertiary and ancillary providers to meet the medical needs of the enrolled population. Also, as part of their medical cost and utilization management strategy, the MCOs control access to specialists by requiring primary care physicians to follow specific referral procedures. For that reason, all MCOs have written policies and procedures for the processes by which members may receive referrals for specialty care.

Pediatricians should be aware that there are usually no referral or preauthorization requirements for well baby and well child care visits when provided by a contracted primary care physician within the member's (insurance plan) network.

References

1. Zeiger R: Food allergen avoidance in the prevention of food allergy in infants and children. *Pediatrics* 111(6):1662-1671, 2003.
2. American Academy of Pediatrics, Work Group on Breastfeeding: Breastfeeding and the use of human milk. *Pediatrics* 115:496-506, 2005.
3. American Academy of Pediatrics, Section on Pediatric Dentistry: Oral health risk assessment timing and establishment of the dental home. *Pediatrics* 111:1113-1116, 2003.
4. Brown CE, Magnuson B: On the physics of the infant feeding bottle and middle ear sequela: Ear disease in infants can be associated with bottle feeding. *Int J Pediatr Otorhinolaryngol* 54:13-20, 2000.
5. American Academy of Pediatrics, Committee on Practice and Ambulatory Medicine: Recommendations for preventive pediatric health care. *Pediatrics* 105:645-646, 2000.

6. American Academy of Pediatrics, Committee on Children with Disabilities: Developmental surveillance and screening of infants and young children. *Pediatrics* 108:192-196, 2001.
7. Hagan JF, Shaw JS, Duncan PM, editors: *Bright Futures: Guidelines for health supervision of infants, children, and adolescents*, ed 3, Elk Grove Village, IL, 2008, American Academy of Pediatrics. Available at http://www.brightfutures. org.

Chapter 20
The 9-Month Well Child Visit

Gina Amoroso DO

Speaking Intelligently

The 9-month visit is an exciting time to observe a child's increasing motor skills, independence, and ability to explore his/her environment. There are continued advances in cognition and communication skills, and the child is interested in everything around him/her. The 9-month-old typically has considerable stranger anxiety and is learning object permanence. This time may be a challenge for parents, because their child now has less interest in being held and cuddled. Discipline and the use of "No" becomes a topic for parents as they are challenged by their baby's energy and activity level and the need to set limits and maintain safety.

Medical Knowledge and Patient Care

History

- **Development.** The 9-month-old is all about exploring, with no awareness of safety. He/she will be "into everything," while frequently turning back to check in with a parent. To assess development, start by asking the parents what new skills they have noticed. He/she has mastered independent sitting and pivoting. The baby should be able to readily transition from sitting to lying and lying down to sitting up. Many 9-month-olds will navigate using a four-point crawl; however, some may "commando" crawl, using their arms to pull themselves forward while remaining prone. This may be a prelude to a traditional four-point crawl, but because traditional crawling is not considered a "mandatory" milestone, be sure to assess for abnormal upper body weakness, hypotonia, or spasticity as a reason for not crawling. Since the advent of "Back to Sleep," (the recommendation that infants sleep supine has resulted in over a 50% decrease in the incidence of sudden infant death syndrome since 1992.) more children are progressing to standing and cruising before crawling. These **motor milestones** correlate with increasing myelination of the central nervous system and cerebellar growth.[1] Some will be pulling to stand and may be cruising on furniture, but all 9-month-olds should be able to bear their full weight when held in standing. Manipulating objects with the hands and mouthing are the principal methods of learning in this **oral motor phase of development.** Though not yet verbal, the child can communicate likes and dislikes clearly using facial gestures and sounds. In the cognitive domain, there is definite stranger awareness; however, the degree of **stranger anxiety** manifested by each infant will vary. **Object permanence,** or understanding that people and things exist that are not currently in sight, has begun to develop. Test for this by hiding a toy under a cloth, and watch the child find it.[1] The 9-month-old loves social interaction and will participate in peek-a-boo and patty-cake. There should be **polysyllabic babbling** and **nonspecific uttering of mama and dada.** Repetition will help children make more sounds. A child's inflections start to mimic spoken language.[1] A 9-month-old can wave goodbye, respond to his/her name, and begin to understand "no." Certain emotions, such as happiness and frustration, will be more evident.[2] The infant may be starting to gesture using the arm, and this will evolve into discrete pointing with an isolated index finger. Simultaneously the grasping of a small object may now be a gross raking motion with progression to a mature pincer grasp using precise finger-thumb apposition. He/she will hold the bottle, and bang two held objects together.

In addition to developmental surveillance, the American Academy of Pediatrics (AAP) recommends administration of a formal developmental screening tool at the 9-month visit. Developmental red flags include absence of babbling or localization to sound, lack of weight bearing, and absence of a bonded relationship with parents and caregivers.

- **Nutrition.** Breast milk or iron-fortified formula is recommended until the first birthday. The typical amount is 6 to 8 ounces, three to four times daily. If not already in use, introduce a cup, with the goal of complete transition to a cup at 1 year for bottle-fed babies. Some infants breastfeed beyond 1 year, and a cup is recommended for all other beverages. Small amounts of juice diluted with water can be offered in a cup. Total daily juice intake should not exceed 6 ounces. **Continue to discourage sleeping with bottles because of the association with dental caries and otitis media.** Encourage regular mealtimes with the child seated in a high chair. At least one serving of iron-fortified cereal daily is recommended. Stage two and three baby foods, which include meats, are served. The baby is now usually taking solids three times a day. Children at this age will typically have two central incisors, and table food can be introduced. Good foods to recommend include small pieces of cheese, cooked egg yolk, noodles, or mashed potatoes. Self-feeding finger foods provides an opportunity to develop a pincer grasp. **Certain foods pose a choking hazard and must be avoided: peanuts, whole grapes, popcorn, candy, and uncut hot dogs.**[3]

- **Sleep.** Sleep hygiene is important and can be a challenge for parents. A bedtime routine is established, which may include a bath and story time. Children should fall asleep and sleep in their crib. The crib mattress is placed on the lowest setting to prevent climbing out. Remove bumper pads because children will use them as steps. A 9-month-old is expected to sleep through the night without awakening for an average of 11 hours. If nighttime awakenings occur, the child should be comforted, but discourage parents from playing with or feeding the child. Because separation anxiety is developing at 9 months, children often have more frequent awakenings without readily putting themselves back to sleep. One to two naps per day is expected, varying from 1 to 3 hours.[4]

    Children may have a transitional object, such as a blanket or stuffed animal, that helps them to sleep. These objects help make the transition from dependence to independence. Transitional objects are effective because they are familiar and harbor the child's scent.[3]

    Discuss how the child spends his/her day. This is a common time for stranger or separation anxiety. Children take comfort when their parents are there and can act differently when they are absent. If day care has just begun, it may be a difficult adjustment for both the child and the parents. Tantrums can be observed at this time of developing increased autonomy.[1]

Physical Examination

Stranger anxiety can make the physical examination challenging. One suggestion is to use a book, which can put the child at ease and allow observation of language and cognitive skills.[1] Anxiety is often lessened when the child is examined while sitting in the parent's lap.[4] Review the growth curves. A drop in percentiles is common, especially in weight. At this age, children develop a long-term growth pattern that may be different from the first few months of life. Hearing and vision screenings are done by observation. A 9-month-old can hear a whisper. Vision resembles that of an adult. Focus should be on observing eye-hand coordination. Some key components of the physical examination include skull shape, checking eye alignment, and examining the teeth.[4] In observing the child standing, parents should be reassured that most children are flat-footed. The arch of the foot is hidden by a fat pad and will usually become evident by 3 years of age. Always note the parent-child interaction during the examination.[4]

Practice-Based Learning and Improvement: Screening and Management of Children With Elevated Blood Lead Levels

Title
Interpreting and managing blood lead levels of less than 10 μg/ dL in children and reducing childhood exposures to lead: Recommendations of the Centers for Disease Control and Prevention Advisory Committee on Childhood Lead Poisoning Prevention

Authors
Binns HJ, Campbell C, Brown MJ, for the Advisory Committee on Childhood Lead Poisoning Prevention

Reference
Pediatrics 120:e1285-e1298, 2007

Historical significance/comments
Although very high lead levels and toxic lead encephalopathy in children are now relatively rare, lead continues to be a common environmental contaminant. There is evidence that surveillance for blood lead levels (BLL) less than 10 mcg/dL is warranted. Both physical and mental development can be affected, and there is an inverse association between BLL and cognitive function measured by IQ. No safe threshold of lead exposure has been identified. Pediatricians screen at either 9 or 12 months, with a possible second screening at age 2 years, when blood lead levels peak. Although precise mechanisms have not been identified, chronic lead exposure can negatively affect cognitive, motor, behavioral, and physical abilities. Legislation in the 1970s to ban leaded gasoline and limit industrial emissions has essentially eliminated most airborne lead. In addition, the removal of lead from paint has markedly decreased interior lead exposure. Current sources of lead exposure include environmental lead dust, contaminated soil, and deteriorating lead-based paint in older homes. In addition, some infants' and children's toys with lead-containing components have been identified.

Those at greatest risk are Medicaid-eligible children, especially the poor and African Americans. Older homes undergoing renovation may expose young children across the socioeconomic spectrum. In addition, immigrant and refugee children, as well as international adoptees, may have sustained lead exposure in their countries of origin. Consistent with Early and Periodic Screening Diagnosis and Treatment (EPSDT) criteria (see Systems-Based Practice below), Medicaid-eligible children should be screened, and pediatricians should obtain an environmental history on all patients. Although the ultimate goal is primary prevention, pediatricians need to improve screening and educate parents and caregivers with appropriate referrals to agencies and sources of information for provision of a lead-free environment.

Interpersonal and Communication Skills

Share Information and Encourage Questions: Highlight Important Aspects of Safety With Emerging Mobility

Providing anticipatory guidance is the most important part of the 9-month well child visit, and is a great opportunity for pediatric trainees to practice and develop effective communication skills. With the infant's emerging mobility, teaching parents how to safely enjoy this new skill is crucial. Suggest that parents crawl around at their child's level to identify safety hazards. **Any object that fits in the opening of an empty toilet paper roll is a choking hazard and should not be within a small child's reach.** Children at this age have no concept of danger and limited memory of warnings. All electrical outlets need to be covered and gates positioned around steps. The hot water heater should be turned down to 120° F. All electrical wires and cords from drapes need to be tied and out of reach because they pose a strangulation hazard. Window screens must be secure.[2] All medicines and caustic cleaning supplies must be kept on high shelves with a lock. Never place a chemical in a plastic juice or soda bottle. Have the local poison control number available in case of ingestion.[1]

Discuss appropriate toys for encouraging walking. Avoid walkers because children can easily tip them over or fall down stairs. Walkers do not strengthen the upper part of the lower extremities and may hinder walking by making getting around easier. Stationary jumping toys and pushing toys work well. Shoes for learning to walk are not necessary. For a first shoe, choose a flexible-sole sneaker or moccasin.[3]

Perhaps the most important part of the visit is dealing with parental questions after anticipatory guidance has been delivered. At this visit, most parents have questions about other potential obstacles or possible dangers in their homes, or they may have questions on how to implement some of the recommendations. Engage in a discussion, answer questions, and then briefly reinforce the most important points that were made at this visit.

Professionalism

Advocacy: Recognizing the Time for Referral

As autonomy begins to emerge, parents need to discipline their child. Many parents are not well prepared to discipline their child effectively. Parents may not know, for example, that punishing or focusing on negative behavior is not an effective form of discipline and that positive reinforcement of desired behaviors is essential,[4] that they should distract and redirect a small child, that rules and discipline need to be consistent in order to be effective, that young children have no concept of "good" or "bad" behavior, and that every child needs freedom to explore his/her environment.

As an advocate for the child, the pediatrician must follow up with parents whom they identify as frustrated and having difficulty with their child's behavior and discipline. Pediatricians must recognize situations in which they cannot devote sufficient time or the situation is beyond their level of experience and expertise. In these cases, when parental skills and coping require additional support, prompt referral to available resources in the community and close follow-up of the family are essential.

Systems-Based Practice

Utilize Government Programs for Your Patients

Early Periodic Screening Diagnosis and Treatment (EPSDT) is a federal program designed to make preventive health care available and accessible to poor children insured by Medicaid up to age 21. This includes regular examinations and screenings for vision, hearing, and dental care, as well as services and durable medical equipment for children with chronic health conditions. Treatment is provided for any condition identified through the screening process, even if it is not a normal component of care covered by the Medicaid insurance. The pediatrician completes a specific EPSDT form documenting the physical examination and screenings performed, including results, for each well visit and any specific referrals generated for problems identified through the screening process.

References

1. Behrman R, Kliegman R, Jenson HB, et al: *Nelson textbook of pediatrics*, ed 17, Philadelphia, 2004, Elsevier, pp 36-38.
2. Boynton RW, Dunn ES, Stephens GR: *Manual of ambulatory pediatrics*, ed 5, Philadelphia, 2003, Lippincott Williams & Wilkins, Philadelphia, pp 59-69.
3. Shevlov S, editor: American Academy of Pediatrics: *Your baby's first year*, New York, 2005, Bantam Dell, pp 295-338.
4. Hagan JF, Shaw JS, Duncan PM, editors: *Bright Futures: Guidelines for health supervision of infants, children, and adolescents*, ed 3, Elk Grove Village, IL, 2008, American Academy of Pediatrics. Available at http://www.brightfutures.org.

Chapter 21
The 12-Month Well Child Visit

Rachel A. B. Dodge MD, MPH

Speaking Intelligently

During the 12-month well visit, I first congratulate parents for successfully navigating 1 year. It is exciting as their infant becomes a toddler who is walking and actively exploring. Important issues to discuss include supervision and safety, stranger anxiety, temper tantrums, bedtime routine and sleep, and parental reaction to their toddler's developing autonomy. Eating issues may arise as the child develops a pincer grasp and wants to self-feed. Overall intake is decreased, as is rate of weight gain, and parents are often concerned. I explain that these changes are normal and reflect increased cognitive awareness and neurodevelopmental maturation. I also reinforce that parents are the mainstay of support as their child explores and learns, and consistency in approach is paramount for a healthy parent-child relationship.

Medical Knowledge and Patient Care

History

The 12-month well child visit marks an important milestone for families—the transition from infancy to toddlerhood. Most 12-month-olds will be cruising (walking while holding onto objects such as a couch) or walking independently—this is an exciting benchmark for parents and the child alike.[1] The child starts to exert his/her independence; **exploration of the environment** becomes the child's main goal. Pediatric residents should become familiar with the physical, cognitive/verbal, social-emotional, and behavioral development occurring during this time. Knowledge about normal development will help with addressing parent concerns and conveying age-appropriate anticipatory guidance. For example, **temper tantrums** and **discipline** are important topics to discuss with parents at the 12-month visit. Independent toddlers are trying to exert their wishes and wants on the world. Yet this world quickly becomes full of "No's." It is no wonder that children want to exert their will with their own "No," and lack of being able to communicate their own wants leads to frustration and the well-known temper tantrum, or as some parents say, "fallout." Dr. Lieberman[2] describes the temper tantrum as "a wonderfully eloquent if seldom appreciated expression of the toddler's inner experience," that is, "throwing oneself on the floor with a mixture of heart-rending crying and angry screaming." Helping parents understand temper tantrums as a normal part of development and giving them advice on handling them will help the parents handle unavoidable parent–child conflicts as they arise.[3] In addition, learning to **support parents in their role as the child's first teacher** is essential.[1] Discipline means to teach[4] and is essentially behavior management, that is, teaching the child how to behave. Knowledge about appropriate discipline techniques such as limit setting and positive reinforcement is important.[4] In addition, the parent should be the toddler's secure base; therefore parents need to be consistent and firm yet loving and encouraging.[2] Toddlers thrive in a safe, secure environment with clear limits and predictable routines.

Physical Examination

The complete physical examination is often carried out in the parent's lap to help reassure and calm the child. Growth parameters, including weight to length ratio are reviewed. Appropriate patient care should also include following health supervision guidelines for this age, for example, giving age-appropriate immunizations; screening for lead exposure, anemia, vision problems, hearing problems; and providing anticipatory guidance.[1]

- **Anticipatory Guidance.** Anticipatory guidance topics that are relevant to the 12-month-old well child visit are mealtime struggles, safety/injury prevention, and counseling on sleep-related issues, all of which are closely tied to the child's developmental stage. In addition, it is important to have knowledge about the child's community to focus your decisions about anticipatory guidance. For example, injuries occurring from home safety are a significant issue among children who live in poverty and socially deprived environments.[5,6] For this population, time to discuss injury prevention is paramount.

Practice-Based Learning and Improvement: Screening for Iron Deficiency

Title
Clinical report: Diagnosis and prevention of iron deficiency and iron-deficiency anemia in infants and young children (0 to 3 years of age)

Authors
Baker RD, Greer FR, Committee on Nutrition, American Academy of Pediatrics

Reference
Pediatrics 126(5):1040-1050, 2010

Problem
Iron deficiency anemia (IDA) and iron deficiency without anemia (ID) in infants and young children is associated with long-term neurodevelopmental and behavioral problems that may be irreversible, even with adequate iron repletion.

Comparison/control (quality of evidence)
Clinical Practice Guideline from the American Academy of Pediatrics with cited references in peer reviewed journal.

Historical significance/comments
Although a causal relationship has not been definitively established, the neurodevelopment deficits associated with ID/IDA are significant enough to warrant aggressive attempts for primary prevention through appropriate dietary iron intake and universal screening to identify ID/IDA. Although the incidence has declined since the introduction of iron-fortified formula and infant cereals in the 1970s, ID/IDA is still prevalent. The guideline outlines iron intake

requirement for infants and toddlers by age and recommended supplementation for preterm infants through 12 months and exclusively breastfed infants at 4 months of age. Universal hemoglobin screening is recommended at 12 months of age, along with a risk factor assessment. Anemia is diagnosed if the hemoglobin concentration is below 11 g/dL. Serum ferritin and C-reactive protein are recommended tests. Ferritin measures total body iron stores, but is also an acute phase reactant. Therefore a C-reactive protein should be simultaneously obtained to exclude inflammation. Alternatively, in cases of mild anemia (hemoglobin 10-11 g/dL), an increase in hemoglobin concentration of 1 g/dL after 1 month of therapeutic iron supplementation supports a diagnosis of ID.

Interpersonal and Communication Skills

Recognizing the Limits of One's Knowledge

The pediatrician should be aware of the limits of his/her knowledge. It is completely appropriate to tell parents that you do not know; however, you should follow up with "but I will find out for you." Use pediatric guidelines, Internet searches, and electronic databases to locate answers. Learn best approaches to providing advice to parents.[10] When you have promised to "find out," set aside time to call parents back on such issues. This will enhance your personal credibility and strengthen the family's trust in your care.

Professionalism

Commitment to Continued Professional Development

Well child care is when pediatricians teach parents about their child's health and development. In order to teach parents effectively the pediatrician must seek training about effective teaching strategies, adult learning theories, motivational interviewing, and behavior change. Pediatricians must also learn about the many resources available to parents for parenting information, such as books, videos, and patient education handouts.

In times of the Internet, these resources continue to multiply, providing opportunities to increase parental understanding. Pointing parents to these resources is clearly beneficial. A pediatrician's knowledge of proper referral sources is associated with higher levels of self-confidence in his/her ability to counsel parents.[7-9]

Systems-Based Practice

Health-Care Technology: Information Systems and Electronic Medical Records

There are three distinct advantages to having a comprehensive office information system. First, complete information access improves quality of care for patients and physician satisfaction. Second, software solutions reduce staff to provider ratios with subsequent cost savings for the practice. Third, improved internal communications help staff to care for patient needs more efficiently.

References

1. Green S, Palfrey JS, editors: *Bright Futures: Guidelines for health supervision of infants, children, and adolescents*, ed 2, Arlington, VA, 2002, National Center for Education in Maternal and Child Health.
2. Lieberman A: *The emotional life of the toddler*, New York, 1993, The Free Press, A Division of Simon & Schuster.
3. Beers NS: Managing temper tantrums. *Pediatr Rev* 24(2):70-71, 2003.
4. Committee on Psychosocial Aspects of Child and Family Health: Guidance for effective discipline. *Pediatrics* 101(4):723-728, 1998.
5. Khambalia A, Joshi P, Brussoni M, et al: Risk factors for unintentional injuries due to falls in children aged 0-6 years: A systematic review. *Inj Prev* 12(6):378-381, 2006.
6. Stone KE, Eastman EM, Gielen AC, et al: Home safety in inner cities: Prevalence and feasibility of home safety-product use in inner-city housing. *Pediatrics* 120(2):e346-e353, 2007.
7. Glascoe FP, Oberklaid F, Dworkin PH, Trimm F: Brief approaches to educating patients and parents in primary care. *Pediatrics* 101(6):E10, 1998.
8. Cheng TL, DeWitt TG, Savageau JA, O'Connor KG: Determinants of counseling in primary care pediatric practice: Physician attitudes about time, money, and health issues. *Arch Pediatr Adolesc Med* 153(6):629-635, 1999.
9. Dodge RA, Cabana M, O'Riordan MA, Heneghan A: What factors are important for pediatric residents' smoking cessation counseling of parents? *Clin Pediatr* 47(3):237-243.

Chapter 22
The 18- and 24-Month Well Child Visits

Mario Cruz MD

Speaking Intelligently

The 18-month-old has relatively well-developed gross motor skills and is actively developing fine motor skills with feeding, manipulating smaller toys, scribbling, and stacking two to three blocks. Language development, both receptive and expressive, begins to accelerate. The 18-month-old understands far more than he/she can say, and by 2 years, many have a vocabulary of 200 words and use 2- and 3-word phrases. The child is gaining social interactive skills but typically engages in parallel play in group settings. Delays in expressive language development may lead to frustration, increased temper tantrums, and aggressive behaviors.

Medical Knowledge and Patient Care

History

The period between 18 and 24 months is characterized by rapid acquisition of developmental milestones. By 18 months, children should be able to remove some of their clothing, speak six words, follow simple commands, scribble with a crayon, self-feed using a spoon, and run. As language develops, the 24-month-old child can speak in 2- to 3-word phrases and speak between 50 and 200 words. At 2 years, 50% of the child's speech should be understandable to strangers. Motor milestones at 24 months include throwing a large ball, jumping, climbing stairs, and running.[1] Up to 18% of children are affected by a developmental delay. Developmental surveillance at 18 and 24 months should use historical information and clinical observation. ***At the 18-month visit, a formal developmental screening tool, such as the Ages and Stages Questionnaire or the Parents' Evaluation of Developmental Status (PEDS) is recommended.***[2] ***In addition, an autism-specific screening tool, such as the Modified Checklist for Autism in Toddlers (M-CHAT) is recommended at both 18 and 24 months.*** (See Chapter 14, Developmental Screening and Surveillance.)

Current estimates of autism prevalence are 6 to 7 per 1000 children. Recent increases in autism diagnosis are related in part to improved awareness of parents and physicians of the early presenting signs (see Chapter 26, Autism). Autistic spectrum disorders are characterized by delays in communication and social interaction and/or restricted behaviors and interests. Impairment in joint attention, the enjoyment in sharing an event with another person by looking back and forth between the two, is one of the earliest indicators of autism. Other red flags include regression, failure to spontaneously use two-word phrases by 24 months, lack of pointing, and absence of emotional responses to engaging stimuli.[2] The "watch and see" approach to developmental delays has proved to be ineffective; although many parents recognize signs of autism before 18 months of age, the mean age at diagnosis is 61 months.[2] Concerns about development should be referred to an early intervention specialist, audiologist, and, if indicated, an autism specialist. Early intervention has the potential to maximize long-term social and academic functioning[2] (see Chapter 25, The Special Needs Child).

- **Discipline strategy.** By 18 months of age, an effective discipline strategy is required. Assess where the parents are with development of this skill. A successful discipline strategy is one that nurtures the child's desire for autonomy while minimizing dangerous behaviors and promoting desirable behaviors. Components of such a strategy include the development of a strong parent-child relationship, positive reinforcement for desirable behaviors, adult role modeling of these behaviors, and the consistent (but not excessive) use of punishment. Despite its widespread acceptance even among some pediatricians, corporal punishment is not a recommended method of discipline. It is associated with various adverse outcomes, including aggressive behavior and violence perpetration. Time-out, the removal of an enjoyable stimulus such as parental attention, in response to negative behavior may be equally efficacious without the adverse consequences of corporal punishment. To be effective, time-out must be used selectively, consistently, and for an appropriate amount of time (approximately 1 minute per each year of age). Practice and patience are required, because the undesired behavior may initially worsen with this technique.[3]

  Temper tantrums are a common response to restrictions on the toddler's autonomy. These are normal responses that peak between 18 and 24 months of age. Successful strategies to manage these angry outbursts include distraction, removal from the environment, and verbal dialogues that encourage the child to use words, instead of tantrums, to express himself/herself.[1] Recognize that children with expressive language delay may experience prolonged or more frequent tantrums because of the inability to effectively communicate with words. Temper tantrums may aggravate parents, especially if they lack social support. Frustrated parents may physically abuse their children as a way to curb these unwanted behaviors. Any suspicion of abuse, such as inadequately explained physical injuries, neglect, or sexualized behaviors should be reported to local child welfare authorities[4] (see Chapter 96, Physical Abuse). Routine screening of female caregivers for domestic violence may serve as an effective screening tool for child abuse.[5]

- **Toilet Training.** Readiness for toilet training may begin as early as 18 months and is manifested by ability to undress, an interest in the potty seat, satisfaction after a bowel movement, increased periods of diaper dryness, and imitation of others using the toilet. Patience is required because attempts to train a child who is not ready will be unsuccessful and lead to frustration. Various toilet-training techniques exist; however, a general rule is to make toilet training a stress-free and enjoyable experience for children. Parents should provide rewards for success and avoid punishment for mistakes.[1]

Physical Examination

During the visit review the growth curves and percentiles. In addition to head circumference and weight, length and weight to length ratio is determined from birth through 24 months. Because obesity can present during early childhood, a BMI-for-age is calculated and plotted for specific age and gender beginning at the 24-month visit. Explain to parents that their child's body fatness will change as he/she grows, and that boys and girls have different degrees of fatness as they mature. Therefore the absolute value of any given BMI percentile will change as the child ages. The ideal BMI is between 5% and 85%, and overweight is defined as greater than 85% but less than 95%. A child with a BMI-for-age greater than 95% is considered obese (see Chapter 39, Weight Gain).

Many 18-month-olds still resist the process of being measured and examined, and the physical examination is typically carried out in a parent's lap. However, by 24 months, many children will sit independently on the examination table with a parent in close vicinity. Examination of the child's doll or mother's throat first may facilitate the process.

Immunizations

Vaccine delays are not uncommon in this age-group. With the 18-month visit, the primary series should be complete and includes four doses of diphtheria and tetanus toxoids and acellular pertussis (DTaP), three doses of poliovirus vaccine inactivated (IPV), four doses of *Haemophilus influenzae* type b (Hib) vaccine, four doses of pneumococcal conjugate vaccine (heptavalent pneumococcal vaccine was administered from 1996 to 2010; 13-valent pneumococcal conjugate vaccine was introduced in 2010), two or three doses of rotavirus, two doses of hepatitis A, one dose each of measles-mumps-rubella (MMR) and varicella, and three doses of hepatitis B. In addition, annual influenza vaccination is provided starting at 6 months of age. It is ideal to plan completion of this primary series at the 18-month visit, and by 24 months at the latest. A routine CBC and lead level are indicated if risk factors exist.[6] Lead-contaminated toys are an emerging risk factor for elevated lead levels.[7] Additional hearing, vision, and laboratory screenings are to be performed if indicated from the history and physical examination. For the current recommended immunization schedules, see Figure 13-9.

Practice-Based Learning and Improvement: Developmental Screening and Surveillance

Title
Selecting developmental surveillance and screening tools

Authors
Drotar D, Stanchin T, Dworkin P, et al

Reference
Pediatr Rev 29:e52-e58, 2008

Historical significance/comments
This article discusses the rationale for screening and contains a list and description of available screening tools.

Developmental surveillance is recommended at all well visits. Its utility is heavily dependent on the health-care professional, and it has been shown to detect less than 30% of developmental problems. (See Chapter 14, Developmental Screening and Surveillance.) Administration of a formal validated developmental screening tool is recommended at the 9-, 18-, and 30-month well child visits. An autism-specific tool is recommended at both the 18- and 24-month visits.

Interpersonal and Communication Skills

Anticipatory Guidance: Injury Prevention, Television Viewing, and Avoidance of Over-the-Counter Cold Medication

Injury prevention is a major issue for children in this age-group. As their ability to run and climb improves, they remain relatively uncoordinated and lack concern for their personal safety. In fact, accidents are a major cause of morbidity and mortality. Motor vehicle accidents are the most common type, followed by drowning and burns. Common nonfatal accidents include falls and toxic ingestions.[8] Anticipatory guidance on injury prevention should specifically address these issues.[9]

Poisons and household cleaning products must be securely locked out of reach. Provide the telephone number of the local poison control center. Inquire about the presence of guns in the home. For homes with guns, counsel that guns should be unloaded and securely locked, with the ammunition locked in a separate location.

Review car seat use, and be sure parents know when to switch to a forward-facing seat (when the child is over 1 year old *and* weighs at least 20 pounds).

Inquire about television viewing. The American Academy of Pediatrics (AAP) recommends no television up to 2 years of age and thereafter up to 2 hours per day of quality programming, ideally prescreened by parents.

Parents of children with upper respiratory tract infections should be counseled to avoid over-the-counter cough and cold preparations.[10]

Professionalism

Addressing the Tardy Doctor, Tardy Patient

Physicians and office staff have a workload and patient flow that are often unpredictable. This means that it is difficult to keep on time when seeing patients, and it is challenging to have a reasonable time lag to the "next available appointment."

However, it is important to remember that patients and families have other commitments to their time and that it is necessary to make every effort to improve access and reduce patient wait times. Apologizing for scheduling inconveniences and wait times, keeping patients apprised and giving explanations when wait times are long, and showing over time that efforts are being made to make an office visit streamlined and satisfying will increase trust in the practice. Patients who arrive late should be treated with consideration and respect. There is a balance between your commitment to care for the individual child, especially if the child is acutely ill or in need of preventive services, and your commitment to the smooth running of patient care in the office. Families who are chronically late or who continually miss appointments constitute a high-risk population. Instead of being disregarded as "noncompliant," they should be screened for biopsychosocial problems that may be interfering with medical care and their children accommodated in the schedule.

Systems-Based Practice

Quality Improvement: NCQA/HEDIS

The Healthcare Effectiveness Data and Information Set (HEDIS) is a set of standardized performance measures designed to assess quality of health care in a systematic way to allow health-care payers and consumers to assess managed care organization performance. The goal is to measure quality of care with the ability to compare performance among insurance companies. HEDIS was developed by the National Committee for Quality Assurance (NCQA), a private not-for-profit organization whose goal is to improve health care through measurement and accountability. Data are collected through surveys, medical charts and insurance claims for hospitalizations, medical office visits, and procedures. Measures include effectiveness of care, access and availability of care, patient satisfaction, and cost. HEDIS measures access to primary and preventive care as a percentage of children covered who have had a visit to a primary care practitioner during a calendar year (http://www.ncqa.org/).

References

1. Dixon SD, Stein MT: *Encounters with children: Pediatric behavior and development*, St. Louis, 2000, Mosby, pp 277-326.
2. Johnson CP, Myers SM, the Council on Children with Disabilities: Identification and evaluation of children with autism spectrum disorders. *Pediatrics* 120(5):1183-12153, 2007.
3. Committee on Psychosocial Aspects of Child and Family Health: Guidance for effective discipline. *Pediatrics* 101:723-728, 1998.
4. Kellogg ND, the Committee on Child Abuse and Neglect: Evaluation of suspected child physical abuse. *Pediatrics* 119(6):1232-1241, 2007.
5. Thackeray JD, Hibbard R, Dowd MD, the Committee on Child Abuse and Neglect, and the Committee on Injury, Violence, and Poison Prevention: Intimate partner violence: The role of the pediatrician. *Pediatrics* 125: 1094-1100, 2010.
6. Committee on Practice and Ambulatory Medicine and Bright Futures Steering Committee: Recommendations for preventive pediatric health care. *Pediatrics* 120(6):1376, 2007.
7. Centers for Disease Control and Prevention: Environmental health: Lead recalls. Available at http://www.cdc.gov/nceh/lead/Recalls/default.htm.
8. Centers for Disease Control and Prevention: Web-based Injury Statistics Query and Reporting System. Available at http://www.cdc.gov/ncipc/wisqars/.
9. Gardner HG, the Committee on Injury, Violence, and Poison Prevention: Office-based counseling for unintentional injury prevention. *Pediatrics* 119(1):202-206, 2007.
10. U.S. Food and Drug Administration: Public Health Advisory: FDA recommends that over-the-counter (OTC) cough and cold products not be used for infants and children under 2 years of age. Available at http://www.fda.gov/Drugs/DrugSafety/PostmarketDrugSafetyInformationforPatientsandProviders/DrugSafetyInformationforHeathcareProfessionals/PublicHealthAdvisories/ucm051137.htm.

Chapter 23
The Annual Well Child Visit

Robert L. Bonner Jr. MD

Speaking Intelligently

As pediatricians, we have a unique position as health-care providers for children. Pediatricians have the opportunity to participate in the growth and development of a child at least once a year from birth through 21 years of age. After age 3, our evaluations and interactions become a yearly meeting at the annual well visit. For otherwise healthy children, this may be the only visit to the pediatrician. The well visit provides a snapshot opportunity for the pediatrician to assess overall health and wellness, detect any illness or developmental issue, promote wellness, and assess school performance, family, and social functioning.

Medical Knowledge and Patient Care

Purpose and Overview

The annual well visit is an integral part of child health supervision. It is designed to develop and maintain a partnership over time for disease prevention and health promotion among the pediatrician, child, and family.[1] Health promotion includes education about nutrition, physical activity, and injury prevention. Achievement of developmental milestones and school performance are monitored, and the pediatrician advocates for the family with assistance from community and health system resources as needed.

With an understanding of normal growth and development, the pediatrician has a foundation to understand all aspects of child health. Nutrition, development, and psychosocial maturity are major components of the annual well visit. Knowledge and competence in management of common pediatric diseases is expected, along with awareness of rare illness.

The pediatrician should be able to recognize the child's nutritional requirements to achieve expected growth. Knowledge of the child's developmental progression in gross motor function, fine motor function, and speech/language will facilitate working with the family to identify areas of concern. The pediatrician must be able to recognize the psychosocial changes and behavior norms in order to identify those children who are taking a path toward future problems.

From ages 3 to 12 years, there is tremendous change that occurs in each area for each individual child.

Growth and Nutrition

Physical growth in early childhood (ages 1 to 4 years) through middle childhood (ages 5 to 10 years) progresses at a steady rate. Both weight gain and linear growth remain constant until 10 to 12 years, when many children in early adolescence begin the pubertal growth spurt. Children's eating habits are a mirror to their growth rate. The young child of early childhood is developing an eating routine with predetermined meals scheduled daily. By middle childhood, the child begins to make food choices, so ensuring the availability of healthy foods becomes important. Consistent daily activity for a child becomes a focus at this time, so balanced meals with the child involved in the decision-making process are beneficial. Children in early adolescence have a heightened growth velocity, so the volume of food intake increases. Maintaining a balance of healthy food choices and consistent physical activity is emphasized. The pediatrician should have a full understanding of pediatric nutrition with focus on caloric needs and healthy food choices.

Development

Because a child's developmental progression is affected by his/her growth and nutritional status, the pediatrician must be aware of these as development is assessed. A child with age-appropriate development will develop skills and knowledge that equip the child to build on these skills and achieve more tasks as he/she matures. Age-appropriate developmental knowledge will allow the pediatrician to inform and educate the child and caregiver about future expected behaviors and abilities. This knowledge will also empower the caregiver to provide structure and discipline as the child becomes more independent. School performance is a means to assess development in early and middle childhood. Understanding potential school problems is essential for an accurate assessment of development. In addition, awareness of appropriate developmental milestones gives the pediatrician knowledge to identify developmental delay or behavior that is not appropriate for the child's age or developmental level.

- **Psychosocial Development.** The psychosocial development of a child will define the individual as growth progresses through adolescence to adulthood. Half of all lifetime cases of mental illness begin by the age of 14, which means that mental disorders are chronic diseases of the young.[2] The pediatrician should have knowledge of the psychosocial changes that occur from early childhood to middle childhood. It is important to be aware of social risk factors, such as poverty or domestic violence, and family risk factors, such as divorce and poor parenting, which can have a significant effect on psychosocial development. Mental health in early childhood is tightly bound to healthy development, healthy relationships within the family, and strong support for both child and family in the community.[3] Knowledge of the norms in development, temperament, and sensory processing by the child and the influences of family and community enable the pediatrician to identify the well-adjusted child and the child with low self-esteem who is at risk for school problems and dysfunctional behavior. The middle childhood to early adolescent child is developing cognitively and seeking more independence. Problems from early childhood may manifest during this time. The pediatrician must have the knowledge to identify at-risk children and educate the child and caregiver about skills to develop for functioning in family and social environments.

This knowledge is incorporated with the skills needed to obtain a complete history, perform a detailed physical examination, and make an informed assessment in providing appropriate and comprehensive patient care. The pediatrician should also develop organizational skills to coordinate longitudinal care plans with families and/or to follow progress with disease processes or problems. During the annual well visit for 3 to 12 year olds, there is a progression in each skill that is influenced by the child's age and development and how the child interacts with his/her family.

During the health assessment the pediatrician will need to assess for risks that could interfere with good healthy outcomes. Performance of a health interview, developmental and educational surveillance, observation of the parent–child interaction, a complete physical examination, screening tests, immunizations, and identification of family and community strengths should occur at every health assessment. Detailed documentation should be recorded in the medical record. Finally, a therapeutic contract[4] should be completed with the child and/or caregiver. There should be agreement on tasks to be performed, who is responsible for the task, and the time to report back on progress and need for further management.

Practice-Based Learning and Improvement

Title
Communicating with children and families: From everyday interactions to skill in conveying distressing information

Authors
Marcia Levetown and the Committee on Bioethics

Reference
Pediatrics 121(5):e1441-e1460, 2008

Historical significance/comments
This article describes health-care communication as a procedure that is neglected and rarely taught in a formal fashion, yet it is integral to providing family-centered quality care to patients and their families. It becomes especially important in the school-age visit because part of the goal of the visit is to begin having the child become more involved in the interview process and the treatment plan. This article provides direction in how to communicate new-onset chronic disease, bad news, therapeutic options, and other pertinent information to parents and children. A useful website is http://www.aap.org/ConnectedKids/.

Interpersonal and Communication Skills

Listen Actively to Children of All Ages

For children of all ages, the pediatrician should engage in active listening, observing intently, making a point not to interrupt. Sitting down is respectful and will create the impression that there is time to discuss their concerns. The interview is age dependent. Children in early childhood will be able to contribute small amounts of information. As children reach 4 to 5 years, they are able to answer simple questions and give information about their health. Children in middle childhood can speak about their health, so the pediatrician's questions can be directed to the child more than to the parent. As children reach the age of 11 years, there may be time allotted to speak with the child without the presence of parents. This will allow discussion of issues the child would like to keep private. The pediatrician should develop skill and comfort asking parents to step out for a brief time during the visit.

Professionalism

Provide Culturally Sensitive Care

The pediatrician must demonstrate sensitivity to cultural issues with children, families, and office staff. "The culturally sensitive clinician realizes that in addition to the pathophysiologic aspects of the disease, the socially defined and culturally relevant meanings and interpretations of illness to the patient are important clinical concerns."[4] The pediatrician should be aware of common beliefs in the patient community being treated. Families being treated should be assessed to determine if these beliefs are in use. The physician should discuss and negotiate an approach and plan of care with the patient and family that is both medically sound and culturally acceptable. In the presence of a language barrier, a qualified interpreter should be used. **Never use a family member or a child to translate because important information may not be disclosed and translation of what the patient or parent says may be filtered and modified.** If at all possible, identify subtle messages from nonverbal communication during the interpretation process.

Systems-Based Practice

Health-Care Economics: Claims, Coding, and Billing

It is important to code correctly and bill for pediatric visits and to apply the *Current Procedural Terminology* (CPT), published by the American Medical Association, and the *International Classification of Disease, Clinical Modifications,* 9th Edition (ICD-9-CM) published by the World Health Organization (WHO). The CPT code tells the insurer "what" was done and the type of visit; whereas the ICD-9 code tells the "why" of the diagnosis. Undercoding of well child visits is highly prevalent in the Medicaid managed care environment because the financial incentive to accurately report events during an office visit is not as strong as in the fee-for-service system.

References

1. Green M, Haggerty RJ, Weitzman M, editors: *Ambulatory pediatrics*, ed 5, Philadelphia, 1999, Saunders.
2. Hagan JF, Shaw JS, Duncan PM, editors: *Bright Futures: Guidelines for health supervision of infants, children, and adolescents*, ed 3, Elk Grove Village, IL, 2008, American Academy of Pediatrics.
3. Goldbloom R, editor: *Pediatric clinical skills*, ed 3, Philadelphia, 2003, Saunders.
4. Spector N, Kelly S, Chanoine P: SCHC resident continuity clinic rotation goals and objectives, 2005, St Christopher's Hospital for Children, Philadelphia.

Chapter 24
The Adolescent Well Visit

Benjamin Alouf MD

Speaking Intelligently

Adolescence spans ages 11 through 21 years and is a time marked by significant physical growth, emotional growth, and pubertal maturation. The adolescent well visit requires a fundamental understanding that the nature and pathogenesis of disease are very different than in younger age-groups. Recognize that most adolescents are healthy and do not require visits to the pediatrician other than for school, camp, or sport physicals.

Medical Knowledge and Patient Care

Background and Adolescent Morbidity

Whereas congenital anomalies and malignant neoplasms are the leading causes of death in childhood, high-risk behaviors manifest during adolescence and place the individual at risk for related morbidities and even mortality.[1,2] In the United States, unintentional injury, homicide, and suicide are leading causes of death among 15- to 19-year-olds. Seventy-one percent of all deaths among persons 10 to 24 years of age result from four causes: motor vehicle crashes, other unintentional injuries, homicide, and suicide.[2] The 2005 Youth Risk Behavior Survey conducted by the Centers for Disease Control and Prevention showed that 10% of high school students had driven a car or other vehicle when they had been drinking alcohol, and close to 20% had carried a weapon. Thirty-six percent of high school students had been in a physical fight during the 12 months preceding the survey, and 8% had attempted suicide.

Psychosocial Problems

Nearly 50% of those surveyed admitted to having had sexual intercourse, and 37% did not use a condom during their most recent sexual intercourse. Half of respondents admitted to drinking alcohol frequently, 20% had used marijuana, and 2% had injected illegal drugs. Feeling sad or hopeless is also common among adolescents. The survey found that during the preceding 12 months, 28.5% of the teens surveyed had felt so sad or hopeless almost every day for 2 or more weeks in a row that they stopped doing some usual activities.[2] Another study found that 4.6% of those 13 to 17 years of age were taking medications to treat attention-deficit/hyperactivity disorder

(ADHD), with 16-year-old males having the highest prevalence of 14.9%.[3]

The two major causes of death in adults, cardiovascular disease and cancer, may in fact have their origins in adolescence, and possibly childhood. During 2005, 25% of high school students had admitted to smoking cigarettes during the 30 days preceding the Youth Risk Behavior Survey. Sixty-seven percent did not attend regular physical education classes, and 13% were overweight.[2]

Phases of Adolescence

Adolescence, a period of tremendous physical growth, is divided into three phases: early (11 to 14 years), middle (15 to 17 years), and late adolescence (18 to 21 years). Weight gain during puberty accounts for about 50% of ideal adult weight, and linear growth during puberty accounts for 20% to 25% of adult height. Up to two-thirds of adult bone mass is accrued during this period. It is also a time of marked divergence in the physical features and body habitus of females versus males that goes beyond gonadal and breast development. Female body fat increases from about 16% to about 27%. When puberty is complete, males have 50% more lean body mass than women, and women have twice the body fat of men. Ninety-five percent of females complete growth by age 16, whereas 95% of males complete growth by age 18.[4]

Menarche occurs and pubertal development goes through predictable stages as outlined in Table 24-1 for girls and Table 24-2 for boys and Figures 24-1 and 24-2.

Table 24-1 Classification of Sexual Maturity Stages in Girls		
Sexual Maturity Stage	**Pubic Hair**	**Breasts**
1	Preadolescent	Preadolescent
2	Sparse, lightly pigmented, straight, medial border of labia	Breast and papilla elevated as small mound; areolar diameter increased
3	Darker, beginning to curl, increased amount	Breast and areola enlarged, no contour separation
4	Coarse, curly, abundant but amount less than in adult	Areola and papilla form secondary mound
5	Adult feminine triangle, spread to medial surfaces of thighs	Mature; nipple projects, areola part of general breast contour

Table 24-2	Classification of Sexual Maturity Stages in Boys		
Sexual Maturity Stage	**Pubic Hair**	**Penis**	**Testes**
1	None	Preadolescent	Preadolescent
2	Scanty, long, slightly pigmented	Slight enlargement	Enlarged scrotum, pink texture altered, enlargement of testes to greater than 2.5 cm in longest axis, excluding the epididymis or a testicular volume of greater than 3 mL.
3	Darker, starts to curl, small amount	Longer	Larger
4	Resembles adult type, but less in quantity; coarse, curly	Larger; glans and breadth increase in size	Larger, scrotum dark
5	Adult distribution, spread to medial surface of thighs	Adult size	Adult size

In addition to pubertal maturation, other adolescent milestones include social and academic competence, connectedness with family, peers, and community; and emotional well-being.[5]

Physical Examination

After eliciting patient and parental concerns and an interim history, a complete physical examination is performed. Blood pressure, hearing, and vision screening results are noted. The height and weight are recorded and body mass index (BMI) is calculated. In this way, teens are screened for being overweight or obese and for the possibility of

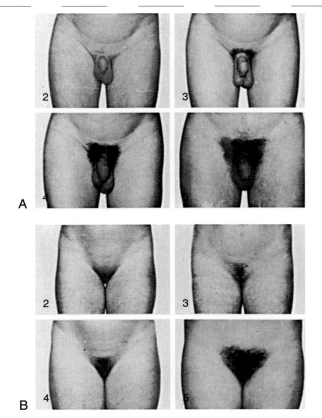

Figure 24-1 Sexual maturity ratings (2 to 5) of pubic hair changes in adolescents. **A,** Boys; **B,** Girls.

an eating disorder. The skin examination should note acne, acanthosis nigricans, nevi, tattoos, piercings, and any sign of abuse or self-inflicted injury. Additional items to note include scoliosis, Sexual Maturity Rating (SMR), and the testicular examination noting hernias and/or hydrocele. The physician should also look for signs of sexually transmitted infection (STI), including warts, vesicles, and vaginal discharge.[5] **See Nelson Essentials 67 and 68.**

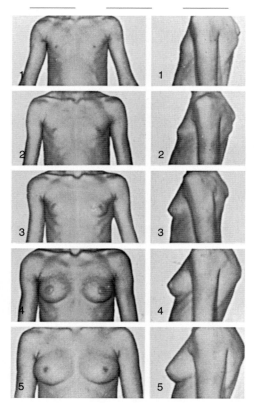

Figure 24-2 Sexual maturity ratings (1 to 5) of breast changes in adolescent girls.

Interpersonal and Communication Skills

Relating to the Adolescent

Understanding the key features of each adolescent stage will facilitate the pediatrician's ability to elicit concerns, assess risk factors, and provide more effective anticipatory guidance.

Early adolescents (11 to 14 years of age) are concrete thinkers who live in the present. They often do not understand that what is done now may affect their future. Appearance is very important to most teens, and some may begin to experiment with drugs and sex. Academic performance may suffer because of the increased demands of middle school, social distractions, and peer pressure. The pediatrician needs to develop trust rather than friendship with the early adolescent. Avoid "talking down" and lecturing. Instead try to engage the patient in a conversation to allow him/her to build confidence in the patient–doctor relationship. Use simple language to create a comfortable environment for sharing, and encourage the adolescent to share his/her feelings and ask questions.

Middle adolescents (15 to 17 years of age) start to develop a better understanding of how things done today will affect them tomorrow. Thinking becomes more abstract. Sense of identity becomes very important, and fitting into a new role in high school can be difficult for some. Despite new responsibilities, increased academic demands, and the need to earn money, striving for independence becomes a focal point. Associating with older teens, driving, and being exposed to more situations in which drugs, alcohol, and sexual activity may appear routine put great pressure on the adolescent to fit in. The pediatrician should position himself/herself as a trusted authority figure who will not be judgmental or reprimand, but rather provide guidance and support where needed.

Late adolescents (18 to 21 years) have adult ability for abstract thinking. They can be intense about beliefs while having the added pressure of going to college, finding a job, and perhaps starting a family. Some may be completely independent, whereas others may live with their parents, maintaining strong physical and emotional family ties. The focus of the visit should be on health promotion, and the pediatrician, who may have known the patient since early childhood, will need to recognize that the child has become a young adult with adult thinking skills and responsibilities. Often by this age, the adolescent will come to the visit alone, which will allow increased individual time for the pediatrician and patient. A discussion on transition to adult care is very important.

Use of a mnemonic such as **HEADS FIRST** to structure the adolescent interview and risk factor assessment will facilitate obtaining a thorough history.

Home—living arrangement
Education
Abuse—physical, verbal, emotional, sexual
Drugs
Safety
Friends
Image—self-esteem
Recreation
Sexuality
Threats—depressed or upset easily, suicidal ideation or attempts, harm to others[6]

Professionalism

Maintain Privacy and Confidentiality: A Particularly Important Value in Adolescent Medicine

In early adolescence the pediatrician should begin to spend part of each well visit alone with the teenager. It is important to explain to both the parent and adolescent why this is important. The goal of a confidential discussion is to allow the child to recognize the pediatrician as a mentor and valuable resource who would like to help with any questions or current issues. These are not necessarily health-care needs, but could be a problem in school, at home, or with friends. Realize that some younger adolescents may not feel comfortable alone with you initially, and their parents also may not feel comfortable having you see their teen alone. Although the expectation is that the conversation will remain confidential, if patients share a plan or desire to hurt themselves or someone else, or report that they have been harmed, **the confidentiality must be breached to secure appropriate help.** These exceptions to maintaining confidentiality should be explained to the adolescent at the beginning of the conversation.

Every state has different laws regarding a minor's rights to consent to health care and make other important decisions. If a teenager presents with a health-related issue, do not assume that a parent must be included in the decision-making process. This is especially true for reproductive and sexual health. Although parental participation is encouraged, the priority is to have the teen cared for promptly without allowing parental consent to become a barrier. The local state health department is a valuable source for checking the laws that govern adolescent health and minors' rights to consent and maintain confidentiality.

Practice-Based Learning and Improvement

Title
Improving adolescent preventive care in community health centers

Authors
Klein JD, Allan MJ, Elster AB, et al

Reference
Pediatrics 107:318-327, 2001

Historical significance/comments
This article looks at the effects of implementing the American Medical Association's Guidelines for Adolescent Preventive Services (GAPS) on health centers. Health center staff were trained and given the resource materials to implement GAPS. It was found that adolescents received more comprehensive screening and counseling,

more health education materials, and had greater access to care after the GAPS implementation. This article's significance stems from the fact that although health-care providers generally provide the best care they know how, implementation of guidelines and standardization of care can improve health-care delivery and avoid missed opportunities for intervention.

Systems-Based Practice

Quality Improvement: Process, Structure, Effectiveness, and Efficiency

The clinical practice improvement model shown to work best is the one that includes leadership engagement, gap and barrier identification, solutions development, and progress monitoring. In one such study, it was found that implementing a clinical practice intervention significantly increased *Chlamydia trachomatis* screening among adolescent females who were patients in a large health maintenance organization (HMO). The authors sought commitment of opinion leaders and established goals and performance measures that were supported by clinical as well as administrative leaders. Successes at meeting these goals were openly acknowledged. Through a process of engaging, team building, redesigning the clinical practice, and sustaining, the authors found that 47% of patients in the clinical improvement intervention practices received *Chlamydia* screening versus 17% in the control clinics.[7]

References

1. Hamilton BE, Minino AM, Martin JA, et al: Annual summary of vital statistics. *Pediatrics* 119(2):345-360, 2007.
2. Youth risk behavior surveillance in the United States, 2005. *MMWR Surveill Summ* 55(SS-5), 2006.
3. Mental health in the United States: Prevalence of diagnosis and medication treatment for attention-deficit/hyperactivity disorder. *MMWR Morb Mortal Wkly Rep* 54(34):842-847, 2005.
4. Joffe A, Blythe MJ (guest editors): Handbook of adolescent medicine. *Adolescent Med State Art Rev* 14(2), 2003.
5. Hagan JF, Shaw JS, Duncan PM, editors: *Bright Futures: Guidelines for health supervision of infants, children, and adolescents*, ed 3, Elk Grove Village, IL, 2008, American Academy of Pediatrics.
6. Goldenring JM, Cohen E: Getting into adolescent heads. *Contemp Pediatr* 5:75-90, 1988.
7. Shafer MB, Tebb KP, Pantell RH, et al: Effect of a clinical practice improvement intervention on chlamydial screening among adolescent girls. *JAMA* 288(22):2486-2852, 2002.

Chapter 25
The Special Needs Child

Maureen C. McMahon MD

Speaking Intelligently

During my first office visit for a child with special health-care needs, I perform a complete assessment. I prioritize by acuity. First, what is the nature of the problem(s)? Is it a genetic disease such as, 22q11 microdeletion syndrome, or a neurodevelopmental disability such as cerebral palsy? Is the child at his/her baseline state of health, or is there a superimposed episodic illness? I review the history, including medications, ongoing treatments, subspecialty care, and home- and school-related issues, and then formulate a problem list and plan.

Medical Knowledge and Patient Care

Background and Definitions

A **special needs child** is one who **has or is at risk for a chronic physical, developmental, behavioral, or emotional condition and requires health and related services not usually required by healthy children with normal development.** Up to 18% of children have special needs, and the prevalence of children at risk is unknown.[1] As a primary care physician, you will encounter a wide variety of chronic childhood conditions. Some examples include Down syndrome, asthma, organ transplantation, childhood cancer, cerebral palsy, autism, attention-deficit/hyperactivity disorder (ADHD), human immunodeficiency virus/acquired immunodeficiency syndrome (HIV/AIDS), and hearing loss. Chronic conditions and special needs occur more often among children who live in poverty and socially deprived environments.[2]

Children with special health-care needs (CSHCN) often have more frequent visits to their primary care doctor. Depending on their diagnosis, they may require subspecialty care, therapies, special education, and/or social services.[1] These therapies may include physical, occupational, speech, feeding, and/or behavioral. Together the pediatrician and family should provide care that meets all the child's needs. Adequate information must be provided to school nurses and educational staff for medically complex children to safely attend school with maximal participation. The pediatrician also communicates with other providers to coordinate care and ensure that needed care is provided. Some pediatric residents and practicing physicians feel a lack of expertise and comfort in caring for the diverse needs of CSHCN.[3] Most primary care offices are set up to provide routine well care and episodic sick visits for otherwise healthy children.[4] In this setting, it is a challenge to provide comprehensive and coordinated care to CSHCN. Studies have shown coordinated care is more efficient and cost-effective, and there is greater family satisfaction. This is a dynamic process because the child and family's need for care and service will vary over time. The need for intervention is usually increased during the diagnostic process, hospital discharge planning, school entry, at transition to adult care, and with any significant change in health status.[5]

The Medical Home

Because many CSHCN see multiple subspecialists and have related services, care can be fragmented. **The medical home** was initially devised as a place to house all health- and service-related records for CSHCN.[6] It has evolved into a model for "a partnership approach with families to provide primary health care that is accessible, family-centered, coordinated, comprehensive, continuous, compassionate, and culturally effective."[7] This **includes traditional primary care, immunizations, and anticipatory guidance, as well as coordinating all other aspects of care related to the child's diagnosis.** For example, you determine the need for subspecialty consultation and communicate with the subspecialist and family about any recommendations. The medical home should be a source of empowerment for families to develop their own advocacy skills. The family is the primary caregiver and decision maker for their child. The pediatrician is the "quarterback" to ensure smooth integration of these services. **A medical home should provide a site for sick and well care, a personal doctor or nurse for each child, easily obtained referrals, and coordinated and family-centered care.**[7] There are specific training programs to facilitate primary care practice transition to a medical home. However, lack of third-party payment for this comprehensive care remains a significant barrier for increased implementation among primary care physicians.[5] This is especially true in community-based private practices.

Screening and Surveillance for Special Needs

Routine surveillance for developmental delays in infants and toddlers occurs during well visits, or anytime a parent expresses a concern. Screening is periodically done, and this may include a parental questionnaire or a screening tool such as the Denver Developmental. Parents should be referred to local early intervention programs for evaluation of any suspected delay. Physical, occupational, and/or speech therapy is provided for documented delays of at least 25%. A complete physical examination and assessment will help determine whether additional workup is needed for an underlying medical condition or genetic syndrome. Delay in more than one area, problems with feeding and growth, or abnormal physical examination findings may require consultation with developmental pediatrics, genetics, or neurology.

Special Education

For school-age children with special needs, cognitive impairment, or significant learning disability who qualify for special education services, an Individualized Education Program (IEP) is formulated. This document is a personalized lesson plan developed at an IEP meeting attended by parents, teachers, therapists, and those who represent any related services needed to support educational achievement. **It describes the child's ability, educational goals, needed accommodations, plans to implement the goals, and methods to measure progress.** Every effort is made for the child to be "mainstreamed" in a typical school setting with age-matched typically developing peers. Although physicians do not usually attend IEP meetings, the pediatrician may be asked to write prescriptions for therapies, medications, nursing care, and durable medical equipment for the school setting. Ask for an updated IEP each year to monitor the child's school progress. Each child with special health-care needs will need a complete history, physical examination, functional assessment, and review of prior medical records, treatments, surgeries, and medications. Your initial assessment will be tailored to the specific chronic condition for each child. A problem list will then be formulated and prioritized according to acuity.

Practice-Based Learning and Improvement

Title
Emergency preparedness for children with special health care needs

Authors
American Academy of Pediatrics Committee on Pediatric Emergency Medicine

Reference
Pediatrics 104:e53, 1999

Historical significance/comments
Formulation of an emergency care plan for CSHCN is described to help ensure identification of key medical issues that may need emergent attention, as well as provide a snapshot view of the child's diagnosis, medications, allergies, and ongoing treatments. It would be ideal to have this form completed in the child's medical record. In addition, the family should have a copy, along with the school, pending parental consent of information release.

Interpersonal and Communication Skills

Listen to Parents Effectively: Develop Empathetic Listening Skills

Empathy is understanding and entering into another's feelings. Understanding the parents' perspective—where they are in the process of understanding and accepting that their child has a chronic condition—will set up good channels of communication and facilitate a sense of partnership with the family. Recognize that parents will experience anxiety through the diagnostic process, and significant lifestyle adjustments may be needed in caring for a child with special needs. Encourage parents to write down questions in preparation for consultation with a specialist. Be available to discuss findings and recommendations. Help parents recognize that the impact of the situation on siblings (who may also be your patients) can be huge: parents spend "excessive" time with the special needs child, and the sibling(s) can feel both unimportant and guilty for being "normal."

Professionalism

Avoid Paternalism

The parents are part of the health-care team and need to "be in the loop" of clinical happenings. Do your best to deliver bad news in stages whenever possible. When seeking subspecialist input, ask focused clinical questions and use their expertise in your case management.

Systems-Based Practice

Federally Mandated Early Intervention and Special Education Services

The Individuals with Disabilities Education Act (IDEA) is the federal special education law. Federal funds are dispensed to each state, and in exchange for federal money, school-age children who qualify receive a Free Appropriate Public Education (FAPE). This is an educational program based on the child's Individualized Education Program (IEP) that should have reasonable expectation for educational progress to be made. In addition, early intervention services for children from birth to 3 years with developmental delay are mandated under IDEA. Most commonly, a 25% delay in one or more areas (gross motor, fine motor, and/or speech) is needed to qualify for service. Services are usually provided by county-based programs, are initiated by parent request for evaluation, and are provided at no cost to the family. Many families are unaware of these programs, and if you provide specific contact information, it will facilitate a family's access to the system as they develop advocacy skills on behalf of their child.[8]

> Consider completing the Emergency Information Form for Children with Special Needs available from the American Academy of Pediatrics with copies to the medical record, school, and home. It provides a snapshot summary of the child's history and emergency needs. See the article discussed in the Practice-Based Learning and Improvement section.

References

1. McPherson M, Arango P, Fox H, et al: A new definition of children with special health care needs. *Pediatrics* 102:137-140, 1998.
2. Newacheck PW, Strickland B, Shonkoff JP, et al: An epidemiologic profile of children with special health care needs. *Pediatrics* 102(1):117-123, 1998.
3. Gupta VB, O'Connor KG, Quezada-Gomez C: Care coordination in pediatric practices. *Pediatrics* 113(5):1517-1521, 2004.
4. Cooley WC, McAllister JW: Building medical homes: Improvement strategies in primary care for children with special health care needs. *Pediatrics* 113(5/S1):1499-1506, 2004.
5. Alexander J, Cartwright JD, Desch LW, et al: Care coordination in the medical home: Integrating health and related systems of care for children with special health care needs. *Pediatrics* 116(5):1238-1244, 2005.
6. Sia C, Tonniges TF, Osterhus E, Taba S: History of the medical home concept. *Pediatrics* 113(5):1473-1478, 2004.
7. Sia C, Antonelli R, Bhushan Gupta V, et al: The medical home. *Pediatrics* 110(1):184-186, 2002.
8. Education Law and Resource Center: Special education, IDEA. 2004. Available at http://www.edlawrc.com.

Chapter 26
Autism

Anne M. Meduri MD

Medical Knowledge and Patient Care

Background and Definitions

Autism is a neurologically based developmental disorder characterized by significant impairment in communication skills and social interactions, along with repetitive and restrictive patterns of behavior. The diagnosis of autism spectrum disorders (ASD) has been increasing at an alarming rate, with the best estimate of the current prevalence at approximately 6 per 1,000 or 1 in 150. Based on a survey completed in 2004, 44% of primary care physicians (PCPs) reported caring for at least 10 children with ASD. It is vitally important therefore that all physicians have awareness and knowledge to better recognize and manage patients with ASD.

Historically, autism was considered a form of schizophrenia. In 1943 Dr. Leo Kanner, a psychiatrist at Johns Hopkins University, described a group of children with extreme aloofness and indifference to other people. These children exhibited features of the disorder from very early in life. In 1944, Dr. Hans Asperger, an Austrian pediatrician, described a similar group of children; however, their cognitive and verbal skills were much higher. **The current criteria for diagnosis of autistic disorder (AD) and Asperger syndrome (AS) can be found in the *Diagnostic and Statistical Manual of Mental Disorders,* fourth edition, text revision (DSM-IV-TR). ASD also includes pervasive developmental disorder–not otherwise specified (PDD-NOS), in which there are subthreshold characteristics that do not meet the full criteria for AD or AS.**

Etiology

The etiology of ASD is not yet fully known. It is most likely multifactorial. There appears to be a strong genetic component but with great complexity involving multiple genes. Estimated recurrence risk is approximately 6% when there is an older sibling with ASD. The rate is even higher if there are two children in the family with ASD. There may also be environmental factors, including advanced paternal and maternal age. There is a male predominance, which suggests a gene located on the X chromosome. Neurogenetic syndromes represent a small percentage of ASD. This includes fragile X syndrome, neurocutaneous disorders, fetal alcohol syndrome, and Rett syndrome. Recent research efforts have been focused on the neurobiologic basis of ASD. Differences exist in brain growth and organization when comparing persons with ASD with their typically developing peers. Children with autism often have an average to below-average head circumference at birth, with acceleration noted in the first year of life.

Clinical Manifestations

Speech delay is often the first deficit noted by parents and brought to the attention of the PCP. This may occur between 15 and 18 months of age. It is important to sort out which children are simply speech delayed. One way to do this is by considering if children are trying to compensate for their lack of verbal skills by communicating via gestures or pointing. Higher-functioning ASD children or those with Aspergers syndrome may have many words that they use; however, they might use them solely for labeling and without communicative intent. These children often have what is described as **"scripted" speech,** reciting volumes of lines from movies and television shows. Children with ASD frequently have **echolalia,** where they repeat portions of another person's speech. It is important to recognize that typically developing children may go through a period of echolalia. In autism, however, the echolalia persists as they grow older. Very early signs of prespeech deficits can include **lack of appropriate gaze, lack of reciprocal vocalizing between infant and parent, lack of response to name, and limited prespeech gestures such as pointing and waving.** A history of **regression or loss of language skills** should be carefully investigated by the PCP because this is reported in approximately 25% of children with ASD.

Deficits in social skills are another key feature of ASD; however, these deficits are not always recognized or reported by the parents. They may describe their babies as very "low maintenance," entertaining themselves for long periods of time or remaining in their cribs without needing attention. They often do not respond or localize when their name is called, and **parents will frequently express a concern about hearing.** When given the opportunity to be around other children, those with ASD are often on the perimeter of activity, unaware and uninterested in what the rest of the group is doing. These social differences become more apparent as children start to participate in group activities such as play groups, preschools, and sports.

Along with assessing speech and social skills, it is important to inquire about and observe a child's **play skills and behavior.** Children with ASD have **difficulty with imaginative or pretend play.** They may become preoccupied with parts of toys and play with them in a repetitive fashion, such as stacking or lining up. They are resistant to any type of imitative tasks. They have intense interest in simple objects, such as pieces of string or spinning fans. They frequently exhibit **repetitive, nonfunctional behaviors** known as **stereotypies.** These can include **hand flapping, finger flicking, jumping, and spinning.** Although these behaviors are not harmful, they can impede development of more appropriate cognitive, communication, and social skills.

Diagnosis of Autism

Early identification of ASD is critical. It is important to carefully consider the diagnostic criteria and to recognize the variation that exists within this set of disorders. As recommended by the American Academy of Pediatrics, developmental surveillance should occur at every well child visit, and screening with a standardized developmental tool should take place at specific intervals or whenever a concern is raised. (See Chapter 14, Developmental Screening and Surveillance.) If warranted, there are a number of **ASD-specific screening tools** that can be administered in the office setting. For children with classic features of autism, the PCP may feel comfortable making the diagnosis and beginning an etiologic workup. Frequently a referral is made to a pediatric subspecialist with experience in diagnosis of ASD. This can include a pediatric neurologist, child psychiatrist, or developmental pediatrician. In addition, a referral to a geneticist may be helpful if there is a family history of ASD or suspicion of a specific genetic syndrome. An **audiologic evaluation** should be considered for any child with a speech/language delay.

Management of Autism

Autism is a chronic neurodevelopmental disability, and there is no "cure." There are a number of treatment modalities, however, that address the core impairments and improve overall outcome. These include **speech therapy, occupational therapy, structured teaching, social skills intervention, and intensive behavioral strategies.** Intervention services are federally mandated for those who qualify under the Individuals with Disabilities Education Act of 2004 (IDEA 2004) and are free of charge. (See Chapter 25, The Special Needs Child, and Chapter 27, Attention Deficit Hyperactivity Disorder.) All physicians who care for patients with ASD should become familiar with how to help families access these services. Services for children in the birth-to-3-years age-group are often managed by counties. They are individualized therapies delivered in a child's "natural environment," with a focus on the family. At the age of 3 years, service delivery shifts to a center-based model, with children attending structured preschool programs within their school district. There are numerous **educational techniques** and **therapy strategies** that have been implemented to treat children with autism, including **applied behavior analysis (ABA); the developmental, individual-difference, relationship-based (DIR) or "floor-time" model; and the Treatment and Education of Autistic and Related Communication Handicapped Children (TEACCH) program,** to name a few. Most community-based programs use an eclectic approach, combining a variety of methods.

Medical care for children with ASD should include the same preventive medicine visits as for their typically developing peers. Also associated with ASD is an **increased prevalence of epilepsy,** a high incidence of **sleep problems,** and a **possible relationship with gastrointestinal problems. Challenging behaviors,** such as **aggression, impulsivity,** and **hyperactivity** may be amenable to pharmacologic management. Referral to a subspecialist may be necessary to treat associated medical and behavioral conditions. **See Nelson Essentials 20.**

Practice-Based Learning and Improvement

Title
Autism and the pervasive developmental disorders, parts 1 and 2

Author
Bauer S

Reference
Pediatr Rev 16:130-136, 1995 and *Pediatr Rev* 16:168-176, 1995

Historical significance/comments
These two articles discuss diagnostic criteria for the autistic
spectrum, including ASD, pervasive developmental disorder, and
Asperger disorder. The importance of screening at age 18 months is
emphasized, as are the differential diagnosis, educational supports,
and benefits of pharmacologic management for some children.

Interpersonal and Communication Skills

**Explore Beliefs, Concerns, and Expectations About the Child's
Health and Illness**

When a physician is concerned about a patient, open and honest
communication is imperative. This is especially true when there
is a concern about a child's development, which will likely have
long-lasting implications. Keep in mind that this is not what the
family expected for their child. They were "counting on" the
typical development you read about in a parenting book. They
will likely want to know about their child's prognosis, but
unfortunately development is hard to predict. It is often a "wait-
and-see" approach. Answer their questions to the best of your
ability. Do not be afraid to say "I don't know." Also problematic
is the fact that a diagnosis of autism is based on a set of
criteria rather than a specific medical test or result. This is very
hard for some people to conceptualize and may seem rather
subjective.

   Autism occurs among people of all races, religions, cultures, and
socioeconomic backgrounds. Discussions must be tailored to fit the
needs of each individual family. It is important to get a good sense
of what the family understands regarding the diagnosis. Have they
ever heard of autism? Do they know anyone with autism? What do
they think autism means? What do they think this means for their
child? It is important to point out that this diagnosis does not
change who their child is, but rather puts things in a framework
to allow him/her to receive needed services to ensure the
best outcome.

Professionalism

Communication and Advocacy: Be Nonjudgmental of Nontraditional Treatments, but an Advocate When Necessary

Families look to their pediatrician or family doctor for information, advice, and support. There are many unanswered questions about the etiology and treatment of ASD. Theories abound on the Internet and in the lay press regarding mercury, immunizations, vitamin deficiencies, and allergies as causative factors. Numerous unproved treatments are touted, including chelation, special diets, and vitamin supplements. It is important for physicians to keep abreast of new developments in treatment and management and to keep an open mind, because traditional medicine does not yet have all the answers. The physician should share his/her critical appraisal of the literature with the family and be careful not to be judgmental when families make choices that he/she feels may not be beneficial. However, when families pursue therapies that have potentially harmful side effects without proved efficacy, the physician, in his/her role as child advocate, should intervene.

Systems-Based Practice

Office-Based Care, Processes, and Structure: Minimize Anxiety for the Child With Autism

The components of successful practice-based care coordination for children with autism include scheduling that ensures access and continuity, office staff training in customer service, medical records integrity and transparency, referrals tracking and coordination, and knowledge of community- and state-based resources and service.

For all physicians involved, it may be necessary to schedule a longer appointment, because patients with autism often have difficulty in the office setting and need time to adjust. Transitions from one area to another can be problematic, so minimizing the number of steps along the way should be considered. Minimizing time spent in the waiting room is also desirable. This may be accomplished by scheduling patients for the first appointment in the morning or after a lunch break.

Chapter 27
Attention-Deficit/ Hyperactivity Disorder (Case 1)

Amanda E. Bennett MD, MPH
and Nathan J. Blum MD

Case: The parent of a 7-year-old boy is concerned about his performance in first grade. He makes careless mistakes and often does not complete his work. He is loud, calls out inappropriately, and makes noise in class and typically does not follow instructions at home or school.

Differential Diagnosis

Attention-deficit/hyperactivity disorder	Learning problems
Other developmental or behavioral problems	Sleep disorder

Speaking Intelligently

When I consider a diagnosis of attention-deficit/hyperactivity disorder (ADHD) in a child with school performance or behavioral problems, I take a history seeking information about the core symptoms of ADHD (inattention, impulsivity, and hyperactivity) as well as other possible medical, emotional, and environmental contributing factors. Specific information about behaviors, including frequency, will help in assessment about whether they are developmentally inappropriate and functionally impairing. Standardized behavior rating scales completed by parents and teachers help in assessing symptom severity. Information on the child's medical history, developmental milestones, sleep schedule, and family and peer relationships helps in assessing for other possible diagnoses.

PATIENT CARE

Clinical Thinking

- Does the child have **difficulty in multiple settings,** both academic and nonacademic?
- Inattention, hyperactivity, and impulsivity are nonspecific symptoms. **Exclude alternative diagnoses** such as seizure disorders, sleep problems, thyroid disorders, hearing and visual deficits, or mental health problems.

History

- Are **parental and teacher reports** on symptoms consistent? If not, evaluation for learning and other behavioral problems will be critical before diagnosing ADHD.
- **Evaluate for specific learning disability** if child has difficulty learning academic skills or has a history of language delays.
- Significant developmental delay or persistent academic problems may warrant subspecialty evaluation.
- **Review sleep history:** Snoring with daytime fatigue suggests obstructive sleep apnea.

Physical Examination

- Vital signs: Plot height, weight, and head circumference for clues to other medical conditions. **Document baseline heart rate and blood pressure** in case medications are considered.
- General **neurologic examination** should be normal. Children with ADHD may have difficulty with coordinating rapid alternating movements or have mirror movements (i.e., moving the right hand when asked to perform sequential finger thumb opposition with the left hand or vice versa).

Tests for Consideration

• **Parent- and teacher-completed behavior rating scale**	Free download
• **Vision screening**	$120
• **Hearing screening**	$250
• **Thyroid function (TSH, free T_4 and T_3) studies in select cases**	$190

Clinical Entities	Medical Knowledge

Attention-Deficit/Hyperactivity Disorder

Pφ **ADHD** is a condition affecting approximately 5% to 10% of school-age children in the United States. There is a strong genetic component, because most children have someone else in the family who has ADHD. Based largely on the medications that are effective in treatment, it is believed that the dopamine and norepinephrine neurotransmitter systems are involved. Neuronal circuits involving the striatum, thalamus, and frontal lobes have also been implicated, yet specific pathophysiology is not well understood.

TP The typical child presents between 6 and 12 years of age with parental and/or teacher concerns about academic and/or specific behavioral difficulties. Symptoms of inattention, hyperactivity, and impulsivity are often first detected between 3 and 7 years of age. Some specific symptoms include difficulty sitting still; poor concentration or daydreaming; acting without thinking; difficulty completing tasks like chores, schoolwork, or homework; and interrupting others or calling out in school.

Dx Diagnosis is usually made by pediatricians, family physicians, psychiatrists, psychologists, neurologists, or clinical social workers, using criteria from the *Diagnostic and Statistical Manual of Mental Disorders,* fourth edition, text revision (DSM-IV-TR). Diagnostic criteria include:
- Six or more symptoms of inattention and/or six or more symptoms of hyperactivity-impulsivity from a diagnostic list of nine inattention and nine hyperactivity-impulsivity symptoms.
- Symptoms are present for at least 6 months.
- DSM-IV-TR states that symptoms must be present before age 7 years and cause impairment in social, academic, or occupational functioning. However, some children with mostly inattentive symptoms are not detected until late elementary or early middle school.
- Impairment from symptoms occurs in two or more settings (e.g., school, home, social settings with peers).
- Symptoms are not better accounted for by another mental disorder.

Diagnosis of ADHD can be divided into three subtypes:
- Attention-deficit/hyperactivity disorder, combined type if both hyperactive-impulsive and inattentive symptoms are present

- Attention-deficit/hyperactivity disorder, predominantly inattentive type if mostly inattentive symptoms are present
- Attention-deficit/hyperactivity disorder, predominantly hyperactive-impulsive type if mostly hyperactive-impulsive symptoms are present—this is seen mostly in children under 6 years of age

Tx	There is strong evidence to support the effectiveness of both stimulant medication and behavioral counseling in the treatment of ADHD. In general, stimulant medications are more effective than behavioral counseling in improving the core symptoms of ADHD, but for most children the most effective treatment is a combination of medication and behavioral counseling. The nonstimulant medications, atomoxetine and guanfacine extended release, are also approved by the Food and Drug Administration (FDA) for the treatment of ADHD. Behavioral counseling can teach parents and teachers to use positive reinforcement to motivate more-appropriate behavior at home or in school. Strategies to support improved organization, such as using a homework notebook, or improved attention, such as making eye contact when giving instructions, are often helpful. Some children with ADHD will qualify for educational interventions under the Individuals with Disabilities Education Act (IDEA) described under learning problems below. **See Nelson Essentials 13.**

Learning Problems (Learning Disability or Intellectual Disability)

Pφ	Severe *intellectual disability* (formerly known as mental retardation) is most commonly caused by genetic abnormalities but occasionally may be caused by an illness, injury, exposure to toxins, or nutritional, social, or cultural deprivation. Mild intellectual disability and specific learning disabilities are caused by a complex interaction of multiple genetic and environmental risk factors.
TP	A child with severe intellectual disability may present as early as infancy with delays in several streams of development that are usually easily detected by parents or physicians. However, some children with mild intellectual disabilities and most children with specific learning disabilities are not identified until they are struggling in school. Some learning disabilities may not become apparent until academic demands increase or specific skill requirements change, such as with the increased demands for reading comprehension that usually occur around the third or fourth grade.

Dx   Diagnosis of intellectual disability includes significantly below average general intelligence (IQ less than 70) accompanied by limitations in adaptive functioning in at least two skill areas (e.g., self-care, functional academic skills, social/interpersonal skills). Learning disorders are diagnosed when achievement in reading, mathematics, or written expression is significantly below that expected for age, education, or level of intelligence.

Tx   There are no specific medical treatments for mental retardation or learning disorders. Small group or individualized instruction may be necessary. IDEA requires schools to develop an Individualized Education Program (IEP) for children with intellectual or learning disabilities. The IEP indicates specific educational goals for the child, as well as the interventions and accommodations the school will provide to help the child achieve these goals (see Chapter 25, The Special Needs Child). **See Nelson Essentials 10.**

Sleep Disorders/Obstructive Sleep Apnea

Pφ   Sleep problems can occur for a variety of reasons, from poor sleep hygiene (e.g., irregular bedtime, TV or light on while trying to fall asleep, loud noises in house) to *sleep disorders* such as *obstructive sleep apnea.* Fatigue and sleep deprivation are associated with a shortened attention span and increased irritability.

TP   Children presenting with obstructive sleep apnea or disordered sleep usually have a history of significant snoring with occasional periods of gasping or choking during the night. They may have enlarged tonsils and adenoids and/or a history of mouth breathing. If children are falling asleep in class or on short car rides, they should be evaluated for a sleep disorder.

Dx   If the history does not suggest poor sleep hygiene as the cause for sleep problems, it is likely that further evaluation using polysomnography (sleep study) will be necessary. Polysomnography measures electroencephalogram (EEG), electrocardiogram (EKG), nasal and/or oral airflow, chest wall movement, leg movement, and blood oxygen saturation.

Tx   Many sleep problems improve if children have a regular bedtime
      and wake-up time, a calming bedtime routine, and do not have
      a TV or light (except a single night-light) on in their room.
      Treatment of obstructive sleep apnea includes surgical removal
      of adenoids and tonsils. Sometimes, especially for children who
      have contraindications to surgery or persistent symptoms after
      adenotonsillectomy, continuous positive airway pressure (CPAP)
      is used to reduce obstruction while sleeping. **See Nelson
      Essentials 15 and 134.**

**Other Developmental/Behavioral Disorder (e.g., Autism Spectrum
Disorders, Oppositional Defiant Disorder, Anxiety, Mood Disorder)**

Pφ   Similar to ADHD, conditions such as autism, depression, and
      anxiety have a strong genetic component, but multiple genes
      interact with environmental factors in ways that are not well
      understood to cause the symptoms.

TP   Children with *autism spectrum disorders (ASD)* diagnosis
      often present with history of difficulty with reciprocal social
      interactions, communication, and/or presence of atypical,
      repetitive, or restricted behaviors or interests. Children with
      oppositional defiant disorder (ODD) present with a history of
      negative, hostile, and defiant behaviors occurring over at least
      6 months and interfering with social, academic, or occupational
      functioning. Children with *anxiety*-related disorders can have
      symptoms including obsessions and compulsions or specific
      phobias or generalized anxiety. Likewise, children with *mood
      disorders* may present with mania, depression, or a cycling of
      symptoms.

Dx   Diagnosis of *developmental/behavioral or mental health
      disorders* is made using criteria from the DSM-IV-TR. There are
      no specific medical tests available at this time to confirm
      diagnosis.

Tx   Treatment of many developmental/behavioral and mental health
      disorders includes a combination of medications and/or
      behavioral therapy, depending on the specific symptoms and
      the severity of the symptoms. When the symptoms are causing
      significant conflict within the family, family therapy may be
      needed. **See Nelson Essentials 8 and 17 to 20.**

ZEBRA ZONE

a. **Tourette's disorder:** Multiple motor tics and one or more vocal tics occurring many times a year nearly every day or intermittently for more than 1 year.

b. **Absence seizures:** Brief episodes of vacant staring, cessation of movement or speech, and eyelid flickering lasting less than 30 seconds followed by resumption of activity without postictal state.

c. **Neurodegenerative disorders:** Early in the course primary symptoms may be inattention and decreasing school performance.

Practice-Based Learning and Improvement

Title
A 14-month randomized clinical trial of treatment strategies for attention-deficit/hyperactivity disorder

Author
The Multimodal Treatment of ADHD Cooperative Group

Reference
Arch Gen Psychiatry 56:1073-1086, 1999

Problem
Comparison of two most commonly used treatments for ADHD

Intervention
14-month treatment program falling into four categories:
(1) community treatment, (2) medication, (3) behavioral therapy,
(4) combined medication and behavioral therapy

Quality of evidence
Multisite randomized clinical trial; strength of evidence: high

Outcome/effect
Treatment using combined medication and behavioral therapy did not significantly differ from treatment using medication alone, and combined or medication management was clinically and statistically superior to behavioral therapy alone or community treatment in improving core ADHD symptoms. Subsequent analysis has demonstrated benefits of combined treatment for some symptoms associated with ADHD.

Historical significance/comments
The MTA study was one of the first to compare evidence-based medical and behavioral treatments in a randomized, controlled fashion using a large sample size and extended trial period.[2]

Interpersonal and Communication Skills

Acknowledge and Respond to Patient's (Family's) Ideas, Feelings, and Values: Recognize and Acknowledge the Impact of ADHD on Family Dynamics

Although ADHD is a diagnosis of the child, it often affects family dynamics significantly. It is important to acknowledge and respond to family concerns and to let the family express their feelings. It is important for patients and families to understand that children with ADHD have more difficulty paying attention and controlling impulses than typical children. However, even children with ADHD can pay attention at times, particularly when they are highly motivated. Thus children with ADHD are often very inconsistent in their performance. This inconsistency can be difficult for parents to understand, and often parents or teachers attribute it to laziness. Physicians need to help parents understand their child's behavior. Parents should be educated on the diagnostic criteria necessary to receive the diagnosis. ADHD is a chronic condition, and the physician will need to help parents understand and learn about potential treatment options. Information on educational rights and parent support groups should be discussed. Communication with the child should include an age-appropriate discussion of the diagnosis and treatment plan.

Professionalism

Respect for Others: Demonstrate Cultural Awareness and Sensitivity to the Impact of a Diagnosis of ADHD

Individuals from different cultures and ethnic backgrounds may have varying opinions on the diagnosis and treatment of behavioral health conditions in general, and about ADHD in particular. Clinicians evaluating and/or treating children with ADHD will need to demonstrate sensitivity to the cultural beliefs of parents and extended family members in terms of assigning a diagnosis to the constellation of symptoms, sharing the diagnosis with other caregivers and school personnel, and treatment by mental health providers.

Systems-Based Practice

Health Law: Federal Laws

Clinicians diagnosing and treating ADHD in children will need to be familiar with policies and federal laws commonly associated with the educational system.

Examples of federal laws addressing the rights of children with identified learning disabilities or cognitive impairments include Section 504 of the Rehabilitation Act of 1973, the Americans with Disabilities Act (ADA), and the Education for All Handicapped Children Act of 1975, renamed the Individuals with Disabilities Education Act (IDEA) reauthorized in 2004.

Section 504 of the Rehabilitation Act of 1973 provides that students with disabilities who are entitled to attend school under state law cannot be excluded from participation in, be denied the benefits of, or be subjected to discrimination under any program or activity receiving federal financial assistance.[3]

The ADA was established by Congress in 1990. The purpose of the law is to end discrimination in the workplace and to provide equal employment opportunities for people with disabilities.

The IDEA is a federal law designed to protect the rights of students with disabilities by ensuring that everyone receives a free appropriate public education (FAPE), equal access, and additional special education services. Children between the ages of 3 and 21 can qualify for services under IDEA if they have 1 of 13 qualifying disabilities: autism, deaf/blind, deafness, hearing impaired, mental retardation, multiple disabilities, orthopedic impairment, serious emotional disturbance, specific learning disabilities, speech or language impairment, traumatic brain injury, visual impairment including blindness, and other health impairment.[4]

References

1. American Academy of Pediatrics: Clinical practice guideline: Diagnosis and evaluation of the child with attention-deficit/hyperactivity disorder. *Pediatrics* 105:1158–1170, 2000.
2. MTA Cooperative Group: A 14-month randomized clinical trial of treatment strategies for attention-deficit/hyperactivity disorder. *Arch Gen Psychiatry* 56:1073–1086, 1999.
3. Office for Civil Rights, US Department of Education: Section 504 of Rehabilitation Act of 1973. Available at http://ed.gov/about/offices/list/ocr/504faq.html, 2009.
4. Office of Special Education Programs, U.S. Department of Education: Individuals with Disabilities Education Act. Available at http://idea.ed.gov.

Chapter 28
Down Syndrome

Kathryn Rausch Crowell MD

Speaking Intelligently

General pediatricians provide care for infants and children with Down syndrome in many different capacities. They may provide prenatal counseling to couples who have received a prenatal diagnosis. The pediatrician may evaluate a newborn who was not diagnosed prenatally but whose appearance and examination are suspicious for Down syndrome in the nursery.[1] In addition to evaluation and care of the baby, it is important to be prepared for the difficult conversation with the parents. Pediatricians also provide ongoing primary care for children with Down syndrome, which will include routine primary care, care needed for specific associated diagnoses, and screening specific to Down syndrome, such as periodic testing for hypothyroidism and monitoring for middle ear effusion.[1]

Medical Knowledge and Patient Care

Background and Definitions

Trisomy 21, or Down syndrome, is a genetic disorder that includes a combination of birth defects. Down syndrome is associated with intellectual disability (formerly known as mental retardation), characteristic facial features, congenital heart defects, visual and hearing impairments, gastrointestinal problems, cryptorchidism, and other health problems, including hypothyroidism. The phenotype is variable, and the severity of these problems is highly variable among affected infants. Down syndrome is one of the most common genetic birth defects, affecting approximately 1 in 800 to 1000 babies.

In Down syndrome there is an extra copy of chromosome 21. Ninety-five percent of cases result from nonfamilial trisomy 21. Three to four percent of cases result from an unbalanced translocation between chromosome 21 and another chromosome, usually 14. Finally, 1% to 2% of cases result from mosaicism. In these individuals, two cell lines are present, one normal and one trisomy 21. **See Nelson Essentials 49.**

Clinical Features

Affected infants may be initially identified by recognizable phenotypic features. Although the phenotype is variable, there is enough consistency to allow an experienced clinician to suspect the diagnosis. The head might appear brachycephalic or microcephalic, and there may be small ears and excessive nuchal skin (i.e., at the nape of the neck). Ophthalmologic examination may reveal epicanthal folds, upward slanting palpebral fissures, and Brushfield spots. The hands typically have a single transverse palmar crease (simian crease), a short fifth finger, and clinodactyly. In addition, examination of the feet may reveal a wide space, often with a deep fissure, between the first and second toes. On neurologic examination, mild to moderate diffuse hypotonia is typical and may contribute to feeding difficulty. **See Nelson Essentials 49.**

- **Feeding Difficulty.** Although all children with Down syndrome have some degree of mental impairment and developmental delay, this becomes more apparent after infancy. In the neonatal period, hypotonia is common and may complicate an infant's ability to effectively orally feed, and inadequate weight gain is common. Consequently, early on, infants need to be followed closely to evaluate for feeding difficulties and weight loss. A speech therapist may be necessary to support feeding techniques. After hospital discharge, all infants with Down syndrome should be referred to early intervention for evaluation by speech, occupational, and physical therapists. Although most children with Down syndrome have delayed acquisition of both fine and gross motor skills, early intervention techniques, education, and vocational training have all been shown to improve the developmental quotient of children with Down syndrome. In later childhood, these children have a tendency to gain excessive weight and are at risk for obesity. They tend to have short stature, and there are specific Down syndrome growth charts to provide height and weight and head circumference data relative to a population of children with Down syndrome.
- **Congenital Cardiac Disease.** These infants have a significantly increased risk for congenital heart defects (50%). An atrioventricular (AV) canal defect is the cardiac lesion most commonly associated with Down syndrome. However, a variety of other defects, such as ventricular septal defects (VSDs) and atrial septal defects (ASDs), also occur. Many infants with congenital cardiac defects will be asymptomatic after delivery and have a normal cardiac examination. Although the diagnosis may sometimes be suspected as a result of physical examination findings, all infants with suspected Down syndrome need to have an echocardiogram in the newborn period. **See Nelson Essentials 49.**
- **Gastrointestinal Problems.** There is increased incidence of gastrointestinal problems, such as duodenal atresia, constipation, and Hirschsprung disease (see Chapter 63, Delayed Meconium Passage). There is a significant increase in the incidence of leukemia among young children with Down syndrome; there is also

increased risk for myeloproliferative disorders and leukemoid reactions, each characterized by a very high white blood cell count and other findings that typically resolve.

- **Hypothyroidism.** Neonates with Down syndrome have an increased risk for congenital hypothyroidism (1%), and the risk for acquired thyroid disease persists for older infants and children (15%). Most neonates with congenital hypothyroidism have a normal physical examination. However, some have more typical neonatal signs of hypothyroidism, including hypotonia, prolonged jaundice, constipation, and macroglossia. Congenital hypothyroidism is usually diagnosed with the newborn thyroid screen. Thyroid screening should subsequently be repeated at 6 months of age, 12 months of age, and then annually for all children with Down syndrome.[1]

- **Hearing Impairment.** These infants and children have an increased risk for hearing loss (75%). It can be sensorineural, conductive, or mixed hearing loss. It is difficult to identify infants with hearing loss by physical examination. Therefore objective testing should be performed in the newborn period (by at least 3 months of age) with either brainstem auditory brainstem response or otoacoustic emission testing.[1] If the initial hearing evaluation results are abnormal, the infant should be referred to an otolaryngologist and audiologist. A behavioral audiogram should subsequently be obtained by 12 months of age in all children (see Chapter 58, Newborn Hearing Screen).

- **Vision Impairment.** Ophthalmology monitoring is also important due to increased incidence of cataracts and strabismus.

Practice-Based Learning and Improvement

Title
Health supervision for children with Down syndrome

Authors
American Academy of Pediatrics, Committee on Genetics

Reference
Pediatrics 107(2):442-449, 2001

Historical significance/comments
This policy statement outlines the recommended guideline for health supervision of infants and children with Down syndrome. In addition, it contains guidelines for counseling families referred with a prenatal diagnosis of trisomy 21. It contains a table summarizing care recommendations by age. It could ideally be incorporated into the child's medical record as a tracking reminder. Interested parents could be given a copy as an adjunct to counseling about necessary testing.

Interpersonal and Communication Skills

Share Information and Check for Understanding When Teaching About Diagnosis and Management

Pediatricians routinely counsel families whose children have genetic disorders. In some instances, pediatricians may be asked to provide prenatal counseling for a family whose fetus has been identified as having Down syndrome. Pediatricians should feel comfortable discussing the prenatal laboratory or fetal imaging studies that lead to the diagnosis, the mechanism for occurrence of the disorder, the potential recurrence rate for the family, as well as the prognosis and manifestations of this diagnosis. Outline the next steps to confirm this possible diagnosis: completion of a karyotype, evaluation by a geneticist, and finally evaluation by a cardiologist. Often parents are overwhelmed by the diagnosis itself and may not retain much of the information that is given in the visit. It is important to check for parental understanding. Asking the parents to repeat back their understanding of what has been discussed is a good way to assess what the parents have actually heard. If key information has been misconstrued by the family, it can be rediscussed at this time. Provide support for the family as they process the information given, and provide hope and guidance for the future.[1,2]

Professionalism

Knowledge of Limits: Recognize That a Multidisciplinary Team of Experts Is Required

The physician alone cannot provide the needed support as a family assimilates information about and comes to terms with the diagnosis of Down syndrome. Emphasizing that the family is not alone and will have a team of medical and lay experts available to them is of paramount importance.

Mobilization of support for the family is the responsibility of the physician. Examples include putting the family in touch with other families with children who have Down syndrome; referral to the local Down syndrome support group; and using the services of clergy, social workers, visiting nurses, and other outreach services.[1]

Systems-Based Practice

Case Management: Use Appropriate Support Services

The mission of the pediatrician and Down syndrome clinic team should be to help each individual with Down syndrome reach his/her full potential and function as independently as possible in all aspects of family, school, and community life. Because patients with Down syndrome are likely to have a variety of illnesses and multiple health screening and social needs, the health-care system has to be very efficient and coordinated. Case managers and social workers from the local health departments or the insurance company must be engaged because they will be a valuable resource to providers and families. They will also provide the following relevant services:

- Information and referral to the local Down syndrome (DS) parent group for family support
- Assistance with application for Supplemental Security Income (SSI), depending on family income
- Help with estate planning and custody arrangements
- Encouraging social and recreational programs with friends
- Discussion of plans for alternative long-term living arrangements such as community living arrangements (CLA) for patients above 18 years

References

American Academy of Pediatrics, Committee on Genetics: Health supervision for children with Down syndrome. *Pediatrics* 107(2):442-449, 2001.
Skotko B: Mothers of children with Down syndrome reflect on postnatal support. *Pediatrics* 115:64-77, 2005.

Chapter 29
Preparticipation Physical Evaluation

Kathleen B. O'Brien MD

Speaking Intelligently

The preparticipation physical evaluation should be designed specifically to ensure the health and well-being of young athletes; that is, to identify medical conditions that put the athlete at risk for sudden death or life-threatening complications. In addition, it strives to identify and rehabilitate prior injuries, as well as provide strategies to prevent these injuries in the future. Currently, 49 of 50 states require a preparticipation physical evaluation (PPE).[1] The requirements of these evaluations, however, vary widely from state to state. For example, some states allow for the PPE to be completed by nonphysician extenders, chiropractors, or even athletic trainers.

Medical Knowledge and Patient Care

Background and Definitions

The history should begin with an understanding of what sport the athlete intends to play. **Sports** have been categorized according to a **grade of contact—low, moderate, or high** (Table 29-1). In addition, activities have been classified based on **dynamic (volume load)** or **static (pressure load)** on the heart (Table 29-2).[2] Understanding these classifications will allow the pediatrician to consider the risks associated with each sport.

History

A review of the general medical history is appropriate, including the use of any medication or supplement that may affect performance. A few conditions deserve special attention. A prior **history of syncope or near-syncope during exercise or palpitations is** especially concerning and should prompt further workup, including evaluation by a pediatric cardiologist. The risk for sudden death in young athletes is estimated to be 1 in 200,000.[3] **Hypertrophic cardiomyopathy** is the most common cause, followed by **congenital coronary artery abnormalities.**[4] Guidelines for athletes with known cardiovascular abnormalities have been supported by the American Heart Association and are based on the 36th Bethesda Conference Guidelines for Participation.[5] **Exercise-induced bronchospasm** and/or **asthma** is relatively common, and a history of wheezing during exercise may need further treatment. **Concussions** occur most commonly with high-impact sports and **need to be taken seriously,** as does a history of "stingers" or "burners." A seizure disorder may not result in disqualification, depending on the sport, but it must be well controlled. Inquiring specifically about a female athlete's menstrual history may uncover primary or secondary amenorrhea and raise concern for the **female athlete triad.** Athletes should be questioned about recent illness, particularly infectious mononucleosis. **Previous musculoskeletal injury is the strongest predictor of sports injury,**[6] and up to 20% of high school athletes will have a musculoskeletal injury that requires medical attention.[7]

Family history should focus on prior **sudden death** and **risk factors** for it, as well as any known cardiac disease. Also important would be a family history of a bleeding disorder or seizure.

Physical Examination

The physical examination begins with vital signs. Hypertension noted in the PPE should be reevaluated on two separate occasions before decisions are made about eligibility and need for further workup. Contagious skin infections can be identified and addressed before the start of the season. The remainder of the examination should focus on areas identified as potential problems by the history, but of course should include a thorough cardiovascular examination. **However, the vast majority of athletes who die of sudden cardiac death were previously asymptomatic and may have a normal cardiac examination.** The musculoskeletal examination should be directed at areas of prior injury, as well as those joints at risk in certain sports (e.g., the shoulder examination in a competitive swimmer).

Testing

There are no specific recommendations for "routine" laboratory tests. Experience in Italy, where federal law mandates an electrocardiogram (EKG) be performed on every athlete as part of their PPE, suggests that sudden cardiac death resulting from hypertrophic cardiomyopathy can be reduced.[8] In the United States, this practice has not been adopted but continues to be debated. For now, EKG testing is at the discretion of the examiner and/or consulting cardiologist.

Table 29-1 Classification of Sport by Degree of Contact		
High Contact/Collision	**Limited Contact**	**Low-Noncontact**
Football	Baseball	Badminton
Ice hockey	Bicycling	Bowling
Basketball	Gymnastics	Golf
Field hockey	Skating	Running
Lacrosse	Skiing	Strength training
Martial arts	Volleyball	Crew
Rugby	Cheerleading	Tennis
Soccer		Swimming
Wrestling		
Diving		

Data from American Academy of Pediatrics, Committee on Sports Medicine and Fitness: Medical conditions affecting sports participation, *Pediatrics* 2001;107:1205.

Table 29-2	Classification of Sport by Demands on the Heart		
High static	Gymnastics	Body building	Cycling
	Martial arts	Skiing	Rowing
	Water skiing	Snowboarding	Speed skating
	Weight lifting	Wrestling	Decathlon
	Field events	Skateboarding	Triathlon
Moderate static	Diving	Football	Basketball
	Equestrian	Figure skating	Ice hockey
	Archery	Rugby	Lacrosse
		Running (sprint)	Running (mid distance)
			Swimming
Low static	Bowling	Baseball/softball	Field hockey
	Golf	Volleyball	Soccer
	Curling	Fencing	Tennis
	Cricket		Running (long distance)
			Cross-country skiing
	Low dynamic	Moderate dynamic	High dynamic

Modified from Baron BJ, Zipes DP: 36th Bethesda Conference: Eligibility recommendations for competitive athletes with cardiovascular abnormalities. *J Am Coll Cardiol* (45):1366, 2005.

Practice-Based Learning and Improvement

Title
Preparticipation examination of the adolescent athlete, parts 1 and 2

Authors
Metzel J

Reference
Pediatr Rev 22:199-204, 2001 and *Pediatr Rev* 22:227-239, 2001

Historical significance/comments
This is a good concise review by one of the leading experts in pediatric sports medicine. It expands on what is presented here, with particular focus in part 2 on the screening for orthopedic injuries.

Interpersonal and Communication Skills

Advocate for the Patient: Base Clearance on PPE Results and Student's Best Interest

At the end of the preparticipation physical examination, plans should be developed with the athlete, and parent, depending on the age of the athlete, to address any identified issues. This may also involve the coach or trainer, keeping in mind patient confidentiality. Adequate follow-up should be ensured. Remember that the parent, coach, and athlete may all have different agendas and expectations concerning the need for follow-up, rehabilitation, and return to play. The physician's role is to advocate for the patient and ensure participation that does not endanger the patient's health. If the patient's health will be jeopardized by participating in a particular sport, it is the physician's job to explain the situation to the parent and athlete.

Professionalism

Self-Improvement: Commitment to Lifelong Learning and Education: Remain Updated Regarding PPE Requirements

Physicians must have the requisite knowledge and skills before they perform PPEs for their patients. A physician must recognize if he/she is not competent to perform the evaluation and seek additional training and education in this area.

Systems-Based Practice

Office-Based Care, Processes, and Structure: Office-Based Versus Station-Based Formats for PPE

Ideally, the PPE would be performed 4 to 6 weeks before the start of the season. This should allow time to address issues and injuries recognized during the PPE. Where to perform the evaluation is at the discretion of both the provider and the school. It typically occurs either in the office or at the school in either a station-based approach with multiple physicians or by an individual provider. Both have their advantages and disadvantages. The station-based or individual provider screening at the school provides the opportunity to screen a large number of athletes at once. It also allows for comparison between students of different ages and skeletal maturity. Because of its setup, however, confidentiality may be compromised, and thus students may not feel comfortable divulging information. In-office screening provides a more comfortable setting for the physician and patient. Because for many young adults this may be the only interaction they have with a health-care provider, this may be a good time to also discuss at-risk behaviors common to adolescents. It is important to remember, however, that the PPE is not a health maintenance visit, and the athlete should be encouraged to schedule one of these as well. A guideline for the PPE endorsed by the American Academy of Pediatrics, American Academy of Family Physicians, American Medical Society for Sports Medicine, American Orthopedic Society for Sports Medicine, and American Osteopathic Academy of Sports Medicine has been developed and is available online at http://www.aap.org/sections/sportsmedicine/spmedeval.pdf.

References

1. Campbell RM, Berger S: Preventing pediatric sudden cardiac death: Where do we start? *Pediatrics* 118:802, 2006.
2. Glover DW, Maron BJ: Profile of preparticipation cardiovascular screening for high school athletes. *JAMA* 279(22):1817-1819, 1998.
3. Maron BJ, Gohman TE, Aeppli D: Prevalence of sudden cardiac death during competitive sports activities in Minnesota high school athletes. *J Am Coll Cardiol* 32(7):1881-1884, 1998.
4. Maron BJ, Thompson MJ, et al: Recommendations and considerations related to preparticipation screening for cardiovascular abnormalities in competitive athletes: 2007 update: A scientific statement. *Circulation* 115:1643-1655, 2007.
5. Maron BJ, Zipes DP: 36th Bethesda Conference: Eligibility recommendations for competitive athletes with cardiovascular abnormalities. *J Am Coll Cardiol* (45):1364-1367, 2005.
6. VanMechelan W, Twisk J, Molenddijk A, et al: Subject related risk factors for sports injury: A 1 year prospective study in young adults. *Med Sci Sports Exerc* 28(9):1171-1179, 1996.
7. DuRont RH, Pendergrast RA, Seymore C: Findings from the preparticipation athletic exam and athletic injuries. *Am J Dis Child* (146):85, 1992.
8. Corrado D, Pelliccia A, Bjornstad HH, et al: Cardiovascular preparticipation screening of young competitive athletes for prevention of sudden death: Proposal for a common European protocol: Consensus statement of the Study Group of Sport Cardiology of the Working Group of Cardiac Rehabilitation and Exercise Physiology and the Working Group of Myocardial and Pericardial Diseases of the European Society of Cardiology. *Eur Heart J* (26):516-524, 2005.

Chapter 30
Sore Throat (Case 2)

Christopher P. Bonafide MD

Case: A 9-year-old with fever, sore throat, and difficulty swallowing for 2 days

Differential Diagnosis

Viral pharyngitis	Group A streptococcal (GAS) pharyngitis	Peritonsillar abscess
Retropharyngeal abscess	Infectious mononucleosis (IM)	

Speaking Intelligently

When I evaluate a child with sore throat, I first check if the airway is patent. Immediate treatment is needed for respiratory distress with airway obstruction. In the absence of respiratory distress, I look for clues such as fever to suggest infection. Asymmetry in the pharynx may indicate a peritonsillar abscess. If it is not a straightforward case of infectious pharyngitis, I consider other etiologies such as a sexually transmitted infection in an abused child or sexually active adolescent. The differential diagnosis broadens for an immunocompromised child. If the history and examination are not suggestive of infection, I ask questions about possible retained foreign bodies, irritants such as dry air or cigarette smoke, postnasal drip, or gastroesophageal reflux.

PATIENT CARE

Clinical Thinking
- Is immediate intervention needed for an **unstable airway?**
- Is this infectious or noninfectious?
- Are there signs of **dehydration** or **systemic illness** that warrant hospitalization?

History
- Rapid onset, fever, rash, conjunctivitis, and sick contacts suggest **infection.**
- Slower onset without signs of infection may indicate **irritative pharyngitis** or **allergic rhinitis.**
- Sore throat with itchy, watery eyes and rhinorrhea without fever and following a seasonal pattern suggests allergy.
- A morning sore throat improved by midday suggests an irritant such as warm dry air from a home heater.
- **Foreign body ingestion** is suggested by history of eating small bones (fish) or ingesting small objects such as a staple.
- Are there indications of **child abuse?**

Physical Examination
- Tachypnea or irregular respirations with increased work of breathing suggests possible respiratory failure with **upper airway obstruction.**
- Tachycardia occurs with **dehydration.**
- Asymmetric tonsils, a fluctuant pharyngeal bulge, and a uvula deviated contralaterally may indicate **peritonsillar abscess.**
- Sandpapery maculopapular rash suggests GAS pharyngitis.
- Hepatosplenomegaly occurs with Epstein-Barr infection.
- Genital lesions raise the possibility of gonococcal pharyngitis.
- A rigid neck without meningitis may suggest **retropharyngeal abscess.**

Tests for Consideration
- **Complete blood count (CBC) with manual differential:**
  Elevated atypical lymphocytes in IM $139
- **Rapid strep antigen:** For GAS $148
- **Throat culture:** If rapid test negative $148
- **Monospot:** Heterophile antibody in IM $175
- **Rapid respiratory panel:** Detects influenza, parainfluenza,
  adenovirus, human metapneumovirus, rhinovirus, and
  respiratory syncytial virus (RSV) $325

IMAGING CONSIDERATIONS

→ **Neck radiograph—Anteroposterior (AP) and lateral
  views:** Foreign body or retropharyngeal abscess $250
→ **Computed tomography (CT) neck:** Retropharyngeal
  abscess $150
→ **Airway fluoroscopy:** Suspected foreign body $225

Clinical Entities   Medical Knowledge

Viral Pharyngitis

Pφ | Many viruses cause pharyngeal inflammation and sore throat: rhinovirus, coronavirus, RSV, adenovirus, influenza, parainfluenza, coxsackievirus, and herpes simplex (HSV). Spread occurs by direct contact with secretions and inhalation of droplets containing virus.

TP | All ages are affected and present with mild sore throat, cough, rhinorrhea, and possibly fever. Associated symptoms such as diarrhea support the diagnosis. Conjunctivitis suggests the pharyngoconjunctival fever syndrome of adenovirus. Summer is peak time for coxsackievirus, which presents with painful papules and vesicles in the posterior pharynx or as part of hand-foot-and-mouth disease with vesicles in the mouth and on palms and soles.

Dx | Diagnosis is clinical. Specific viral testing may be done in select cases.

Tx | Treatment is supportive with particular attention to pain control and hydration. **See Nelson Essentials 103.**

Group A Streptococcal Pharyngitis

Pφ	Sore throat is caused by local invasion of the posterior pharynx with the help of streptokinase and hyaluronidase and release of exotoxins causing pain and fever. M protein, the major virulence factor of **GAS**, acts by preventing activation of complement, protecting the organism from phagocytosis. Spread occurs via direct contact with secretions and inhalation of bacteria-containing droplets.
TP	Abrupt onset of sore throat and fever with headache and abdominal pain is typical. Classic examination findings include red inflamed tonsils with exudates, a red swollen uvula, palatal petechiae, and tender anterior adenopathy. In addition, the fine sandpapery maculopapular rash and strawberry tongue may occur, and 5- to 11-year-olds are most commonly affected.
Dx	Perform a throat swab for GAS antigen, with culture performed if the rapid point of care test is negative. Diagnosis can be confusing in GAS "carriers."
Tx	Oral penicillin or amoxicillen for 10 days is the treatment of choice. For penicillin allergic children who have had mild (non-type I hypersensitivity) reactions to penicillins, a 10-day course of a first-generation cephalosporin is appropriate. For children with immediate (type I) hypersensitivity reactions to penicillins, a 10-day course of clindamycin or a 5-day course of azithromycin are alternative regimens. Treatment will shorten the course and reduce incidence of peritonsillar or retropharyngeal abscess, cervical adenitis, and rheumatic fever. **See Nelson Essentials 103.**

Peritonsillar Abscess (PTA)

Pφ	**PTA** is a suppurative complication of GAS pharyngitis, infectious mononucleosis, or viral pharyngitis. Usually unilateral and located near the superior pole of the tonsil, the most likely organisms are GAS, other streptococci, staphylococci including *Staphylococcus aureus,* or anaerobes.
TP	Adolescents are more commonly affected and present with fever, sore throat, painful and difficult swallowing, difficulty opening the mouth (trismus), drooling, and a muffled "hot potato" voice. On examination there is an asymmetric posterior pharynx with a unilaterally enlarged tonsil and contralateral deviation of the uvula, with possible peritonsillar fluctuance.

Dx	Diagnosis is clinical. Cultures of the abscess fluid following drainage may identify the organism(s) and allow targeted treatment.
Tx	Initial treatment is with intravenous antibiotics. Clindamycin will cover GAS, most methicillin-resistant *S. aureus* (MRSA), and many anaerobes and is a reasonable first-line therapy. Ampicillin/sulbactam is another option but does not cover MRSA. Otolaryngology consultation is obtained for drainage. Adequate hydration and analgesia should be maintained. **See Nelson Essentials 135.**

Retropharyngeal Abscess

Pφ	*Retropharyngeal abscess* may follow acute pharyngitis. The fluid collection accumulates between the wall of the posterior pharynx and the prevertebral fascia. Responsible organisms are similar to PTA.
TP	Toddlers and young children are usually affected. Signs and symptoms include those of PTA, and, in addition, these children often resist movement of their neck and prefer a hyperextended position, mimicking meningismus. There may be stridor and respiratory distress in severe cases with airway obstruction.
Dx	Anterior bulging of the posterior pharyngeal wall may be appreciated. A lateral neck radiograph in the hyperextended position demonstrates a widened prevertebral space at the level of C2. Normally, **the prevertebral space is less than half the width of the vertebral body.** CT scan of the neck with contrast will delineate the collection and aid in the decision regarding need for surgical intervention.
Tx	As in PTA above. **See Nelson Essentials 135.**

Infectious Mononucleosis

Pφ	*IM* is most commonly due to Epstein-Barr virus (EBV); spread is via close contact with saliva. Lymphocytes are infected, which can produce multiple-system involvement, but acute pharyngitis is most common. Viral shedding can persist for months after symptom resolution.

TP	The typical patient is an older child presenting with sore throat, headache, fever, and fatigue. Examination reveals exudative pharyngitis, palatal petechiae, and tender cervical lymphadenopathy. Splenomegaly is common, and there may be hepatomegaly. Although the sore throat, headache, and fever usually resolve within 1 to 3 weeks, the fatigue may persist for 8 weeks or longer. Co-infection with GAS is not uncommon. Occasionally, a morbilliform rash may develop after amoxicillin given for GAS. This classic reaction may be related to an elevated level of benzylpenicilloyl-specific IgM antibodies in patients with IM and should not be considered an allergy.
Dx	Diagnosis is made by history, examination, along with supportive laboratory data. CBC demonstrates atypical lymphocytosis greater than 10%, which along with a positive heterophile antibody or Monospot is diagnostic. Monospot may be negative under 4 years of age, and serologic testing for EBV is also available; the IgM against viral capsid antigen may be most helpful in these cases.
Tx	Treatment is supportive. Spleen size should be monitored by the pediatrician, and contact sports avoided until the spleen is no longer palpable, because of the risk for life-threatening rupture. Corticosteroids may be helpful if there are severe symptoms, including airway compromise or massive splenomegaly. There is no evidence to support use of corticosteroids in uncomplicated cases. There is a theoretical risk that corticosteroid therapy may contribute to eventual development of EBV-associated malignancies, so they should be used only after careful consideration of risk and benefit. **See Nelson Essentials 99.**

ZEBRA ZONE

a. **Lemierre syndrome:** Life-threatening pharyngitis and septic thrombophlebitis of the internal jugular vein caused by *Fusobacterium necrophorum*

b. **Non-Hodgkin lymphoma:** Rarely presents as unilateral tonsillar enlargement

Practice-Based Learning and Improvement

Prevention of rheumatic fever: Treatment of preceding streptococcic infection

Authors
Denny F, Wannamaker LW, Brink WR, et al

Reference
JAMA 143:151-153, 1950

Problem
Rheumatic fever was noted to follow streptococcal pharyngitis in some patients.

Intervention
Treatment of exudative pharyngitis with intramuscular penicillin G

Quality of evidence
A study of 1634 patients at an air force training base who had exudative pharyngitis. Half received intramuscular penicillin, and half received no treatment.

Outcome/effect
The Jones criteria were used to determine which patients developed acute rheumatic fever. Of the 798 patients who received penicillin, definite acute rheumatic fever developed in only 2 patients, whereas of the 804 in the control group, 17 developed acute rheumatic fever ($p = 0.0006$).

Historical significance/comments
This is one of the seminal papers that demonstrated a reduction in the incidence of rheumatic fever by treating streptococcal pharyngitis.

Interpersonal and Communication Skills

Communicate Privately With Teenagers

Effective, developmentally appropriate communication is essential even when approaching a topic that seems, on the surface, as benign as a sore throat. That means developing a therapeutic relationship and asking the tough questions when appropriate to the clinical scenario. If there is concern about abuse or risky sexual behavior that makes gonococcal pharyngitis a consideration, the next appropriate step is asking the parent to step out for a few minutes so you can talk with the child alone. This can be difficult and requires taking into account the socioeconomic and cultural background of the family. Some offices tell parents that once the child reaches his/her teenage years, they will always ask the parent to step out of the room for a few minutes so the doctor and child can speak privately. With this office routine it is easier to coax the parent to leave for discussion of sensitive issues.

Professionalism

Reliability and Responsibility: Follow Up and Communicate Laboratory Results

If a throat culture is sent to an outside laboratory, the ordering physician is responsible for following up the result and notifying the family. Physicians who work in a group must make sure that they communicate to each other those tests results that need to be retrieved and dealt with when they are off duty. The onus should not be on families or patients to call the office to find out the results.

Systems-Based Practice

Quality Improvement: NCQA/HEDIS Criteria for Diagnostic Testing in Acute Pharyngitis.

One of the Healthcare Effectiveness Data and Information Set (HEDIS) measures required as part of the National Committee for Quality Assurance (NCQA) accreditation process for commercial and Medicaid health plans is *appropriate testing for children with pharyngitis*. This process quality measure is used to assess the percentage of children 2 to 18 years of age who were diagnosed with pharyngitis, were dispensed an antibiotic, and received a GAS test during episodes of care in which pharyngitis was diagnosed and an antibiotic was prescribed. The rationale for this measure is that GAS pharyngitis is one of the only upper respiratory infections whose diagnosis can easily be established using a widely available test. Failure to test for GAS suggests the overprescription of antibiotics without appropriate testing, which may contribute to the development of resistance. This measure serves as an important indicator of appropriate antibiotic use among all respiratory tract infections.

Reference

1. National Quality Measures Clearinghouse, National Committee for Quality Assurance Measure Summary: Appropriate testing for children with pharyngitis. Available at: http://www.guideline.gov/content.aspx?id=14937.

Chapter 31
Cough (Case 3)

Aaron S. Chidekel MD

Case: A 5-year-old has a tight, nocturnal cough for 4 weeks with posttussive emesis.

Differential Diagnosis

Infection	Asthma	Foreign body
Suppurative lung disease	Aspiration/dysphagia/gastroesophageal reflux	

Speaking Intelligently

In evaluating a child with cough, my first step is a quick clinical assessment. If the child is ill or in respiratory distress, the immediate focus is stabilization of the ABCs (airway, breathing, and circulation). Otherwise, the evaluation is individualized based on history and physical examination to avoid unnecessary testing. Although protracted cough is a significant parental stress and may disrupt family life, any treatment should focus on the underlying cause. It is critical to communicate the relative ineffectiveness of cough suppressants and the potential danger of adverse effects in young children and reported abuse by adolescents.

Cough is a vagally mediated reflex. An intact cough is critical to airway protection and clearance, and some normal children cough daily. Temporally cough is acute (<2 weeks), subacute (2 to 4 weeks), or chronic (>4 weeks). It may be part of an underlying illness or syndrome, such as cystic fibrosis (CF) or immunodeficiency, or more commonly a manifestation of an intercurrent viral infection. Rarely, there is a life-threatening problem such as foreign body aspiration. In cases of acute or even protracted cough associated with viral infection, no testing may be needed. For chronic cough, chest radiography and spirometry are recommended. Additional evaluation may include allergy testing, otolaryngologic evaluation, and sweat chloride analysis.

PATIENT CARE

Clinical Thinking

- **If the child is acutely ill or in respiratory distress, consider foreign body aspiration, pertussis in a young infant, severe laryngotracheitis (croup), bacterial tracheitis, or an asthma exacerbation.**
- Viral infection is the most common cause of acute coughing-related illness, whereas asthma and rhinosinusitis predominate in subacute and chronic cough.
- Environmental tobacco smoke (ETS) exposure is common and itself may cause chronic cough.
- A chronic productive or moist cough suggests underlying suppurative lung disease such as cystic fibrosis, or more commonly persistent bacterial bronchitis.
- A specific cause may not be determined, and despite this the cough will resolve.

History

- Consider **duration** and symptoms of acute or chronic illness.
- Evaluate potential respiratory **irritants, particularly ETS.**
- Review **vaccination status** and risk for exposure to infectious agents.
- Review of systems should be tailored, yet comprehensive enough to evaluate for systemic symptoms as well as emotional, neurologic, or other factors.
- *Common cough syndromes and clinical clues include:*
  - Asthma: Wheezing
  - Foreign body: Unequal breath sounds, wheezing
  - Pertussis: Paroxysmal coughing/inspiratory whoop
  - *Chlamydia:* Staccato cough/conjunctivitis
  - Croup: Barky cough/stridor
  - Tracheomalacia: Barky cough/stridor
  - Dysphagia/gastroesophageal reflux (GER)/aspiration: Cough may be associated with feeding
  - Suppurative lung disease*: Wet cough/clubbing/poor growth
  - Habit-cough syndrome: Honking sound/absent during sleep

Physical Examination

- Vital signs: Temperature, respiratory rate, oxygen saturation, and weight; **fever suggests infection, weight loss suggests more serious underlying illness.**
- Assess **work of breathing** (see Chapter 44, Difficulty Breathing).
- Characteristics of cough, if heard, should be described.
- Carefully examine head and neck to identify rhinosinusitis, which may be allergic or infectious (see Chapter 36, Fever).

*Examples include CF, ciliary dyskinesia, and immunodeficiency. (Modified from Landau LI: Acute and chronic cough, *Paediatr Respir Rev* 7S:S64-S67, 2006.)

- Assess chest wall symmetry and configuration
- Evaluate breath sounds for clarity and equality.
- Evaluate for clubbing of extremities.

Tests for Consideration

- **Complete blood count (CBC):** Lymphocytosis in pertussis; eosinophilia in *Chlamydia* — $139
- **Serology:** For *Mycoplasma* and hypersensitivity pneumonitis — $196 each
- **Immunoglobulin levels:** If suspected immunodeficiency — $167
- **Spirometry:** For asthma or other obstructive lung disease — $1352
- **Sweat chloride analysis:** If suspect CF — $125
- **Nasopharyngeal (NP) swab for pertussis polymerase chain reaction (PCR)** — $168
- **NP swab for viral studies:** Influenza, parainfluenza, adenovirus, RSV, metapneumovirus — $325
- **Tuberculin skin testing:** If exposure or risk factors — $174
- **Radioallergosorbent test (RAST), ImmunoCAP, or specific allergen skin testing:** If suspected allergy — $400
- **Bronchoscopy:** If foreign body aspiration, chronic infection, or suspected structural airway abnormality — $1400
- **pH probe or impedence probe testing:** In select cases to document GER — $5585
- **Endoscopy:** Is gold standard for GER diagnosis—consider in difficult-to-manage cases — $1313

IMAGING CONSIDERATIONS

→ **Chest radiograph** posteroanterior (PA) and lateral views: If chronic cough or suspected pneumonia or asthma complication — $231

→ **Lateral neck radiograph:** For suspected croup or epiglottitis — $150

→ **Sinus computed tomography (CT):** In select cases — $1716

→ **Airway fluoroscopy:** If foreign body aspiration — $225

→ **Chest CT:** If suspect suppurative lung disease — $1941

→ **Barium swallow:** If suspect anatomic abnormality such as vascular ring or H-type tracheoesophageal (TE) fistula — $840

→ **Videofluoroscopic swallow study:** If suspect dysphagia and/or aspiration — $840

→ **Nuclear medicine gastric emptying (milk scan):** If suspect GER; will quantify gastric emptying, and may document aspiration — $1118

Clinical Entities	Medical Knowledge

Infection

Pφ	The differential diagnosis is broad; however, viral *infection* is the most common cause of acute and subacute cough. Upper respiratory infection (URI)–associated coughing is related to direct mucosal infection and injury with exposure of cough receptors. This injury and cough receptor hypersensitivity can cause protracted cough.
TP	Cough with typical URI symptoms is most common. There are well-described infection-associated cough syndromes for pertussis, *Chlamydia*, croup, and bronchiolitis. Bacterial pneumonia often presents with high fever and respiratory distress, with cough a less-prominent feature. Acutely ill children may have respiratory distress and hypoxemia. See Chapter 44, Difficulty Breathing, and Chapter 36, Fever.
Dx	Diagnosis is usually clinical. Specific tests for pertussis and *Chlamydia* are available. If illness is severe or the child is immunocompromised or has an underlying disorder such as asthma, specific testing for viral agents may be indicated.
Tx	Treatment of viral infection is supportive. Treatment of a specific infection such as pertussis or *Chlamydia* should be instituted if strongly suspected pending confirmatory testing. Cough suppressants are typically ineffective and not recommended in children. A trial of bronchodilators or inhaled steroids may be initiated in select cases of protracted viral cough or acute bronchiolitis, but their use is not well supported by medical evidence. **See Nelson Essentials 102, 107, 108, 109, and 110.**

Asthma

Pφ	See Chapter 44, Difficulty Breathing.
TP	Chronic cough with recurrent wheezing is typical. Asthmatic coughing tends to be dry and tight, may be associated with posttussive emesis, and occurs more frequently after midnight with sleep disruption.

Dx	In children who can perform lung function testing, spirometry is the diagnostic gold standard. In young children the diagnosis is made clinically with appropriate signs and symptoms, after eliminating other potential diagnoses. A diagnostic/therapeutic trial of inhaled corticosteroids (ICSs) and bronchodilators for up to 4 weeks with avoidance of specific triggers may be a reasonable approach.
Tx	Treatment involves daily use of a low-dose ICS, and a bronchodilator to relieve acute symptoms. See Chapter 87, Status Asthmaticus. **See Nelson Essentials 78.**

Foreign Body

Pφ	Coughing secondary to *foreign body* aspiration occurs with partial airway obstruction, which may progress to complete obstruction and possible respiratory arrest.
TP	See Chapter 44, Difficulty Breathing. **See Nelson Essentials 136.**

Suppurative Lung Disease

Pφ	CF, primary ciliary dyskinesia (PCD), non-CF bronchiectasis, and immunodeficiency are examples of *suppurative lung disease.* Although the specific pathogenesis varies widely, within the lung, retention of secretions with resultant infection and inflammation leads to a vicious cycle leading to progressive lung damage. A more recently described condition, protracted bacterial bronchitis, which involves neutrophilic inflammation and bacterial infection in an otherwise healthy child, was the most common cause of subacute and chronic cough in a recent Australian study.
TP	The chronic cough begins early in life, occurs daily, and is wet or productive. It is often worse in the morning. There is risk for chronic airway infection, which must be aggressively sought and treated. CF, PCD, and immunodeficiency states are multisystem disorders, whereas non-CF bronchiectasis may be identified in isolation. CF is classically associated with failure to thrive, PCD with recurrent sinopulmonary infection and severe ear disease, and significant immunodeficiency with recurrent severe infections in multiple sites.

Dx	Specific testing will confirm the suspected diagnosis. Sweat chloride testing remains the gold standard in CF, but genetic testing and newborn screening have become more common. PCD is suspected with chronic or recurrent sinopulmonary infections and otitis and may be associated with situs inversus (Kartagener's syndrome). Biopsy of airway epithelium (nose or carinal trachea) and electron microscopy will confirm ultrastructural ciliary abnormalities.
Tx	Specific treatment is beyond the scope of this text. However, principles in management of any patient with chronic suppurative lung disease include close clinical monitoring, aggressive airway clearance, early diagnosis and treatment of respiratory tract infection, and possible chronic suppressive antibiotic therapy. Good nutrition and complete vaccination are also critical. Protracted bacterial bronchitis is treated with a single 2-week course of antibiotics. **See Nelson Essentials 73, 74, 75, 136, and 137.**

Aspiration/Dysphagia/Gastroesophageal Reflux

Pφ	The proximity of the respiratory and digestive tracts provides the basis of the pathogenesis of cough related to swallowing dysfunction and *gastroesophageal reflux (GER).* Direct entry of foreign material into the larynx or even the airway itself will cause cough. Chronic *aspiration* may become silent over time. The pathophysiology and frequency of cough related to GER are more complex and controversial. The mechanism is straightforward if reflux is severe enough to stimulate upper airway cough receptors with microaspiration and upper airway inflammation. However, the cause of respiratory symptoms attributed to isolated GER is less clear and most often attributed to vagal reflexes transmitted from the GI tract to the airway.
TP	Cough with aspiration and *dysphagia* is usually associated with feeding, most commonly thin liquids. There is often a predisposing underlying neurologic condition, neuromuscular disease, or prematurity.
Dx	Aspiration and dysphagia may be diagnosed by videofluoroscopic swallow study with a speech pathologist in attendance. GER may be detected in several ways, and the optimal study remains unclear. Upper endoscopy and prolonged esophageal monitoring with either a pH or impedance probe are highly sensitive, but invasive. Imaging studies such as nuclear medicine scanning (GER or milk scan) or an upper gastrointestinal series may be sufficient. GER is frequently diagnosed clinically.

Tx   Treatment should be individualized. Cold, thickened feeds can often overcome dysphagia and aspiration. Invasive tube feedings may be required, although every attempt is made to promote oral feeding. Initial management of GER is reflux precautions: small, frequent, thickened feedings with upright positioning after feeds. Medical management begins with acid blockade, or proton pump inhibitors in more severe cases. See Chapter 40, Feeding Difficulty. **See Nelson Essentials 128 and 136.**

ZEBRA ZONE

a. **Habit cough syndrome:** Severe cough in an otherwise well child that is absent during sleep and bothers everyone except the person coughing. Suggestion therapy and hypnosis may be indicated.

b. **H-type tracheoesophageal fistula:** See Chapter 75, Tracheoesophageal Fistula.

Practice-Based Learning and Improvement

Title
Evaluation and outcome of children with chronic cough

Author
Marchant JM

Reference
Chest 129:1132-1141, 2006

Problem
How to accurately diagnose etiology of chronic cough in children

Intervention
An adult-based diagnostic algorithm was applied to a cohort of 108 young children that included early flexible bronchoscopy.

Outcome/effect
The top three diagnoses in these children were (1) protracted bacterial bronchitis with airway neutrophilia, (2) natural resolution of the cough, and (3) bronchiectasis.

Historical significance/ comments
The three most common causes of cough in adults, namely, asthma, rhinosinusitis (upper airway cough syndrome), and gastroesophageal reflux, were uncommon in this cohort.

Interpersonal and Communication Skills

Use Open-Ended and Closed-Ended Questions Appropriately

Although it is desirable to conduct the history with open-ended questions, once the history has been obtained and you have begun to think through the differential diagnosis, it is appropriate to ask a few closed-ended questions to help narrow the possibilities. For the chief complaint of cough, some examples of closed-ended questions that might be appropriate include: Is it possible that the child could have choked on a toy or food? Have you noticed any abnormal noises when the child is breathing? Have you noticed any color change of the lips or skin when the child coughs? Use of closed-ended questions once the initial history has been taken will help prioritize items in the differential list.

Professionalism

Altruism: Balancing Personal and Professional Obligations

Case scenario: You are about to leave the office a little earlier than usual on a Friday afternoon when a mother calls begging for her child with asthma to be seen for what seems to be an acute flare. She does not want to go to the emergency department because she has had bad experiences with long waits and "too many chest x-rays." You are reluctant to treat this child over the telephone because she has needed hospital admission and intensive care unit (ICU) care on several occasions in the past. The family lives 5 minutes away.

Discussion: Being devoted to the welfare of your patients is part of professional responsibility. Physicians feel flattered when a patient or family wants to see only them because they have developed a relationship of trust. However, it is important to recognize when patients have become too dependent on you and are making unreasonable demands on your time.

In this scenario the telephone call is made during office hours and it seems reasonable to stay and see this patient because the patient can be in the office quickly. However, would the decision be different if the family lived farther away? If you were leaving the office because you had a social event to go to, would it be inappropriate to refuse the request? If you were leaving because of an important family event, would it be appropriate to refuse the request?

Balancing work and family/home life is one of the greatest challenges physicians face. Most of the time we sacrifice our own needs for those of our patients, but we face burnout and dysfunctional family relationships if we put no limits on our altruistic behavior. A healthy family and social life is essential for personal balance, which, in turn, is essential for being a good and effective clinician and caregiver.

Systems-Based Practice

Disclose Relevant Information to the Patient

Patients and parents need to be well informed about their medical conditions to enhance understanding and health-care decision making, decrease fear, and increase overall satisfaction with care. The **American College of Physicians** *Ethics Manual* outlines that physicians should disclose to patients information about procedural or judgment errors made during care, as long as the information is material to the patient's well-being. An error made by a physician or other member of the health-care team may not be negligent or even medically significant. Nonetheless, when reviewed retrospectively, the failure to disclose pertinent information in a timely manner may be considered problematic. If a physician is uncertain or feeling uncomfortable with any aspect of disclosure to a family, advice and guidance can be obtained from risk management. The pediatrician should also take cues from the family about the desired amount and depth of information presented.

Reference

1. Snyder L, Leffler C, for the Ethics and Human Rights Committee, American College of Physicians: *Ethics manual,* ed 5. *Ann Intern Med* 142(7): 560-582, 2005.

Chapter 32
Headache in Childhood (Case 4)

Marcy E. Yonker MD, FAHS

Case: An 8-year-old child with episodic headaches

Differential Diagnosis

Migraine	Tension-type headache	Acute sinusitis

Speaking Intelligently

When I evaluate a child with headache, I first determine the pattern of the headaches (episodic, daily with headache-free periods, daily without headache-free periods), and the tempo of the complaint (stable or progressive). If a child has progressively worsening headaches, I am more concerned about a serious cause. I inquire about the specific headache symptoms: location, nature, severity, duration, associated symptoms, exacerbating and ameliorating features to further refine whether this is a *primary headache disorder* such as migraine or tension-type headache, or if it may be *secondary to a neurologic problem* causing increased intracranial pressure like a brain tumor, venous sinus thrombosis, or pseudotumor cerebri. Most headache diagnoses are made clinically by taking a thorough history and performing complete medical and neurologic examinations. I rarely obtain an imaging study in a patient with episodic headaches and a normal examination.

PATIENT CARE

Clinical Thinking
- Healthy patients with episodic headaches and normal examinations rarely have a serious neurologic problem.
- **Migraines** in children are moderate to severe headaches that cause disability and are associated with light and sound avoidance and/or nausea/vomiting, and are usually relieved by sleep. Duration may be as short as 1 hour. Patients with infrequent migraines need only as-needed therapy. Patients with frequent (more than three to four disabling headaches per month) need both preventive and abortive therapy.
- Children with **progressive headaches** without significant migrainous features, or with concerning neurologic symptoms/signs such as intellectual deterioration, gait ataxia, double vision or seizures, need urgent evaluation and imaging.
- **Sinus headaches** are caused by acute obstruction of the osteomeatal complex and are associated with nasal discharge, postnasal drip and/ or chronic cough. Chronic sinus disease that does not obstruct the drainage of nasal secretions usually does not cause headache (see Chapter 36, Fever).

History
- Note onset of headaches and any inciting incidents (head trauma, illness, change in medications such as oral contraceptives, stressful events). Emergent evaluation and neuroimaging may be required for head trauma to exclude intracranial hemorrhage or concussion syndrome (see Chapter 86, Trauma).
- Note nature of headaches: gradual versus sudden onset of pain, description of pain, severity of pain, location, exacerbating/ ameliorating features.

- Note presence of migraine-associated symptoms such as light sensitivity, sound sensitivity, nausea, vomiting, exacerbation by or avoidance of routine physical activities.
- Note presence of migraine aura preceding or during headache, such as flashing lights, black spots, vertigo, or paresthesias, that clears within 1 hour.
- Headaches that awaken a patient from sleep or reach maximal intensity abruptly are concerning for a headache caused by an intracranial process such as increased intracranial pressure or intracranial bleed.
- Headache, stiff neck, vomiting, and/or change in mental status is concerning for meningitis (see Chapter 49, Meningitis).

Physical Examination
- Vital signs: Systolic hypertension may be secondary to ongoing headache pain or increased intracranial pressure. Obesity is associated with pseudotumor cerebri.
- A thorough general examination including inspection of the tympanic membranes and oropharynx and palpation of the face to exclude otitis media, mastoiditis, and sinusitis
- A complete neurologic examination including visualization of the optic discs and observation of venous pulsations to help rule out increased intracranial pressure is mandatory.
- Neurologic examination should exclude any focal neurologic abnormalities such as focal weakness, dysmetria, ataxia, or focal sensory loss.

Tests for Consideration
- **Lyme titers:** If an endemic area or other symptoms such as fever, erythema migrans rash, arthritis $180
- **Lumbar puncture:** With measurement of opening pressure
  - **Enterovirus cerebrospinal fluid (CSF) polymerase chain reaction (PCR)** $300
  - **Lyme CSP PCR** $180
  - **Gram stain CSF** $180
  - **Culture CSF** $152
  - **Cell count CSF** $150
  - **Glucose CSF** $75
  - **Protein CSF** $75

IMAGING CONSIDERATIONS

→ Urgent **magnetic resonance imaging (MRI) scan of the brain:** If papilledema, abnormal neurologic examination, or seizures $1331

→ Urgent **computed tomography (CT) scan of the brain:** Followed by lumbar puncture if abrupt onset of severe headache symptoms suggestive of intracranial hemorrhage $1827

→ **Sinus CT** in select cases $1716

Clinical Entities	Medical Knowledge

Migraine

Pφ	The exact cause of *migraine* is not known, though it is typically inherited as an autosomal dominant disorder with variable penetrance. Several genes have been identified for a rare type of migraine—familial hemiplegic migraine.
TP	Children typically present with episodes of headache associated with avoidance of light and sound and/or nausea or vomiting. They stop their routine activities and seek isolation. They sleep, and when they awaken, the headache has typically resolved. Their neurologic examinations are typically normal unless they suffer from another, unrelated neurologic condition.
Dx	Diagnosis is made with clinical findings and appropriate history. Imaging is typically unnecessary.
Tx	Treatment may consist of as-needed medications such as over-the-counter nonsteroidal medications given at an appropriate mg/kg dose, antiemetics, or migraine-specific medications such as 5-HT-1 agonists (triptans) or ergotamines. Patients with frequent migraines may require a period of prophylaxis. Agents used include cyproheptadine, tricyclic antidepressants, beta-blockers, calcium channel blockers, and anticonvulsants such as valproic acid or topiramate. **See Nelson Essentials 180.**

Tension-Type Headache

Pφ	The cause of *tension-type headache* is unknown.
TP	Tension-type headaches differ from migraines in that they are described as bandlike headaches across the frontal region that are mild to moderate in intensity, without migraine-associated symptoms and not aggravated by routine physical activities.
Dx	Diagnosis is clinical with a normal examination
Tx	Treatment may include reassurance, identification and avoidance of the stressor, psychotherapy, biofeedback training, and avoidance of nonsteroidal medication overuse (more than twice a week). Patients with chronic tension-type headache (more than 15 days per month) may also benefit from low-dose tricyclic antidepressant therapy. **See Nelson Essentials 180.**

Acute Sinusitis	
Pφ	See Chapter 36, Fever.
TP	Older children may complain of head pain in the sinus regions in addition to congestion, cough, and possibly fever.
Dx	Diagnosis can be made on clinical grounds although imaging may be supportive in select cases.
Tx	See Chapter 36, Fever. **See Nelson Essentials 104.**

ZEBRA ZONE

a. **Pseudotumor cerebri:** Increased intracranial pressure without a mass or obstructive hydrocephalus or other pathology. There is elevated opening pressure (>200 mm Hg) on lumbar puncture (LP) and normal neuroimaging. LP is both diagnostic and therapeutic. It may be idiopathic or associated with obesity or some medications: tetracyclines, human growth hormone, oral contraceptives, tretinoin (Retin-A), and hypervitaminosis A and D. Imaging of the brain's venous drainage in addition to MRI is done to exclude venous sinus thrombosis causing decreased cerebrospinal fluid (CSF) absorption resulting from back pressure. Acetazolamide is prescribed if the initial LP is not curative.

b. **Posterior fossa tumors:** Classically cause occipital headache, papilledema, palsy of cranial nerves III and VI, and a wide-based gait with obstructive hydrocephalus.

Practice-Based Learning and Improvement

Title
Practice parameter: Evaluation of children and adolescents with recurrent headaches

Authors
Lewis DW, Ashwal S, Dahl G, et al

Reference
Neurology 59:490-498, 2002

Practice parameter with review
Review of the evidence for evaluation of children with headaches

Outcome/effect
Most children with recurrent headache do not require diagnostic workup.

Historical significance/comments
Refutes the need for electroencephalogram (EEG) in the evaluation of headache, formerly a common clinical practice

Interpersonal and Communication Skills

Provide Reassurance and Acknowledge Fear of "Worst-Case Scenario"

Many patients and their parents are concerned about brain tumors even when headaches are infrequent. Reassurance regarding this issue is important in any child with headaches. Patient education regarding healthy habits such as diet and exercise and proper use of prescribed medications will improve patient satisfaction and outcome.

Professionalism

Understanding the Impact of School Absence

Although migraines are not a life-threatening problem, many patients with migraine suffer from severe disability and discomfort at the time of their attack. Many patients are unfairly accused of shirking school responsibilities or being depressed because they have frequent headaches. Acknowledging this and helping the patient and parents deal with this prejudice are important in implementing the treatment plan.

Systems-Based Practice

Compliance With Clinical Practice Guidelines

A pediatrician may be inclined to obtain an imaging study of a child with recurrent headache because of fear of malpractice and/or parental worry about a bad diagnosis causing the headache. The American College of Radiology (ACR) Appropriateness Criteria on Headache-Child outlines criteria recommended by their expert panel for determining appropriate imaging examinations in children with headache. Headaches are common, but intracranial pathology is relatively rare. In isolated nonprogressive headache or migraine without neurologic signs, an imaging study is not recommended.

Features such as vomiting, awakening from sleep or headache on rising, or intense prolonged headaches without a family history of migraine, presence of seizure, or abnormal findings on examination such as nystagmus, papilledema, or abnormal gait all increase the likelihood of a positive scan.[1]

Computed tomography (CT) is associated with increased radiation exposure when compared with conventional radiology, and the effects are cumulative. Epidemiologic data to support increased risk for cancer from typical doses of radiation incurred in CT scans are derived from cancer incidence and mortality data among atomic-bomb survivors. Children are more vulnerable to these adverse effects given the greater number of dividing cells and increased longevity compared with adults, providing more time for latent cancers to develop.[2] As data accumulate about latent risk from CT radiation, it is imperative to be aware of guideline recommendations (and the quality of their evidence base) to optimize safe care and diagnostic accuracy.

References

1. Strain JD: ACR appropriateness criteria on headache-child. *J Am Coll Radiol* 4:18-23, 2007.
2. Brenner DJ, Hall EJ: Computed tomography: An increasing source of radiation exposure. *N Engl J Med* 357:2277-2284, 2007.

Chapter 33
Eye Pain and Discharge (Case 5)

Lisa Humphrey MD

Case: 12-year-old boy with right eye pain and discharge

Differential Diagnosis

Conjunctivitis	Orbital cellulitis		Preseptal cellulitis
Corneal abrasion		Foreign body	

Speaking Intelligently

In evaluating a child with eye pain, I first check for a history of trauma. My focus is on visual acuity, extraocular mobility, and the state of the eyelid, sclera, and pupil. If there has been trauma, I quickly assess for immediate problems such as foreign body, hyphema, or corneal abrasion. More serious trauma (e.g., penetrating injuries) will rarely present in the outpatient setting. If there is no trauma history, I evaluate for infection by taking a history for fever, sinusitis, herpes, chickenpox, or other etiology. Most cases of eye pain and discharge are due to conjunctivitis and treated symptomatically or with a topical antibiotic.

PATIENT CARE

Clinical Thinking
- Evaluate for **trauma** such as globe rupture or penetrating **foreign body,** both ophthalmologic emergencies that mandate immediate consultation. Delay in definitive diagnosis and treatment could result in permanent impairment of vision or blindness.
- A child with **suspected orbital cellulitis requires immediate evaluation** for extension of infection to the central nervous system (CNS).
- Children hate to have their eyes examined, especially when they are already in pain and afraid. It can be difficult to make even simple diagnoses, and consultation with an ophthalmologist may be required.

History
- Is there a history of trauma or foreign body?
- Has there been any contact with children with similar symptoms? Is there fever or other systemic signs of illness?
- Are there signs of upper respiratory illness?
- Is there local skin infection (e.g., impetigo)?
- Can the pain be localized (i.e., lid, conjunctiva)?
- How quickly have symptoms evolved?

Physical Examination
- Fever suggests infection.
- Rash may point to a systemic illness.
- Evaluate for meningeal signs; if the eye pain is due to orbital cellulitis, there could be extension to the brain.
- Always try to assess/document **visual acuity** in each eye.
- Are there signs of trauma or lesions of the globe, sclera, conjunctiva, or eyelids?
- Is there decreased visual acuity, impaired extraocular mobility, impaired pupillary response, or proptosis?
- Are eyelids edematous or discolored?

- Are the **conjunctivae inflamed?** If there is discharge, what is the nature?
- Are there local skin lesions (e.g., an insect bite) as the source of contiguous infection?

Tests for Consideration

- **Fluorescein examination:** Of the sclera for abrasions, or dendritic or ulcerative lesions consistent with keratitis $110
- **Complete blood count (CBC) with differential:** If ill-appearing $116
- **Blood culture:** If febrile and/or toxic appearing with concern for preseptal or orbital cellulitis $152
- **Erythrocyte sedimentation rate (ESR):** To monitor response to therapy in orbital cellulitis $85
- **C-reactive protein (CRP):** To monitor response to therapy in orbital cellulitis $69
- **Slit-lamp examination:** If concern for uveitis   Variable cost by ophthalmology
- **Visual acuity testing** $180

IMAGING CONSIDERATIONS

→ **CT scan with contrast of the orbits, sinuses, and brain:** For suspected orbital cellulitis $1827

Clinical Entities   Medical Knowledge

Conjunctivitis

Pφ   Two thirds of pediatric **conjunctivitis** ("pink eye") is due to bacterial organisms, with viral infections accounting for the rest. Nontypable *Hemophilus influenzae* (HiNT) are the most common bacterial isolates, followed by *Streptococcus pneumoniae* and *Moraxella catarrhalis*. *Neisseria gonorrhoeae* and *Chlamydia trachomatis* occur rarely in neonates who have received prophylaxis. Adenovirus is the most common viral etiology. Enteroviruses cause epidemics of acute hemorrhagic conjunctivitis. Infectious agents are usually inoculated by contaminated hands or aerosolized droplets.

TP   There is conjunctival erythema, discharge, and mild discomfort, and possible photophobia or chemosis (conjunctival edema). Bacterial conjunctivitis is typically acute in onset, with mucopurulent exudate. The onset of a viral infection is typically unilateral, often subacute with clear discharge, but either bacterial or viral infections may be unilateral or bilateral. There may also be otitis media in infants and toddlers.

Dx   The diagnosis is usually clinical—significant injection of the
      palpebral conjunctiva helps to distinguish conjunctivitis from
      other entities. Infants and toddlers should be checked for otitis
      media. Cultures may be indicated with suboptimal response to
      therapy. Cultures (requiring specialized medium/collection) are
      warranted in neonates if chlamydia, gonorrhea, or herpes
      simplex virus is suspected, along with evaluation for systemic
      infection.

Tx   Bacterial conjunctivitis is self-limiting but responds faster with
      topical ophthalmic antibiotics such as polymyxin B/
      trimethoprim. Quinolone drops are effective but more expensive
      and reserved for difficult-to-treat cases. Drops are easier to
      instill and better tolerated than ointments. For conjunctivitis-
      otitis, oral antibiotics alone are generally adequate. Caution
      patients to avoid letting the tip of the bottle contact the
      conjunctiva and contaminate topical medications.
          Practically speaking, the difficulty of distinguishing viral
      from bacterial conjunctivitis in addition to school/day care
      policies prohibiting return until "on treatment," results in
      routine treatment of presumed viral conjunctivitis with topical
      antibiotics. Children with active discharge and symptoms should
      avoid school until clear, given the contagiousness of
      adenovirus. If symptoms worsen or fail to improve, a slit-lamp
      examination should be considered. If neonatal chlamydia is
      suspected, oral or intravenous erythromycin is required to
      prevent pneumonia. Neonatal gonococcal ophthalmias is treated
      with parenteral antibiotics. **See Nelson Essentials 119.**

Orbital Cellulitis

Pφ   *Orbital cellulitis* most often results from extension of ipsilateral
      sinusitis causing subperiosteal abscess or phlegmon and can
      involve inflammation of all tissues posterior to the orbital
      septum. The most common organisms are those found in acute
      and chronic sinusitis: pneumococcus, HiNT, *M. catarrhalis*,
      Staphylococcus aureus, and respiratory tract anaerobes.

TP   Classically, there is prodrome of upper respiratory infection
      (URI), followed by sudden onset of unilateral eyelid edema and
      erythema, with complaints of eye pain, especially with eye
      movement. Fever is common, and the child may appear quite
      ill. There may be proptosis, decreased visual acuity, diplopia,
      abnormal pupillary reflexes, and impaired extraocular muscle
      movement. These findings may be difficult to ascertain on
      examination due to patient anxiety and lid swelling with
      inability to open the eye.

Dx	History and physical examination findings will prompt a computed tomography (CT) scan of the orbits to confirm the diagnosis and typical preexisting sinusitis. White blood cell (WBC) count and acute phase reactants are typically elevated. Blood cultures are usually negative.
Tx	This is an ophthalmologic emergency, and intravenous antibiotics such as ampicillin/sulbactam are empirically administered. Clindamycin is used if methicillin-resistant *S. aureus* (MRSA) is a concern. Otolaryngology and ophthalmology are consulted for consideration of surgical intervention. Surgery is indicated for abscess drainage, significant impairment of visual acuity, or worsening of clinical symptoms on intravenous antibiotics. Following clinical improvement, therapy is changed to a comparable oral antibiotic with close outpatient follow-up. If a blood or surgical culture yields an organism, antibiotic coverage may be altered accordingly. Duration of therapy is individualized based on severity of presentation, the organism, and overall response to treatment. **See Nelson Essentials 104 and 119.**

Preseptal Cellulitis

Pφ	***Preseptal or periorbital cellulitis*** is infection of the eyelid and surrounding soft tissues, commonly due to contiguous skin infection or break in the integrity of the skin. It can extend to, but not past, the orbital septum. Before *H. influenzae* type b (Hib) vaccine licensure, the cause was usually hematogenous spread of typable *H. influenzae*. In ipsilateral acute sinusitis, there may be sterile inflammatory changes from venous stasis in the preseptal area. These conditions are always unilateral. There is no paralysis of extraocular movement or proptosis with a preseptal process. It may be difficult to distinguish orbital from periorbital cellulitis on examination, but they have distinctly different mechanisms and microbiology.
TP	See Table 33-1.
Dx	Physical examination can be challenging and inconclusive because children are likely to be uncooperative, and edema may prevent adequate assessment of extraocular eye movements. There is significant likelihood that CT will be required.
Tx	See Table 33-1. **See Nelson Essentials 104 and 119.**

| Table 33-1 | Diagnosis and Management of Preseptal Cellulitis | | | |
Etiology	Presentation	Pathogens	Diagnosis	Treatment
Preseptal cellulitis Trauma/contiguous skin infection	Often acute redness, swelling of lids, not systemically ill; entry site may not be visible	Group A beta-hemolytic streptococcus (GAS) S. aureus	Culture from wound if available	Often parenteral, because of rapid progression: MRSA and GAS coverage
Bacteremic periorbital cellulitis	Acute onset following URI, high fever, sometimes toxic child	Historically, H. influenzae, type b; now, S. pneumoniae	Elevated WBC, CRP, ESR; blood culture sometimes positive	Parenteral antibiotics active against S. pneumoniae
Preseptal inflammatory edema resulting from sinusitis	Subacute onset, URI symptoms; usually well appearing	Periorbital tissues are sterile; acute paranasal sinuses infected with: S. pneumoniae, HiNT, M. catarrhalis	Sinus radiographs show ipsilateral changes of sinusitis	Attempt oral antibiotic directed at acute sinus pathogens if well appearing

Corneal Abrasion

Pφ	This is superficial trauma to the corneal epithelium.
TP	There may be a foreign body sensation in the eye or pain with or without eye movement. In addition, there will be lacrimation, photophobia, and conjunctival erythema. There is often a history of antecedent eye trauma.
Dx	Fluorescein dye illuminated with ultraviolet light will demonstrate the corneal defect. A slit-lamp examination may be indicated if more extensive damage is suspected.
Tx	Topical antibiotics are used until the lesion is healed. Protective patching is no longer advised. Simple **corneal abrasions** should have outpatient follow-up with expected healing in approximately 24 hours.

Foreign Body

Pφ	An object or substance is imposed in the cornea or deeper, typically by trauma.
TP	There may be a sensation of something in the eye or focal eye pain, tearing, photophobia, and scleral injection.
Dx	Identification is by gross visual inspection or slit-lamp examination.
Tx	Some **foreign bodies** can be flushed out with irrigation or with a cotton-tip swab. However, some need to be removed by an ophthalmologist, requiring urgent consultation.

ZEBRA ZONE

a. **Infectious keratitis:** Deep corneal infection with bacterial or viral etiology that is most common in contact lens wearers and others with local or systemic risk factors. Rare, but has the potential to cause blindness—an ophthalmologic emergency.

b. **Endophthalmitis:** Intraocular infection resulting from bacteria or fungi that is often secondary to surgery or trauma—an ophthalmologic emergency.

c. **Uveitis:** Intraocular inflammation causing pain and redness, most often resulting from autoimmune diseases (e.g., juvenile idiopathic arthritis [JIA]).

Practice-Based Learning and Improvement: Evidence-Based Pediatrics

Title
Medical management of orbital cellulitis

Authors
Starkey CR, Steele RW

Reference
Pediatr Infect Dis J 20:1002-1005, 2001

Problem
Could orbital cellulitis be managed with fewer surgical interventions, given the availability of better imaging studies?

Outcome/effect
Prospective study showed greater than 90% of cases could be managed nonsurgically.

Historical significance/comments
Like many other abscesses, more orbital abscesses can be managed nonsurgically with the use of accurate serial imaging studies (e.g., CT scans).

Interpersonal and Communication Skills

Communicate Accurately With Consultants

When a patient needs emergent care, the primary physician needs to effectively and efficiently obtain the necessary support to care for the patient. This requires an effective toolbox of interpersonal skills to be able to communicate the patient's needs in a professional but convincing manner. If a patient with probable orbital cellulitis arrives in the emergency department at midnight on a weekend, the patient merits imaging by the radiology technician, imaging interpretation by the radiologist, and consultation by ophthalmology. These personnel may not be present on site. Before calling a consult, review your facts, generate your clinical question, and then make a concise presentation. By taking this pause, you ensure that you have clarity on what you are asking your consultant, which will ensure that he/she will be able to help answer your question appropriately.

Professionalism

Honesty in Discussing Clinical Outcomes

The course and outcome of medical emergencies such as globe rupture are dependent on many variables, only some of which can be controlled. Although a clinical outcome may be uncertain, information must be provided to the patient and family in a way that gives neither false hope nor an overly pessimistic prediction for what the outcome might be. A physician may be tempted to describe a worse-than-expected outcome so that he/she will "look like a hero" when the actual outcome is better or in the belief that this course of action might avoid a lawsuit.

Physicians must always be honest and straightforward with patients. Returning to a family and patient to discuss a poor outcome is always a difficult conversation but should never be avoided or delegated.

Systems-Based Practice

School Attendance Policy and Physician Prescribing Patterns

The cost of bacterial cultures as well as the time required to obtain results makes this method of determining etiology of conjunctivitis in the common pediatric population relatively impractical and not cost-efficient.[1]

Very often, social factors, including the need for children to attend day care or school and for parents to go to work, contribute to the decision to prescribe antibiotics for children with acute infective conjunctivitis. Understanding these issues and changing school policies in line with national guidance may reduce pressure on physicians to prescribe for this condition.[2]

References

1. McNier ML: The physician's ability to clinically differentiate between bacterial and viral conjunctivitis is poor unless additional physical findings of otitis media or pharyngitis are present. Critically appraised topic. Available at http://www.med.umich.edu/pediatrics/ebm/cats/conjdx.htm
2. Rose PW, Ziebland S, Harnden A, et al: Why do general practitioners prescribe antibiotics for acute infective conjunctivitis in children? Qualitative interviews with GPs and a questionnaire survey of parents. *Fam Practice* 23(2):226-232, 2006. Available at http://fampra.oxfordjournals.org/cgi/content/full/23/2/226

Chapter 34
Diarrhea (Case 6)

Daniel Walmsley DO

Case: A 2-year-old boy with 2 days of vomiting, fever, and diarrhea. He attends day care and has been less active, drinking and voiding less than usual.

Differential Diagnosis

Viral gastroenteritis	Bacterial gastroenteritis	Protozoan and parasitic infections
Pseudomembranous colitis	Malabsorption	Inflammatory bowel disease (IBD)

Speaking Intelligently

Diarrhea in infants and children is usually infectious. When evaluating a child with diarrhea, I first check for signs of dehydration. Key findings that may lead to further investigation of the cause include gross blood in the stool, a toxic appearance, or diarrhea following antibiotic use. Gross blood may indicate a bacterial etiology. It is important to pay close attention to infants under 2 months of age and toxic-appearing children, because they are more likely to become dehydrated. Most acute episodes of diarrhea last 14 days or less; therefore illness duration is an important consideration in forming a differential diagnosis. A thorough assessment is done to determine the degree of dehydration, the child's ability to tolerate oral fluids, and whether intravenous fluid administration is required.

PATIENT CARE

Clinical Thinking
- Is the dehydration significant enough to require IV fluid administration, or will the parents be able to orally rehydrate?
- Is there a bacterial cause?
- Are there electrolyte abnormalities that require specific interventions?

History
- **Assess hydration status:** Inquire about the number of stools, emesis, frequency and amount of urination, and overall activity level.

Tx   Treatment of all infectious diarrhea is basically the same.
      Supportive care with fluid repletion is the mainstay. The type
      of fluid rehydration depends on the degree of dehydration,
      with severely dehydrated children requiring IV repletion. Oral
      rehydration therapy (ORT) with glucose- and electrolyte-
      containing solutions such as Pedialyte or Infalyte is considered
      the best option but may not be possible in children who are
      not tolerating fluids, are excessively vomiting, or are severely
      dehydrated. ORT should initially be given in frequent small
      volumes and advanced slowly. A child who is significantly
      dehydrated may benefit from initial IV fluids followed by an
      oral challenge to see if the child can be maintained without
      continued IV fluids. Early refeeding has been shown to result in
      faster resolution. Antidiarrheal medications such as loperamide
      can delay transit time and prolong the diarrhea, and should be
      avoided. Probiotics such as lactobacillus have been shown to
      reduce stool output and duration of diarrhea by altering
      intestinal flora. **See Nelson Essentials 112.**

Bacterial Gastroenteritis

Pφ   Several pathologic mechanisms produce bacterial diarrhea.
      These include enterotoxin production and direct cell invasion
      and destruction. This destruction leads to an impaired ability to
      absorb certain foods and digest complex carbohydrates,
      resulting in both a secretory and osmotic form of diarrhea.
      Some bacteria like *Staphylococcus aureus* and enterotoxigenic
      Escherichia coli, the cause of traveler's diarrhea, produce
      cytotoxins that directly cause intestinal cell damage resulting
      in diarrhea. Salmonella, in particular, may cause systemic illness
      by invading enterocytes and subsequently entering the
      bloodstream, which may lead to bacteremia, osteomyelitis, or
      meningitis. Other bacterial pathogens include *Campylobacter,
      Salmonella, Shigella, Vibrio cholerae, Bacillus cereus, Aeromonas
      hydrophila,* and *Clostridium difficile.*

TP   There are diarrhea and fever, but vomiting is less common.
      The diarrhea may be bloody. There may be a history of travel
      or abdominal pain. The incubation period can range from
      1 to 7 days. The presentation of *Yersinia* infection may mimic
      appendicitis.

Dx   A stool culture will identify the specific pathogen. Fecal
      leukocytes on Wright stain suggests a bacterial etiology, but
      they may also be present in IBD or milk protein intolerance in
      infants.

Tx   See treatment of viral gastroenteritis above. Fluid and
     electrolyte resuscitation is provided as needed. Antibiotics
     should not be routinely used in acute bloody diarrhea until the
     specific pathogen is identified by culture. Antibiotics are
     indicated for certain infections, such as *Campylobacter* and
     Shigella in all ages, for *Salmonella* in infants under 3 months of
     age, and in any age with bacteremia. **See Nelson Essentials
     112.**

Protozoan and Parasitic Infections

Pφ   These organisms invade enterocytes, leading to intestinal
     inflammation, villous atrophy, and malabsorption. The
     protozoans typically invade intestinal cells in the trophozoite
     stage. Examples include *Giardia lamblia, Entamoeba histolytica,
     Cryptosporidium parvum,* and *Isospora belli.*

TP   Symptoms may vary depending on the organism. There may be
     gradual onset of colicky abdominal pain with flatulence and
     frequent stools and profuse diarrhea containing blood or mucus.
     Foul-smelling diarrhea, abdominal distention, gastroesophageal
     reflux, and frequent loose stools accompany *Giardia* infections.
     The diarrhea is often chronic, lasting more than 14 days. Travel
     to an endemic area such as a tropical country is a risk factor.
     Cryptosporidium should be considered in immunocompromised
     patients and those in day care.

Dx   Stool for ova and parasites should be sent for 3 consecutive
     days. *Giardia* can also be identified in a specific stool antigen
     test.

Tx   Supportive care with fluid repletion is the cornerstone of
     treatment. Many protozoan and parasitic infections are also
     treated with metronidazole. **See Nelson Essentials 112.**

Pseudomembranous Colitis

Pφ   Antibiotic-associated diarrhea is due to the overgrowth of
     toxin-producing *Clostridium* organisms in the bowel. Antibiotics
     are the culprit because they often disrupt the normal intestinal
     flora, leading to this bacterial overgrowth. *C. difficile* organisms
     then release enterotoxins that lead to mucosal injury and
     inflammation, resulting in formation of a shallow ulcer on the
     mucosal surface, which characterizes the colonic
     pseudomembrane. It can also be transmitted as a primary
     pathogen.

TP	There are acute watery diarrhea with lower abdominal pain, fever, and leukocytosis.
Dx	Identification of the *C. difficile* cytotoxins A and/or B is diagnostic.
Tx	Fluid repletion is administered as needed. Metronidazole is the primary treatment. The inciting antibiotics should be stopped. Severe infection or bowel perforation may require surgery. Probiotics can help replete normal intestinal flora. **See Nelson Essentials 112.**

Malabsorption

Pφ	*Malabsorption* typically occurs as an osmotic diarrhea in which an added absorbable solute is not absorbed properly. This solute draws water into the gut lumen by altering its concentration gradient. This additional solute results from the inability to break down certain complex carbohydrates such as lactose, which can occur because of a lactase deficiency or from a lack of pancreatic enzymes as in cystic fibrosis. Celiac disease also results in malabsorption secondary to villous atrophy resulting from gliadin intolerance.
TP	There is usually chronic watery diarrhea. Other systemic findings include failure to thrive, frequent respiratory infections, or anemia suggesting the overall disorder. Lactase deficiency is a transient problem in younger children, often secondary to an episode of gastroenteritis in which mucosal injury leads to the deficiency. Older children may develop a primary lactase deficiency. A child with cystic fibrosis may present with failure to thrive and a history of frequent respiratory infections. Celiac disease can present as chronic diarrhea and anemia, or more commonly is asymptomatic.
Dx	Tests for stool-reducing substances will detect complex carbohydrates in the stool. In addition, specific tests for cystic fibrosis, celiac disease, or lactase deficiency can be pursued based on clinical suspicion.
Tx	Treatment of the underlying disorder will correct the diarrhea. In cystic fibrosis specific pancreatic enzymes are taken with each meal. Celiac disease is treated by avoidance of gluten, and lactase deficiency by avoidance of lactase-containing products. **See Nelson Essentials 126, 129, and 137.**

Inflammatory Bowel Disease

Pφ The exact mechanism of *IBD* is unknown, but the common final pathway is inflammation. Inflammation leads to ulceration, edema, and bleeding. Ulcerative colitis involves the colonic superficial mucosa and always involves the rectum with a variable degree of proximal involvement. Crohn's disease is a transmural disease, affecting anywhere from the mouth to the anus, and is characterized by skip lesions and noncaseating granulomas.

TP The first episode may present as acute bloody diarrhea. There is often a history of weight loss, poor growth, recurrent abdominal pain, aphthous ulcers, arthritis, and anal skin tags. In addition, a prolonged duration of bloody diarrhea suggests IBD. In rare cases, a child will present with growth failure without gastrointestinal symptoms.

Dx Either ulcerative colitis or Crohn's disease should be suspected based on clinical signs such as growth failure, anemia, abdominal pain, or bloody diarrhea. Laboratory testing may show increased white blood cells, platelets, sedimentation rate, and C-reactive protein in addition to decreased albumin. There may be fecal leukocytes. Precise diagnosis is confirmed by colonoscopy and endoscopy with biopsy and visualization of characteristic features.

Tx Treatment involves management of flares in addition to preventive therapy that is specific to the disease. Most treatment involves immunomodulators such as corticosteroids, aminosalicylates, methotrexate, and infliximab. Any concurrent infection is also treated, usually with metronidazole. **See Nelson Essentials 129.**

ZEBRA ZONE

a. **Hemolytic uremic syndrome:** May follow an infection, typically *E. coli* O157:H7 with hemolytic anemia, thrombocytopenia, and renal failure.

b. **Toddler's diarrhea:** Is a common benign condition associated with excessive fluid intake, especially juice.

Practice-Based Learning and Improvement

Title
Oral versus IV rehydration of modestly dehydrated children: A randomized, controlled trial

Authors
Spandorfer P, Alessandrini EA, Joffe MD, et al

Reference
Pediatrics 115:295-301, 2005

Problem
Oral rehydration therapy (ORT) is recommended as the first-line treatment in mild to moderate dehydration secondary to viral gastroenteritis, but is infrequently used in emergency departments.

Intervention
Young children with viral gastroenteritis randomized to receive ORT or intravenous (IV) IV fluids over 4 hours in an emergency department setting

Outcome/effect
ORT is as effective as IV fluids for rehydration of moderately dehydrated children.

Interpersonal and Communication Skills

Check for Parental Willingness to Follow the Treatment Plan: Check for Understanding and Ability to Follow Treatment Plan

Important information to share with families in regard to diarrhea is signs and symptoms of dehydration and how to orally rehydrate a child at home. It is important to verify that the family understands the plan and is willing to follow the instructions at home, or the child will shortly be back in your office or the emergency department.

Professionalism

Impact of the Physician-Family Relationship on Compliance

Diarrhea is an illness that calls for parents to spend a lot of time and energy changing diapers and ensuring that their child is hydrated. Your job as the physician is to give the information and recommendations to manage this illness and prevent complications such as significant dehydration. A recent study showed that patients who felt more connected to their primary care physician were more likely to follow their doctor's recommendations.[1] Building a relationship with children and parents at well visits will help build their trust in your care and hopefully lead to their following your recommendations during episodes of illness.

Reference

1. Atlas SJ, Grant RW, Ferris TG, et al: Patient-physician connectedness and quality of primary care. *Ann Intern Med* 150(5):325-335, 2009.

Chapter 35
Constipation (Case 7)

Gerald M. Fendrick MD

Case: A 6-year-old boy with infrequent bowel movements, every 6 to 7 days. Stools are large, hard, and painful to pass and have clogged the toilet. There are frequent soiling and malodor. Embarrassment in school prompted this visit. Abdominal examination was positive for what appeared to be large amounts of stool in the lower left abdomen.

Differential Diagnosis

| Functional constipation | Hirschsprung disease | Hypothyroidism |

Speaking Intelligently

When I evaluate a patient with constipation, the term has to be defined. Is the definition based on frequency of stools or quality of the stool? Once it is established that constipation is really present, I ask myself if the history and physical examination lean toward a diagnosis of **functional** or **organic** constipation. There is a long differential diagnosis for constipation; however, functional constipation, which is the etiology in 95% of cases, must be considered first. Questions should be asked about the time of the first bowel movement after birth (which most parents will not know or recall), toilet training history, bowel history, treatment attempted for the problem, and medications and dietary habits. Constipation may also be accompanied by complaints of abdominal pain, decreased appetite, irritability, and occasionally vomiting.

PATIENT CARE

Clinical Thinking
- Is there fecal impaction?
- Does the history or physical examination suggest an organic etiology?
- What are the course and duration of constipation?

History
- Is time of first meconium passage known?
- Did constipation begin around toilet training?
- Did constipation begin with attendance at preschool or grade school?
- Have there been any dietary changes?
- A recent viral syndrome may cause transient ileus.
- Is the child on medications (including over-the-counter preparations), such as calcium, iron, antihistamines, anticholinergics, diuretics, or opiates?
- Are symptoms present to suggest an endocrine, metabolic, or neuromuscular problem?
- Are there any associated gastrointestinal (GI) abnormalities, such as failure to thrive or gastroesophageal reflux disease (GERD)?
- **Functional constipation can be accurately diagnosed with history and physical examination, and *additional testing is usually not indicated*.**

Physical Examination
- Note general well-being and overall nutritional status, looking for signs of systemic disease.
- Review height, weight, body mass index (BMI), and prior growth pattern.

- Palpate the neck for thyromegaly.
- Perform an abdominal examination with particular attention to overall contour, bowel sounds, and palpation and percussion for presence of masses or stool. Note quality of abdominal musculature.
- Inspect the perianal, perineal, and lumbosacral areas for fissures, anatomic abnormalities (anteriorly placed anus), dimples, tufts of hair, masses, or hemangiomas.
- **In functional constipation, digital anorectal examination will be positive for a large rectal vault filled with hard stool, whereas in Hirschsprung disease the sphincter tone is tight with an empty narrow vault.**

Tests for Consideration

- **Rectal suction biopsy:** For Hirschsprung disease $606
- **Anorectal manometry:** To evaluate for Hirschsprung disease $555
- **Urinalysis:** If impaction present $95
- **Urine culture:** If impaction present $148
- **Complete blood count (CBC):** If failure to thrive $116
- **Celiac panel:** If failure to thrive $225
- **Thyroid-stimulating hormone (TSH), triiodothyronine (T_3), and free thyroxine (T_4):** If concern for hypothyroidism $194
- **Electrolytes, including calcium and magnesium:** If decreased fluid intake or metabolic abnormalities suspected $290

IMAGING CONSIDERATIONS

→ **Single view abdominal radiograph:** Can demonstrate degree of fecal retention, rectal and colonic dilation $170
→ **Unprepped barium enema:** To demonstrate narrow aganglionic segment in Hirschsprung disease and locate transition zone $530

Clinical Entities   Medical Knowledge

Functional Constipation

Pφ   Decreased stool frequency and voluntary stool withholding may be triggered by painful defecation. The colon absorbs water from the retained stool; stool hardens and becomes larger and hence more difficult and painful to evacuate. Over time, the colon and rectum lose tone and dilate, and there is decreased sensation of rectal fullness. There are no pathologic findings of organic disease.

TP   As large, hard stool accumulates, a vicious cycle ensues. Stool passage is difficult and painful and may result in an anal fissure, which in turn increases pain with passage, and further retention may result. Fecal incontinence can occur as loose stool leaks around a large, hard fecal mass. Surprisingly, often the parent calls not for constipation, but for the involuntary passage of stool and soiling.

Dx   Criteria for functional constipation are at least two of the following six findings in a child with a developmental age of at least 4 years with insufficient criteria for diagnosis of irritable bowel syndrome: (1) two or fewer defecations in the toilet per week, (2) at least one episode of fecal incontinence per week, (3) history of retentive posturing or excessive volitional stool retention, (4) history of painful or hard bowel movement, (5) presence of a large fecal mass in the rectum, (6) history of large-diameter stools that may obstruct the toilet. Criteria should be met at least once a week for 2 months.

Tx   The best treatment is prevention and requires discussion of diet and bowel patterns at each health maintenance visit. Excessive cow's milk intake is discouraged. Minimum daily fiber intake should equal the child's age in years plus 5 grams.
      Early constipation in infants can be treated with sorbitol-containing juice (apple, pear, or prune), sorbitol syrup, or lactulose syrup, 1 to 3 mL/kg/day. If necessary, polyethylene glycol (PEG) 3350 1 g/kg/day is used.
      In children older than 2 years, disimpaction may be done with a sodium phosphate enema (6 mL/kg up to 135 mL). Other rectal alternatives include saline, 5 to 10 mL/kg, or mineral oil, 15 to 30 mL/year of age (up to 240 mL). Orally, PEG 3350 1 to 1.5 g/kg/day for 3 days may be used. Maintenance PEG 3350 up to 1 g/kg/day is taken until there have been regular soft, painless daily stools for a good period of time and then slowly tapered, with monitoring for recurrence. Mineral oil 1 to 3 mL/kg/day may be administered as ongoing maintenance. Regular toilet sitting, especially after meals, is an important adjunct to the treatment regimen. If no progress is made, referral to a gastroenterologist is indicated. If encopresis, with voluntary passage of stool, rather than soiling from leakage is present, mental health consultation may be necessary. **See Nelson Essentials 14 and 126.**

Hirschsprung Disease

Pφ   This is a neuromuscular disorder of the colon resulting from failure in embryonic migration of neural crest cells, resulting in absence of ganglionic cells in the affected segment. The affected segment begins most distal at the external anal sphincter with a varying degree of proximal progression. The aganglionic segment fails to relax, producing a functional obstruction. In approximately 75% of patients, a short segment in the rectosigmoid is affected. Cases identified in childhood are usually short or ultrashort segment. See Chapter 63, Delayed Meconium Passage.

TP   Hirschsprung disease is usually suspected in the newborn period with failure to pass meconium within 48 hours. In the first few months it may present as enterocolitis with fever, diarrhea, and vomiting. With later diagnosis there will be a history of chronic constipation with abdominal distention and poor response to medical management.

Dx   Digital rectal examination will reveal a tight external anal sphincter with an empty ampulla (except in some cases of short segment disease). On withdrawal of the examining finger, there may be forceful release of loose stool. Rectal biopsy is the definitive test, demonstrating an absence of ganglion cells in the submucosal plexus. Anorectal manometry is especially useful in short segment disease. Barium enema is usually unnecessary after infancy, although it may be useful in locating the transition zone.

Tx   Treatment is surgical with excision of the aganglionic segment, often with a colostomy proximal to the affected site. If short segment disease is not diagnosed until adulthood, medical management with osmotic laxatives may be attempted. **See Nelson Essentials 126 and 129.**

Hypothyroidism

Pφ   The most common cause in children is chronic lymphocytic thyroiditis (Hashimoto thyroiditis). This is an autoimmune condition, and antithyroid antibodies—antithyroglobulin and antithyroperoxidase—are present. There may be goiter with no symptoms, or clinical signs of hypothyroidism, or rarely, a period of hyperthyroidism.

TP   Signs of hypothyroidism include cold intolerance, bradycardia, weakness, anorexia, weight gain, constipation, lethargy, edema of face and eyelids, dry coarse skin, and alopecia.

Dx	TSH is elevated. In compensated hypothyroidism the free T_4 is normal, and in uncompensated hypothyroidism the free T_4 is low with increased TSH. The antibodies listed above are elevated.
Tx	Thyroid hormone replacement for acquired hypothyroidism is with thyroxine starting at 2.5 mcg/kg/day should be initiated for acquired hypothyroidism. The free T_4 and TSH are followed to guide dose adjustment to the euthyroid state. Laxatives as described above may be required until normal thyroid hormone levels are established. **See Nelson Essentials 175.**

ZEBRA ZONE

a. **Infant botulism:** Ingestion of *Clostridium botulinum,* which elaborates a toxin blocking the release of acetylcholine at the neuromuscular junction, causing diffuse hypotonia

b. **Spinal cord abnormalities:** Myelomeningocele with abnormal or absent colonic innervation and peristalsis

c. **Intestinal pseudo-obstruction:** Signs of intestinal obstruction without an anatomic lesion, either primary or secondary to another disorder, and includes abdominal distention, vomiting, constipation, and urinary retention

d. **Lead poisoning**

Practice-Based Learning and Improvement

Title
Evaluation and treatment of constipation in infants and children: Recommendations of the North American Society for Pediatric Gastroenterology, Hepatology and Nutrition

Authors
Baker SS, Liptak GS, Colletti RB, et al

Reference
J Pediatr Gastroenterol Nutr 43:e1-e13, 2006

Problem
Review of diagnosis and treatment of constipation in infants and children

Comparison/control (quality of evidence)
Extensively referenced review article by the NASPGHAN Constipation Guideline Committee

Interpersonal and Communication Skills

Explain Time Course for Expected Improvements

Functional constipation with fecal impaction and rectal dilation takes weeks to months to develop. In developing a therapeutic plan, explain to the parents that it will take weeks to months to reverse. Medication will be needed until the rectum reverts to normal size, which will be evidenced by daily stools of normal caliber. A clear understanding of the process may facilitate compliance with the regimen.

Professionalism

Demonstrate Compassion and Empathy When Managing Encopresis

The child experiencing involuntary fecal soiling in school will experience embarrassment and may be teased or shunned by other children. The family experiences both stress and anxiety. Therefore, although encopresis may not be a major medical illness, it is potentially devastating to the family. Acknowledge this and create a mutually agreed-upon action plan. Arrange close follow-up to monitor progress, and offer support and reassurance through the disimpaction and maintenance phases. This will enable the family and child to cope with and resolve this difficult condition.

Systems-Based Practice

Physician Compliance With Clinical Practice Guidelines

Clinical practice guidelines (CPGs) have been developed by a multitude of government, subspecialty, and local organizations in an attempt to reduce undesirable variations in care and to improve the quality of care. CPGs are evidence based to the extent possible. The level of evidence is a numeric grading (one through five) of quality, and recommendations are graded (A to D) according to both quality and quantity of the evidence. In instances when evidence is lacking, expert consensus opinion is provided.

In order for guidelines to improve care, they must influence the decisions that physicians and other health-care providers make as they care for patients on a day-to-day basis. Physicians demonstrate variable acceptance of CPGs. Some reasons include lack of awareness of a particular guideline, clinical inertia with current practice methods, disagreement with guideline recommendations, and a perception that CPGs are too time consuming and limit the use of personal judgment and experience.[1]

Reference

1. Cabana MD, Rand CS, Powe NR, et al: Why don't physicians follow clinical practice guidelines. *JAMA* 282(15):1458-1465, 1999.

Chapter 36
Fever (Case 8)

Justin F. Lynn MD, MPH

Case: A 24-month-old with fever of 38.8° C (102° F) for 24 hours who is cranky and not feeding or sleeping well

Differential Diagnosis

Upper respiratory infection	Acute otitis media	Acute bacterial sinusitis
Bronchiolitis and pneumonia	Viral syndrome	Urinary tract infection

Speaking Intelligently

Fever is generally defined as a body temperature greater than 38° C (100.4° F). Recognize that fever is common in children and by itself is not a diagnosis. It is a reset of the body's thermostat in response to a stimulus, and the goal of evaluation is to find the stimulus. If the exact cause is not identified, serious causes need to be excluded. Using both the history and physical examination, it is helpful to take the outside-in approach and start with a general sense of the child's well-being and then narrow in on specific signs or symptoms. Most children with fever have a benign self-limited viral illness or a bacterial cause identified on examination. Antipyretics will decrease the temperature but are not always necessary, and treatment of the underlying condition (if possible) is the priority. In the office setting, the extent of laboratory evaluation is guided by the child's age, immunization status, overall appearance, and the physician's ability to make a clinical diagnosis.[1] (See Chapter 46, Neonatal Fever).

PATIENT CARE

Clinical Thinking
- ***Does the child's appearance raise concern for serious bacterial infection?*** Does the child look significantly better after a dose of antipyretics and/or fluids?

- Are there localizing signs or symptoms that can lead to diagnosis?
- Is there specific treatment, such as penicillin for group A streptococcal pharyngitis?
- What caregiver education is needed for supportive care and need for follow-up?
- Is additional testing such as urine, blood, or chest radiograph indicated?
- Season may be important: Coxsackie hand-foot-and-mouth disease and Lyme disease occur in spring/summer, whereas bronchiolitis and influenza have a fall/winter occurrence.

History

- Is there history of exposure to other febrile children? Does the child attend day care or school?
- *A child with normal activity level and oral intake has a decreased likelihood of a serious infection.*
- Are **vaccinations** current?
- Prolonged fever may indicate an unresolved infection or an inflammatory disease.
- Poor linear growth and weight gain may occur with inflammatory disease.
- Change in mental status is concerning for meningitis/encephalitis.
- A fever developing once an illness has started is concerning for secondary bacterial infection, such as acute otitis media with upper respiratory infection (URI).
- Fever and tachypnea may indicate pneumonia if tachypnea persists after administration of an antipyretic and decreased temperature.

Physical Examination

- Note general sense of well-being. Is the child toxic, somnolent, or irritable appearing?
- Vital signs: Note tachypnea or tachycardia out of proportion to fever. Include pulse oximetry if respiratory symptoms.
- Note **hydration status:** Assess activity level, oral intake, urine output, presence of tears, and fluid losses from vomiting or diarrhea.
- Is there rhinorrhea?
- Bulging fontanelle occurs in infants with meningitis; classic meningeal signs occur in older children. See Chapter 46, Neonatal Fever, and Chapter 49, Meningitis.
- Bulging tympanic membrane with inflammation and acute onset of symptoms occur in acute otitis media.
- On lung examination, note overall aeration, respiratory rate, and retractions as well as auscultation findings.
- A careful skin examination for rashes may provide diagnostic clues. Distribution and pattern may suggest an etiology. Petechiae below the nipple line should raise concern about meningococcemia, generalized erythroderma with toxin-mediated bacteremia, a discrete fine

maculopapular sandpaper rash in group A streptococcal infection, and a polymorphous rash in viral exanthems.

Tests for Consideration

- **Complete blood count (CBC):** Leukocytosis with a left shift supports bacterial etiology, though early on viral processes may be neutrophil predominant. $116
- **Urinalysis:** Nitrites and leukocyte esterase indicate infection; infants may only have increased microscopic white blood cell count. $95
- **Urine culture:** Confirms infection. $148
- **Blood culture:** If toxic appearing. $152
- **Erythrocyte sedimentation rate (ESR):** Marked elevation with bacterial infection; can be used to follow response to treatment. $85
- **C-reactive protein:** Elevated with infection and inflammation. $69
- **Metabolic panel:** If concern for dehydration, renal function, or hepatitis. $174
- **Rapid respiratory panel:** Respiratory syncytial virus (RSV), influenza, parainfluenza, adenovirus, human metapneumovirus. $325
- **Rapid antigen for *Rotavirus.*** $170

IMAGING CONSIDERATIONS

Sinus computed tomography (CT) scan: In refractory cases or if concern for underlying anatomic abnormality $1716

Chest radiograph: If concern for pneumonia $231

Bone scan: In select cases with fever of unknown source to check for osteomyelitis $1512

Clinical Entities

Upper Respiratory Infection

Pφ In the common cold, nasal epithelium is infected by virus particles with an acute cytokine response and inflammatory cell infiltrate to produce the symptoms of rhinosinusitis. Obstruction of the osteomeatal complex or eustachian tube can lead to secondary bacterial sinusitis or acute otitis media. Up to 50% of cases are due to rhinovirus. Other pathogens include RSV, coronavirus, adenovirus, influenza, parainfluenza, and enterovirus. Spread occurs via small- or large-particle aerosols and direct contact (see Chapter 30, Sore Throat).

TP   A sore, scratchy throat is followed by nasal congestion and rhinorrhea, with onset of cough 1 to 2 days later. The nasal secretions are initially clear and may progress to opaque and then green. Green nasal discharge does not indicate bacterial superinfection. Fever may occur initially and is more common in infants and toddlers. Later-onset fever suggests a complication such as otitis media, sinusitis, or pneumonia. Children may have increased fussy periods, disrupted sleep, and decreased fluid intake. A URI is a common asthma trigger. Symptoms last 7 to 14 days, and for many there is prolonged cough (see Chapter 31, Cough).

Dx   Diagnosis is clinical with history being key. There are generally few examination findings: nasal congestion, rhinorrhea, erythematous pharynx, serous middle ear fluid, and cough.

Tx   Because most colds are self-limiting, treatment is supportive and includes maintenance of hydration with analgesia for pain control and antipyretics as needed. In addition, monitor for complications such as pneumonia, acute otitis media, acute sinusitis, or an asthma exacerbation. Parents should be counseled about expected time course and when and if a follow-up visit is needed. Antibiotics are not indicated for viral URIs, and part of treatment may include caregiver education in this regard. **See Nelson Essentials 102.**

Acute Otitis Media

See Chapter 37, Ear Pain, and Chapter 38, Teaching Visual: Examination of the Middle Ear.

Acute Bacterial Sinusitis

Pφ   Before pneumatization of the sinuses, true bacterial sinusitis does not occur. The maxillary and ethmoid sinuses are pneumatized at birth, and the sphenoid sinus is pneumatized by 6 years, but the frontal sinuses are not reliably pneumatized until adolescence. There is usually a preexisting viral URI. Normal sinus drainage and cilia function are impaired when the ostia are blocked by mucosal inflammation and thickened secretions. Negative pressure develops when the osteomeatal complex is blocked, bacterial pathogens proliferate with mucosal thickening, edema, and inflammation. The chief pathogens are those with acute otitis media; namely, *Streptococcus pneumoniae,* nontypable *Haemophilus influenzae,* and *Moraxella catarrhalis.*

TP   There are three typical presentations. One is the "cold that won't go away" with persistent congestion and rhinorrhea beyond 14 days. The second is a cold that is improving by day 7, with sudden recurrence of fever, increased nasal secretions, and worsening cough. The third is acute onset of high fever (temperature greater than 39° C [102.2° F]) with purulent nasal discharge for at least 3 days. Young children do not usually have headache or face pain.

Dx   Diagnosis is challenging, and history is key. Clarify if there have been congestion-free periods, which may lend support to sequential viral infection rather than a developing sinusitis. Diagnosis is usually clinical. Sinus tenderness is not a reliable sign. CT scan or magnetic resonance imaging (MRI) will demonstrate mucosal thickening and air-fluid levels, but will not clarify a viral versus bacterial etiology. Plain radiography lacks sensitivity and specificity for acute sinus changes. Imaging is most helpful with recurrent disease, suspected anatomic abnormality, or complications.

Tx   Antibiotics are prescribed for 10 to 21 days, depending on clinical response. If improvement is noted after the first few days, a 10-day course may suffice. Initial therapy to target intermediate-resistance pneumococcus, the predominant culprit, is with amoxicillin 80 to 90 mg/kg/ day. Amoxicillin (80 to 90 mg/kg/day)/clavulanate (6.4 mg/kg/day) may be required for beta-lactamase–producing *H. influenzae* and *M. catarrhalis,* or if poor response to amoxicillin. In some cases, amoxicillin/ clavulanate is prescribed as first-line therapy. Alternative choices include cephalosporins such as cefdinir and cefuroxime, and azithromycin if both penicillin and cephalosporin allergic. Additional therapy includes saline nasal irrigation and nasal steroid spray. Recheck if symptoms do not improve, because chronic sinusitis is caused by *Staphylococcus aureus* and anaerobes. **See Nelson Essentials 104.**

Bronchiolitis and Pneumonia

See Chapter 31, Cough, and Chapter 44, Difficulty Breathing.

	Viral Syndrome
Pφ	A virus infects epithelial cells, typically respiratory or gastrointestinal tract mucosa, and then replicates. Cell necrosis and viremia may ensue, with seeding of another site, such as the pharynx. There may be secondary findings such as an exanthem, which may be nonspecific or provide specific clues to etiology. Viremia results in fever, fatigue, myalgias, and other systemic illness manifestations.
TP	The presentation can vary widely, and infants and young children are typically affected. Some common presentations include fever alone or fever with myalgias, malaise, increased fussiness, rhinorrhea, nasal congestion, cough, conjunctivitis, diarrhea, or exanthema (rash). There may be a nonspecific viral exanthem (typically diffuse, blanching erythematous macular or papular). Some viruses have a specific rash, enabling a precise diagnosis. Some examples include roseola and erythema infectiosum, caused by human herpesvirus 6 (HHV-6) and parvovirus B19, respectively. Hand-foot-and-mouth disease, caused by coxsackievirus A, has a specific macular papular exanthem on the palms and soles, in addition to pharyngeal vesicles (an enanthem). Adenovirus has several presentations; one is a constellation of rhinitis, pharyngitis, fever, and conjunctivitis. Respiratory viruses are discussed in Chapter 30, Sore Throat; Chapter 31, Cough; and Chapter 44, Difficulty Breathing. Gastrointestinal viruses are discussed in Chapter 34, Diarrhea.
Dx	In otherwise healthy children, the diagnosis is clinical, but a thorough physical examination is done to exclude a bacterial cause of fever and hence the need for specific treatment, along with an assessment of hydration status. Immunofluorescence testing is available for respiratory viruses and rotavirus but these are used infrequently in the outpatient setting.
Tx	Treatment is supportive with attention to comfort and hydration, and antipyretics as needed. Parents should be educated that fever alone will not harm their child and may actually help fight the infection. Precise instructions for follow-up should be given regarding hydration, prolonged fever, or worsening symptoms. **See Nelson Essentials 97.**

Urinary Tract Infection
See Chapter 41, Dysuria, and Chapter 46, Neonatal Fever.

ZEBRA ZONE

a. **Occult bacteremia:** Bacteremia with body temperature of 39° C (102.2° F) or higher without localizing signs in relatively well-appearing 3 to 36 month olds that usually clears spontaneously, but can rarely seed serious bacterial infection such as meningitis. It is now uncommon (risk <1%) with vaccination against *H. influenzae* (type b) and *S. pneumoniae*.

b. **Periodic fever, aphthous ulcers, pharyngitis, and adenopathy (PFAPA syndrome):** A predictable cycle of fevers with the accompanying findings. Corticosteroids administered at the onset will result in shorter duration of fever.

Practice-Based Learning and Improvement

Title
Urine testing and urinary tract infections in febrile infants seen in office settings

Authors
Newman TB, Bernzweig JA, Takayama JI, et al

Reference
Arch Pediatr Adolesc Med 156:44-54, 2002

Problem
Evaluation of febrile infants younger than 3 months old

Comparison/control (quality of evidence)
Prospective cohort study of 3066 febrile infants. The participating physicians, members of the Pediatric Research in Office Settings (PROS) Network, were from 219 practices in 44 states.

Outcome/effect
Up to 10% of young febrile infants have UTIs; hence routine urine testing is recommended. This study found that many physicians do urine testing selectively, being more likely to test younger and sicker-appearing infants and those without a fever source. Of those tested, higher fever was associated with having a UTI. However, those at highest risk—uncircumcised boys, girls, and those with fever longer than 24 hours—were not readily tested. Only 2 of 807 infants who did not receive initial urine testing or antibiotic treatment actually had a UTI, and none had bacteremia.

Historical significance/comments
Clinical judgment with selective urine testing is probably a safe approach for the experienced clinician who provides close patient follow-up.

Interpersonal and Communication Skills

Elicit the Family's Concerns and Dispel Fever Phobia

Fever is a major concern of parents; for example, some parents fear that fever may cause brain damage or that all fevers need to be treated with antibiotics. In the evaluation of fever be sure to understand the parents' concerns, so that you can better address them. This will help build trust in the relationship and guide your discharge instructions. Be sure to explain to parents what to watch out for and when they should to return to the office.

Professionalism

Self-Awareness: Follow Through on Your Clinical Suspicions

Although you always rely on training, experience, and practice guidelines, do not ignore your instincts—that gut feeling that tells you that something is just not right. Never hesitate to take a closer look at a seemingly minor symptom, and never ignore a symptom that does not fit with the normal or expected pattern of presentation of a particular illness.

Systems-Based Practice

Cost-Effective Evaluation of Fever Without Localizing Signs

The typical general pediatrician works in a high-volume, low-acuity setting, in which many patients are seen daily. Of those who present with fever as the chief complaint, the vast majority have a benign self-limited viral illness. In the post–Hib (*H. influenzae* type b) vaccine and post-PCV-7 (7-valent conjugated pneumococcal vaccine; note the 13-valent formulation was introduced in 2010) era, a fully immunized well-appearing child from 3 to 36 months of age with a fever to 39° C (102.2° F) or higher without localizing signs has a <1% risk for occult bacteremia. Therefore it is reasonable to weigh the consequences of testing and treatment for fever, including the discomfort to the child, related financial costs, and unintended consequences of false-positive results, against the small risk for serious bacterial infection and potential liability. Many pediatricians have become less aggressive in the laboratory evaluation of these children and instead perform a careful evaluation, give careful instructions to the caregiver, and arrange for a timely follow-up for reexamination.[2]

References

1. Finkelstein JA, Christiansen CL, Platt R: Fever in pediatric primary care: Occurrence, management, and outcomes. *Pediatrics* 105(1 Suppl):260-266, 2000.
2. Avner JR, Baker MD: Occult bacteremia in the post-pneumococcal conjugate vaccine era: does the blood culture stop here? *Acad Emerg Med* 16(3):258-260, 2009.

Chapter 37
Ear Pain (Case 9)

Jacquelyn M. Aveta MD, FAAP

Case: A 22-month-old with ear pain

Differential Diagnosis

Otitis media	Foreign body
Traumatic ear injury	Otitis externa

Speaking Intelligently

When asked to evaluate a child with ear pain, I first obtain the history. If there has been trauma or a foreign body inserted in the canal, I will check the tympanic membrane (TM) for perforation. For an embedded ear piercing, it is critical to determine presence of infection and cartilaginous involvement. Facts such as recent congestion, previous otitis media, or day care attendance followed by onset of fever suggest acute otitis media (AOM), or possibly acute pharyngitis with referred ear pain. Physical examination and history are key to distinguishing AOM from otitis media with effusion (OME), or fluid in the middle ear space that is not acutely infected.

PATIENT CARE

Clinical Thinking
- Ear pain is usually not an emergency; but pain control is a high priority.
- When evaluating the middle ear, **distinguish AOM from otitis media with effusion.**

History
- Are there preexisting symptoms such as rhinorrhea, sore throat, or cough; or was there abrupt onset of ear pain?
- Is the child playful or fussy or somnolent?
- Any fever?
- Any ear drainage? Specify if purulent or sanguinous or clear.

- Any history of objects in the ear or nose?
- Has the child been swimming?
- Are there ear piercings? Any associated swelling or redness?
- Has there been recent otitis media? What was the treatment? Was there a follow-up examination after treatment?
- Are there craniofacial anomalies, immunodeficiencies, or cochlear implants to increase risk for otitis media or mastoiditis?
- Any dental problems, such as unfilled caries or abscess?

Physical Examination
- Note general appearance. Most with ear pain will be calm or perhaps crying, but should not be lethargic.
- Check vital signs, and note presence of **fever.** Tachycardia occurs with pain and/or fever.
- Are the ears symmetric, or is one pushed forward as in mastoiditis?
- Is there pain on tugging the tragus?
- Is there drainage in the canal to suggest AOM with TM perforation?
- Using an otoscope, evaluate the canal for erythema, drainage, and foreign body.
- **Use pneumatic otoscopy to identify middle ear effusion (MEE).** Distinguish effusion from acute infection by the additional presence of erythema and pus in acute infection (see Chapter 38, Teaching Visual: Examination of the Middle Ear).
- Complete the oral examination using a tongue blade and otoscope with appropriate support to position the child to maximize your examination and minimize discomfort.
- Assess the neck for any lumps, swelling, or tenderness.

Tests for Consideration
- **Culture of ear drainage:** Indicated if chronic and unresponsive to therapy $152
- If suspect group A streptococcus:
  - **Rapid streptococcal antigen test** $148
  - **Throat culture** $148
- **Tympanometry:** Indicated to confirm presence of MEE $125

IMAGING CONSIDERATIONS

→ **Computed tomography (CT) scan for mastoiditis**	$1965
→ Magnetic Resonance Imaging (MRI) for mastoiditis	$2308

| **Clinical Entities** | **Medical Knowledge** |

Otitis Media

Pφ An antecedent viral upper respiratory infection (URI) may be followed by fever. The eustachian tube, which normally allows ventilation between the nasal airway and middle ear, becomes blocked, creating negative pressure leading to accumulation of serous fluid. The fluid subsequently becomes infected with either a virus or bacteria. *Streptococcus pneumoniae,* nontypable *Haemophilus influenzae,* and *Moraxella catarrhalis* are the most common bacteria. Rapid growth of the infectious agent and the resultant inflammatory reaction leads to pain and pressure on the TM, which may perforate. Since introduction of the heptavalent pneumococcal conjugate vaccine in 2000, there has been an overall decrease in *S. pneumoniae,* with emergence of some nonvaccine strains and an increase in nontypable *H. influenzae.* The 13-valent pneumococcal conjugate vaccine was approved in 2010, and ongoing alteration in causative bacteria may continue to emerge.[2]

TP Infants may only have URI symptoms, or there may be fever, irritability, poor oral intake, and/or sleep disruption. Toddlers may tug the ear or seem less balanced when walking. Older children will usually verbalize ear pain and may perceive decreased hearing.

Dx The diagnosis is made using pneumatic otoscopy. The American Academy of Pediatrics 2004 diagnostic criteria for AOM are:
1. Abrupt onset of signs and symptoms
2. Presence of MEE
3. Signs and symptoms of acute inflammation that include erythema of the TM, bulging of the TM, immobility, and/or otalgia interfering with normal activity

MEE occurs in both AOM and OME, but in acute infection there is abrupt onset of signs and symptoms as described above. OME occurs following acute otitis media or with viral upper respiratory infection and eustachian tube dysfunction.[1] (see Chapter 38, Teaching Visual: Examination of the Middle Ear).

Tx Pain control is a top priority. Acetaminophen and ibuprofen, and topical agents such as benzocaine, in a nonperforated TM are effective. Codeine with acetaminophen is effective for severe pain. Because up to 80% of ear infections may spontaneously resolve, the need for antibiotic treatment is assessed.[1,2] Infants under 6 months should be treated. With a certain diagnosis in the 6- to 24-month-old, or an uncertain diagnosis with severe pain or temperature above 39° C (102.2° F), an antibiotic is prescribed. Children over 24 months with severe pain or temperature above 39° C (102.2° F) should be treated. Otherwise healthy children can be observed for 48 to 72 hours. With worsening or failure to improve, treatment is initiated. Amoxicillin 80 to 90 mg/kg/day for up to 10 days is first-line therapy. For a severely ill child or suspected antimicrobial resistance, amoxicillin (90 mg/kg/day)/clavulanate (6.4 mg/kg/day) is prescribed. Ceftriaxone (50 mg/kg) is an alternative for the toxic-appearing child. Azithromycin is prescribed in those with type I hypersensitivity reaction to penicillin. If treatment fails after 48 to 72 hours, options include amoxicillin/clavulanate, cefdinir, ceftriaxone, or clindamycin. Studies have shown a modest benefit with prompt antibiotic treatment, but there is increased incidence of rash and diarrhea as well as concern about antibiotic resistance in the long term. Cases that benefit from prompt antibiotic therapy include bilateral AOM, ruptured tympanic membrane, children under 6 months of age, and those with severe pain or high fever.[2] **See Nelson Essentials 105.**

Foreign Body
Pφ A foreign body can be either a piercing or a foreign body placed in the ear canal. *Staphylococcus aureus* and *Pseudomonas aeruginosa* are the pathogens in secondary bacterial infection of embedded piercings, especially with cartilaginous involvement.
TP For an embedded piercing there is often significant redness and/ or swelling. If the foreign body is in the ear canal, the child may be able to verbalize what was placed (e.g., a bead). If there is intermittent severe pain, especially in the morning, the culprit may be an insect.
Dx Diagnosis is made with visual inspection, using otoscopy. For embedded piercings, it is critical to determine if cartilage is involved, because systemic antibiotic therapy may be warranted.

Tx   Removal of the object from the ear canal will require careful
      secure positioning of the child. If the TM is intact, anesthetic
      drops can be instilled, because removal may be painful. Removal
      is accomplished with a curette, forceps, or irrigation (with an
      intact TM and the foreign body will not swell with water).
      Antibiotic drops are used if irritation or trauma to the
      epithelium is noted. Removal of a mildly embedded piercing
      can be accomplished with pressure after removal of the earring
      back. The degree of pain and swelling may necessitate
      otolaryngology consultation. Administration of IV antibiotics
      to cover *P. aeruginosa* is indicated with significant cartilage
      involvement.

Otitis Externa

Pφ   Water is retained in the ear canal after swimming, or there may
      be trauma from a cotton swab. Bacterial growth is followed by
      inflammation, with *P. aeruginosa* the most common pathogen.

TP   This occurs more commonly in older children, with an insidious
      onset over several days, often associated with itching or
      discharge.

Dx   Classically, there is increased pain with traction on the tragus.
      Otoscopic examination reveals debris in the canal (usually
      white), and often the TM is incompletely visualized. However,
      the TM may be red, but middle ear effusion is not present.

Tx   If possible, gently clean the ear canal. An ear wick may be
      placed to help deliver antibiotic drops deeper into the canal.
      Treatment is with topical antibiotic drops, such as ofloxacin or
      an antibiotic plus corticosteroid–containing drop for severe
      pain. Severe or refractory cases may warrant otolaryngologic
      consultation. **See Nelson Essentials 106**.

Traumatic Ear Injury

Pφ   External trauma is caused by direct blunt force to the ear.
      Middle ear trauma is commonly caused by overzealous ear
      cleaning with a cotton swab, causing injury to the canal or TM.
      The child may have placed another object into the ear,
      resulting in trauma. Loud noise may cause inner ear trauma.

TP	Trauma may have occurred during sports, a fight, or a fall along with bleeding. With middle ear injury, the caregiver or child will usually admit to sticking something in the ear. Typically, those with inner ear trauma have been exposed to loud noise or music.
Dx	External ear injuries consist of lacerations or bruising. A hematoma appears as a bluish swelling disrupting the normal ear contour. Abrasions on the canal wall may be present with middle ear trauma. Hemorrhage or perforation may be noted with TM injury. There may be vertigo, hearing loss, or facial nerve paralysis. Hearing loss on audiometry may be the only finding with trauma from sound.
Tx	Ear lacerations should always be closed by someone with expertise, especially with cartilaginous involvement. Hematomas require immediate evacuation to avoid necrosis of the cartilage. Bruising of the ear and canal abrasions will typically self-resolve. Tympanic membrane perforations usually spontaneously heal within 3 weeks; otolaryngology (ENT) consultation is indicated for large and persistent perforations. Immediate ENT consultation is needed for vertigo, hearing loss, or facial nerve paralysis. For noise trauma, there is usually self-resolution if exposure is discontinued.

ZEBRA ZONE

a. **Eosinophilic granuloma:** A destructive lesion of the temporal bone causing otalgia, otorrhea, hearing loss, and abnormal tissue in the ear canal, treated with local excision and/or radiation

b. **Rhabdomyosarcoma:** A mass or polyp of the middle ear or ear canal with bleeding from ear, otalgia, otorrhea, facial paralysis, and hearing loss

Practice-Based Learning and Improvement

Title
Tympanostomy tubes and developmental outcomes at 9 to 11 years of age

Authors
Paradise JL, Feldman HM, Campbell TF, et al

Reference
N Engl J Med 356:248-261, 2007

Problem
It was long believed that middle ear effusion (MEE) in otherwise healthy children was a cause of conductive hearing loss and delayed

expressive language development, but unclear whether prompt insertion of myringotomy tubes compared with delayed insertion after 9 months of persistent MEE would have a positive impact on long-term developmental outcome.

Intervention

A prospective randomized controlled trial of 6350 children enrolled in early infancy was monitored for development of MEE. Of these, 429 before 3 years of age with persistent MEE were assigned to prompt insertion of myringotomy tubes versus delayed tube placement after up to 9 months of persistent MEE. At 9 to 11 years of age, literacy, attention, social skills, and academic achievement were assessed in 391 of the children.

Comparison/control (quality of evidence)

Mean scores on 48 developmental measures in children who received early insertion of myringotomy tubes did not differ significantly from scores in those with delayed insertion of tubes.

Historical significance/comments

This landmark study found that in otherwise healthy young children with persistent middle ear effusion, prompt insertion of myringotomy tubes in infants and young children does not result in improved developmental outcomes at 9 to 11 years of age.

Interpersonal and Communication Skills

Summarize and Confirm Agreement With Treatment

Once the diagnosis has been established and you have decided on an appropriate therapeutic course of action, it is time to make sure that the parents agree and will carry out the plan. State the diagnosis and the likely cause. Explain your therapeutic choice and what will be required to carry it through. For example, if you feel you must use a particular antibiotic that does not taste good, you will need to proactively discuss this with the parents and offer suggestions to make delivery easier. It is important to summarize the plan and get parental "buy-in" for the plan to be successfully carried through at home.

Professionalism

Provide Timely Appointments for Patients With Ear Pain

For many families ear pain constitutes an emergency, and they often seek care in the emergency department (ED). This is an inappropriate use of ED services and drains resources. Educating parents to call the office first for ear pain—and similar conditions—is important.

However, physicians must make sure that parents experience a quick response time when they call. During office hours there must be adequate space in the schedule to provide a same-day acute care visit appointment if deemed necessary. After office hours physicians must not only respond promptly to patient calls, but also triage patients with uncomplicated ear pain away from the ED, call in medications for pain control, and follow up closely.

Systems-Based Practice

Identify Areas for Practice Improvement in Monitoring and Documenting Findings for Children With Acute or Chronic Otitis Media

In 1996, the American Academy of Pediatrics' Ambulatory Care Quality Improvement Program (ACQIP) formulated a self-assessment exercise for outpatient pediatricians.[3] It contains 22 questions that assess adequacy of documentation of history and key physical examination findings. The pooled results were published to identify self-reported practice patterns in the nation and to enable practitioners to compare their own practice with that of the group, and suggest a standardized format for documenting and tracking. Key features such as fever, TM mobility, presence or absence of fluid or pus and notation about hearing, treatment, and prior episodes of acute otitis media (AOM) are included. This format allows standardization of the approach and documentation of AOM diagnosis and treatment. In addition, the exercise asked about prescription of prophylactic antibiotics and referral to otolaryngology for asymptomatic middle ear effusion. Despite the changes in management since 1996 (i.e., fewer otolaryngology consults for myringotomy tube placement for asymptomatic middle ear effusion and no longer prescribing antibiotic prophylaxis), this format remains valuable (with updated modifications) as a tool to standardize documentation and tracking of children with both acute and chronic otitis media.

References

1. American Academy of Pediatrics: American Academy of Family Practice and the American Academy of Otolaryngology-Head and Neck Surgery: Diagnosis and management of acute otitis media. *Pediatrics* 113(5):1451-1465, 2004.
2. Coker TR, Chan LS, Newberry SJ, et al: Diagnosis, Microbial epidemiology, and antibiotic treatment of acute otitis media in children, *JAMA* 304(19):2161-2169, 2010.
3. Sebring RH, Staff of the Division of Quality Care: Quality improvement: An ACQIP exercise on the management of otitis media. *Pediatr Rev* 17(7):251-256, 1996.

Chapter 38
Teaching Visual: Examination of the Middle Ear

Maureen C. McMahon MD

Objectives

- Define otitis media with effusion and acute otitis media.
- Describe use of pneumatic otoscopy and interpretation of findings in the normal ear, acute otitis media, and otitis media with effusion.
- Describe two positioning techniques for visualization of the middle ear in infants and young children.

MEDICAL KNOWLEDGE

Ear pain, fever, and concern for possible ear infection are among the most common reasons for visits to the pediatrician; thus identification of the normal tympanic membrane (TM) and accurate distinction between acute otitis media (AOM) and otitis media with effusion (OME) is essential to correct management.[1]

The normal tympanic membrane (TM) is translucent gray, and the handle of the malleus is visible along with a cone-shaped light reflex (Figure 38-1).

- Connect the dashed line outlining the handle of the malleus.
- Connect the dotted lines that outline the area of the expected light reflex on the tympanic membrane.

Figure 38-1 Tympanic membrane. *Red dashed line,* Handle of the malleus; *green dotted line,* light reflex.

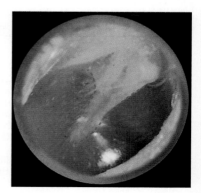

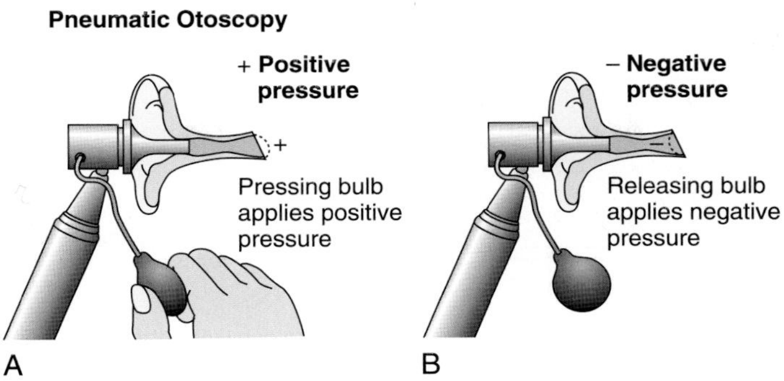

Pneumatic Otoscopy

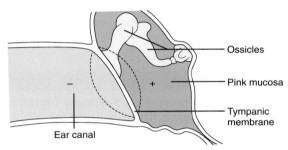

Figure 38-2 Pneumatic otoscopes.

Figure 38-3 Pnematic otoscopy with normal tympanic membrane.

Note that with pneumatic otoscopy the normal ear drum moves in response to both positive and negative pressure gently applied with an insufflation bulb (Figure 38-2).

■ Complete the dotted line to demonstrate movement of the normal tympanic membrane with positive pressure (Figure 38-3).
■ Complete the dashed line of normal movement with negative pressure.

In AOM there is purulent middle ear effusion (MEE) and signs of inflammation that include otalgia or erythema of the TM. The TM is full and bulged outward, and there is no movement with insufflation (Figure 38-4).[1] By contrast, in otitis media with effusion (OME), there is fluid in the middle ear space without signs of acute infection.[2]

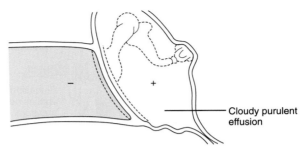

Figure 38-4   Pnematic otoscopy with acute purulent otitis media.

■ Complete the dashed and dotted lines demonstrating relative immobility in acute purulent otitis media. See Figure 38-5 for photographs of acute suppurative otitis media, otitis media with air-fluid level, and otitis media with effusion. Note that the distinction between and proper management of AOM and OME is discussed in Chapter 37, Ear Pain.

Patient Care

Positioning for Accurate Examination, Safety, and Comfort

To facilitate the examiner's visualization of the TM and prevent possible discomfort with sudden movement, the child may need to be securely positioned. Older infants and toddlers may be examined in the caregiver's lap.[3] Figure 38-6, *A*, shows the child sitting upright in the caregiver's lap, facing forward. If necessary to enhance stabilization, the child's legs are secured between the caregiver's legs. The caregiver wraps his/her arms around the child in a secure hug. Using his/her nondominant hand, the examiner will position and lean the child's head to the child's left, securely against the caregiver's chest, as demonstrated in Figure 38-6, *B*. This same hand will pull the child's right pinna up and out. The otoscope is held using the dominant hand with the insufflator bulb in the palm, secured against the otoscope shaft and gently introduced in the external ear canal. Regardless of the technique used for visualizing the TM, the examiner must ensure stabilization of the hand holding the otoscope against the child's face or skull to avoid trauma when the child attempts to move away as speculum is placed in the ear canal.

For young infants, or toddlers who strongly resist being held in the caregiver's lap, positioning on the examination table as shown in Figure 38-6, *C*, is an alternative. The child is supine with the

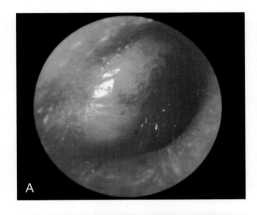

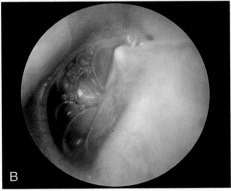

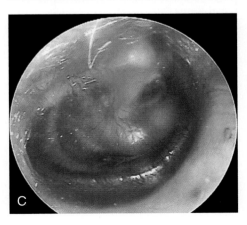

Figure 38-5
A, Photograph of acute suppurative otitis media. **B,** Photograph of otitis media with air-fluid level.
C, Photograph of acute serous otitis or otitis media with effusion.

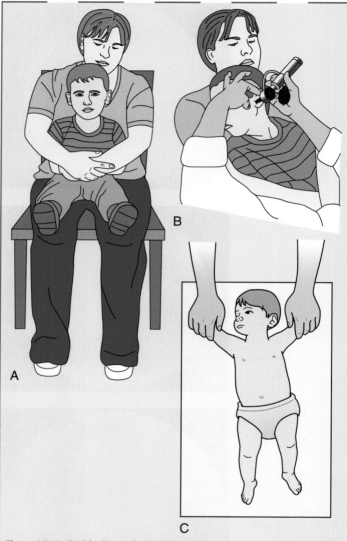

Figure 38-6 Positioning techniques for middle ear examination. **A,** Young child seated in caregiver's lap. **B,** Head stabilization for pneumatic otoscopy. **C,** Supine placement of infant.

caregiver next to the child's head. The caregiver extends the child's arms overhead, holding them securely on the table, being sure to anchor the elbows. This provides stabilization and allows the child to see and be verbally comforted by the caregiver. The examiner gently leans over the child's chest, and examines the left ear by turning the child's head to the child's right, proceeding with the examination described above. If additional help is needed to hold the child still, a third person can hold the child's legs. In very young infants, the pinna is pulled down and posterior because of the high cartilage component of the canal.

To achieve a good seal for visualization and pneumatic otoscopy, use the largest speculum that fits comfortably in the ear canal.[3] Note any erythema or drainage in the external canal. Note if the TM is translucent, and if the malleus and cone of light are present. Next, perform pneumatic otoscopy, and describe the examination findings.

Interpersonal and Communication Skills

Teach Parents About the Need for Accurate Diagnosis and Appropriate Use of Antibiotics Using Understandable Language

It is not uncommon for parents to suspect that their young child with a fever, irritability, congestion, and poor sleeping has an acute ear infection. In many instances, their hunch is correct. Parents may call the office or have you paged after hours asking that "an antibiotic be called in." It may be a challenge to persuade parents to bring a child to the office for an examination. The parents are likely distressed about the child's discomfort and perhaps their lack of sleep. Nonetheless, it is important to examine the child to correctly establish the diagnosis and treatment plan, and discuss whether antibiotic treatment is indicated. Explain that ear infections are a leading reason for prescription of antibiotics in children, and an accurate diagnosis with an assessment of need for prompt antibiotic treatment will limit unnecessary prescriptions. This is important because *Streptococcus pneumoniae*, a common cause of AOM, has developed penicillin resistance. Carefully selected children with AOM may be monitored off antibiotics for 3 days and observed for resolution (see Chapter 37, Ear Pain). Many times the fussy child with congestion may have fever from viral upper respiratory infection or incidental fussiness related to another factor, such as teething.

References

1. American Academy of Family Physicians, American Academy of Otolaryngology-Head Neck Surgery, and American Academy of Pediatrics Subcommittee on Otitis Media with Effusion: Clinical practice guideline. Otitis media with effusion. *Pediatrics* 113(5):1412-1429, 2004.
2. American Academy of Pediatrics and American Academy of Family Physicians Subcommittee on Management of Acute Otitis Media: Diagnosis and management of acute otitis media. *Pediatrics* 113(5):1451-1465. 2004.
3. Algranti PS: The pediatric patient: *An approach to history and physical examination*, Baltimore, MD, 1992, Williams & Wilkins.

Chapter 39
Weight Gain (Case 10)

Sandra Gibson Hassink MD, FAAP

Case: A 9-year-old has gained 20 pounds in the past year, with a body mass index (BMI) greater than 95% for age. His parents have recently separated, and the joint custody arrangement leaves little opportunity for physical activity. He attends a new school and has made few friends. His nighttime sleep is restless with snoring, and on examination you note acanthosis nigricans and elevated blood pressure. Family history is positive for type 2 diabetes mellitus.

Differential Diagnosis

Environmental causes of obesity	Psychosocial stressor and obesity
Growth hormone deficiency	Cushing disease

Speaking Intelligently

When evaluating a child with excessive weight gain, I inquire, "What has changed?" This often leads to discussion of the impact of nutrition, activity and inactivity, and identification of what can be changed. I explain that significant weight gain may be associated with changes in health status, family circumstances, or stress. A complete review of systems and careful physical examination help delineate comorbid conditions and identify the need for prompt intervention in conditions such as pseudotumor cerebri. The first encounter includes assessment of readiness to change.

PATIENT CARE

Clinical Thinking

- **Measure** height and weight, **calculate** BMI, **classify by** BMI percentile: less than 5%, underweight; 5% to 84%, normal weight; 85% to 94%, overweight; greater than 95%, obese; and greater than 99%, morbid (severe) obesity.
- Is there an underlying medical condition predisposing to weight gain such as hypothyroidism?
- Are there **coexistent medical conditions** such as poorly controlled asthma?
- Use family history, review of systems, and physical examination to gather critical information and establish the case for intervention.
- Identify comorbid conditions and any need for intervention. Signs and symptoms of obesity-related comorbidities help **assess disease risk and burden,** and delineate the urgency and intensity of the intervention.
- **Open-ended questions and motivational interviewing** techniques are used to establish a working partnership to facilitate change.

History

- Medications such as oral corticosteroids, antidepressants, antiepileptic and psychotropic agents may contribute to weight gain and also provide insight into conditions affecting potential for lifestyle change (e.g., depression, asthma, or seizure disorder).
- Check for family history of obesity, diabetes, cardiovascular disease and hypertension, and early death from myocardial infarction or stroke.
- **Assess lifestyle:** Eating behaviors; including fast food and eating out; diet history; amount of physical activity; daily screen time; and readiness for change.
- Short stature, linear growth deceleration, and delayed puberty are **clues to an endocrine disorder.**
- Psychosocial factors such as parental divorce play a role in causality and affect treatment.
- Environmental factors such as food exposure, income, culture, and ethnicity are variables that are crucial to understanding the nutritional/activity environment and individualizing interventions.

- **Screen for signs of comorbid conditions:**
  - Headache, vomiting, or visual field cuts in pseudotumor cerebri.
  - Snoring, restless sleep, heavy breathing, orthopnea, frequent night awakening, enuresis and apnea at night, morning headache, daytime tiredness, napping, poor school performance, and irritability with obstructive sleep apnea syndrome (OSAS).
  - Type 2 diabetes presentations can range from asymptomatic glycosuria to ketonuria or ketoacidosis with dehydration and weight loss.
  - Slipped capital femoral epiphysis (SCFE) may present with knee, hip, groin, or thigh pain, loss of internal rotation, flexion and abduction of the hip.
  - Blount disease presents with tibial bowing and possible tenderness of proximal tibia, abnormal gait, and leg length discrepancy.
  - Nonalcoholic fatty liver disease (NAFLD): Signs may be absent or subtle: mild abdominal pain and fatigue with progression to pruritus, anorexia, nausea, and cirrhosis.
  - Polycystic ovary syndrome (PCOS): Menstrual irregularity, hirsutism, and acne.
  - Hypertension.
  - Asthma under poor control may lead to decreased activity and deconditioning, and excess use of systemic steroids will predispose to further weight gain.
  - Insulin resistance and metabolic syndrome.
  - Mental health: Depression, anxiety, and low self-esteem.

Physical Examination
- Vital signs should always include blood pressure, taken seated in the right arm using the proper size cuff.
- Anthropometric measurements such as waist circumference to further define body composition.
- Sensitivity to using proper size gowns and to self-consciousness about body size and shape is crucial.
- Tanner staging is included to ascertain onset and pace of puberty.
- Acanthosis nigricans suggests insulin resistance.
- Striae occur in Cushing syndrome.
- Hirsutism in females with PCOS.
- Tonsillar hypertrophy in OSAS.
- Goiter may occur in hypothyroidism.
- Abdominal tenderness and hepatomegaly may indicate NAFLD.
- Limited hip range of motion may indicate SCFE.

Tests for Consideration
- If BMI is 85% to 94% with no risk factors: **Fasting lipid profile.** $156

- If BMI is 85% to 94% with risk factors in history or physical
  examination:
  - **Fasting lipid profile** $156
  - **AST, ALT** $132
  - **Fasting glucose** $70
- If BMI is greater than 95%:
  - **Fasting lipid profile** $156
  - **AST, ALT** $132
  - Fasting glucose $70
  - Bun/creatinine $174
  can be obtained if indicated.
- **Night polysomnography:** For suspected obstructive
  sleep apnea $9657
- **Urine free cortisol:** For suspected Cushing disease $170
- **Locu-dose dexamethasone suppression test:** For suspected
  Cushing disease $400
- **Insulin-like growth factor-I (IGF-I):** For suspected growth
  hormone deficiency. $194
- **Insulin-like growth factor–binding protein 3 (IGFBP-3):**
  For suspected growth hormone deficiency $177
- **Luteinizing hormone (LH)** and **follicle-stimulating
  hormone (FSH):** For suspected PCOS $168
- **Thyroid-stimulating hormone (TSH), triiodothyronine (T_3),
  and free thyroxine (T_4):** If goiter or suspected
  hypothyroidism. $194
- **Urine glucose and ketones:**
- For suspected type 2 diabetes:
  - **Urine glucose and ketones** $95
  - **Insulin level** $137
  - **Hemoglobin A_{1c}** $128
  - **Fasting plasma glucose** $70
  - **Two-hour oral glucose tolerance test** $375

IMAGING CONSIDERATIONS

→ **A/P and frog hip radiograph:** For suspected slipped
  capital femoral epiphyses $230
→ **Bone age radiography:** For suspected growth hormone
  deficiency $151
→ **Magnetic resonance imaging of brain:** For suspected
  hypothalamic etiology or pseudotumor cerebri $2331
→ **Abdominal ultrasound:** for suspected cholelithiasis or
  steatohepatitis $846
→ **AP** and **lateral radiograph of tibia:** For suspected
  Blount disease $219

| Clinical Entities | Medical Knowledge |

Environmental Causes of Obesity

Pφ	Environmental causes of energy imbalance operate via energy intake and energy expenditure interacting with genetic predisposition to create weight gain. Excess consumption of sugar-containing beverages, fast food, increased portion sizes, snacking, and breakfast skipping have been shown to contribute to weight gain. Screen time promotes a sedentary lifestyle and increased exposure to media advertisements for energy-dense foods. In addition, decreased outdoor play, physical education time, and overall fitness levels contribute to decreased energy expenditure.
TP	The typical child without organic disease usually presents with one of the high-risk behaviors listed above. Families may underappreciate how these factors contribute to weight gain. Behavioral issues around hunger, food sneaking, food seeking, and emotional eating may also contribute. Environmental factors such as fast food restaurants, corner stores, school vending machines, meals, snacks, safety issues, and lack of outdoor play opportunities can all contribute to obesity. Family microenvironments are key, and family lifestyle change is essential.
Dx	Careful daily dietary and exercise records coupled with a history can identify most of the environmental risk. Because families may not initially appreciate the factors contributing to weight gain, specific questions should be used to elicit as much information about the daily routine of the child as possible.
Tx	Motivational interviewing techniques and brief focused negotiation can be used for goal setting, and assessment of willingness and barriers to change are recommended to allow families to "own" the desired behavior change. Families need to be prepared to change together. Self-monitoring and frequent follow-up are strategies that promote optimal results.[2] **See Nelson Essentials 29.**

Psychosocial Stress and Obesity

Pφ	Depression has been found to be a precursor to obesity. Obesity can also occur after a family or child stressful experience such as death of a parent, difficult school change, or move of a household. Mechanisms for weight gain are unclear; however, changes in eating and activity patterns often accompany these stressors.

TP	One clue to a stress-induced weight gain is the presence of an inflection point on the growth curve, with a period of rapid weight gain that temporally coincides with the stressors. Attention to school functioning, family and peer relationships, and mood can also alert the clinician that a child is in a stressful situation.
Dx	Diagnosis is determined by history, depression inventories, and/or family stress scales.
Tx	Often realization of the connection between weight gain and a child/family stressor is enough to start the "change" conversation. Understanding how nutrition and activity patterns altered in response to the stressor can give valuable information about the direction of lifestyle change.[3]

Cushing Disease

Pφ	Hypercortisolism, or Cushing disease, is the result of excess cortisol secretion due to pituitary adenoma secretion of adrenocorticotropic hormone (ACTH), nonpituitary tumors secreting ectopic ACTH, or adrenal tumors. An inherited form of Cushing disease, primary pigmented micronodular adrenal disease, can occur in children and young adults. Multiple endocrine neoplasia type I can also cause Cushing syndrome. Prolonged therapy with corticosteroids or ACTH is a common cause of Cushing syndrome. Inappropriate use of topical corticosteroids has been a reported cause of Cushing disease in infants. The excess cortisol levels result in increased protein breakdown and gluconeogenesis, hence favoring fat biosynthesis.
TP	Truncal obesity and linear growth deceleration are the most common signs of cortisol excess. Additional signs include striae, fatigue, hypertension, increased blood glucose, irritability, and depression. Hirsutism and missed or irregular periods can occur in females.
Dx	Clinical findings and a 24-hour urinary free cortisol and/or low-dose dexamethasone suppression test are used to diagnose Cushing disease and differentiate it from primary adrenal hypercortisolism. Additional testing is performed to localize the source of ACTH or cortisol production.
Tx	Depending on the cause, surgical excision of a pituitary adenoma or surgery and/or chemotherapy are used to treat an ectopic ACTH-secreting tumor. **See Nelson Essentials 178.**

Growth Hormone Deficiency

Pφ	There is a paucity or lack of growth hormone, which may be idiopathic, or the direct result of a variety of mutations, absence of the pituitary gland, central nervous system (CNS) trauma, or a tumor.
TP	Key findings include linear growth deceleration, short stature, weight gain, increased waist circumference, headaches, polyuria, polydipsia, and delayed or absent menstruation.
Dx	Bone age is delayed, IGF-1 and IGFBP-3 levels are decreased, and there are an abnormal growth hormone stimulation test results.
Tx	Treatment is growth hormone replacement with close monitoring of linear height progression by an endocrinologist. **See Nelson Essentials 173.**

ZEBRA ZONE

a. **Prader-Willi Syndrome (PWS):** Deletion of chromosome 15q11-q13, resulting from uniparental disomy. Infants are hypotonic with severe feeding difficulties, which reverts to hyperphagia with food seeking and lack of satiety in childhood. Delayed cognitive and motor development, **hypogonadism,** and short stature are characteristic.

b. **Hypothalamic obesity:** This is due to hypothalamic dysfunction secondary to an insult such as brain tumor, CNS radiation, or injury.

Practice-Based Learning and Improvement: Evidence-Based Pediatrics

Title
Ten year outcomes of behavioral based family-centered treatment for childhood obesity

Authors
Epstein LH, Valosky A, Wing RR

Reference
Health Psychol 13(5):373-383, 1994

Problem
Childhood obesity

Intervention
Lifestyle behavior change with family support and education and lifestyle education

Comparison/control (quality of evidence)
Randomized controlled treatment studies

Outcome/effect
At 10 years, 34% decreased percentage overweight by 20% or more, and 30% were not obese.

Historical significance/comments
This study is significant for long-term success in a family-based behavioral program based on lifestyle change. It identified important factors correlated with success such as lifestyle, exercise versus calisthenics, importance of family involvement, self-monitoring, family meals, family and friend support.

Interpersonal and Communication Skills

Use Motivational Interview Technique to Encourage Lifestyle Change

Motivational interview techniques are useful when working with patients and families to identify motivation for change and resolve ambivalence through a nonjudgmental approach. Reflective listening, assessing readiness for change, and brief focused negotiation are important skills to encourage lifestyle change. Accepting families and patients "where they are" and partnering with them by supporting achievement of incremental steps toward the goals of improved nutrition and activity is important in helping them succeed.

Professionalism

Be Self-Aware of Prejudice Toward Obese Patients

Societal attitudes and prejudices about obesity may lead to obese children enduring unkind comments from adults and teasing and bullying by peers. These experiences often leave obese children vulnerable with low self-esteem. Clinicians must be self-aware of the impact societal attitudes and prejudices have on patients of all ages. Physicians must examine their own feelings about working with this group of patients, and make sure that they provide compassionate and nonjudgmental care.

Systems-Based Practice

Using the Chronic Care Model in Obesity Management

The chronic care model includes six elements: Decision support, self-management support, clinical information systems, delivery system design, health-care organization, and linkages with community resources (Figure 39-1).

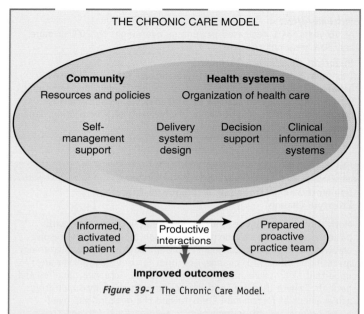

Figure 39-1 The Chronic Care Model.

Comprehensive Care Through Use of the Chronic Care Model

The Chronic Care Model (CCM) identifies the essential elements of a health-care system that encourage high-quality chronic disease care. These elements are the community, the health system, self-management support, delivery system design, decision support, and clinical information systems. Evidence-based change concepts under each element, in combination, foster productive interactions between informed patients who take an active part in their care and providers with resources and expertise.

The model can be applied to a variety of chronic illnesses, health-care settings, and target populations. The bottom line is healthier patients, more satisfied providers, and cost savings.[4]

References

1. Hassink S: *A clinical guide to pediatric weight management and obesity*, 2006, Lippincott Williams & Wilkins.
2. Hassink S: *Pediatric obesity: Prevention, intervention and treatment strategies for primary care*, Elk Grove Village, IL, 2006, American Academy of Pediatrics.
3. Hassink S, editor: *A parent's guide to childhood obesity: A road map to health*, Elk Grove Village, IL, 2006, American Academy of Pediatrics, (Book for pediatricians and parents)
4. Robert Wood Foundation: Chronic Care Model. Available at http://www. improvingchroniccare.org/index.php?p=The_Chronic_Care_Model&s=2

Chapter 40
Feeding Difficulty (Case 11)

Deborah M. Consolini MD

Case: An otherwise healthy 12-month-old boy with frequent emesis and feeding difficulties since birth has poor weight gain and food refusal.

Differential Diagnosis

Behavioral/environmental/ etiologies	Gastrointestinal disorders	Chronic illness or disability

Speaking Intelligently

Feeding problems occur in healthy children, those with gastrointestinal disorders, and in those with chronic illness or disability. The etiology is usually multifactorial, involving medical, behavioral, and environmental factors. Even with a clear organic etiology, maladaptive feeding behaviors can develop and persist after resolution of the organic problem. Feeding difficulty in a child is seldom limited to the child alone; it is a family problem. Parental child-rearing skills, nutritional knowledge, emotional stability, and feeding competency can both precipitate and maintain feeding difficulties. Given the multifactorial nature, assessment and treatment are done best by an interdisciplinary team that may include the pediatrician, a nutritionist, an occupational and/or speech therapist, and often a gastroenterologist and a developmental/behavioral specialist. Intervention should be comprehensive and include treatment of underlying medical conditions, behavioral modification to alter learned maladaptive feeding behaviors, and education and training in appropriate parenting and feeding skills. Most feeding problems can be resolved or greatly improved with medical, oromotor, and behavioral therapy.

PATIENT CARE

Clinical Thinking
- **Take parental concerns about their child's feeding difficulty seriously.**
- Is there failure to thrive or weight loss requiring urgent intervention?

- Feeding difficulties are often the first clue of a gastrointestinal disorder causing pain, discomfort, appetite suppression, and/or reduced motivation to feed.

History
- Information about feeding environment, consistency of caregivers, feeding practices, availability of food, child temperament, and food preferences may identify *inappropriate mealtime behavior or environment, food selectivity,* or *food refusal.*
- Choking, gagging, and/or coughing with feeds, frequent respiratory infections or a history of aspiration pneumonia, multiple swallows, or noisy breathing, especially during eating, may signal *swallowing dysfunction.*
- Irritability with feeds, frequent emesis, arching, epigastric pain, or heartburn is suggestive of *gastroesophageal reflux (GER)/ esophagitis.*
- Abdominal pain, early satiety, nausea, vomiting, abdominal distention, excessive belching or flatulence, or abnormal stool pattern may indicate *constipation, food allergy or intolerance, malabsorption,* or *motility disorder.*
- Underlying conditions such as *central nervous system (CNS) disorders* (cerebral palsy), *genetic syndromes* (Prader-Willi and Down syndromes), and *developmental disabilities* (autism and prematurity) predispose children to feeding difficulties.

Physical Examination
- Review growth parameters (weight, height, head circumference [<3 years], weight for height, and/or body mass index [BMI]) to **assess nutritional status** and severity of feeding disorder.
- Noisy breathing, stridor, respiratory distress, increased work of breathing, and/or wheezing suggest *swallowing dysfunction* or **GER** with recurrent aspiration.
- Abdominal tenderness or distention or palpable stool suggest a *gastrointestinal disorder.*
- Abnormal tone, focal neurologic deficits, or dysmorphic features may suggest an underlying *CNS disorder* or *genetic syndrome.*

Tests for Consideration
If concerned about nutritional status, vitamin/mineral deficiency, consider:

- **Complete blood count (CBC)** $116
- **Comprehensive metabolic panel** $237
- **Prealbumin** $117
- **Ferritin** $177
- **Zinc level** $135
- **Lead level** $34
- **Specific vitamin levels** $150-250

If concerned for gastrointestinal disorder, consider:

- **pH or impedance probe** $5585
- **Endoscopy** $1313
- **Stool for occult blood** $170
- **Sweat test** $25
- **Celiac panel** $225
- **Fecal fat studies** $210

If concerned about underlying genetic syndrome, consider:

- **High-resolution chromosomes** $500
- **Fragile X testing** $250
- **DNA methylation test for Prader-Willi syndrome** $250

IMAGING CONSIDERATIONS

→ **Modified barium swallow:** If concern for swallowing dysfunction $840
→ **Upper gastrointestinal series (UGI):** If frequent emesis to rule out gastric outlet obstruction or malrotation $840
→ **Gastric emptying scan:** If concern for delayed gastric emptying or GER $1118

Clinical Entities   Medical Knowledge

Behavioral/Environmental

Pφ   Healthy normal children often develop transient feeding difficulties. Occasionally these progress to lasting inappropriate feeding behaviors. Significant nutritional deficiencies are rare unless the problem is long term or food selectivity is severe. Feeding difficulties in healthy children are linked to a variety of causes, including environmental disruption, parental incompetencies, and child temperament. For example, some children are more easily distracted from feeding in a highly stimulating environment. Parents with poor knowledge of nutrition and development and their own emotional or feeding disorders may reinforce inappropriate feeding behaviors. As children move toward independence over what, when, and how much they eat, some parents may be intolerant of their child's messiness while feeding, may not encourage self-feeding for fear that inadequate food will be consumed, and may not pace the meal properly because of time pressures. Parents may try to coax, threaten, or even force-feed their child, which may strengthen the child's resolve to avoid eating.

TP   There may be limited intake of food, food refusal, food selectivity by type or texture, disruptive mealtime behaviors, and excessive meal duration. Examination rarely shows signs of significant growth failure, nutritional deficiency, or developmental concerns.

Dx   Testing is not a priority unless malnutrition or vitamin/mineral deficiencies are suspected. Observation of feeding in the child's natural environment can provide critical information in understanding the parent's competency, feeding schedules and routines, child temperament and food/texture preferences, available resources, and the settings that affect the child's feeding behaviors.

Tx   Treatment should focus on teaching the parent to understand the child's temperament, set limits, and facilitate the child's internal regulation of feeding to improve the parent-child relationship and produce mutually satisfactory mealtimes. Consultation with nutrition, occupational, and/or speech therapy may be necessary. **See Nelson Essentials 27 and 28.**

Gastrointestinal Disorders

Pφ   Gastrointestinal disorders cause pain, discomfort, appetite suppression, and reduced motivation to feed. Repeated pairing of pain with feeding can lead to food refusal or selectivity, which may persist after resolution of the organic problem. Dysphagia, or swallowing disorder, can be caused by congenital, acquired, or functional factors and can involve the oral, pharyngeal, or esophageal phase of swallowing (e.g., cleft lip/palate, enlarged tonsils and adenoids, esophagitis). Multiple medical procedures involving the face and mouth (e.g., dental work, repeated nasogastric tube passage, oral suctioning, and tracheostomy) can result in conditioned dysphagia, with hypersensitivity to touch in these areas and defensive posturing when food is brought to the mouth.

TP   Children with dysphagia may present with food refusal, swallowing refusal, cough, gag or aspiration when swallowing, multiple swallows, drooling, difficulty handling oral secretions, and frequent respiratory infections. Defensive behaviors seen with conditioned dysphagia can include crying, gagging, throwing up, turning away, and batting at food. **GER** may present with gagging, choking, emesis, irritability, arching/posturing, pain, and food aversion/refusal. Feeding difficulties caused by food allergies/intolerance, malabsorption, or motility disorders may present with early satiety, nausea, vomiting, belching, abdominal pain/cramping, and diarrhea as well as limited food intake. Examination findings depend on the specific disorder and its severity and duration.

Dx   A modified barium swallow is critical if dysphagia is suspected to determine the aspiration risk before instituting feeding therapy. Further testing is determined by the clinical presentation and suspected disorder.

Tx   Because most children have both medical and behavioral issues, an interdisciplinary team approach is best. Treatment of dysphagia may include surgical correction of underlying structural deficits, followed by skill shaping and reinforcement and systematic desensitization to develop functional swallowing. Nutritional therapy includes fortification of foods to get the most calories in the smallest volume of food and modification of food taste, temperature, texture, and consistency to stimulate salivation and aid swallowing. Medical management of digestive disorders should be timely and aggressive to avoid the development of secondary maladaptive behaviors. Increasing intake is critical because feeding behavior may improve with an improved nutritional state. Enteral tube feedings or parenteral nutrition may be necessary but, to avoid iatrogenic feeding problems, should be initiated only after a trial of oral feeding therapy fails, unless the child is severely malnourished or oral feedings are medically contraindicated. Because reinstituting oral feeds is often difficult due to poor oromotor skills, maladaptive behaviors and difficulty identifying hunger/satiety cues, even when nonoral feeding is medically necessary, oral feeding should be maintained to some degree whenever possible. Behavioral therapy may also be necessary. **See Nelson Essentials 127 and 128.**

Chronic Illness or Disability

Pφ   Virtually any pediatric medical problem can set the stage for poor feeding. Illness reduces motivation to feed. Children who are ill may have reduced energy, experience discomfort and pain, deal with distortions of taste and smell, and suffer from fatigue and stress. Certain diagnoses that are "red flags" for feeding problems include CNS disorders, genetic disorders, developmental disabilities, and prematurity. Feeding difficulties in children with these diagnoses are usually attributed to abnormalities in tone or sensation, oromotor dysfunction, immature feeding and communication skills, associated gastrointestinal disorders such as reflux, and maladaptive feeding behaviors.

TP   Children with CNS disorders (e.g., cerebral palsy) may demonstrate oromotor dysfunction, postural tone abnormalities, and oral tactile sensitivity. When presented with foods in a manner they cannot handle, they may react vigorously by turning their head, spitting food, and making vocalizations, and they expend a tremendous amount of time and energy in feeding. Some genetic syndromes (e.g., Down syndrome) are associated with hypotonia and poor coordination of breathing, sucking, and swallowing. These children tend to be poor feeders and are slow to acquire feeding skills. Children with developmental disabilities (e.g., autism) may demonstrate increased or decreased oral tactile sensitivity. Hyposensitivity can affect swallowing, diminish taste, and interfere with feeding skills and motivation. With hypersensitivity, the slightest advancement in texture may be met with refusal, leading to a very limited food repertoire. Examination may reveal signs of growth failure or nutritional deficiency.

Dx   Children with neurologic impairment are especially at risk for swallowing dysfunction and esophagitis, and therefore a modified barium swallow to assess for aspiration with a variety of textures and endoscopy should be strongly considered.

Tx Because most children have both medical and behavioral issues, an interdisciplinary team approach is best. Occupational and speech therapy are essential, with a nutritionist as needed. Behavioral therapy should be considered for maladaptive feeding behaviors. In addition to addressing ongoing medical issues, treatment of feeding problems in children with special needs requires careful attention to proper seating and positioning, modulation of the sensory environment, appropriate textures for easy chewing and swallowing, and utensils designed for the child's physical capabilities. Fortification of foods to get the most calories in the smallest volume reduces the amount of food the child has to eat, the time taken to feed, and the effort needed in feeding. **See Nelson Essentials 10, 20, and 49.**

ZEBRA ZONE

a. **Food phobia:** Children may react with extreme anxiety after a choking episode and develop an intense fear of eating, often panic when forced to eat, and demonstrate rapid weight loss and social withdrawal.

b. **Medications:** Medications may impact feeding through appetite suppression, nausea and vomiting, dysphagia, and abdominal pain. Commonly implicated medications include nonsteroidal antiinflammatory drugs (NSAIDs), anticholinergics, antibiotics, antiseizure medications, stimulants used for attention-deficit/hyperactivity disorder (ADHD), and atypical antipsychotics used in behavioral/developmental disabilities.

Practice-Based Learning and Improvement

Title
Pediatric feeding disorders

Authors
Manikam R, Perman JA

Reference
J Clin Gastroenterol 30:34-46, 2000

Problem
Review of feeding disorders in children

Comparison/control (quality of evidence)
Review article with cited references in peer-reviewed journal

Interpersonal and Communication Skills

Communicate Effectively With Consultants and Therapists When Managing Complex Feeding Issues

Given the multifactorial nature of feeding problems, an interdisciplinary approach often works best in evaluating these problems. This often includes an initial evaluation by the pediatrician, nutritionist, and occupational and/or speech therapist. Other specialists such as a gastroenterologist or a developmental/behavioral pediatrician may be consulted as needed. Ongoing involvement by some or all of these people will be needed depending on what the cause of the feeding problem is felt to be. This interdisciplinary team approach necessitates frequent and effective communication either through regularly scheduled team meetings or written encounter notes to keep all team members abreast of the child's progress as well as ongoing medical, behavioral, and psychosocial issues.

Professionalism

Communicate to Empower Parents

Parents are often reluctant to acknowledge the importance of their own psychosocial factors in their child's feeding difficulties, and professionals may find it challenging to explain to parents that their stress is influencing their child's feeding behavior. Effective management of feeding disorders should always be seen as a partnership between the parents and the interdisciplinary team. Providing parents with proper training as well as realistic goals, regular instruction for home practice, and the expectation for periodic setbacks can instill in the parent a feeling of competence and help the child and the parent reap the most benefit from feeding intervention.

Systems-Based Practice

Managed Care: Member Benefits and Services Requiring Authorization

The American health-care system is a mix of both private and public insurance plans. By far, the most important source of coverage for the nonelderly population is through employers. The medical benefit coverage (what procedures or services get covered) will vary among insurance companies. Many of those not covered through private insurance or federal programs are covered through state-run programs, primarily Medicaid, or the State Children's Health Insurance Program (SCHIP). Health insurance coverage for children and spending on services for this population vary considerably among states. Physicians need to be aware that in order to control cost, most insurance companies will require medical necessity review and authorization before specialized services like feeding programs are rendered.

Chapter 41
Dysuria (Case 12)

Carolyn Milana MD

Case: A 4-year-old girl with dysuria and frequency for 1 day

Differential Diagnosis

Urinary tract infection	Trauma
Sexually transmitted infection/child abuse	Nonvenereal vulvovaginitis

Speaking Intelligently

Dysuria is pain while voiding that results from irritation of the bladder, urethra, or surrounding perineal tissues. Urinary tract infection (UTI) is the most common potentially serious cause. My first step in evaluation of a patient with dysuria is to perform a thorough history and physical examination. Laboratory work should be based on clinical impressions gleaned from the initial evaluation.

PATIENT CARE

Clinical Thinking

- Bacterial cystitis can progress to pyelonephritis with possible risk for sepsis, renal scarring, and/or hypertension.
- Dysuria is more common in females because of the presence of a short urethra, thin prepubertal vaginal mucosa, and urethral proximity to the anus.
- Sexually transmitted infection (STI) in children should be aggressively pursued for management and reporting to appropriate child protective services.

History

- **Systemic signs or symptoms:** fever, vomiting, anorexia, abdominal or flank pain?
- **Localizing signs:** urgency, frequency, hesitancy, hematuria, enuresis, or nocturia?
- History of **prior UTI, vesicoureteral reflux (VUR),** or **antibiotic prophylaxis?**
- Constipation?
- Environmental exposures: poor hygiene, new bath products, or wearing tight or wet clothing?
- Trauma?
- For adolescent girls, are they **sexually active?** For the younger child, is there **suspicion of molestation?**

Physical Examination

- Vital signs: Note fever, weight loss, hypertension or hypotension.
- Abdominal examination: Note abdominal or costovertebral angle (CVA) tenderness; palpate for bladder distention and tenderness; check for palpable fecal masses.
- Inspect external genitalia and urethra; note vaginal discharge, foreign bodies, discoloration, swelling, excoriations, trauma, perineal lesions.

Tests for Consideration

- **Urine dipstick:** *Any* nitrite or moderate leukocyte esterase (LE) is highly specific for UTI (98%, 99%). $95
- **Urinalysis (U/A):** Adds little to diagnosis of UTI; consider if blood or significant protein. $95
- **Urine culture and antibiotic sensitivity:** Gold standard for UTI diagnosis: urethral catheterization or suprapubic aspiration (SPA) if in diapers; clean catch midstream (CCMS) urine if toilet-trained. Diagnosis of UTI is dependent on the method of urine specimen collection. $148
  - *CCMS specimen:* In males, ≥10,000 CFU/mL of a single organism; in females, ≥100,000 CFU/mL of a single

organism. Pure growth of fewer pathogens may be
significant in appropriate clinical settings. $148

- *Urethral catheterization specimen:* Per the American Academy of Pediatrics (AAP) guideline: ≥10,000 CFU/mL of a single pathogen is considered positive. Other authors have noted that ≥50,000 CFU/mL are more likely to correspond to true pathogens, and hence UTI, and a repeat catheterized specimen is suggested for 10,000 to 50,000 CFU/mL.[1,2]
- *SPA specimen:* **Any** growth of a gram-negative rod (GNR) or more than a few thousand CFU/mL of gram-positive cocci is considered positive.

- **Cervical/vaginal cultures:** For gonorrhea (GC), chlamydia, or bacterial vaginosis if indicated $290
- **Urine polymerase chain reaction (PCR):** For gonorrhea and chlamydia if indicated $250
- **Culture or direct fluorescent antibody test for herpes simplex virus:** If genital ulcers $289
- **Electrolytes, blood urea nitrogen (BUN), and creatinine:** If concern for renal function $174
- If febrile and ill appearing
  Complete blood count $116
  Blood culture $152

IMAGING CONSIDERATIONS

→ **Renal ultrasound:** Was routine with most first UTIs to identify anomalies; this practice is currently under scrutiny given prenatal ultrasound and low yield in identifying treatable conditions (see Chapter 64, Antenatal Hydronephrosis). $590

→ **Radiographic voiding cystourethrography (VCUG):** To detect and grade vesicoureteral reflux (VUR). Radionuclide cystogram identifies VUR without grading. The relevance of VCUG for first UTIs is also being investigated. $600

→ **Renal scintigraphy with dimercaptosuccinic acid (DMSA):** If indicated to identify acute pyelonephritis and chronic scars. $1524

→ **Computed tomography (CT) scan of abdomen/pelvis:** If diagnosis in doubt or suspect renal calculi. $1691

Clinical Entities	Medical Knowledge

Urinary Tract Infection

Pφ   A *urinary tract infection* is bacteria in the urinary tract with an inflammatory response (pyuria). Cystitis involves the lower-tract with focal symptoms, whereas in pyelonephritis there is upper tract (kidney) involvement with a systemic inflammatory response. Pyelonephritis results from ascending infection, and it is difficult to distinguish upper from lower tract infection in infants and young children. Anomalies such as hydronephrosis, VUR, duplication of ureters, or posterior urethral valves in males are predisposing risk factors. Eighty percent of first community-acquired UTIs are due to *Escherichia coli*. Other organisms include *Klebsiella pneumoniae, Proteus, Enterobacter, Proteus vulgaris,* and enterococcus. Rare pathogens tend to emerge with prior treatment, hospitalization, instrumentation, or urinary tract anomalies.

TP   Dysuria is the typical chief complaint in cystitis without fever or other systemic signs. There may be suprapubic pain along with urinary frequency, urgency, and hesitation; young children may have daytime enuresis. Toilet-trained children may have poor toilet hygiene, constipation, and/or dysfunctional voiding. Examination is generally unremarkable, but check for CVA or suprapubic tenderness (both more common in upper tract infection) and signs of fecal retention. Children with pyelonephritis may be quite ill or toxic-appearing and have fever, chills, vomiting, and dehydration, along with generalized abdominal or flank pain. Infants typically have fever and may lack other signs or may be irritable, with poor feeding. Risk factors in infants are white females, uncircumcised males, fever >39° C (102.2° F), and fever for at least 2 days.[3]

Dx   Urine dipstick is the initial screen, and findings may include nitrites, leukocyte esterase, blood, and/or protein. Microscopic examination of urine may demonstrate white blood cells (WBCs) greater than 5 to 10 per high power field, WBC casts, and/or bacteria. Urine culture is diagnostic. Specimen collection and diagnostic criteria are discussed above. Renal ultrasound can be done at any time. Although VCUG is presently the subject of a large clinical study, the AAP as of this writing recommends VCUG in all children with first UTI between the ages of 2 months and 2 years; however, its utility has been questioned.[4] A VCUG is also advised for school-age girls with two or more UTIs and any male with a UTI regardless of age.

Tx   Empirical antibiotic therapy is recommended in suspected UTI pending culture results. Third-generation cephalosporins such as cefixime or cefdinir are recommended first-line agents for febrile UTI in the outpatient setting. Nitrofurantoin is good empirical treatment for cystitis. Amoxicillin and trimethoprim-sulfa may be less useful because of resistance patterns. Intravenous treatment, such as ampicillin and gentamicin to cover gram-negative pathogens and enterococci, is indicated if the child is toxic appearing or unable to tolerate oral therapy. Coverage is narrowed based on sensitivities. Duration of therapy varies by age and level of infection. Under 12 years of age, guidelines recommend treatment for 7 to 10 days, whereas in adolescents a 3-day course for cystitis may suffice. Infants and children with pyelonephritis are treated for 10 to 14 days. Standard of care has been antimicrobial prophylaxis after treatment is complete, pending VCUG. With documented VUR, prophylaxis is continued with annual VCUG until resolution, or in cases of significant anatomic abnormalities or high-grade reflux, surgical correction. The utility of prophylaxis to prevent recurrent UTI/ renal scarring is currently being questioned. Furthermore, the practice may predispose to infection with resistant organisms (See Practice-Based Learning and Improvement and Chapter 46, Neonatal Fever). **See Nelson Essentials 114.**

Trauma	
Pφ	Straddle injury is the most common traumatic cause of dysuria. However, other mechanisms of injury to the genitourinary area are always of concern and should elevate concern for abuse. The history of injury should be consistent with physical examination findings.
TP	Girls present with pain, bruising, dysuria, and difficulty voiding. Boys may have blood at the meatus or penile bruising and swelling. Examination of the testes for swelling or hematoma is important. Check for bladder distention because severe pain may cause urinary retention.
Dx	Imaging is usually not required; however, with concern for compromised blood flow, particularly to the testes, a scrotal ultrasound is recommended.
Tx	Treatment is supportive. For female straddle injuries, ice packs and analgesics generally suffice. Consultation with urology is indicated for extensive injury.

Sexually Transmitted Infection/Child Abuse

Pφ Some **STIs** that cause dysuria include gonorrhea (GC), chlamydia, and herpes simplex. Gonorrhea is caused by *Neisseria gonorrhoeae*, a gram-negative diplococcus. *Chlamydia trachomatis* is an obligate intracellular parasite, and herpes simplex (HSV) is a double-stranded DNA virus, with genital infection more commonly resulting from type 2 HSV.

TP Chlamydia and gonorrheal infections may be asymptomatic or present with vaginal or urethral discharge and dysuria. Fever and other systemic symptoms are usually absent. Herpes simplex is suspected with vesicular or ulcerative genital lesions.

Dx Urine nucleic acid amplification tests (NAATs) have made diagnosis of chlamydia and GC faster and simpler. However, cervical cultures and pelvic examination to exclude pelvic inflammatory disease (PID) may be warranted. Pathogen-specific cultures are still considered the gold standard for forensic evidence in child abuse; adherence to specimen collection requirements is critical in such cases.

Tx Treatment is tailored toward the organism. Current treatment for chlamydia is a 5-day course of azithromycin; gonorrhea is treated with a single dose of ceftriaxone. The CDC website is the best source for current recommendations. Mandatory public health reporting is required for many STIs. STIs in young children should always be reported to the appropriate child welfare agencies. **See Nelson Essentials 22 and 116.**

Nonvenereal Vulvovaginitis

Pφ Pediatric **nonvenereal vulvovaginitis** has multiple causes, and the most common is nonspecific inflammation resulting from poor hygiene in young toilet-trained girls. Adolescents may experience transient dysuria from perineal irritation following sexual intercourse.

TP Other causes include chemical irritation from bubble bath, retained foreign body, group A beta-hemolytic streptococcus (GAS) infection, pinworm infestation, or candidal infection.

Dx Diagnosis is clinical. Check for poor hygiene. Chemical irritation presents with vulvar redness and possible excoriations. Vaginal foreign bodies cause persistent foul-smelling discharge. Florid, well-circumscribed inflammation of the perineum in girls occurs with group A streptococcus (GAS). Monilial infections cause diaper rash in infants and pruritus, redness, and vaginal discharge in adolescents.

Urine dip may show leukocyte esterase. Pinworm infection is diagnosed by parental visualization or the cellophane tape test. GAS is diagnosed by culture. KOH prep and/or culture will confirm monilial infection in teens. Recurrent or refractory inflammation should prompt further investigation, such as STI or occult foreign body. Rarely, examination under anesthesia may be necessary to exclude a foreign body, tumor, and/or to obtain valid cultures.

Tx   Supportive treatment may include sitz baths and topical treatment for itching. Elimination of inciting factors and correction of hygiene practices is key. Failure to respond in several days to conservative therapy should prompt reevaluation. Specific therapy is instituted against specific pathogens. **See Nelson Essentials 115.**

ZEBRA ZONE

a. **Bladder Sphincter Dyssynergy** and other disorders of voiding and enuresis often associated with constipation.

b. **Urolithiasis:** Hypercalciuria may lead to stone formation and severe dysuria while passing a stone.

Practice-Based Learning and Improvement

Title
Recurrent urinary tract infections in children: Risk factors and association with prophylactic antimicrobials

Author
Conway PH, Cnaan A, Zaoutis T, et al

Reference
JAMA 298(2):179-186, 2007

Intervention
Prospective study of a primary care cohort of children after a first UTI with documented vesicoureteral reflux (VUR) to identify risk factors for recurrent UTI, the association between antimicrobial prophylaxis and recurrent UTI, and the risk factors for resistant infections.

Outcome/effect
White race, age 3 to 5 years, and grade 4 to 5 VUR were associated with increased risk for recurrent UTI. Antimicrobial prophylaxis was not associated with lower risk for recurrent UTI, but prophylaxis was associated with increased risk for resistant infections.

Historical significance/comments
Current practice of antimicrobial prophylaxis to prevent recurrent UTI in children with VUR may offer little benefit.

Interpersonal and Communication Skills

Explain Diagnostic Procedures in a Focused and Sensitive Manner

Evaluation of a patient with dysuria requires insightful and sensitive communication with the patient and parents. Once the examination is complete, you may find yourself recommending tests and procedures that may cause discomfort, such as urethral catheterization or VCUG. The importance of these tests should be conveyed to the parents and patient in a concise, logical manner. Without parental understanding of the importance of testing and the impact of a positive test on the patient's future care, you may face a family who refuses the testing.

Professionalism

Advocacy: The Obligation to File for Suspected Child Abuse

If the physician suspects that a child with dysuria may have been sexually abused, this must always be immediately addressed with the parents/family. It is a clinician's legal obligation to file a child abuse report when child abuse is suspected clinically. It is not the clinician's job to prove or disprove the allegation of abuse; this is the job of child protective services and law enforcement agencies. Physicians are protected from slander laws when they file child abuse reports in good faith.

Systems-Based Practice

Inappropriate Use of the Emergency Department for Nonurgent Problems

Children insured by Medicaid visit emergency departments (EDs) for nonemergent care more frequently than do those with commercial insurance. A Center for Health Care Policy and Evaluation (CHCPE) study from 2000 showed that of all encounters for which UTI was listed as the primary diagnosis, the rates of ED visits were substantially higher for those insured by Medicaid than the rates for those insured commercially. Interventions in pediatric EDs aimed at decreasing subsequent ED utilization for nonurgent care can be effective, resulting in a modest decrease in the cost of health care for a Medicaid population. Interventions included information from either a health professional or a clerical employee about the importance of a primary care provider and assistance with making an appointment with the provider of their choice.[5,6]

References

1. American Academy of Pediatrics: Practice parameter: The diagnosis, treatment, and evaluation of the initial urinary tract infection in febrile infants and young children. *Pediatrics* 103(4, pt 1):843-852, 1999.
2. Hoberman A, Wald ER, Reynolds EA, et al: Pyuria and bacteriuria in urine specimens obtained by catheter from young children with fever. *J Pediatr* 124:513-519, 1994.
3. Gorelick M: Urinary tract infection. In Bergelson JM, Shah SS, Zaoutis TE, editors: *Pediatric infectious diseases: The requisites in pediatrics*, Philadelphia, PA, 2008, Mosby Elsevier, pp 191-197.
4. Hoberman A, Charron M, Hickey RW, et al: Imaging studies after a first febrile urinary tract infection in young children. *N Engl J Med* 348:195-202, 2003.
5. National Kidney and Urologic Diseases Information Clearinghouse (NKUDIC). Available from http://kidney.niddk.nih.gov/statistics/uda/Urinary_Tract_Infection_in_Children-Chapter13.pdf
6. Grossman LK, Rich LN, Johnson C: Decreasing non-urgent emergency department utilization by Medicaid children. *Pediatrics* 102(1):20-24, 1998.

Professor's Pearls
Section II: The Outpatient Office
Rosemary Casey MD

Consider the following clinical problems and questions posed. Then refer to the discussion of these issues by Rosemary Casey MD, Associate Professor of Pediatrics, Department of Pediatrics, Jefferson Medical College, Philadelphia, Pennsylvania.

1. **Case:** A mother brings her 5 year-old daughter to your office with a history of fever and a sore throat for 3 days. She could barely open her mouth because of pain. Several children in her class have had streptococcal infections. What further history would be helpful? What specific findings would you look for on physical examination, and what laboratory studies would you order to manage this patient?

2. **Case:** A-20-month-old is brought to your office for evaluation of limping for a few days. Her mother is concerned about her swollen right knee. The mother cannot recall seeing her toddler fall or injure that knee, despite an apparent bruise. The child has not had a fever, recent illness, or immunization. She appears stiff, and the limp is particularly noticeable when she gets out of bed in the morning. Do you want further history? What radiographs or laboratory studies would you obtain to make a diagnosis for this child?

3. **Case:** A 6-year-old boy presents to your office for follow-up after an emergency department (ED) visit the day before, in which he was seen for fever, nausea, and progressive swelling and redness of his right eye. At the time of the ED evaluation he had right-sided periorbital erythema and edema, full extraocular movements (EOM), and conjunctival injection. A computed tomography (CT) scan showed periorbital or preseptal cellulitis and bilateral ethmoid sinusitis. How would you manage this child?

4. **Case:** You have been consulted by the parents of an 11-year-old girl with poor appetite, vague abdominal pain, and fatigue for several months. The patient denies diarrhea or constipation and says the pain varies from day to day and has never been crampy. She has never had any blood in her stool. Her parents describe her as an honors student who is a perfectionist, and she has been "having difficulty handling stress." They consulted a nutritionist who found that her caloric intake is at least 150 calories below the number expected per day. They do not have a family history of celiac disease or inflammatory bowel disease, but they do have a strong family history of constitutional short stature. She has not gained weight since her last visit 6 months ago, and her height has decreased to below the 5th percentile. On physical examination the child appears depressed and teary eyed. She has no rashes, her mucous membranes are clear, and her chest is clear to auscultation. Cardiac examination is normal with no murmurs. The abdomen is soft, flat, and nontender. Bowel sounds are normal. The perianal area is normal. Breasts and pubic hair are Tanner 1. How would you approach the diagnostic workup for this child?

Discussion by Rosemary Casey MD, Associate Professor of Pediatrics, Department of Pediatrics, Jefferson Medical College, Philadelphia, Pennsylvania.

1. **Discussion:** Pharyngitis is a common pediatric illness. It can be caused by a number of different viruses, as well as group A beta-hemolytic streptococcus. Further history for this patient should include the child's oral intake, respiratory status, and whether the child can open her mouth. On physical examination, she appeared very uncomfortable, and findings included bilateral tender anterior cervical lymphadenopathy and erythematous pharynx with asymmetrically enlarged tonsils. Her left tonsil was bulging and inflamed with exudate, although her airway was patent. The rapid strep test was positive. This child could not open her mouth because of trismus. The asymmetric tonsils and trismus make a diagnosis of uncomplicated strep pharyngitis unlikely; one must consider the possibility of peritonsillar abscess. CT scan is the preferred imaging study and is helpful in distinguishing a peritonsillar abscess from a retropharyngeal abscess. CT scan confirmed the diagnosis of a peritonsillar abscess.

Peritonsillar abscess requires immediate treatment because the complications include airway obstruction, septicemia, thrombosis, and rupture. She was treated with intravenous clindamycin and dexamethasone and responded quickly. Surgical drainage is sometimes necessary because of poor antibiotic penetration into the peritonsillar space.

2. **Discussion:** The differential diagnosis of a swollen joint includes fracture, septic arthritis, Lyme disease, serum sickness, and juvenile idiopathic arthritis (JIA) (formerly juvenile rheumatoid arthritis). After obtaining a detailed history you learn that the family lives in an area where deer are endemic, although the patient does not have a history of a recent tick bite. Family history is remarkable for a grandmother and a cousin with rheumatoid arthritis. On physical examination, she has an antalgic gait. Her right knee is swollen but nontender, without erythema. Range of motion is limited, and the patella is ballotable. The rest of her examination is unremarkable. A radiograph demonstrates a joint effusion but no fracture. Laboratory studies should include a complete blood count (CBC) with differential, erythrocyte sedimentation rate (ESR), C-reactive protein (CRP), and Lyme titers. Infection is unlikely in this child because she has been afebrile and the joint is not red or tender. In most children presenting with a joint effusion, antinuclear antibody (ANA) and rheumatoid factor measurements are not necessary; they should be considered for this child because of her positive family history. Her laboratory studies included a CBC showing a leukocytosis with a normal differential, ESR elevated at 61 mm/hour, Lyme titer negative, ANA and rheumatoid factor negative. The patient was diagnosed with inflammatory juvenile arthritis. Ophthalmologic examination was normal and was performed because uveitis is the most serious complication of pauciarticular JIA. It is often asymptomatic initially; by the time the child complains of poor vision, permanent irreversible damage may already have occurred.

The arthritis was considered an inflammatory arthritis, and the patient responded well to naproxen. Two months later she complained of wrist and hand pain, prompting referral to a rheumatologist, who diagnosed her as having pauciarticular JIA. Criteria for the classification of JIA include age at onset <16 years, arthritis in one or more joints, and duration of symptoms at least 6 weeks. Pauciarticular JIA involves no more than four joints and usually affects one of the lower extremity joints, such as the knee or ankle, as was the case with this patient. Elevated ANA titers are present in 40% to 85% of children with pauciarticular or polyarticular JIA. Although the degree of elevation of white blood cell count (WBC) and ESR correlate with inflammatory joint activity, a positive ANA is associated with increased risk for development of uveitis. Although this child's ANA was negative, girls developing JIA before age 6 are at risk for chronic uveitis, regardless of the severity of arthritis. Although her ophthalmologic examination was normal, she will be followed every 6 months.

3. **Discussion:** The most common organisms causing preseptal cellulites include *Streptococcus pneumoniae, Staphylococcus aureus*, other *Streptococcus* species, and anaerobes. This child was over 1 year of age and was up to date on immunizations, including *Haemophilus influenzae* type b and *S. pneumoniae*. Standard management for this boy is a broad-spectrum oral antibiotic with a daily follow-up examination. He had received two doses of Augmentin at the time of the follow-up visit. On physical examination his right eye was swollen shut, and the erythematous soft tissue swelling, tenderness, and warmth had extended below the right eye, across the nasal bridge, and up to the right frontal area. It was impossible to see the pupil or assess EOM movement. A CT scan confirmed orbital or postseptal cellulitis with a large subperiosteal collection of pus and an orbital abscess. Although this child's initial outpatient treatment is the usual management, his course underscores the need for close follow-up. Sinusitis is the most common risk factor for orbital cellulitis and is present in more than 70% of cases. This child presented with bilateral ethmoid sinusitis. The abcess required surgical drainage and the patient was treated with 3 weeks of intravenous ampicillin/sulbactam. Orbital cellulitis has a 1% to 2% mortality rate and a 3% to 11% rate of vision loss. This child made a complete recovery.

4. **Discussion:** Short stature, poor weight gain, and delayed puberty raise the possibility of hypothyroidism. Celiac disease and inflammatory bowel disease should be considered because of the intermittent abdominal pain. This child could also be depressed and showing signs of an eating disorder, but organic disease should be ruled out first. Screening laboratory tests for this patient revealed a microcytic anemia, an elevated ESR, and hypoalbuminemia. Her thyroid function tests were normal, and celiac panel was negative. Her bone age was delayed at 8 years 10 months. Hemoccult test results were positive. This child was referred to gastroenterology. Her endoscopy showed chronic gastritis with granulomas, active duodenitis, severe terminal ileitis, and left colitis with granulomas. Biopsy results showed transmural inflammation and confirmed a diagnosis of Crohn's disease. Although fatigue and prolonged diarrhea with abdominal pain and bleeding are the classic symptoms of Crohn's disease, poor growth is a common presentation in children. Patients can have nonspecific symptoms resembling irritable bowel syndrome for years before a diagnosis of Crohn's disease. This child had been suffering from a chronic disease for at least 6 months and was showing signs of emotional distress because she was unable to function at her normal pace.

Section III
THE INPATIENT WARD

Section Editor

David I. Rappaport MD

Chapter 42
Family-Centered Care

David I. Rappaport MD

Speaking Intelligently

Family-centered care has been defined as "an approach to the planning, delivery, and evaluation of health care that is grounded in mutually beneficial partnerships among health-care patients, families, and providers."[1] It means care for a person—not a condition. It means care for a person with a family, culture, and goals—a person whose family should be allowed to actively participate whenever possible and desired by the patient. You will know family-centered care when you see it.

Medical Knowledge and Patient Care

Definition and Rationale

Provision of family-centered care carries particular importance in pediatrics because of most children's dependence on family members. Most young children cannot provide accurate medical, family, or social histories. Most cannot drive themselves to the doctor, take medicines, convince their parents to quit smoking, or avoid abusive situations. The American Academy of Pediatrics[2] recognizes that pediatricians must provide family-centered care to achieve ideal clinical outcomes.

Asthma: An Example

An example of the family's role in pediatric care involves children with asthma. Asthma, the most common chronic disease of childhood, affects roughly 9 million children, disproportionally affecting those who are poor, African American, and without consistent medical care. Addressing a child's respiratory problems—even with a clearly delineated asthma action plan—without targeting such factors as the child's physical environment, access to health care, and the family's level of health-care literacy will have limited effectiveness.

Scope

Although this chapter focuses on hospitalized children, family-centered care should be provided to patients of all ages in all contexts. This approach requires discussion of such "nonmedical" issues as transportation, parental employment, and family dynamics. These issues are generally addressed as outpatients but may also carry importance during a hospital admission. Families generally want to be involved in the inpatient plan so they will follow it as outpatients. Family members may even provide direct care during the hospitalization. In one pediatric cardiovascular center, parents of children undergoing cardiac surgery provide "nursing care" as early as the first postoperative day; outcomes have been excellent and families highly satisfied.[3]

Parental Expectations

What do families want from family-centered care? Most want good communication and information sharing. Parents specifically do not wish to request information—they want providers to offer it, both verbally and in writing.[4] They want providers to be open to flexibility and negotiation, not paternalistic, including allowing them to be present during procedures performed on their child.[5] However, parents vary in the extent to which they wish to participate in hands-on care[6]; recognition of such variations represents a key aspect of family-centered care. Adolescents represent a special population in pediatrics, and their autonomy should be considered.

Cultural Competence

Care cannot be family-centered without cultural competence. Culturally competent providers "demonstrate behaviors, attitudes, policies, and structures that allow them to work cross-culturally."[7] Cultural competence requires flexibility to present information differently to different families. The increasing proportion of minority populations in the United States renders cultural competence more complex and more important. Cultural competence in health care may help address the significant health-care disparities among minority populations and is an important component of patient safety.[8]

Special Needs

Provision of family-centered care to children with special health-care needs (CSHCN) is likewise difficult and important. The complex maze of health care required by many CSHCN often leads to fragmented care of poor quality. Improved survival of medically fragile children, especially ex-preemies or other CSHCN, has required many parents or caregivers to care for children dependent on technologies such as gastrostomy tubes, tracheostomies, and ventilators. Health care simply cannot be effective for these children with complex health issues without understanding the family's role in the care of the child. Recognition of wide variation among individuals with a given condition is crucial, and parents of CSHCN usually know their child better than anyone. This is especially true for patients who are admitted to the hospital frequently. For instance, a patient with cerebral palsy may have mild motor weakness with intact cognition or be totally debilitated. Seizures may be difficult to recognize in an unfamiliar patient. Familiarity with a child's previous reaction to problems or therapies can avoid unhelpful or even harmful strategies (see Chapter 25, The Special Needs Child).

Team Approach

Family-centered care requires a team approach. Nurses, therapists, nutritionists, and social workers all contribute significantly to the care plan and must communicate with each other and the family. An additional team member unique to inpatient pediatrics, the child life specialist, may be especially helpful with anxious children or those undergoing procedures. Child life specialists have been recognized as an indicator of excellence in the care of children[9] and generally may be consulted similarly to medical or surgical specialists. Cases in which child life involvement has precluded the need for pharmacologic sedation are plentiful.

Family-centered care in the hospital often includes family-centered rounds, in which the health-care team rounds in conjunction with the family[10]; and this is now the most common way for pediatric hospitalists to conduct inpatient rounds.[11] Family-centered care recognizes the important contributions that all members of the health-care team—and the family—make to the care of the patient. Today's demographic, financial, and medical realities demand family-centered care to ensure a safe, healing, and collaborative experience for providers, patients, and families. At its best, it is warm, personable, efficient, and flexible. Know it when you see it.

Practice-Based Learning and Improvement

Title
Family-centered bedside rounds: A new approach to patient care and teaching

Authors
Muething SE, Kotagal UR, Shoettker PJ, et al

Reference
Pediatrics 119:829-832, 2007

Historical significance/comments
This article summarizes implementation of family-centered rounds (FCR) at Cincinnati Children's Hospital, one of the first institutions to embrace this approach. The article addresses concerns about FCR's effects on teaching and efficiency. In this study, more than 85% of families chose the FCR model. FCR were also associated with earlier discharge times.

Interpersonal and Communication Skills

Acknowledge Role of Family Members and Integrate Their Input

When conducting daily rounds in a family-centered care model, the health-care team and the family often will be in the room together. Each member of the health-care team has a different role and concerns; these different perspectives help clarify information for the family. Ask family members to add their perspective or correct the presentation as necessary. Family-centered rounds ensure that all members of the health-care team understand the plan and that the family hears one message from their team.

Professionalism

Be Aware of Your Knowledge and Limitations

- Develop a healthy balance between confidence and humility.
- Integrate other members of the team such as nurses and therapists into the care plan.
- Be honest if unsure about how to approach a problem or answer a question, and ask for help.

Systems-Based Practice

Quality Improvement Through Use of Patient-Centered Outcomes

Quality and safety are hallmark principles of the medical home as outlined in the Joint Principles of the Patient-Centered Medical Home from February 2007 by American Academy of Family Physicians (AAFP), American Academy of Pediatrics (AAP), American College of Physicians (ACP), and American Osteopathic Association (AOA). More specifically, (1) patient-centered outcomes should be based on partnership between physicians, patients, and the patient's family; (2) decision making should rely on evidence-based medicine; (3) physicians should voluntary engage in quality improvement activities; (4) information technology should be used appropriately; and (5) patients and families also engage in quality improvement activities at their primary care physician's office.[12]

References

1. What is patient- and family-centered health care? Institute for Family-Centered Care, Patient-Centered Primary Care Collaborative. Available at http://www.familycenteredcare.org.
2. American Academy of Pediatrics Section on Hospital Care and Institute for Family-Centered Care: Family-centered care and the pediatrician's role. *Pediatrics* 112(3):691-696,2003.
3. Turley KM, Higgins SS: When parents participate in critical pathway management following pediatric cardiovascular surgery. *Am J Matern Child Nurs* 21(5):229-234, 1996.
4. Lam LW, Chang AM, Morrissey J: Parents' experiences of participation in the care of hospitalized children: A qualitative study. *Int J Nurs Studies* 43:535-545, 2006.
5. Neill SJ: Parent participation 2: Findings and their implication for practice. *Brit J Nurs* 5(2):110-117, 1996.

6. Coyne IT: Parental participation in care: A critical review of the literature. *J Adv Nurs* 21:716-722, 1995.

7. National Center for Cultural Competence. http://www11.Georgetown.edu/research/gucchd/nccc/index.html.

8. Flores G, Ngui E: Racial/ethnic disparities and patient safety. *Pediatr Clin North Am* 53:1197-1215, 2006.

9. National Association of Children's Hospitals and Related Institutions: *Pediatric excellence in health delivery systems*, Alexandria, VA, 1996, NACHRI, pp 9-10.

10. Mittal VS, Siegrest T, Ottolini MC, et al: Family-centered rounds on pediatrics wards: A PRIS Network Study of US and Canadian Hospitalists. *Pediatrics* 126:37-43, 2010.

11. Muething SE, Kotagal UR, Shoettker PJ, et al: Family-centered bedside rounds: A new approach to patient care and teaching. *Pediatrics* 119:829-832, 2007.

12. Joint Principles of the Patient Centered Medical Home. The Patient-Centered Primary Care Collaborative. Available at http://www.pcpcc.net/node/14.

Chapter 43
Fever and Rash (Case 13)

Kate L. Fronheiser MD

Case: A 2-year-old boy presents with a 3-day history of fever and a rash "all over."

Differential Diagnosis

Meningococcemia	Henoch-Schönlein purpura (HSP)	Toxic shock syndrome (TSS)
Rocky Mountain spotted fever (RMSF)	Kawasaki disease (KD)	

Speaking Intelligently

Distinguishing a benign cause of fever and rash from a potentially life-threatening one is of utmost importance but may be difficult. Serious bacterial illness tends to progress quickly, becoming fulminant in hours. An ill-appearing febrile child with a progressive petechial or purpuric rash or diffuse erythema (erythroderma) suggests a serious infection. Prompt assessment and stabilization of the ABCs (airway, breathing, and circulation) are the first step. Meningococcemia, RMSF, and TSS can cause inadequate perfusion and hypotension, requiring fluid resuscitation. Laboratory studies are drawn, and intravenous targeted antibiotic therapy is quickly initiated. If the likely cause is relatively benign, the workup may proceed with less urgency. In an immunocompromised child, however, even "mild" infections can be serious, and these children typically receive empirical broad-spectrum antibiotics. Realize that most cases of fever and rash in children are due to benign viral processes; however, in addition to serious bacterial infection, one must occasionally consider rheumatologic, immune-mediated, and oncologic etiologies.

PATIENT CARE

History
- Review symptom onset and progression. Include activity level, fluid intake, and urination to assess **hydration status** and determine clues to etiology.
- Is there a community outbreak? Any ill family members or close contacts?
- Consider opportunistic etiologies in an immunodeficient child.
- An **incompletely immunized child** may be at risk for a vaccine-preventable disease such as varicella or measles.
- Timing of the rash may suggest etiology (e.g., several days of fever precedes rash in RMSF and roseola).
- Elicit **rash distribution** and **progression.** Scarlet fever rash begins on the face and spreads caudally. The lesions of RMSF begin on the distal extremities, involve palmar and solar surfaces, and spread centripetally. Morphology is also important. A maculopapular rash that becomes petechial or purpuric within several hours suggests meningococcemia.
- **Mental status changes** suggest a life-threatening bacterial infection, such as meningococcemia, RMSF, or toxic shock syndrome.

Physical Examination
- **Evaluate ABCs.** Note general appearance, color, and mental status. Check for increased work of breathing; assess perfusion by checking capillary refill and pulses.
- Vital signs: Tachycardia is a sign of compensated **shock.** Hypotension signifies decompensated shock (see Chapter 84, Shock).
- A nontoxic appearance is reassuring, but be cautious of rapid deterioration in **meningococcemia.**
- Pay close attention to oral mucosa. Bright red lips or strawberry tongue suggest **Kawasaki disease.** Ulcerative lesions of erythema multiforme (EM) or vesicles of enterovirus are diagnostic clues.
- Note altered mental status (confusion, agitation, or lethargy) and meningeal signs such as a positive Kernig or Brudzinski sign.

- Perform a complete joint examination. There may be a painless joint effusion in **Lyme disease.** Joint swelling, warmth, morning stiffness or pain may occur in rheumatologic processes such as juvenile idiopathic arthritis (JIA).
- The rashes of RMSF, ehrlichiosis, erythema multiforme, Stevens-Johnson syndrome, enterovirus, group A streptococcus, Kawasaki disease, and drug reactions may involve **palms and soles.**

Tests for Consideration

- **Complete blood count (CBC) with differential:** Leukopenia suggests overwhelming infection or viral suppression; leukocytosis and thrombocytosis are nonspecific for infection; thrombocytopenia in sepsis, RMSF, and ehrlichiosis; and thrombocytosis in Kawasaki disease — $116
- **Blood culture:** If ill-appearing — $152
- **Complete metabolic panel:** Hyponatremia occurs in RMSF and other tick-borne illnesses — $237
- **Liver transaminase levels:** Elevated levels may signal organ inflammation or inadequate perfusion — $132
- **RMSF acute and convalescent titers** — $349
- **Group A streptococcus antigen** — $148
- **Rapid respiratory panel to check for adenovirus** — $325
- **Lumbar puncture if clinically indicated:**
  - **Enterovirus polymerase chain reaction (PCR)** — $300
  - **Lyme PCR** — $180
  - **Gram stain** — $180
  - **Culture** — $152
  - **Cell count** — $150
  - **Glucose and protein** — $75
- **Urinalysis:** To check for hematuria, proteinuria, or casts — $95
- **Urine culture** — $148
- **Prothrombin time (PT) and partial thromboplastin time (PTT):** If petechiae and/or purpura — $105
- **Erythrocyte sedimentation rate (ESR):** To monitor inflammatory response in HSP or Kawasaki disease — $85
- **Renal biopsy:** For persistent HSP — $1325

IMAGING CONSIDERATIONS

→ **Head computed tomography (CT):** Before lumbar puncture if altered mental status — $1827
→ **Echocardiogram in Kawasaki disease:** To identify coronary artery aneurysms — $1630
→ **Abdominal ultrasound:** If suspect Henoch-Schönlein purpura with intussusception — $846

| Clinical Entities | Medical Knowledge |

Meningococcemia

Pφ *Neisseria meningitidis* is a gram-negative bacterium that colonizes the nasopharynx of approximately 5% of the population, and transmission is via respiratory droplets. Bacteremia and meningitis are forms of invasive disease with a mortality rate up to 10%. Meningococcal endotoxins cause extensive capillary injury, which results in the characteristic hemorrhagic rash and can progress to uncompensated shock and death. Extremity necrosis is a common and devastating sequela of fulminant *meningococcemia.*

TP Peak incidence occurs under 1 year and in middle to late adolescence. A brief nonspecific febrile prodrome precedes high fevers, mental status change, petechial or purpuric rash, and hypotension.

Dx Diagnosis is supported by gram-negative cocci on Gram stain of the blood or spinal fluid, and cultures are confirmatory.

Tx Supportive treatment consists of ventilation, oxygenation, and hemodynamic support. Ceftriaxone and vancomycin are preferred empirical therapy. If cultures confirm meningococcemia, coverage can be narrowed to penicillin G for 7 to 14 days.[1] **See Nelson Essentials 100.**

Rocky Mountain Spotted Fever

Pφ *RMSF* is a tick-borne illness caused by *Rickettsia rickettsii,* a gram-negative coccobacillus that infects the small vessels of all tissues and organs, producing an infectious vasculitis. Host immune response contributes to diffuse vascular damage.

TP This entity is commonly confused with meningococcemia; clinical presentation is quite similar. Clues to distinguish RMSF from meningococcemia are high fevers preceding rash for several days, distal extremity petechial rash spreading centrally to include palms and soles, and travel to an endemic area. High prevalence areas in the United States include the mid-Atlantic, Southern, and south-central states. RMSF has a seasonal predilection for April through September.

Dx Diagnosis is often made clinically with supportive laboratory data, such as hyponatremia, hypoalbuminemia, elevated transaminases, anemia, and thrombocytopenia. Antibody titers to *Rickettsia* species are insensitive; comparative acute and convalescent antibody titers may be more helpful.

Tx	Doxycycline is the treatment of choice for this life-threatening illness and should be started once RMSF is suspected, with supportive treatment as needed.[1] **See Nelson Essentials 122.**

Toxic Shock Syndrome

Pφ	Gram positive bacteria, typically *Staphylococcus* and *Streptococcus* species, produce toxins that cause a characteristic "erythroderma" rash, fever, tachycardia, and possibly hypotension as a result of toxin-mediated vasodilation.
TP	Patients present with a diffuse red macular tender rash (which later undergoes desquamation), fever, and possible alteration of mental status or other signs of inadequate perfusion, such as oliguria. Females may have a history of tampon use.
Dx	Diagnosis is clinical; namely, fever, the specific appearance of the rash, and signs of compensated shock (tachycardia), or decompensated shock (hypotension). Creatinine and liver transaminases may be elevated. Bacterial cultures are rarely positive, because toxins are responsible for clinical manifestations.
TX	Intravenous antibiotics are promptly begun with a two-drug regimen: A bactericidal agent interfering with cell wall synthesis, such as a beta-lactam, and another targeting ribosomal toxin production, such as clindamycin. Intravenous fluids and cardiorespiratory monitoring are provided as needed.[1] **See Nelson Essentials 97.**

Kawasaki Disease

Pφ	**KD** represents a febrile multisystem vasculitis with preferential involvement of medium-size arteries. Inflammation may involve all three layers of the vessel wall, with possible aneurysm formation. An infectious etiology has been postulated.
TP	The child is extremely irritable. In classic Kawasaki disease, there is fever for at least 5 days, with at least four of the following: 1. Bilateral nonexudative conjunctivitis 2. Erythema of oral and pharyngeal mucosa with strawberry tongue, dry cracked lips 3. Edema and erythema of hands 4. Rash 5. Cervical lymphadenopathy, unilateral >1.5 cm

In incomplete or atypical Kawasaki disease, patients present with 5 days of fever and fewer than four additional findings. This is more common in infants under 1 year, in whom diagnosis is more difficult but who have higher rates of coronary artery aneurysms. Also possible are myocarditis, hydrops of the gallbladder, mild hepatitis, aseptic meningitis, arthritis, and urethritis.

Dx   Diagnosis is clinical, and there are three phases:
1. Acute febrile phase lasts 1 to 2 weeks: fever and other signs and symptoms, including perineal desquamation
2. Subacute phase lasts 2 to 4 weeks. Fever and other symptoms have resolved, but irritability, anorexia, and conjunctivitis persist; new periungual desquamation of fingers and toes, marked thrombocytosis of up to $1,000,000/mm^3$, and coronary artery aneurysm formation.
3. Convalescent phase up to 8 weeks from onset; all symptoms resolve. ESR and C-reactive protein (CRP) are normal. Echocardiogram is done at diagnosis and if normal, is repeated at 2 to 3 weeks and again 6 to 8 weeks after onset.

Tx   Intravenous immunoglobulin (IVIG) 2 g/kg within 10 days of onset decreases symptoms and markedly reduces coronary artery aneurysm formation. Children with KD are also treated with high-dose aspirin (antiinflammatory dosing) for 14 days, or until afebrile for 3 to 4 days, followed by low-dose aspirin (antithrombotic dosing) until 6 to 8 weeks from onset. Persistent or recurrent disease may require a second course of IVIG. Factors associated with poor outcome include male gender, age <1 year, prolonged fever, or fever recurrence after an afebrile period.[1] **See Nelson Essentials 88.**

Henoch-Schönlein Purpura

Pφ   *HSP* is an immune-mediated, diffuse small vessel vasculitis of unknown cause, with the skin, gastrointestinal (GI) tract, joints, and kidneys most commonly involved. Immunofluorescence demonstrates IgA deposits in skin and renal glomeruli. The vasculitis results in cutaneous bleeding, producing petechiae, palpable purpura, and soft tissue edema without thrombocytopenia.

TP   An upper respiratory prodrome (viral or group A streptococcus) occurs about 1 to 3 weeks before onset of a maculopapular blanching rash that may be pruritic. It becomes petechial with palpable purpura, classically on the buttocks and posterior thighs, and recurrent crops occur over several weeks. Low-grade fever and malaise are common. Colicky abdominal pain with heme-positive stools, diarrhea, and possible vomiting occur along with arthritis in the knees and/or ankles. Intussusception, typically ileoileal, may occur. Renal involvement with hematuria, proteinuria, casts, and hypertension occurs in half of cases. Fewer than 1% have ongoing renal involvement, and end-stage renal disease is rare. The typical course lasts 6 weeks (but may be up to 1 year), and most recover fully.

Dx   Diagnosis is clinical with supporting laboratory data, including mild leukocytosis, elevated ESR, and anemia if significant bleeding. Platelets, PT, and PTT are normal. With renal involvement, there is hematuria, proteinuria, and casts. There may be guaiac-positive stools or frank hematochezia. Cutaneous biopsy can help confirm diagnosis, and renal biopsy is done for persistent urine abnormalities and hypertension. Abdominal ultrasound may confirm a suspected intussusception.

Tx   Treatment is supportive with hydration, acetaminophen for fever and pain, and bland diet. Steroids are used for intestinal complications. Blood pressure, urinalysis, and stool for guaiac are monitored at least weekly for 6 weeks, and monthly for up to 6 months. A nephrologist is consulted for children with persistent renal involvement. **See Nelson Essentials 87.**

ZEBRA ZONE

a. **Leukemia:** With fever and ecchymosis or petechiae, a CBC with differential should be checked to detect white cell precursors (blast cells) or cytopenias, suggestive of leukemia.

b. **Acute rheumatic fever (ARF):** Is characterized by fever and evanescent rash in addition to carditis, chorea, subcutaneous nodules, and arthritis caused by an immune response after recent untreated group A streptococcal pharyngitis.

Practice-Based Learning and Improvement

Title
Life-threatening rashes: Dermatologic signs of four infectious diseases

Authors
Drage LA

Reference
Mayo Clin Proc 74(1):68-72, 1999

Problem
Review of dermatologic findings in RMSF, meningococcemia, staphylococcal TSS, and streptococcal TSS

Historical significance/comments
Review article with cited references in peer-reviewed journal

Interpersonal and Communication Skills

Role Modeling Is a Powerful Means of Communication

A child admitted to the inpatient ward with fever and rash with an uncertain diagnosis will require close monitoring of his/her clinical status and perfusion. A team approach that includes communication with the nursing staff is very important. Sharing an understanding that the child requires close monitoring of mental status, vital signs, and urine output by both nursing and physicians will facilitate a collaborative approach and acknowledge the valuable role of hands-on nursing care. Physicians should set a positive example with strict hand washing and, where indicated, maintenance of isolation precautions.

Professionalism

Commitment to Learning and Education Through Maintenance of Certification

The American Board of Pediatrics (ABP) Maintenance of Certification (MOC) program requires pediatricians to recertify every 7 years and is designed to promote ongoing learning, maintenance of skill level, and assessment of competence in each of the six Accreditation Council for Graduate Medical Education (ACGME) competencies. Revision and reformulation of residency education goals have influenced the ongoing certification process, and pediatricians are expected to evaluate how they satisfy the following competencies every 7 years: medical knowledge, systems-based practice, patient care, interpersonal skills and communication, professionalism, and practice-based learning and improvement. The emphasis for recertification continues to broaden beyond demonstration of didactic medical knowledge.

Systems-Based Practice

Careful Evaluation to Avoid a Missed Diagnosis and Malpractice Litigation

Misdiagnosis of children with sepsis and meningitis is among the most common and costliest reasons for medical malpractice suits in emergency medicine.

Quoting directly from its website (http://www.aap.org/visit/coml.htm), The Committee on Medical Liability and Risk Management (COMLRM) is a group of pediatricians appointed by the AAP Board of Directors to address emerging medicolegal issues affecting pediatrics. These are nationally recognized experts in risk management, professional liability insurance, and trends in medical malpractice claims. The Committee on Medical Liability is committed to:

1. Alerting pediatricians and pediatric medical and surgical specialists to common causes of malpractice actions and how to prevent medical errors
2. Educating pediatricians on risk management and loss prevention strategies
3. Equipping pediatricians to make sound business decisions when purchasing professional liability insurance
4. Reforming the medical liability tort system to be just and fair
5. Helping pediatricians survive a medical liability crisis

For additional information, please call the Division of Health Care Finance and Quality Improvement (847-434-7662).

Although the message of this System-Based Practice box is not to espouse the general practice of "defensive medicine," there are certain situations, such as the case of a child with fever and a petechial rash, in which physicians must take particular caution in their diagnostic evaluation.

References

1. American Academy of Pediatrics: *Red Book: 2009 Report of the Committee of Infectious Diseases*, Elk Grove Village, IL, 2009, American Academy of Pediatrics.

2. Selbst S: The febrile child: Missed meningitis and bacteremia. *Clin Pediatr Emerg Med* 1(2):164S-171S, 2003.
3. AAP Committee on Medical Liability and Risk Management: Available from http://www.aap.org/visit/coml.htm on 3/15/2010.

Chapter 44
Difficulty Breathing (Case 14)

Rachel Wohlberg Friedberg MD *and Suzanne Swanson Mendez* MD

Case: A 26-month-old presents with respiratory distress, tachypnea, and hypoxia.

Differential Diagnosis

Croup	Bronchiolitis		Pneumonia
Asthma		Foreign body (FB)	

Speaking Intelligently

The first step is assessment of the child's degree of distress. The ABCs (airway, breathing, and circulation) are always top priority to evaluate airway patency, adequacy of respiration, and tissue oxygenation. Second, stabilizing measures are instituted, including changing position to maintain airway patency and administering oxygen for hypoxemia or significantly increased work of breathing. For poor air movement or wheezing, administer inhaled albuterol or racemic epinephrine. Assisted ventilation is provided for respiratory failure. Reassessment after each intervention is critical. After stabilization, determine etiology and institute specific treatment.

PATIENT CARE

Clinical Thinking
- What is my first impression? *A child who is pink, breathing, and mildly hypoxic but talking is mildly distressed. A child who has rapid shallow breathing, deep retractions, or appears tired is severely distressed.*
- What is the degree of activity and interaction? A well toddler will generally resist being examined, but if in significant distress may offer no objection.
- Is there stridor to suggest extrathoracic obstruction, such as in croup, or expiratory wheezing to suggest intrathoracic obstruction?
- Are there any neurologic impairments or swallowing difficulty to raise concern for aspiration?

History
- Fever suggests infection.
- Clarify onset, duration, and immunization status.
- Any known triggers, association with feeds, time of day, or season?
- **Does the child have asthma?**
- Any prior episodes of difficulty breathing? Any hospitalizations, prior intubation, or intensive care admissions?
- Any tobacco smoke exposure?
- Is there a personal or family history of atopy?

Physical Examination
- Assess overall sense of well-being and **the ABCs.**
- Check vital signs: Elevated temperature for infection, respiratory rate and pulse oximetry to assess oxygenation, heart rate and blood pressure for perfusion.
- Focus on the **respiratory examination:** Note respiratory effort, adequacy of ventilation, any asymmetry, nasal flaring, and presence of retractions (subcostal, intercostal, or supraclavicular). Check for drooling and note child's position of comfort (e.g., sitting up, tripod position).
- Inspiratory stridor suggests upper airway/laryngeal obstruction.
- Biphasic stridor indicates obstruction at the level of the distal larynx/ trachea. Upper airway rhonchi, suggesting nasal or postnasal congestion, may also be biphasic.
- Expiratory wheezes, crackles, or diminished aeration indicate lower airway disease.
- Dullness to percussion suggests an effusion or mass, although these findings are often difficult to localize in infants and toddlers.
- Dysmorphic features, micrognathia, or macroglossia may have associated airway involvement.
- Heart murmur or pericardial rub may suggest cardiac dysfunction.
- Hepatomegaly may indicate congestive heart failure.

Tests for Consideration

- **Complete blood count (CBC) with differential:**
  Leukocytosis in infection $116
- If concern for infection:
  - **Blood culture** $152
  - **Urine culture** $148
- **Electrolytes, blood urea nitrogen (BUN), and creatinine:**
  If concern for dehydration $174
- **Arterial blood gas levels:** If concern for rising P_{CO_2} $222
- **Electrocardiogram (EKG):** If concern for cardiac etiology $217
- **Viral respiratory panel:** For cohorting hospitalized patients $325

IMAGING CONSIDERATIONS

→ **Chest radiograph:** If concern for pneumonia,
  pneumothorax, pleural effusion, cardiomegaly,
  or mediastinal mass $231
→ **Neck radiograph:** For severe croup or to assess degree of
  adenoidal hypertrophy $150
→ **Upper gastrointestinal (GI) studies:** If concern for
  anatomic abnormality $840
→ **Airway fluoroscopy:** For radiolucent foreign body,
  tracheomalacia, or laryngomalacia $225
→ **Chest computed tomography (CT):** For pneumonia with
  significant parapneumonic effusion $1941

Clinical Entities   Medical Knowledge

Croup

Pφ   *Croup,* or laryngotracheobronchitis, is a viral infection causing
     edema and inflammation in the subglottis, most commonly
     resulting from parainfluenza. Other causes include adenovirus,
     respiratory syncytial virus (RSV), human metapneumovirus
     (HMPV), and influenza. Spasmodic (noninfectious, typically
     allergic) croup presents acutely, usually in the middle of the
     night without a viral prodrome or fever. It tends to recur, and
     the etiology is unclear.

TP   Children with croup are typically 6 months to 3 years of age
     and present with acute onset of inspiratory stridor, hoarseness
     and barky cough a few days after onset of upper respiratory
     symptoms. Symptoms are worse at night and with agitation.
     There may be high fever and significant respiratory distress with
     supraclavicular retractions, tachypnea, and hypoxemia.

Dx	The classic triad is inspiratory stridor, barky cough, and hoarseness. Clinical severity is determined using a croup severity score, which assesses inspiratory stridor, retractions, air entry, cyanosis, and level of consciousness. Although not typically indicated, a posteroanterior neck radiograph may demonstrate subglottic narrowing (steeple sign).
Tx	Humidity, cool night air, nebulized racemic epinephrine, corticosteroids (a single dose of dexamethasone [0.6 mg/kg IM or PO]) and supplemental oxygen are administered as needed. The need for hospitalization is assessed based on severity of presentation, response to acute treatment, and availability of follow-up. **See Nelson Essentials 107.**

Bronchiolitis

Pφ	In *bronchiolitis,* a virus infects distal bronchiolar epithelium, causing inflammation, bronchiolar cell necrosis, ciliary disruption, airway edema, mucus production, and sloughed epithelial cells, which all contribute to airway obstruction and atelectasis. The resulting ventilation-perfusion mismatch leads to hypoxemia with increased work of breathing. RSV is the most common cause. Others include HMPV, adenovirus, influenza, parainfluenza, rhinovirus, and human bocavirus.
TP	Occurring up to 2 years of age, the initial symptoms are nasal congestion, rhinorrhea, low-grade fever, and decreased feeding. With lower airway involvement there is wheezing and a tight cough, tachypnea, accessory muscle use with retractions, nasal flaring, and/or grunting. In more severe cases there may be hypoxemia or apnea. More severe cases occur in children under 6 months. Distinguishing viral-induced wheezing from an asthma exacerbation can be difficult. With increased work of breathing and hypoxemia, infants may have difficulty maintaining adequate oral intake and risk dehydration.
Dx	Diagnosis is made clinically and includes assessing illness severity. Specific viral testing may be helpful for admission cohorting. Chest radiograph may show hyperinflation with peribronchial thickening and subsegmental atelectasis. Focal densities occur in severe cases. Risk factors for severe disease include prematurity, age less than 12 weeks, congenital heart disease, neurologic disorders, immunodeficiencies, and pulmonary disease.

Tx   Supportive care is the mainstay of therapy. Consider supplemental oxygen, inhaled albuterol or racemic epinephrine, and continue if improvement is noted. Small feeding volumes may reduce gastric distention. Respiratory status, age, and duration of illness will determine need for hospitalization. With outpatient management, young infants and those early in the course need frequent office visits to monitor hydration status and work of breathing. **See Nelson Essentials 109.**

Pneumonia

Pφ   ***Pneumonia*** is a lower tract infection involving the bronchioles, alveoli, and/or interstitium, and the most common bacterial causes are *Streptococcus pneumoniae* and increasingly *Staphylococcus aureus*. Viruses and atypical bacteria *(Mycoplasma pneumoniae)* infect airway epithelial cells, producing a diffuse interstitial pattern. Pneumonia may occur via several mechanisms: as a primary infection of the lower tract, in association with an upper tract infection (common cold), from aspiration, or via hematogenous spread. Parapneumonic effusions and empyema are more common with streptococcal and staphylococcal infections, particularly community-acquired methicillin-resistant *S. aureus* (CA-MRSA). Likely pathogens vary based on age, environment, and risk factors (see Chapter 31, Cough, and Chapter 46, Neonatal Fever).

TP   A child with bacterial pneumonia typically presents with fever, tachypnea, and cough, and often malaise, headache, and abdominal pain. On examination focal crackles and/or wheezing may be heard. Interstitial pneumonia presents with fever, cough, and diffuse lung findings, though differentiation of "typical" from "atypical" pneumonia may be difficult. Young infants may have fever and tachypnea without localizing lung findings.

Dx   Diagnosis can be made clinically in a nontoxic child with classic physical findings. Focal consolidation on radiograph often reflects bacterial pneumonia. Aspiration more commonly occurs in the right upper lobe. Dullness to percussion suggests an effusion. Decubitus chest radiograph, ultrasound, or CT scan further delineates pleural fluid. Viral pathogens and atypical bacteria usually produce a diffuse interstitial pattern.

Tx   Antibiotics that cover gram-positive organisms should be started. High-dose amoxicillin/ampicillin targets intermediately resistant pneumococcus. Macrolides may be used in penicillin-allergic patients and in suspected *M. pneumoniae*. Antibiotics are not indicated for viral processes. Persistently febrile and ill-appearing children should have a repeat chest radiograph to exclude parapneumonic effusion or empyema. With sizeable collections, drainage with video-assisted thoracoscopy (VATS) or chest tube placement may be needed. Cell count, Gram stain, and culture guide antibiotic treatment. Aspiration pneumonia requires coverage of gram-negative and perhaps anaerobic organisms. MRSA is usually treated with clindamycin, vancomycin, or linezolid, depending on illness severity and regional sensitivity patterns. **See Nelson Essentials 110.**

Asthma
Pφ   *Asthma* is characterized by recurrent reversible airflow obstruction, inflammation, and hyperresponsiveness of the lower airways. Common triggers are viral respiratory infections, environmental tobacco smoke, and allergens such as dust mites, animal dander, molds, and pollen. Airway edema with mucus plugging causes air trapping with hyperinflation and atelectasis, resulting in ventilation–perfusion mismatch.
TP   Presentation varies, but typical findings are polyphonic bilateral expiratory wheezing and cough, although wheezing may be inspiratory or absent with severely compromised airflow. Wheezing is absent in cough-variant asthma.
Dx   Diagnosis is made clinically, based on symptoms and physical examination findings, along with response to bronchodilator therapy. Baseline peak expiratory flow (PEF) is decreased during an exacerbation, as is forced expiratory volume (FEV_1) on spirometry. There may be atopic findings such as eczema and seasonal allergies. There is overlap in presentation between asthma and bronchiolitis in children under 2 years. A prior history of wheezing and a family history of asthma or atopy can help solidify the diagnosis.

Tx   First-line treatment, after assessing the ABCs and providing supplemental oxygen, is to reverse bronchoconstriction. Albuterol, a short-acting beta agonist, is most commonly used, either by nebulization or inhaler. An aerosolized anticholinergic such as ipratropium may be useful on initial presentation. Additional medications include terbutaline, epinephrine, and intravenous magnesium sulfate. Inflammation is treated with systemic corticosteroids. Consider a chest radiograph if concern for complications: pneumonia, pneumothorax, pneumomediastinum, or significant atelectasis. All patients should be discharged with an asthma action plan and close follow-up (see Chapter 31, Cough, and Chapter 87, Status Asthmaticus). **See Nelson Essentials 78.**

Foreign Body

Pφ   Most *foreign bodies* are lodged in the bronchi, most commonly in the right lung. A laryngotracheal FB causes significantly higher morbidity and mortality than bronchial aspirations. Common aspirates include seeds, nuts (especially peanuts), and small toys.

TP   Respiratory distress or altered mental status require immediate intervention with bronchoscopy and appropriate respiratory support to relieve airway obstruction. Cyanosis, hoarseness, stridor, and acute respiratory distress suggest laryngotracheal aspiration. Nonemergent presentations are more common: following the acute event, after coughing and gagging have subsided, the child may be asymptomatic; thus an accurate history is key in making the diagnosis. This is especially true with a bronchial FB, in which the classic triad of wheeze, cough, and diminished breath sounds occurs in only 50% of cases. Cough or wheeze that fails to resolve should raise concern for an aspirated FB.

Dx   Radiopaque objects such as coins may be seen on the radiograph, though most objects are radiolucent. With a bronchial FB, radiographic findings include hyperinflation, atelectasis, mediastinal shift, and pneumonia. A lateral decubitus chest film may demonstrate persistent air trapping in the dependent lung.

Tx   Bronchoscopy is the treatment of choice. After removal of the FB, the airway is evaluated for smaller fragments and general inflammation. Gram stain and culture of fluid are performed to excludea secondary pneumonia. Antibiotics should be started accordingly. **See Nelson Essentials 136.**

ZEBRA ZONE

a. **Myocarditis with congestive heart failure:** A viral infection of the myocardium with dilated cardiomyopathy.

b. **Tracheoesophageal fistula:** Direct communication between esophagus and trachea can precipitate respiratory distress with feeds (see Chapter 75, Tracheoesophageal Fistula).

c. **Epiglottitis:** A bacterial infection, most commonly caused by *Haemophilus influenzae*. This is an airway emergency requiring emergent intubation by an anesthesiolgist.

Practice-Based Learning and Improvement

Title
A randomized trial of nebulized epinephrine vs albuterol in the emergency department treatment of bronchiolitis

Authors
Mull CC, Scarfone RJ, Ferri LR, et al

Reference
Arch Pediatr Adolesc Med 158(2):113-118, 2004

Problem
Management of moderately ill infants with bronchiolitis in an urban emergency department (ED)

Intervention
Double-blind administration of either nebulized albuterol or racemic epinephrine

Outcome/effect
No clinical significant difference was found between groups.

Historical significance/ comments
These results suggest that both medications lead to similar improvements and rates of discharge from the ED in moderately ill infants.

Interpersonal and Communication Skills

Recognize the Role of the Nurse and Respiratory Therapist in the Management of the Child in Respiratory Distress

A child admitted with an acute asthma exacerbation will be cared for by both nurses and respiratory therapists who spend a great deal of time caring for the patient, including administering treatments and monitoring respiratory status. Acknowledge that they will often be the first to recognize an acute change in the patient's status that may require an intervention such as transfer to the intensive care unit.

Professionalism

Advocate With Third-Party Payers to Optimize Asthma Management

Physicians must be willing and prepared to advocate, when appropriate, for additional services for children with asthma. These might include a home visit to assess environmental triggers, asthma education programs, and supplies and equipment for home environmental control. Speaking with the insurance company, requesting a case manager, writing letters of medical necessity, and referral to community resources would be typical ways to advocate and improve asthma control in the child with poorly controlled disease.

Systems-Based Practice

Coordination of Asthma Management in the School-Aged Child

Asthma is a chronic inflammatory disorder that requires ongoing management at home, with the primary medical provider, and at school.

As summarized in the 2007 National Heart Lung Blood Institute (NHLBI) guidelines (http://www.nhlbi.nih.gov/guidelines/asthma/), there are two major goals in controlling asthma and in meeting patient and family expectations of asthma care.

1. *Reduction of impairment:* Optimizing the number of symptom-free days and minimizing the use of rescue medications.
2. *Reduction of Risk for Hospitalization:* Reducing the risk for hospitalization (and reducing school absenteeism) and reducing the risk for side effects from the medications used for asthma control. Asthma care must be coordinated between the caregiver and primary medical provider, and, for school-aged children, this may also involve the school nurse. For children who have been hospitalized, the inpatient medical provider should coordinate with the primary medical provider to ensure a smooth transition to home and back to school. Every child should be discharged with an asthma action plan, and a copy of this should be placed in his/her medical chart. In appropriate cases, a copy should be taken to school by the child or parent and given to the school nurse (after obtaining appropriate parental consent).

Chapter 45
Anemia (Case 15)

Hal C. Byck MD

Case: A 15-month-old girl with pneumonia is noted to have a hemoglobin level of 8 g/dL.

Differential Diagnosis

Iron deficiency anemia	Glucose-6-phosphate dehydrogenase (G6PD) deficiency	Thalassemia trait
Hereditary spherocytosis (HS)	Lead poisoning	

Speaking Intelligently

When evaluating a child with anemia, I first check for signs of blood loss and assess hemodynamic stability. Anemia is a clinical sign; my task is to determine the cause and institute treatment where indicated. The mean corpuscular volume (MCV) classifies the anemia as normocytic, microcytic, or macrocytic. A careful history, including diet and ethnicity, is important. A reticulocyte count helps assess production and destruction of red blood cells. Infections such as pneumonia or viral syndromes can cause transient bone marrow suppression and anemia.

PATIENT CARE

Clinical Thinking
- **Does the child need immediate support or transfusion?**
- Are there signs of congestive heart failure?
- If neither of the above is true, there is time to consider the differential and plan the workup.
- Hemoglobin levels vary by age, and in adolescents, by gender (Table 45-1).
- **Physiologic anemia of infancy** (resulting from multiple factors related to transition to extrauterine life) results in a progressive drop in hemoglobin in the first 8 weeks of life in term infants to 9 to 11 g/dL. In preterm infants, the drop occurs in the first 3 to 6 weeks and is more severe—to 7 to 9 g/dL. No treatment is required: iron stores are adequate, and recovery occurs as erythropoietin increases.

Table 45-1	Age-Specific Hemoglobin
Age	**Hemoglobin (g/dL)***
1-3 days	18.5 (14.5)
2 weeks	16.6 (13.4)
1 month	13.9 (10.7)
2 months	11.2 (9.4)
6 months	12.6 (11.1)
6 months-2 years	12 (10.5)
2-6 years	12.5 (11.5)
6-12 years	13.5 (11.5)
12-18 years	
Male	14.5 (13)
Female	14 (12)
Adult	
Male	15.5 (14)
Female	14 (12)

*Data are mean (−2 SD).
Data from Oski FA, Naiman JL: *Hematological problems in the newborn infant,* Philadelphia, Saunders, 1982; Nathan D, Oski FA: *Hematology of infancy and childhood,* Philadelphia, Saunders, 1998; Matoth Y et al: Postnatal changes in some red cell parameters. *Acta Paediatr Scand* 1971;60:317; and Wintrobe MM: *Clinical hematology,* Baltimore, Williams & Wilkins, 1999.

History

- Review **newborn screen** results: note G6PD deficiency, sickle cell disease, or Bart's hemoglobin (indicating α-thalassemia trait).
- What is the child's diet? Is there excessive intake of whole milk (≥24 ounces daily)?
- Any family history of anemia?
- What is the child's ethnicity? African, Asian, and Mediterranean ancestry is associated with β-thalassemia trait; and Southeast Asian, Chinese, and African heritage with α-thalassemia trait.
- Is there family history of splenectomy or cholecystectomy?
- Does the child live or attend day care in an old house or one being renovated?
- Have any siblings had lead poisoning?
- Is there pica?
- Has the child had prior episodes of anemia or any treatment?
- Has there been a recent respiratory or gastrointestinal illness?
- Is there evidence of **blood loss** such as tarry stools, hematochezia, or hematemesis?
- Has there been fever, poor appetite, weight loss, or other **constitutional symptoms?**
- Is there bone pain?
- Does the child bruise easily?

Physical Examination
- Vital signs: Check for tachycardia and hypotension (a very late finding) with blood loss.
- Assess capillary refill.
- Note pallor or pale sclerae.
- A systolic flow murmur is common and not indicative of cardiovascular compromise.
- Signs of heart failure (gallop, hepatomegaly, crackles) suggest severe anemia.
- Bruising, petechiae, or significant lymphadenopathy suggest an oncologic etiology.
- Splenomegaly occurs with hereditary spherocytosis, splenic sequestration, or malignancy.
- Jaundice suggests a hemolytic process.

Tests for Consideration
- **Complete blood count (CBC) with differential:** To check hemoglobin, MCV, platelets, and white blood cells to distinguish anemia from pancytopenia $116
- **Peripheral blood smear:** To check red blood cell (RBC) shape, central pallor $75
- **Reticulocyte count:** To check bone marrow response; increased with hemorrhage, hemolysis, or recent treatment of iron deficiency $74
- **Ferritin:** To check tissue iron stores; may be falsely elevated with any inflammatory process $177
- **Hemoglobin electrophoresis:** To identify abnormal hemoglobin (see Table 45-1) $135
- **Lead level** $34
- **Coombs test:** For autoimmune hemolysis $87
- **Osmotic fragility test:** For hereditary spherocytosis $954
- If macrocytic anemia:
  - Vitamin B_{12} $196
  - Folate $491
- **Stool guaiac:** To detect occult blood loss $170
- **Bone marrow biopsy:** If decreased production or infiltrative process $756

IMAGING CONSIDERATIONS

→ **Abdominal ultrasound:** If hemolytic process and concern for splenomegaly $846
→ **Abdominal radiograph:** If suspect paint chip ingestion/acute lead poisoning $266

| Clinical Entities | Medical Knowledge |

Iron Deficiency Anemia

Pφ **Iron deficiency** usually results from inadequate intake and increased demand. By 6 months of age, prenatal stores are depleted. Iron is preferentially used as a catalyst in synthesis of heme from free erythrocyte protoporphyrin (FEP), and significant iron deficiency develops before anemia, which is microcytic and hypochromic with a depressed reticulocyte count.

TP From 6 months to 2 years of age, and again in adolescence, iron deficiency is common. Toddlers often drink excessive amounts of cow milk (>24 ounces/day). Unless severe, clinical manifestations of iron deficiency are limited, although iron deficiency impairs attention, alertness, and learning, and cognitive changes may persist after repletion of iron stores. There may be a history of pica (ingestion of nonfood substances) with pallor and a systolic flow murmur noted on examination.

Dx Diagnosis is usually suggested by history and low hemoglobin for age. Additional tests include iron to total iron-binding capacity (TIBC) ratio, ferritin, and reticulocyte count. Because ferritin is an acute phase reactant, obtaining a simultaneous C-reactive protein will exclude inflammation as the cause of a normal or elevated ferritin level.

Tx A trial of ferrous sulfate (4 to 6 mg/kg/day of elemental iron) is prescribed. The reticulocyte count should increase within 1 week. The hemoglobin is rechecked in 1 month. If increased, iron is continued for 1 month to replete stores. An inadequate response to iron requires additional evaluation.[1]
See Chapter 21, The 12-Month Well Child Visit. **See Nelson Essentials 150.**

Glucose-6-Phosphate Dehydrogenase Deficiency

Pφ **Glucose-6-phosphate dehydrogenase deficiency** is an RBC enzyme deficiency causing hemolytic anemia, most commonly precipitated by exposure to an oxidative stress such as infection, sulfa medications, or aspirin. Inheritance is X-linked. Heterozygous females show resistance to falciparum malaria. Over 100 enzyme variants of G6PD have been isolated. The anemia is normocytic and normochromic.

TP	The typical patient is of African, Mediterranean, or Asian descent. Children with chronic hemolysis are generally asymptomatic, and those with hemolysis in response to oxidative triggers are asymptomatic between episodes. Severe hemolysis may produce pallor, jaundice, fatigue, hemoglobinuria, and abdominal pain. The extent of hemolysis is inversely proportional to the active enzyme level and will also vary with the oxidative trigger. Most episodes resolve shortly after the offending agent is discontinued.
Dx	G6PD activity in RBCs of <10% suggests the diagnosis. After an acute hemolytic episode, the reticulocyte count is elevated. In some G6PD variants, young cells have higher G6PD activity; thus diagnostic testing should be deferred for a few weeks.
Tx	Avoidance of triggers is important; families should be provided with a list of offending agents. Acute hemolytic episodes require supportive care with evaluation for transfusion as needed.[2] **See Nelson Essentials 150.**

Thalassemia Trait

Pφ	Normal hemoglobin is a tetramer of two pairs of globin chains. *Thalassemia trait* involves decreased synthesis of α- or β-globin chains; clinical α-thalassemia trait generally involves two gene mutations (of the four loci responsible for α-globin production), whereas β-thalassemia trait involves a single gene mutation (of the two loci responsible for β-globin production). In α-thalassemia trait there is decreased synthesis of α chains, whereas β-thalassemia trait involves decreased production of β chains.
TP	Most patients are asymptomatic and detected via screening. A family history of mild anemia may be suggestive, especially among those of Mediterranean or African descent with β-thalassemia trait, and Southeast Asian or African descent with α-thalassemia trait.

Dx   Diagnosis is supported by mild microcytic anemia in a patient
      of typical ethnicity. Microcytosis is generally greater than that
      seen in iron deficiency. In β-thalassemia trait, electrophoresis
      demonstrates increased δ (delta) chains (HbA$_2$), and elevated
      HbF. Hemoglobin is reduced about 2 g/dL with marked decrease
      in MCV to about 65 fL. α-Thalassemia trait has mildly decreased
      hemoglobin and MCV, with normal HbA$_2$ and HbF levels.
      α-thalassemia trait is typically diagnosed after exclusion of iron
      deficiency and β-thalassemia trait, or the newborn screen may
      demonstrate hemoglobin Bart's (γ4) chains. The red cell
      distribution width (RDW) is normal in thalassemia trait, but
      increased in iron deficiency anemia.

Tx   No treatment is required; in fact, iron therapy will not increase
      the hemoglobin, and chronically administered iron may cause
      iron overload. However, iron deficiency and thalassemia trait
      can coexist. If microcytic anemia persists, but the RDW corrects
      after a course of iron, check parental indices for microcytosis,
      or hemoglobin electrophoresis in the patient.[1] **See Nelson
      Essentials 150.**

Hereditary Spherocytosis

Pφ   ***Hereditary spherocytosis*** is an RBC membrane abnormality that
      alters cell shape from the normal biconcave disc to a round
      spherocyte. There is reduced membrane surface area and
      deformability, so cells are trapped and prematurely destroyed in
      the spleen. Inheritance is classically autosomal dominant, but
      new mutations may occur.

TP   Newborns may have severe hemolysis with significant jaundice
      and anemia. In infancy and childhood, presentation varies from
      asymptomatic to severe anemia with pallor, jaundice, fatigue,
      and exercise intolerance. Splenomegaly develops in early
      childhood, and bilirubin gallstones occur in untreated children.

Dx   Blood smear demonstrates spherocytes (round RBCs with
      decreased central pallor) and reticulocytes. The reticulocyte
      count and indirect bilirubin are elevated. There is splenomegaly
      and usually a positive family history. The osmotic fragility test
      shows swelling and lysis of spherocytes in hypotonic saline. The
      MCV is normal, but the mean corpuscular hemoglobin
      concentration (MCHC) is usually elevated.

Tx   Treatment is supportive during hemolytic episodes, with
      transfusion provided for severe hemolysis. Splenectomy may be
      curative. Cholecystectomy may be indicated for bilirubin
      gallstones.[1] **See Nelson Essentials 150.**

Lead Poisoning

Pφ	Environmental lead exposure from contaminated dust, paint chips, water in lead pipes, or contaminated soil, coupled with typical hand-to-mouth behavior, is the source of lead acquisition in young children. Lead may produce anemia because of inhibition of three enzymes in the heme synthetic pathway. In addition, lead exposure produces symptoms in the gastrointestinal tract and central nervous system.
TP	Most children are asymptomatic and detected on routine screening.
Dx	Blood lead level (BLL) is elevated. CBC demonstrates microcytic, hypochromic anemia with basophilic stippling. Free erythrocyte protoporphyrin (FEP) is elevated because of inhibition of ferrochelatase, the last enzyme in the heme synthetic pathway. Screening for iron deficiency and hemoglobin electrophoresis should be considered. Abdominal radiographs may demonstrate lead paint chips in acute poisoning.
Tx	Treatment is dependent on BLL but at minimum requires sufficient dietary iron and calcium, which compete with lead for binding sites in the gut, as well as family education about hand washing and assessment of living conditions. Environmental evaluation performed by governmental agencies to assess the source of the exposure is required. BLL is followed until resolution. See Chapter 20, The 9-Month Well Child Visit. **See Nelson Essentials 150.**

ZEBRA ZONE

a. **Autoimmune hemolytic anemia:** An antibody-mediated hemolysis, usually idiopathic, presenting suddenly with pallor, fever, icterus, and dark urine. Treatment involves corticosteroids and avoidance of transfusion when possible.

b. **Transient erythroblastopenia of childhood (TEC):** Self-limited red cell aplasia that may follow a viral illness. Treatment is supportive with transfusion as necessary.

c. **Anemia of chronic disease:** Iron may be trapped in tissue macrophages in inflammatory diseases, preventing its transport to erythroid precursors. Erythropoietin is elevated, and the diminished bone marrow response to anemia is thought to involve inflammatory cytokines.

Practice-Based Learning and Improvement

Title
A practical approach to the evaluation of the anemic child

Authors
Hermiston ML, Mentzer WC

Reference
Pediatr Clin North Am 49(5):877-891, 2002

Problem
A systematic approach to the evaluation of childhood anemia

Quality of evidence
Review article with cited references in peer-reviewed journal

Significance to the student/resident
I keep such references handy in my office and consult them frequently for specific issues for example, determining the etiology of anemia and when a consultation with a pediatric hematologist is warranted.

Interpersonal and Communication Skills

Obtain a Focused History for Clues to Etilolgy

When a child is found to be anemic, the physician must determine a definitive etiology. A careful history and physical examination may reveal important clues to the cause. A complete diet history, family history, and social history will be necessary, and this is time consuming to do correctly. Ensure that the parent remains on topic by gently steering the conversation back to the topic at hand. For example, the physician might say, "That is interesting, but I want to ask you more about . . ." Be organized, and manage your time efficiently by keeping the conversation on target.

Professionalism

Self-Awareness of Counseling on the Importance of Adequate Iron Intake

It is important for the physician to reflect on whether nutritional anemia could have been prevented with appropriate supplementation of iron or improved anticipatory guidance. Discussion about adding iron to the diet of the exclusively breastfed infant at 6 months or the consumption of whole milk in the toddler can be easily overlooked during a well-child visit, especially if there are many other issues and concerns to discuss. Reflection about the role the physician may have played in a particular outcome allows for improvements in practice.

Systems-Based Practice

Informed Consent: Obtaining Consent for Transfusion of Blood or Blood Products in Children and Adolescents

There is significant concern in the public domain because of potential infectious and noninfectious risks associated with transfusion of blood and blood products since the first documented transfusion transmission of human immunodeficiency virus (HIV) in 1982. The risk for viral infection is now quite minimal because of donor screening and extensive testing of donated blood. Some noninfectious risks include incorrect donor-recipient matching with ABO incompatibility (immune hemolytic reaction), allergic reactions ranging from simple to anaphylaxis, volume overload, iron overload, graft-versus-host disease (GVHD), transfusion-related acute lung injury (TRALI), and febrile nonhemolytic reactions.

In 1996 the Joint Commission on Accreditation of Healthcare Organizations mandated documentation of informed consent for transfusion with a specific institution–approved informed consent form. There are unique considerations regarding consent in children: the parent or surrogate provides informed permission, and the assent of the child is sought whenever possible. To ensure that parents and patients have the information necessary to make an informed choice, an explanation of why transfusion is recommended and the expected benefit(s), a review of all infectious and noninfectious risks, and a description of alternative treatment(s) along with risk and benefits should be included. The expected outcome without transfusion should be discussed.[3-5]

References

1. Segel GB, Hirsh MG, Feig SA: Managing anemia in pediatric office practice, part I. *Pediatr Rev* 23(3):75-83, 2002.
2. Segel GB, Hirsh MG, Feig SA: Managing anemia in pediatric office practice, part II. *Pediatr Rev* 23(4):111-121, 2002.
3. American Academy of Pediatrics Committee on Bioethics: Informed consent, parental permission, and assent in pediatric practice. *Pediatrics* 95:314-317, 1995.
4. American Association of Blood Banks Standards Program Committee: *Standards for blood banks and transfusion services*, ed 23, Bethesda, MD, 2004, American Association of Blood Banks Press.
5. Sazama K: Practical issues in informed consent for transfusion. *Am J Clin Pathol* 107:S72, 1997.

Chapter 46
Neonatal Fever (Case 16)

Jennifer R. Rosenthal MD

Case: A 17-day-old presents with a fever.

Differential Diagnosis

Sepsis	Urinary tract infection (UTI)
Bronchiolitis	Meningitis or encephalitis

Speaking Intelligently

When evaluating a febrile neonate, I remember that fever may be the only sign of a significant underlying infection. A history of fever at home should be taken seriously, even if the infant is afebrile on presentation. Fever is defined as a rectal temperature of 38°C (100.4° F). Distinguishing between neonates (from birth to 28 days) and young infants (29 to 60 days) is important, because neonates face greater risk for systemic infections, and even a thorough physical examination is unreliable. The term "rule out sepsis" (or "rule out serious bacterial infection" [SBI]) is used to describe the standard workup of a febrile neonate. Neonates hospitalized since birth have higher risk for infections, including nosocomial infections, than neonates admitted from home. Nonetheless, a complete workup is indicated, and some cases of SBI will be identified (see Chapter 77, Neonatal Sepsis).[1]

PATIENT CARE

Clinical Thinking
- The workup for febrile **neonates** is relatively straightforward. A **complete diagnostic evaluation,** IV antibiotic administration, and hospital admission are all considered standard practice. In some cases, a positive rapid test such as respiratory syncytial virus (RSV) may change decision making.
- **Young infants** are approached differently. Here clinical judgment is used. For well-appearing febrile infants, **laboratory testing** is

necessary **to determine which patients are at risk for SBI.** Any ill-appearing infant should be admitted for empirical antibiotics, regardless of initial laboratory results.

- Well-appearing infants who are discharged to home should have a follow-up examination and laboratory results checked within 24 hours.
- In a well-appearing infant (over 28 days), a lumbar puncture (LP) may be considered optional. However, if antibiotics are administered, an LP should be performed.
- Criteria for differentiation of high-risk patients (i.e., Rochester, Philadelphia, Boston) may be used to guide therapeutic decision making, although these were developed before the heptavalent (now 13-valent) *Streptococcus pneumoniae* vaccine.

History
- A detailed birth history is crucial.
- Gestational age?
- Prolonged rupture of membranes?
- Prenatal laboratory results, including group B streptococcus? Adequate treatment?
- Nursery course and any complications?
- Any sick contacts?
- Inquire about activity level.
- Alert or lethargic? (Use "lethargic" with caution; it describes a baby who is not just sleepy, but difficult to arouse.)
- Is the baby feeding normally?
- Increased irritability? Consolable?

Other symptoms:

- Upper respiratory symptoms?
- Vomiting?
- Diarrhea?
- Decreased wet diapers and/or foul-smelling urine?
- Has the fever been treated?
- Any factitious cause for fever such as excessive bundling, high ambient temperature, or inaccurate thermometer?

Physical Examination
- Vital signs: Rectal temperature, heart rate, respiratory rate, oxygen saturation, and growth parameters (weight, length, head circumference).
- General appearance: Does the infant appear toxic? Realize a seriously ill neonate may not be ill appearing.
- Cardiovascular: Is perfusion adequate? Note capillary refill and pulses.
- Respiratory: Good air movement? Retractions? Sounds on auscultation?
- Abdomen: Distended? Bowel sounds?

- Skin: Rashes? Look specifically for vesicles, petechiae, or evidence of cellulitis or abscesses such as mastitis.
- Neurologic: Alert? Irritable? Bulging fontanelle? Floppy?

Tests for Consideration
- **Complete blood count (CBC) with manual differential.** $116
- Low-risk criteria include a white blood cell count (WBC) >5000 and <15,000 μL
- Number of bands on the differential should be $<1.5 \times 10^9$ cells/L
- **Blood culture** $152
- **Urine dipstick** $95
- **Urinalysis and urine culture** $243
- **Lumbar puncture for cerebrospinal fluid (CSF):** Cell count, glucose, protein, Gram stain, and culture
- A herpes simplex virus (HSV) polymerase chain reaction (PCR) should be sent for neonates who have risk factors for HSV, abnormal neurologic examination, or suspicious skin findings or are ill-appearing $300
- **Rapid respiratory panel** $325
- **Coagulation studies: Prothrombin time and partial thromboplastin time** $105

IMAGING CONSIDERATIONS

→ **Chest radiograph:** If respiratory symptoms $231

Clinical Entities   Medical Knowledge

Sepsis

Pφ   ***Sepsis*** is the systemic response to pathogens or their toxins. Physical and chemical barriers to infection are functionally deficient in the newborn period. Sepsis in the first week of life is usually acquired transplacentally or via the birthing process. After 1 week sepsis is usually environmentally acquired, with the exception of late-onset group B streptococcus infection, which may be transmitted vaginally or environmentally. Group B streptococcus, *Escherichia coli, Listeria monocytogenes,* and *Staphylococcus aureus* are the most common bacterial culprits. However, *Chlamydia pneumoniae, Haemophilus influenzae,* and *Enterobacter* have also been identified.

TP   Unfortunately, there is no "typical" presentation of a septic infant. Sepsis can present with fever or hypothermia; tachypnea or apnea; tachycardia or bradycardia if prolonged; poor feeding; vomiting and/or diarrhea; oliguria or anuria; jaundice or pallor; petechiae, purpura, or bruising; hypoperfused extremities; irritability or lethargy; seizures; or change in tone. You may hear a septic infant described as simply "not looking right."

Dx   Diagnosis is made with clinical presentation and laboratory data. Vital signs are extremely important in diagnosis. CBC with manual differential is done for quick clues, whereas blood culture takes longer. CBC may show leukocytosis with bandemia—or of greater significance in a neonate, leukopenia and/or thrombocytopenia. Coagulation studies are useful if considering diffuse intravascular coagulation (DIC). Urine culture and lumbar puncture are done, and a chest radiograph when history and/or symptoms warrant.

Tx   Treatment begins with the ABCs (airway, breathing, and circulation). Ensuring a patent airway, providing supplemental oxygen, assisted ventilation (bag-valve-mask), IV access, and volume resuscitation are all vital. If the infant is hypoglycemic, correct the blood glucose level with 0.5 to 1 g/kg of IV dextrose. Empirical antibiotics should be started; these generally include ampicillin with an aminoglycoside or cefotaxime. **See Nelsons Essentials 65.**

Urinary Tract infection

Pφ   **UTI** is defined as the presence of an inflammatory response anywhere along the urinary tract with bacteriuria. The mechanism in otherwise normal infants is typically ascending infection, although in young infants pyelonephritis may occur from hematogenous seeding of the kidneys. There may be predisposing urinary tract abnormalities, including hydronephrosis, posterior urethral valves, and urethral obstruction/stenosis, which may increase the risk for UTI.

TP   The presentation in this age-group is nonspecific. Fever with vomiting, poor feeding, and/or irritability should raise concern for UTI. In addition, there may be abdominal distention, poor weight gain, and malodorous urine.

Dx   Diagnosis is made by either bladder catheterization or suprapubic aspiration. Culture is the diagnostic gold standard. If urinalysis shows at least 5 WBCs per high-power field, leukocyte esterase, nitrites (indicating nitrate-splitting bacteria), and bacteria on Gram stain, the culture will likely be positive. *E. coli* is the cause of 75% to 90% of all UTIs, followed by *Klebsiella, Enterococcus* spp, *Proteus,* group B streptococci, *Enterobacter, Pseudomonas, Serratia* spp., and *S. aureus.* Per the American Academy of Pediatrics guideline, ≥10,000 colony-forming units (CFU/mL) of a single pathogen on a catheterized specimen may be considered positive. Other authors, have noted that ≥50,000 CFU/mL are more likely to correspond to true pathogens and UTI, and repeat catheterization is recommended if bacterial counts are 10,000 to 50,000 CFU/mL.[2] On a suprapubic specimen, any growth of a gram-negative rod (GNR) or more than a few thousand CFU per milliliter of gram-positive organisms is considered positive. A renal ultrasound to identify structural abnormalities after febrile UTI has been routinely obtained; however, this practice is currently being questioned in a large clinical trial, especially with a third-trimester ultrasound.

Tx   Neonates and infants under 60 days of age are admitted for IV antibiotic therapy. Initial therapy should be ampicillin plus either gentamicin or a third-generation cephalosporin. Once culture and sensitivities are available, therapy can be narrowed. Controversy surrounds duration of parenteral therapy in this age-group, because recent studies suggest that 72 hours of IV antibiotics or less may be sufficient if there is good clinical response.[3] Total duration of antibiotic therapy (IV and PO) should be no less than 10 days. A voiding cystourethrogram (VCUG) is typically done to assess for urinary reflux, although routinely obtaining this study is under scrutiny as the role of antimicrobial prophylaxis in prevention of repeat UTI is studied.[4] See Chapter 41, Dysuria. **See Nelson Essentials 114.**

Meningitis or Encephalitis

Pφ | *Meningitis* results from inflammation of the meninges that surround the brain and spinal cord. Neonates and infants to a lesser degree have a high risk for hematogenous spread of bacterial infections because of an immature immune system and blood-brain barrier. In neonates, the most likely organisms are group B streptococcus, *E. coli, and L. monocytogenes. S. pneumoniae* rises in predominance during the second month and is the major pathogen by the third month of life.

TP | Headache, vomiting, and nuchal rigidity may be absent or difficult to assess in young infants. Altered mental status can manifest as irritability or lethargy. A bulging fontanelle may suggest increased intracranial pressure. Seizures may suggest HSV infection.

Dx | CSF fluid is diagnostic. Bacterial meningitis is suggested by a CSF protein >150 mg/dL, glucose level <30 mg/dL, >25 leukocytes/mL, and a positive Gram stain. Lymphocyte predominance suggests viral etiology. Culture is confirmatory.

Tx | Ampicillin and gentamicin or cefotaxime provide empirical coverage pending culture results. In an older infant, a third-generation cephalosporin will suffice. Acyclovir is added if herpes simplex virus is suspected. See Chapter 49, Meningitis. **See Nelson Essentials 100 and 101.**

Bronchiolitis

See Chapter 44, Difficulty Breathing.

Practice-Based Learning and Improvement

Title
Practice guideline for the management of infants and children 0 to 36 months of age with fever without source

Authors
Baraff L, Schriger D, Bass J, et al

Reference
Pediatrics 92;1-12, 1993

Problem
Specific practice guidelines were needed to manage infants with fever without a source, because standard of care at that time was to treat all infants age 0 to 36 months, with varying presenting symptoms, all the same.

Intervention

The National Library of Medicine Medline bibliographic database from 1977 through August 1991 was used to search for all publications concerning the management of febrile infants and children. A meta-analysis was performed to combine the results of multiple studies when more than one report addressed a single topic area of interest. An algorithm was then created with decision "nodes" where various management strategies were proposed. The algorithm, as well as a summary of the literature search and meta-analysis, were submitted to an expert panel to circulate, review, and formulate practice guidelines.

Outcome/effect

All toxic-appearing infants and febrile infants less than 28 days of age should be hospitalized for parenteral antibiotic therapy. Febrile infants 28 to 90 days of age who are defined as low risk by specific clinical and laboratory criteria may be managed as outpatients if close follow-up is ensured.

Historical significance/comments

This article employed what is known as the "Rochester criteria" to stratify febrile infants into high- versus low-risk categories. Infants older than 28 days who were considered low risk were the most significantly impacted; the study demonstrated that they do not require hospitalization.

Interpersonal and Communication Skills

Provide Reassurance and Explain the Rationale for Laboratory Testing in the Febrile Neonate

An important aspect of a pediatrician's job is to provide reassurance! Parents of a febrile newborn are usually anxious, especially if it is their first child. Make sure they understand what will be done to their baby. If the baby appears seriously ill, they should be told this. However, the majority of neonates with fever look well on admission, and initial laboratory studies do not reveal serious abnormalities. In this case, assure the family that the tests are routine and do not indicate a high suspicion of a serious illness. They will be comforted by the fact that antibiotics are empirical and initiated before culture results return. Answer their questions, and report all laboratory results carefully and promptly.

Professionalism

Self-Improvement: Remain Current on Recommendations for Management of Fever in the Neonate and Young Infant

The recommended management of febrile infants under 3 months of age has changed dramatically over the last 25 years as data from research studies have been published. Data from future research will continue to inform the content of new, updated practice guidelines. It is the physician's responsibility to keep abreast of these developments in order to provide optimal care to this group of patients.

Systems-Based Practice

Quality Improvement: Benchmarking

The Institute of Medicine's 1999 report on medical errors stated that 44,000 to 98,000 deaths occur annually because of adverse patient events, at a national cost of $17 billion to $29 billion. Hospital-acquired infections (HAIs) are estimated to represent 50% of this human and economic burden. Surveillance in combination with infection control programs can prevent up to one third of HAIs by organizing and implementing focused prevention interventions. The National Nosocomial Infections Surveillance (NNIS) system, created by the Centers for Disease Control and Prevention in 1970, establishes and monitors national benchmarks for HAI rates, based on standardized definitions and validated methodology, and facilitates comparative quality assessments for individual hospitals. Estimates of the burden of HAIs on hospitalized children can vary widely from less than 1% to greater than 20%, depending on the patient's host factors or extrinsic exposures, the methodology used to ascertain infections, and the denominator used to calculate rates. It is useful to have benchmark rates, such as those determined through the NNIS system, that reflect consistently collected data over time and for large populations of patients. The data provided by the NNIS system (incidence data) and the Pediatric Prevention Network—a collaboration between the National Association of Children's Hospitals and Related Institutions and the Hospital Infections Program at the Centers for Disease Control and Prevention—(prevalence data) surveys are important contributors to the overall understanding of the epidemiology of HAIs in pediatric patients.[5]

References

1. American College of Emergency Physicians Clinical Policies Subcommittee on Pedia: Clinical policy for children younger than three years presenting to the emergency department with fever. *Ann Emerg Med* 42(4):530-545, 2003.
2. Hoberman A, Wald ER, Reynolds EA, et al: Pyuria and bacteriuria in urine specimens obtained by catheter from young children with fever, *J Pediatr* 124:513-519, 1994.
3. Hoberman A, Wald E, Hickey RW, et al: Oral versus intravenous therapy for urinary tract infections in young febrile children. *Pediatrics* 104(1):79-86, 1999.
4. American Academy of Pediatrics: Practice parameter: The diagnosis, treatment, and evaluation of the initial UTI in febrile infants and young children. *Pediatrics* 103:843-852, 1999.
5. Sohn A, Jarvis W: Benchmarking in pediatric infection control: Results from the National Nosocomial Infections Surveillance (NNIS) system and the pediatric prevention network. *Semin Pediatr Infect Dis* 12(3):254-265, 2001.

Chapter 47
Seizure (Case 17)

Cynthia Gibson MD, FAAP

Case: A 6-month-old presents with extremity shaking for 10 minutes and is now sleepy.

Differential Diagnosis

Infection	Epilepsy	Metabolic and electrolyte disturbances
Trauma	Toxic ingestion	Tumor

Speaking Intelligently

Acute management of seizures includes assessment and stabilization of airway, breathing, and circulation (ABCs) before administration of antiseizure medication, typically a benzodiazepine. Persistent seizures and those in neonates are often treated with phenobarbital, which requires monitoring for respiratory depression and hypotension. Therapy should be implemented while simultaneously investigating etiology. Febrile seizures are the most common type of childhood seizure and typically carry an excellent prognosis (see Chapter 87, Status Epilepticus).

PATIENT CARE

Clinical Thinking

- Support the ABCs.
- Is the patient stable, or is intensive care required?
- Seizures have many possible causes, which will dictate treatment. A detailed history and examination may suggest **infection, toxic ingestion, or trauma.** If the seizure recurs or does not respond to antiepileptics, other correctable causes must be considered.
- Review **treatable causes** such as hypoglycemia or hyponatremia.
- Are there preexisting neurologic abnormalities?
- **Diagnoses that mimic seizures** include benign paroxysmal vertigo, breath holding, syncope, shuddering attacks, narcolepsy, night terrors, pseudoseizures, benign myoclonus of infancy, and tics.
- Proceed in a stepwise fashion to avoid unnecessary testing.

History

- Obtain a detailed description, including circumstances, prodrome, focality, duration, frequency, and postictal state.
- Fever in an otherwise healthy child may suggest **febrile seizure** or central nervous system (CNS) infection.
- Recent trauma and rapid symptom progression suggest **intracranial hemorrhage.**
- Obtain detailed history of possible ingestion, including all household medications.
- Localizing neurologic signs point to an **intracranial mass.**
- Dehydration or metabolic disorder may suggest an electrolyte abnormality.

Physical Examination

- Assess and stabilize the ABCs.

Vital signs:

- Realize that heart rates, blood pressure, and respiratory rates vary with age.
- Hypertension, tachycardia, and arrhythmias may manifest during a seizure.
- Assess hydration status.
- **Thorough neurologic examination** includes: mental status, cranial nerves, reflexes, muscle strength and tone. Focal findings such as weakness or paralysis may localize a lesion.

- Fontanelle size and character in infants can be helpful but are inconsistent.
- Funduscopic examination may reveal **retinal hemorrhages or papilledema.**
- Assess for dysmorphology and neurocutaneous lesions.

Tests for Consideration

- **Complete blood count (CBC):** Leukocytosis with infection $116
- **Electrolytes:** Sodium, calcium, magnesium, phosphorous, and blood glucose levels are correctable abnormalities that may provoke seizure $392
- **Blood culture:** If concern for infection $152
- **Lumbar puncture:** If concern for meningitis/encephalitis; includes Gram stain, cell count, protein level, glucose level, culture, enterovirus polymerase chain reaction (PCR), herpes PCR $1028
- **Electroencephalogram (EEG):** To evaluate seizure character or abnormal brain activity $727
- If suspected undiagnosed metabolic disorder:
  - **Serum amino acids** $322
  - **Urine organic acids** $609
- **Serum lactate** $211

IMAGING CONSIDERATIONS

→ **Head computed tomography (CT) noncontrast:**
To assess for intracranial hemorrhage or mass $1827
→ **Magnetic resonance imaging (MRI) (when clinically stable):** More definitive for brain structure $2331

Clinical Entities   Medical Knowledge

Infection

Pφ   CNS *infections* are commonly caused by bacteria or viruses and may result in meningitis, encephalitis, and occasionally intracranial abscesses. These infections typically occur via direct injury or inflammation of neurons or their supportive structures. Seizures may develop from infection-related inflammation and/or cell death.

TP   CNS infections may present with symptoms of fever, altered consciousness (lethargy or irritability), headaches, vomiting, bulging fontanelle, widened sutures, and papilledema. Signs of systemic illness, such as petechiae in *Neisseria* meningitis, may occur over hours to days. About 20% of patients with meningitis will have seizures; 80% of those will be complex seizures.

Dx	In meningitis, lumbar puncture is usually diagnostic; in encephalitis it may be unrevealing. Special cerebrospinal fluid polymerase chain reaction (CSF PCR) studies may be required to confirm etiologies such as herpes simplex virus (HSV) and enterovirus. In some cases EEG or imaging findings—such as paroxysmal lateralizing electrical discharges (PLEDs) on EEG associated with herpes infections—will suggest the diagnosis.
Tx	Treatment includes antimicrobial and supportive therapy. Initially, broad-spectrum antibiotics are appropriate pending culture results. Causative microorganisms differ according to age. In neonates, the most common organisms are *Escherichia coli*, other gram-negative organisms, and group B streptococcus. After 4 to 6 weeks of age, *Streptococcus pneumoniae* and *Neisseria meningitidis* occur more commonly (see Chapter 46, Neonatal Fever, and Chapter 49, Meningitis). **See Nelson Essentials 100 and 101.**

Toxic Ingestion

Pφ	Many drugs of abuse, household substances, or medications taken inappropriately or accidentally cause seizures via direct excitatory or sedative-hypnotic effects on the brain. Seizures may also result from medication side effects such as hypoglycemia.
TP	There may not be a history of ingestion. Knowing which medications are present in the household may provide a clue. Intentional ingestions are more common in adolescents; accidental ingestions typically occur in toddlers. Many drugs have characteristic symptoms called toxidromes. Poison control centers are useful in these cases. Common causes of toxin-induced seizures can be remembered using the mnemonic OTIS CAMPBELL: <ul><li>**O**rganophosphates</li><li>**T**ricyclic antidepressants</li><li>**I**soniazid, insulin</li><li>**S**ympathomimetics</li><li>**C**amphor, cocaine</li><li>**A**mphetamines</li><li>**M**ethylxanthines</li><li>**P**CP (phencyclidine hydrochloride), propranolol</li><li>**B**enzodiazepine withdrawal, botanicals</li><li>**E**thanol withdrawal</li><li>**L**ithium, lidocaine</li><li>**L**indane, lead</li></ul>

Dx Presence of a toxidrome can make a diagnosis. Many laboratories offer a quick screen for drugs of abuse, and a comprehensive toxicology screen, including many medications, may also be available. Other studies include electrocardiogram (EKG) for arrhythmias; abdominal radiography for radiopaque drugs; electrolytes; liver function tests, and arterial blood gas.

Tx Typical treatment for toxic ingestion includes:
   • Assessment and management of the ABCs
   • Prevention/reduction of absorption: gastric lavage (rarely used), activated charcoal, whole bowel irrigation
   • Enhancement of excretion: urinary alkalinization, neutral diuresis, hemodialysis
   • Administration of antidotes: only for specific toxins
   • Control of seizures with medications until the toxin has cleared. **See Nelson Essentials 45.**

Epilepsy

Pφ *Epilepsy* is characterized by recurrent unprovoked seizures and requires two or more afebrile seizures. Children with developmental delay, learning disability, cerebral palsy, or neuroanatomic lesions face increased risk for epilepsy. The underlying pathophysiology is not clearly understood. The excitatory neurotransmitters glutamate and aspartate may play a role via excitation of specific neuronal cell receptors.

TP Seizures of epilepsy present in many ways. They may be partial—either simple or complex involving motor, sensory, autonomic, or psychic manifestations—or generalized. Generalized seizures may be divided into absence, tonic-clonic, tonic, clonic, myoclonic, atonic, or infantile spasm varieties. Children with brain injuries may be predisposed to epilepsy. There may be a positive family history.

Dx Assessment for dysmorphology and neurocutaneous lesions may help diagnose an underlying neurologic abnormality. Consultation with a neurologist and an EEG may determine seizure type. MRI should be considered in patients with unexplained neurologic abnormalities or cognitive or motor impairments.

Tx   Antiepileptic therapy is usually required in epilepsy. Many medications exist; some control certain types of seizures more effectively than others. A neurologist guides the choice of long-term medications. Some examples include carbamazepine, levetiracetam, oxcarbazepine, and valproic acid.
Nonpharmacologic therapies include ketogenic diet, vagal nerve stimulators, and surgery. **See Nelson Essentials 181.**

Trauma

Pφ   *Trauma* can cause hemorrhage in the epidural, subdural, or subarachnoid spaces—or in brain parenchyma. Epidural bleeding occurs with arterial injury, exerting a mass effect on brain tissue beneath. Subdural bleeding occurs with injury to the bridging veins between the dura and brain surface. Subarachnoid and intraparenchymal bleeding can occur from a variety of sources.

TP   Nontraumatic hemorrhages can develop from severe dehydration, anatomic abnormalities (arteriovenous malformations or aneurysms), and metabolic and hematologic disorders such as sickle cell disease. Bleeding disorders may predispose children to hemorrhages with minor or no trauma. A history of trauma is almost always present. Symptoms often occur abruptly and include altered mental status. Intracranial bleeding without history of trauma should raise suspicion of child abuse.

Dx   Noncontrast head CT is typically diagnostic for intracranial hemorrhage. Anatomic abnormalities, such as arteriovenous malformations or aneurysms, may require MRI.

Tx   Treatment is often supportive. Some cases require neurosurgical intervention. Risk for herniation may be high. If there are signs of herniation, intervention is required to decrease intracranial pressure while awaiting neurosurgical intervention. Immediate management includes respiratory and hemodynamic support, osmotherapy, and adequate sedation and pain control. Seizures should be aggressively treated (see Chapter 81, Raised Intracranial Pressure, and Chapter 86, Trauma). **See Nelson Essentials 184.**

Metabolic and Electrolyte Disturbances

Pφ	***Disturbances of electrolytes,*** including glucose, sodium, calcium, magnesium, and phosphorous, can cause seizures by affecting neurotransmitters. Glucose and sodium affect the osmolarity of brain cells. ***Metabolic disorders,*** such as maple syrup urine disease, organic acidurias, and urea cycle disorders, can include neurologic manifestations.
TP	Seizures due to electrolyte disturbances typically resolve with correction of the abnormality and rarely require subsequent anticonvulsants. Pertinent physical signs include dehydration, cardiac arrhythmias, tetany, or hyperreflexia. A history of poor or unusual oral intake, poor growth, unusual odors, or family history of neonatal deaths, may suggest an inborn error of metabolism.
Dx	Test for glucose, sodium, calcium, magnesium, metabolic acidosis, lactate, and urine ketones, as well as liver and renal function. Quick glucose analysis can be done at the bedside. Quantification of serum amino acids and urine organic acids should be performed. Physical features may characterize some metabolic disorders. Consultation with a geneticist or metabolism specialist may guide evaluation and treatment of a suspected inborn error of metabolism.
Tx	Stabilize the ABCs. Correction of dehydration and electrolyte abnormalities is the only way to stop the seizures. Infusion of glucose quickly treats hypoglycemia. With a metabolic crisis, an infusion of dextrose and lipids will avoid catabolism. Severe cases may require hemofiltration to treat hyperammonemia. **See Nelson Essentials 35, 36, and 37.**

Tumor

Pφ	Seizures may occur with primary or metastatic CNS ***tumors,*** meningeal leukemia, or from chemotherapy. Children who have received cranial irradiation also face an increased risk for seizures.
TP	In oncologic processes, neurologic symptoms may be acute or chronic and may include headache, dizziness, lethargy, or visual disturbances. Seizures may be focal if emanating from a specific lesion or generalized if resulting from global effects of chemotherapy, leukemia, or irradiation.

Dx   The history will guide diagnosis and management. An EEG and CT scan may reveal an underlying cause. A primary CNS tumor may be apparent on CT; however, MRI may be needed if it is small or in the brainstem. Electrolyte abnormalities occur commonly in children undergoing chemotherapy.

Tx   Prolonged seizures may require anticonvulsants and/or correction of metabolic disturbances. Valproic acid and carbamazepine may be contraindicated because of bone marrow suppression. Prolonged or repetitive seizures often require long-term therapy. Antibiotics are appropriate for those with signs or symptoms of meningitis or those at increased risk for meningitis (fever and neutropenia). **See Nelson Essentials 157.**

ZEBRA ZONE

a. Infantile spasms: A specific type of generalized seizures that begin between 4 and 8 months of age, characterized by brief symmetric contractions of the neck, trunk, and extremities and featuring hypsarrhythmia on EEG. They are associated with tuberous sclerosis and West syndrome.

b. Neurocysticercosis: Pork tapeworm cysts *(Taenia solium)* in the brain that may cause seizures and obstructive hydrocephalus; the host response may produce signs and symptoms of meningitis.

Practice-Based Learning and Improvement

Title
Magnetic resonance imaging and electroencephalographic findings in a cohort of normal children with newly diagnosed seizures

Author
Doescher JS, deGrauw TJ, Musick BS, et al

Reference
J Child Neurol 21(6):491-495, 2006

Problem
How to evaluate otherwise healthy children with new-onset seizures

Comparison/control (quality of evidence)
This study looks at healthy, school-age children with normal intelligence and new-onset seizures and attempts to describe the relationship between EEG and MRI findings.

Outcome/effect

Abnormal MRIs were found in children with normal EEGs.

Historical significance/comments

Normal EEGs cannot be used to predict a low-risk group who do not require brain MRI.

Interpersonal and Communication Skills

Communicate Effectively With Subspecialists in the Care of the Child With Complex Medical Issues

Establishing seizure etiology will determine which subspecialists become involved. With ongoing seizures, critical care may be necessary for airway support. Early contact with a neurosurgeon may be lifesaving. A hematologist-oncologist will need to be involved if cancer or a bleeding disorder is suspected. A neurologist may be required to characterize the seizure and its etiology and to determine long-term therapy. Long-term care may involve a developmental pediatrician, a physiatrist, and speech, occupational, and/or physical therapy. Child abuse specialists and child protective services may be necessary if there is suspicion for abuse. Clear communication and medical record documentation will help optimize management of medically complex children (see Chapter 25, The Special Needs Child).

Professionalism

Demonstrate Responsiveness to the Family in an Emergency

A child with a seizure is a frightening emergency situation for a parent. Parents need to know they can quickly and reliably contact their doctor's office in the event of an emergency. Physicians must have an adequate telephone response time not only during office hours but also after hours. Even if parents have accessed the 911 emergency services, they often need the comfort and assurance of speaking to someone who is from their primary-care practice.

Systems-Based Practice

Quality Improvement: Patient Safety

Confusing drug names is a common system failure. Many drug names can look or sound like other drug names, which may lead to potentially harmful medication errors. In addition, factors such as poor handwriting or poorly communicated oral prescriptions can exacerbate the problem. In 2001, The Joint Commission published a

Sentinel Event Alert on look-alike and sound-alike drug names. Two of The Joint Commission's 2010 National Patient Safety Goals (NPSGs) for the hospital setting address safety of using medications and medication reconciliation across the continuum of care.

As noted on The Joint Commission website (http://www. jointcommission.org/SentinelEvents/SentinelEventAlert/sea_19.htm), prescribers can do the following to avoid medication errors:

- Maintain awareness of look-alike and sound-alike drug names as published by various safety agencies.
- Clearly specify the dosage form, drug strength, and complete directions on prescriptions. These variables may help staff differentiate products.
- With name pairs known to be problematic, reduce the potential for confusion by writing prescriptions using both the brand and generic names.
- Include the purpose of medication on prescriptions. In most cases, drugs that sound or look similar are used for different purposes.
- Alert patients to the potential for mix-ups, especially with known problematic drug names. Advise ambulatory care patients to insist on pharmacy counseling when picking up prescriptions and to verify that the medication and directions match what the prescriber has told them.
- Encourage inpatients to question nurses about medications that are unfamiliar or look or sound different than expected.
- Give verbal or telephone orders only when truly necessary, and never for chemotherapeutics. Include the drug's intended purpose to ensure clarity.
- Encourage staff to read back all orders, spell the product name, and state its indication.

Reference

1. http://www.jointcommission.org/SentinelEvents/SentinelEventAlert/sea_19. htm.

Chapter 48
Apparent Life-Threatening Event (Case 18)

Craig C. DeWolfe MD, MEd

Case: A 1-month-old infant presents with an episode in which he turned blue, went from stiff to limp, and may have stopped breathing.

Differential Diagnosis

Respiratory infections	Choking resulting from gastroesophageal reflux (GER) disease/aspiration	Seizure
Idiopathic apparent life-threatening event (ALTE)	Intentional trauma	

Speaking Intelligently

An apparent life-threatening event (ALTE) is not a diagnosis; it is a description of an event with many potential causes. A National Institutes of Health Consensus Statement defines it as an episode that is frightening to the observer and characterized by some combination of apnea (central or occasionally obstructive), color change (usually cyanotic or pallid but occasionally erythematous or plethoric), marked change in muscle tone (usually limpness), choking, or gagging. Our goal is to determine the underlying cause and/or risk for harm. I carefully reconstruct the event, because a detailed history usually saves immeasurable time, testing, and anxiety. I try to understand what frightened the parents, and what resuscitation, if any, was needed. Causes are typically self-limited and benign, but life-threatening events and diagnoses do occur. I highlight the myriad of possible tests and need for a judicious yet thorough evaluation. Ideally, the extent of my evaluation will match the parents' level of concern. The evaluation of each case is individualized; there are no clinical practice guidelines for ALTE evaluation and management.

PATIENT CARE

Clinical Thinking
- First evaluate the **airway, breathing, and circulation (ABCs).** Ensure the infant is stable and on a cardiorespiratory monitor.
- Reconstruct the presentation from the primary witness.
- Was there **apnea?** Apnea is defined as cessation of breathing for 20 seconds or longer.
- The type and distribution of color change will help differentiate significant hypoxia from less-concerning etiologies. Isolated cyanosis around the lips and extremities is not indicative of true desaturation, whereas cyanosis of the lips, tongue, face, and/or trunk is considered **central cyanosis.**
- Methodically approach a differential diagnosis, considering central, obstructive, or mixed apnea events.
- Consider child abuse.

History
- Note any change in tone, rhythmic shaking, and its distribution.
- Was there choking, gagging, coughing, or vomiting? Was milk noted at the mouth? Was the infant recently fed?
- Any loss of consciousness?
- Is there fever or hypothermia to suggest infection?
- Is there a prior history of trauma, intentional or unintentional?
- What was the location and/or sleep position?
- What type of resuscitation was required, and by whom? Include initial cardiorespiratory assessment details.
- Review prehospital emergency medical service records.
- What is the infant's current condition, and how long did it take the child to return to baseline?
- Any prior history of ALTE? What intervention was required? Is there a home apnea monitor?
- Review birth history. Is the infant premature?
- Identify preexisting medical conditions, such as GER or seizures.
- Has the infant or breastfeeding mother taken any medications?
- Any family history of ALTE, sudden infant death syndrome (SIDS), or infant death?

Physical Examination
- Evaluate ABCs, and check vital signs, including pulse oximetry.
- Determine the infant's general arousal and state.
- Search for dysmorphic features to suggest a metabolic or genetic condition. Pay special attention to craniofacial abnormalities.
- Obtain growth curves, including head circumference, which may suggest microcephaly or hydrocephalus.
- Check tympanic membranes for hemotympanum, eyes for pupil reactivity, and funduscopic examination for retinal hemorrhages.

- Examine the head, skin, and musculoskeletal system for evidence of trauma.
- Focus on the neurologic examination for tone, degree and symmetry of movement, deep tendon reflexes, and developmental milestones.

Tests for Consideration
- If concerned about a history of poor perfusion or a metabolic disorder:
  - **Blood gas** $222
  - **Lactate** $211
- **Complete blood count (CBC):** Leukocytosis or leukopenia in infection; hemoglobin if traumatic $116
- An occult urinary tract infection has been linked to patients presenting with an ALTE with no fever and/or residual clinical manifestations. Occult bacteremia and meningitis have been documented much less frequently. If concerned about infection:
  - **Blood culture** $152
  - **Urine culture** $148
  - **Cerebrospinal fluid (CSF) culture** $152
  - **CSF Gram stain** $180
  - **CSF cell count** $150
  - **CSF protein and glucose** $75
  - **Herpes simplex virus polymerase chain reaction (PCR)** $300
- **Electroencephalogram (EEG):** If concern for seizure $727
- **Electrolytes, glucose, calcium, and magnesium:** If concerned for seizure $392
- **Electrocardiogram (EKG):** To check QTc interval $217
- **Pneumogram:** If the event was serious, occurred during sleep, and cannot be easily explained by history/examination $5585
- **Rapid respiratory panel:** If the history or congestion suggests a viral source such as respiratory syncytial virus (RSV) $325
- **Pertussis polymerase chain reaction (PCR):** If the congestion or cough suggests an infectious source $168

IMAGING CONSIDERATIONS

→ **Chest radiograph:** If concern for bronchiolitis, pneumonia, or cardiac disease $231
→ **Head computed tomography (CT):** If concern for trauma $1827
→ **Skeletal survey:** If concern for trauma or hydrocephalus $500
→ **Nuclear medicine milk/gastric emptying scan or pH probe:** To assess gastroesophageal reflux $1118
→ **Five-channel video fluoroscopic swallow study:** To assess swallowing function $840

| Clinical Entities | Medical Knowledge |

Viral Respiratory Infection

Pφ   Respiratory syncytial virus (RSV), human metapneumovirus, influenza, and other viruses infect airway epithelium and cause upper and lower airway edema with mucus production and airway plugging. These viruses may also cause central apnea, perhaps by altering the sensitivity of laryngeal chemoreceptors to regurgitated gastric contents. Pertussis and bacterial pneumonias may present in a similar fashion and can be manifest as obstructive or central apnea.

TP   Infants present with nasal congestion, cough, and often have difficulty feeding. With lower airway involvement there is wheezing, increased work of breathing, and hypoxemia. Coughing and gagging may worsen gastroesophageal reflux because of increased intra-abdominal and intrathoracic pressure.

Dx   Diagnosis is based on clinical findings. Specific viral or pertussis testing is available. A chest radiograph may be beneficial in diagnosing a bacterial pneumonia.

Tx   Supportive care includes cardiorespiratory monitoring, suctioning, supplemental oxygen, smaller-volume frequent feeds, and intravenous fluids as needed. Inhaled albuterol or racemic epinephrine may help in select cases. Antibiotics would be warranted for pertussis or bacterial pneumonia (see Chapter 44, Difficulty Breathing, and Chapter 46, Neonatal Fever). **See Nelson Essentials 109.**

Choking due to Gastroesophageal Reflux Disease or Aspiration

Pφ   A choking episode secondary to gastroesophageal reflux (GER) results from the regurgitation of stomach contents through the lower esophageal sphincter into the oropharynx or lower respiratory tract, causing obstructive apnea. Central apnea may occur when regurgitated contents trigger the laryngo-chemoreceptor reflex, in which the infant stops breathing to protect the airway. An infant might also choke on oropharyngeal secretions.

TP   GER classically occurs shortly after a feed but can occur any time. It commonly manifests as regurgitation and can involve choking, coughing, gagging, or other symptoms. Recurrent reflux episodes may cause vocal cord edema with stridor. Prolonged choking may result in a vagal response, whereby the infant becomes limp and "resets" the respiratory pattern.

Dx   Diagnosis can be made by history alone if regurgitation and/or aspiration are witnessed. There may be a history of reflux, back arching (Sandifer syndrome), and/or decreased feeding. In subtle cases, a radioisotope scan can grade reflux, quantify aspiration, and assess gastric emptying. Additional tests, including pH probe or esophageal impedance, may be especially useful when performed with a sleep study. An upper GI scan will delineate anatomy but offers low sensitivity for detection of GER. Beware of labeling too many cases of ALTE as secondary to GER, because reflux commonly occurs in many healthy infants.

Tx   Reflux precautions include smaller frequent feeds, frequent burping, upright postprandial positioning, and thickened feeds using rice cereal for bottle-fed infants. Histamine-2 blockers and proton pump inhibitors can prevent caustic effects of regurgitated materials. Prokinetic drugs such as metoclopramide or erythromycin may improve gastric emptying with varying effectiveness and may be considered in difficult to manage cases. In select cases a Nissen fundoplication and/or gastrojejunostomy tube may be considered. **See Nelson Essentials 128.**

Seizure

Pφ   A *seizure* is a paroxysmal disturbance of brain wave propagation often leading to abnormal motor activity, behavioral abnormalities, and sensory and/or autonomic dysfunction. Not a diagnosis itself, a seizure may occur with many types of central nervous system (CNS) pathology, including infection, fever, metabolic derangements, toxins, CNS malformations, trauma, or epilepsy.

TP   Seizures do not usually generalize in neonates because of immature neuronal connections and myelination. Tone may be increased or decreased, and movements may be clonic or tonic-clonic. Apnea may occur in all ages.

Dx   Determining the underlying etiology is most important. Studies usually include glucose, blood urea nitrogen (BUN), and electrolytes, including calcium and magnesium. In addition, one should consider cultures of blood, urine, and cerebrospinal fluid (CSF) and CSF herpes simplex virus polymerase chain reaction (PCR) for encephalitis. Brain imaging will evaluate for congenital or traumatic lesions such as hemorrhage. An EEG and neurology consultation are usually indicated.

Tx   Treatment is based on underlying etiology. Recurrent seizures may require long-term antiepileptic therapy, usually managed by a neurologist (see Chapter 47, Seizure). **See Nelson Essentials 181.**

Idiopathic Apparent Life-Threatening Event

Pφ   This is a diagnosis of exclusion and is used to describe at least 25% of all cases when the history, examination, or workup does not provide an underlying diagnosis. These patients typically have no residual examination findings or subsequent events.

TP   There are variable presentations.

Dx   Diagnosis is clinical.

Tx   An initial period of observation and reassurance, if appropriate, are indicated. Anticipatory guidance for sleep position, the natural history of ALTE, and a review of ABC management techniques should be provided. The use of a home apnea monitor may be discussed, but monitors have never been shown to alter the natural course of the underlying condition. **See Nelson Essentials 134.**

Intentional Trauma

Pφ   Studies have demonstrated that intentional suffocation, shaken baby syndrome, and Munchausen syndrome by proxy may manifest with nonspecific symptoms and few, if any, clinical signs.

TP   These children face continued risk if they return to an unsafe environment. One study identified shaken baby syndrome as a disproportionately important cause of death in infants presenting with ALTEs, whereas another documented deliberate suffocation in over 10% of patients referred to an apnea center after active resuscitation and in which the team had suspicion for intentional trauma.

Dx   Diagnosis and treatment are individualized on a case-by-case basis.

Tx   Stabilize the infant. Involve child and family services in order to provide a safe environment upon discharge. **See Nelson Essentials 16 and 22.**

ZEBRA ZONE

a. **Congenital central hypoventilation syndrome (Ondines curse):** Sleep-induced hypoventilation with severe hypercapnia and hypoxemia, likely as a result of severe autonomic dysregulation. Mechanical ventilation is required during sleep.

Practice-Based Learning and Improvement: Evidence-Based Pediatrics

Title
Cardiorespiratory events recorded on home monitors: Comparison of healthy infants with those at increased risk for SIDS

Authors
Ramanathan R, Corwin MJ, Hunt CE, et al

Reference
JAMA 285(17):2199-2207, 2001

Problem
Do infants with idiopathic ALTE requiring resuscitation, preterm infants, and SIDS siblings have a greater risk for cardiorespiratory events than healthy infants?

Intervention
Researchers compared home apnea monitor data to identify subpopulations of infants at increased risk for cardiorespiratory events.

Comparison/control (quality of evidence)
Prospective, multicenter, cohort study of 1079 infants

Outcome/effect
Twenty-second apnea events, previously considered pathologic, were found in 41% of all populations, including healthy infants. Only preterm infants less than 43 weeks post–conceptual age had a statistically increased risk for apnea >30 seconds.

Historical significance/comments
This study raised doubts about the need for home monitors in infants with idiopathic ALTE requiring some resuscitation/stimulation. Of note, the age of greatest risk for prolonged apnea spells was younger than patients who tend to die of SIDS, suggesting that prolonged apnea spells are likely not a significant predeterminant of SIDS.

Interpersonal and Communication Skills

Formulate an Individualized Management Plan for the Infant With an Apparent Life-Threatening Event (ALTE)

A careful and detailed history can be therapeutic. Most parents prefer to discuss the episode and the practitioner's rationale for observation/reassurance or a limited evaluation rather than subject their child to a battery of tests. Acknowledge that parents may fear another ALTE or even SIDS. Reassure them that ALTEs have not reliably been found to cause SIDS. Also explain that home apnea monitors have not reduced the rate of SIDS, but that the Back to Sleep campaign has decreased the occurrence of SIDS by 30% to 50%. It is also wise to have the family learn cardiopulmonary resuscitation.

Professionalism

Demonstrate Self-Awareness: Ask for Consultation or Assistance When Needed

Do not order tests based on an incomplete history or your level of anxiety. Rather, develop comfort with the presentation and natural history of ALTE, and appreciate the value of observation. Remember, our job is to do no harm. An exhaustive battery of tests yielding findings of questionable clinical significance or false-positive results may lead to more family anxiety and unnecessary, expensive, and invasive procedures.

Systems-Based Practice

Home Care: Home Apnea Monitoring

When the physician orders home apnea monitoring, a hospital case manager must obtain approval from the patient's insurance company. Each insurance company generally has a contractual arrangement with a durable medical equipment (DME) company to deliver the monitor to the hospital. The monitor is applied to the infant before discharge while the primary caregivers are taught application, care, and interpretation of alarms (i.e., disconnected lead versus true alarm). Monthly downloads are interpreted by the physician group (often a pulmonologist or neonatologist) contracted by the DME company. Results are communicated directly to the family through a sleep clinic or through the primary care physician. Duration of monitoring is based on overall patient progress. Specific criteria are applied for discontinuance, such as 2 months without an event requiring stimulation.

Chapter 49
Meningitis (Case 19)

Rebecca Tenney-Soeiro MD

Case: A 2-year-old boy with fever, vomiting, and irritability is found to have meningitis.

Differential Diagnosis

Bacterial meningitis	Aseptic meningitis

Speaking Intelligently

When I suspect a child has meningitis, I quickly assess clinical status to determine if antibiotics are urgently needed. Does the child need resuscitation? Is a head computed tomography (CT) scan needed before a lumbar puncture (LP)? After this assessment, I perform an LP, and the cerebrospinal fluid (CSF) is evaluated for cell count, glucose, protein, and Gram stain and culture. For suspected bacterial meningitis, empirical antibiotic therapy is begun. Beyond the neonatal period, treatment includes vancomycin and a third-generation cephalosporin such as cefotaxime. The child's age, immunization status, season, and recent illness or sick contacts are important considerations. Distinguishing between viral and bacterial meningitis at presentation, and hence the need for hospitalization and treatment, can sometimes be difficult. The Bacterial Meningitis Score may help to differentiate aseptic from bacterial meningitis in patients over the age of 2 months. Patients have a low risk for bacterial meningitis if they demonstrate *all* of the following: (1) negative CSF Gram stain, (2) CSF absolute neutrophil count (ANC) less than 1000 cells/μL, (3) CSF protein less than 80 mg/dL, (4) peripheral blood ANC less than 10,000 cells/μL, and (5) no history of seizure before or at the time of presentation.

PATIENT CARE

Clinical Thinking

- Support the airway, breathing, and circulation **(ABCs).**
- Is the intensive care unit needed?
- Begin **empirical treatment with broad-spectrum antibiotics** and narrow coverage once the organism and sensitivities are known.
- **Monitor for complications** of bacterial meningitis: change in level of consciousness, increased intracranial pressure (ICP), seizures, acidosis, coagulopathy, syndrome of inappropriate antidiuretic hormone (SIADH), abscess, or subdural empyema.

History

- Was onset sudden, or have symptoms developed gradually?
- Have there been seizures (an important prognostic indicator)? Early generalized **seizures** may be due to cortical inflammation or SIADH. Focal or later-onset generalized seizures are suggestive of a suppurative complication or permanent brain damage (see Chapter 47, Seizure).
- Review **immunization status;** specifically *Streptococcus pneumoniae* and *Haemophilus influenzae* vaccines, and in adolescents, *Neisseria meningitidis.*
- A recent upper respiratory infection (URI) or gastroenteritis may suggest aseptic meningitis.
- Has there been recent treatment with antibiotics? If so, consider a partially treated meningitis and limited reliability of culture results.
- Any ill contacts?

Physical Examination

- Assess ABCs.
- Vital signs: Fever in most cases, but can have temperature instability in young infants. Tachycardia will occur if febrile, dehydrated, or in shock. Note hypotension if in shock. **Cushing triad** of hypertension, bradycardia, and respiratory depression indicates increased intracranial pressure.
- What is the general appearance? Is the child alert and talking? Lethargic? Irritable? Unconscious or disoriented?
- Head, eyes, ears, nose, throat (HEENT): In infants, assess fontanelle size. Measure head circumference under 24 months of age. Any photophobia? Any signs of URI? Is there otitis media?
- Neck: Is there nuchal rigidity? Are **Kernig or Brudzinski signs** present? These may be unreliable in young infants.
- Skin: Infants may be jaundiced. Is there a rash, particularly petechial or purpuric? Vesicles?
- Neurologic: Any mental status changes? Any **cranial nerve palsies** to suggest increased ICP?

Tests for Consideration

- **Complete blood count (CBC) with differential** $116
- **Blood culture** $152
- **Electrolytes, blood urea nitrogen (BUN), and creatinine:** To evaluate hydration status, SIADH $174
- **CSF glucose level:** Approximately half the plasma level in bacterial meningitis $75
- **Coagulation studies:** Prothrombin time/partial thromboplastin time (PT/PTT) if petechiae or purpura $105
- **CSF fluid studies:** Cell count with differential, protein, glucose, Gram stain for immediate assessment in determining bacterial versus aseptic meningitis (Table 49-1) $405
- **CSF culture and sensitivity:** Gold standard for diagnosis of bacterial meningitis $152
- **CSF herpes simplex virus (HSV) polymerase chain reaction (PCR):** If concern for herpes meningoencephalitis $300
- **CSF enterovirus PCR** $350

IMAGING CONSIDERATIONS

→ **Head CT before LP:** If concern for herniation. Indications include recent head trauma or neurosurgery, history of hydrocephalus, CSF shunt, coma, or focal neurologic signs or to define later complications, such as abscess. $1827
→ **Brain magnetic resonance imaging (MRI):** Usually indicated during illness or recovery to define potential complications such as abscess. $2331

Table 49-1	Normal CSF Values by Age		
	WBC cell count/µL	Protein (mg/dL)	Glucose (mg/dL)
Preterm newborn	0-25	65-150	24-63
Term newborn	0-22	20-170	34-119
Infant and child	0-7	5-40	40-80

CSF, Cerebrospinal fluid; WBC, white blood cell count.

Clinical Entities   Medical Knowledge

Bacterial Meningitis

Pφ Meningitis results from inflammation of CSF in the subarachnoid space, including the cerebral ventricles and arachnoid space. Each organism may have a specific route of infection. *N. meningitidis, H. influenzae,* and *S. pneumoniae* may first enter the nasopharynx. *S. pneumoniae* may enter the central nervous system (CNS) through direct extension across a skull fracture. *Listeria monocytogenes* first enters through the gastrointestinal (GI) tract or across the placenta. Coagulase-negative staphylococci are found on the skin or are associated with foreign bodies. *Staphylococcus aureus* may be spread secondary to bacteremia, or from dermal or foreign body exposures. Gram-negative rods have various entry points.
    Bacterial etiologies vary by age.

<1 month	1 month to 2 years	2 years to young adults
Group B streptococcus	*S. pneumoniae*	*N. meningitidis*
L. monocytogenes	*N. meningitidis*	*S. pneumoniae*
E. coli	Group B streptococcus	*H. influenzae*

TP Most children present with fever and signs and symptoms of CNS involvement such as nausea, vomiting, irritability, back pain, headache, nuchal rigidity, or change in mental status. Symptoms usually develop more rapidly than in patients with aseptic meningitis. See Chapter 46, Neonatal Fever, for neonatal presentation.

Dx Diagnosis is made via history, physical examination, and CSF analysis. In bacterial meningitis, CSF white count and protein are elevated and glucose is low (see Table 49-1). Gram stain may be positive for bacteria and white cells. CSF culture is confirmatory.

Tx Treatment includes broad-spectrum antibiotics (usually a third-generation cephalosporin and vancomycin) until an organism and susceptibilities are known, at which time antibiotic coverage can be narrowed. Duration of therapy is based on the specific organism, clinical improvement, and development of complications. The ABCs should always be monitored. Dexamethasone administration is controversial. The patient should be closely monitored for complications, such as prolonged fever, abscess formation, seizures, and SIADH. A hearing test should be performed before discharge or during follow-up. A developmental evaluation should be performed early along with referral to early intervention, because many children have long-term neurologic sequelae.

Organisms and Their Specific Antibiotics

Group B streptococcus	Uniformly sensitive to penicillin. Treat with ampicillin or penicillin and aminoglycoside until blood and CSF sterile then penicillin G monotherapy.
S. pneumoniae	If susceptible to penicillin, continue cephalosporin alone or change to penicillin. If not susceptible to penicillin, but susceptible to cefotaxime and ceftriaxone, use these alone. If also not susceptible to cephalosporins, continue vancomycin and cephalosporin and consider addition of rifampin.
N. meningitidis	Penicillin G; cefotaxime, ceftriaxone, and ampicillin are alternatives. If penicillin/cephalosporin allergic, chloramphenicol is recommended.
Escherichia coli	Ampicillin if susceptible; if resistant, use expanded-spectrum cephalosporin and aminoglycoside.
L. monocytogenes	Ampicillin and gentamicin until CSF sterilized and patient is improved clinically, then ampicillin alone.
H. influenzae	Cefotaxime or ceftriaxone. Meropenem is an alternative. Ampicillin and chloramphenicol are other alternatives

See Nelson Essentials 100.

Aseptic Meningitis

Pφ **Aseptic meningitis** represents meningeal inflammation from a nonbacterial cause, most commonly viral, with at least 80% caused by an enterovirus. Viruses infecting the CNS usually first infect mucosal surfaces of the respiratory and/or GI tracts, with subsequent replication in local lymph nodes followed by a primary viremia that seeds other organs. The virus then replicates in these organs, and a second viremia occurs that leads to CNS infection. HSV infection causes meningoencephalitis (see Chapter 46, Neonatal Fever, and Chapter 77, Neonatal Sepsis). Other etiologies include Lyme disease caused by *Borrelia burgdorferi*. Noninfectious causes of aseptic meningitis include Kawasaki disease and intravenous gamma globulin.

TP The presentation of viral meningitis may closely resemble that of bacterial meningitis, although signs and symptoms typically develop more gradually. There are specific criteria for Kawasaki disease (see Chapter 43, Fever and Rash). With Lyme disease, there may be the rash of erythema migrans, papilledema, Bell palsy, and/or history of a tick bite.

Dx Diagnosis is made via history, physical examination, and CSF analysis. Early viral infection may show a neutrophil-predominant CSF followed by lymphocyte predominance, usually without prominent elevation of protein and low glucose. PCR testing for enterovirus and herpes simplex is highly specific and faster than culture. Erythema migrans and papilledema help differentiate Lyme from viral meningitis, which is important because Lyme requires prolonged antibiotic treatment. Serum testing may be negative in Lyme meningitis; the CSF shows lymphocytes, although CSF PCR for *B. burgdorferi* lacks sensitivity.

Tx Treatment is mainly supportive with the ABCs as top priority. HSV infections are treated with acyclovir, although a significant number of patients with treated HSV suffer long-term neurologic sequelae. Lyme disease is treated with ceftriaxone, and full recovery is expected. Kawasaki disease is treated with intravenous gamma globulin with full resolution expected. **See Nelson Essentials 100.**

ZEBRA ZONE

a. **Tuberculous meningitis:** Caused by *Mycobacterium tuberculosis*.

b. **Syphilis-aseptic meningitis:** Caused by *Treponema pallidum* and treated with penicillin G.

c. **Malignancy:** Leukemic cells or other tumor metastases may be recovered from CSF and require specific therapy.

Practice-Based Learning and Improvement

Title
Development and validation of a multivariable predictive model to distinguish bacterial from aseptic meningitis in children in the post-*Haemophilus influenzae* era

Authors
Nigrovic L, Kuppermann N, Malley R

Reference
Pediatrics 110:712-719, 2002

Problem
Distinguishing bacterial from aseptic meningitis to avoid unnecessary hospitalization

Intervention
Development of a Bacterial Meningitis Score to identify children at low versus high risk for bacterial meningitis

Comparison/control (quality of evidence)
Retrospective peer-reviewed cohort study

Outcome/effect
Accurate identification of low-risk cases that can potentially be managed as outpatients

Historical significance/comments
Most meningitis cases are aseptic, and accurate identification will prevent admissions and costly antibiotic use and decrease development of bacterial resistance.

Interpersonal and Communication Skills

Communicating Effectively With Families

Morbidity and mortality are quite high in bacterial meningitis, particularly when not recognized and treated early. Even when treated appropriately, mortality may range from 0% to 15% depending on the etiology. Neurologic sequelae occur in about 15%, with deafness, spasticity and/or paresis, seizures, and intellectual disability being most common. Potential consequences should be discussed openly with a family from the time the diagnosis is made. Families should be informed that the patient is being monitored closely for complications, although treatment does not always prevent morbidity. The prognosis cannot always be ensured at the time of discharge, and follow-up should be with primary care, audiology, and other specialties as needed.

Professionalism

Compassion and Empathy: Understanding Children's Reaction to Pain

Never forget adequate pain control when performing procedures, such as a lumbar puncture, on children. Depending on their developmental stage, children have no or limited understanding of what happens in a medical setting compared with adults. The fear aroused by being ill, in a hospital, and surrounded by strangers will all increase a child's experience of pain. Parents should be allowed to be with their child during procedures whenever possible.

Systems-Based Practice

Home Care: Selection of Patients for Outpatient Treatment of Bacterial Meningitis

For carefully selected patients with meningitis, completion of intravenous (IV) antibiotic treatment at home can lead to improved health-care effectiveness and efficiency because of shortened duration of hospitalization, decreased risk for acquiring nosocomial infection, and increased quality of life.[1]

A retrospective chart review identified the factors outlined here to consider in selecting patients with CNS infection for outpatient parenteral antimicrobial therapy (OPAT): Factors to consider in evaluating a patient with:

- *Infection:* Establish the pathogen when possible; the patient must be afebrile with a clinically stable or improving condition.
- *Antimicrobial:* The first dose given under medical supervision and without adverse reaction.
- *Other disease(s):* Stable, improving, or no significant need for nursing care.
- *Vascular access:* There is a reliable intravenous line and infusion device.
- *Neurologic state:* Risk for seizures; need for medications; neurologic dysfunction have been carefully evaluated.
- *Follow-up:* Plan for physician visits, nurse visits, laboratory monitoring, and emergencies are identified and feasible.

- *Family support:* Able to assist in care, infusions, transportation, and emergencies; domestic problems.
- *Home environment:* Safe environment; telephone, utilities, adequate food, refrigerator.
- *Patient abilities:* Cooperative and willing to participate in OPAT.[2]

References

1. Waler JA, Rathore MH: Outpatient management of pediatric bacterial meningitis. *Pediatr Infect Dis J* 14:89-92, 1995.
2. Tice AD, Strait K, Ramey R, et al: Outpatient parenteral antimicrobial therapy for central nervous system infections. *Clin Infect Dis* 29:1394-1399, 1999.

Chapter 50
Teaching Visual: Lumbar Puncture

*Patrice Kruszewski DO and
Glenn R. Stryjewski MD, MPH*

Objectives

- Visualize spinal anatomy to enhance understanding of the lumbar puncture (LP)
- Describe preparation and performance of a lumbar puncture
- Obtain informed consent from patient and/or family for performing a lumbar puncture

MEDICAL KNOWLEDGE

Before Starting the Procedure
Contraindications to performing an LP:

- **Increased intracranial pressure (ICP):** If there is clinical suspicion of increased ICP, LP should not be performed. Fundoscopic examination of the eye, as well as a CT scan of the head, may be required to rule out intracranial mass lesions. A negative CT scan of the head does not rule out increased ICP definitively, but it does help to rule out the risk for herniation.

- **Thrombocytopenia:** Most clinicians will not perform an LP if the patient's platelet count is less <50,000.
- **Unstable patient:** For example, if the patient is unable to be safely positioned for the LP because of compromised respiratory status

If the above conditions have been excluded, it should be safe to proceed with the procedure.

Beginning the Procedure
Obtain an LP procedure kit, and position items where they are easily reached without contaminating your sterile field:

- Spinal needle
- Sterile cerebrospinal fluid (CSF) collection tubes (at least three, and more if needed)
- Sterile gloves: antiseptic solution
- Sterile gauze pads
- Sterile drape
- Band-Aid

Positioning the Patient
There are two ways of positioning patients for an LP (Figure 50-1):

- Lateral recumbent position
  - An assistant helps by flexing the patient's neck and drawing the patient's knees to the patient's chest.
  - Remember to keep the patient's shoulders and hips perpendicular to the bed. This keeps the spinal column in alignment.
- Sitting position
  - This position may be used for older patients.

An imaginary line between the iliac crests should intersect the midline just above the L4 vertebra (see Figure 50-1).

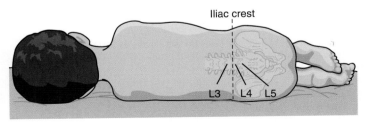

A

Figure 50-1 Positioning the patient. **A,** Lateral recumbent position.
Continued

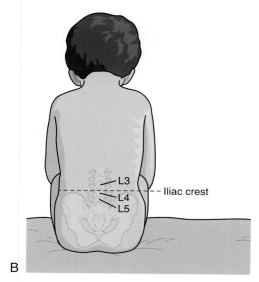

Figure 50-1, cont'd. **B,** Sitting position.

Prepping the Area
- Remove any anesthetic cream (e.g., EMLA) if it was applied.
- The clinician wears sterile gloves and cleanses the area with povidone-iodine–soaked sterile sponges at least three times.
- The skin and subcutaneous tissues are then infiltrated with 1% lidocaine for local anesthesia.

Performing the Procedure
- The needle is then inserted into the spinal space. In Figure 50-2, connect the dots to visualize the needle's trajectory.
- Needle size is determined by age. In the neonate to 2 year old, use a 22-gauge 1½-inch needle. In children 2 to 12 years old, use a 22-gauge 2½-inch needle, and over 12 years old, use 20- or 22-gauge 3½-inch needle.
- In the lateral recumbent position the needle is inserted slightly cephalad toward the umbilicus and caudad if the patient is in the sitting position.
- The needle is advanced through the skin (initially with resistance) and then with less resistance when the clinician penetrates the ligamentum flavum.
- There is further resistance as the dura mater (literally "tough mother") is penetrated, and a "pop" may be sensed as this is accomplished. Once the pop is appreciated, the needle's stylet may be removed and the CSF may be obtained from the patient.

(If a pop is not felt, the stylet should be removed after the needle is advanced 1 to 2 cm in infants younger than 6 months of age.)
- The needle is supported with one hand throughout the entire procedure.
- In some cases it may be necessary to obtain CSF opening pressure. This is obtained before the CSF collection.

Once the free flow of CSF is obtained, the pressure manometer is attached to the needle hub via a three-way stopcock. CSF measurement is recorded as the highest level reached by the fluid in the column. It is helpful to have an assistant support the column by holding it at its top.

- The CSF is collected in sterile collection tubes for Gram stain and culture, glucose and protein, and cell count—usually in three tubes. The *third* tube should be the tube sent for cell count.

The stylet is then reinserted in the needle hub, and the needle is removed from the patient. The clinician holds gentle pressure at the site for at least 2 minutes. The area is then cleansed of the povidone-iodine, and a Band-Aid is placed over the site.

Interpersonal and Communication Skills

Before the Procedure

- It is helpful to explain that you as the clinician are concerned that the child may have a central nervous system (CNS) infection and that a lumbar puncture is the only way to accurately assess whether the child has this type of infection. Parents may be reluctant to give consent for an LP because they feel it is an invasive procedure or unnecessary. It is helpful to explain to the parents that untreated CNS infections may lead to serious long-term sequelae, including brain damage, seizures, or hearing loss and for this reason, the procedure is strongly recommended.
- For parents of infants and young children it is important to point out that physical examinations in this age-group may be unreliable and that children are often are unable to communicate to others if they have pain or a headache. CNS infections in these children may have very subtle findings.
- To older children and their parents, you should explain that although these patients have more reliable reporting of symptoms, symptom perception not highly accurate, especially when the child is ill.
- For children of every age-group, you should explain to the parents and patient that the risks of not performing the LP may be far greater than the risks of performing it. *(From the clinician's*

Lumbar puncture

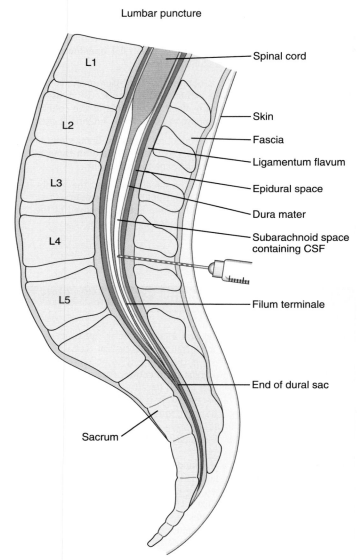

Figure 50-2 Connect the dotted line overlying the needle and note that it traverses the (1) skin, (2) interspinous ligament, (3) ligamentum flavum, and (4) dura mater. As you complete the *dashed line* of the needle, pay attention to the sequential penetration of the skin, interspinous ligament, ligamentum flavum, and dura mater.

standpoint, if you are concerned enough to think about doing an LP, you should do it.)

- You should also explain to parents that the patient's vital signs are continuously monitored during the procedure to ensure the patient's safety.
- Once the indications and potential complications are fully explained, obtain written consent for the LP. The written consent should have the indications, benefits, and potential adverse effects of the procedure. These should include:
  □ Rare adverse effects include bleeding, infection, and nerve damage.
  □ More commonly, there may be headache following the procedure, which is easily treated with mild analgesics.
  □ Be sure to explain the risks of *not* performing the procedure. Sign and date the consent.
  □ A witness should be present in the room as you discuss the consent with the patient and parent(s).

During the Procedure

- You may allow the parent to stay in the room or leave while the procedure is completed. If the parent stays in the room, it is best to request that the parent sit down while watching. (Parental empathy often leads to a vaso-vagal reaction!) Explain what you are doing as you perform the procedure.
- It is essential to have another medical person present in the room to assist with positioning and provide the child with calming thoughts.

After the Procedure

- When the procedure has been completed, explain to the parents (and the child, if appropriate) that the preliminary results (CSF Gram stain, glucose, protein, and cell count) should be completed in about 1 hour.
- It is helpful to reassure the parent and patient that the child tolerated the procedure well.
- If the procedure is unable to be completed after two attempts, the procedure should be terminated and attempted at another time.

Reference

1. Henretig F: *Textbook of pediatric emergency procedures*. Baltimore, MD, 1997, Williams & Wilkins, pp 541-548.

Chapter 51
Skin and Soft Tissue Infections (Case 20)

Lindsay Chase MD *and Gary Frank* MD, MS

Case: A 5-year-old boy has a "rash" on his right thigh. A bug bite from several days earlier has enlarged and become painful. On examination there is a 5- × 7-cm tender, swollen, erythematous lesion.

Differential Diagnosis

Cellulitis	Abscess	Necrotizing fasciitis
Pyomyositis	Erysipelas	Superficial thrombophlebitis

Speaking Intelligently

Most skin and soft tissue infections can be treated with oral antibiotics in the outpatient setting. However, you need to always carefully check for evidence of systemic infection. Vital signs are "vital"—check for fever, tachycardia, and blood pressure abnormalities (elevations with pain or hypotension with sepsis and shock). I assess perfusion by checking quality of pulses and capillary refill along with mental status. Think about underlying structures, because the infection can descend from the skin or could have started deeper and spread to the skin. An important consideration is methicillin-resistant *Staphylococcus aureus* (MRSA). Given the high prevalence of community-acquired MRSA, it is prudent to act as if all skin infections are caused by MRSA until proved otherwise by culture.

PATIENT CARE

Clinical Thinking
- Measure and **mark** the area of erythema to monitor progression.
- Check for pus (fluctuance), because cellulitis may be accompanied by abscess. Pus often requires drainage.

- **Culture, culture, culture.** If possible, obtain Gram stain and culture of pus before starting antibiotics.
- Know local bacterial susceptibility patterns and the patient's risk factors.
- Are there underlying structures to worry about such as in osteomyelitis?
- Consult specialists if needed.
- Are there any special circumstances to suggest unusual organisms (nail through tennis shoe, diabetes)?
- Imaging studies are not usually needed, but may be helpful for infections overlying a joint or near the eyes, to evaluate for penetration into deeper structures, and to evaluate for drainable abscesses.

History
- Are there any special circumstances to suggest unusual organisms (nail through tennis shoe, diabetes)?
- Any family history of recent abscess or skin infection?

Physical Examination
- With isolated cellulitis with or without abscess, vital signs are usually normal. ***Signs of systemic infection*** include fever, tachycardia, hypotension, brisk capillary refill with bounding pulses (warm shock), prolonged capillary refill (cool shock), or altered mental status.
- First assess airway, breathing, and circulation. Evaluate heart, lungs, abdomen, and mental status.
- If the patient is stable, evaluate the skin—all of it! Look for erythema, warmth, edema, tenderness, drainage, abrasions, lacerations, and ulcers.
- Mark the area of erythema to monitor progression and resolution.
- Palpate for fluctuance.
- If there is extreme sensitivity to light touch, consider compartment syndrome or necrotizing fasciitis.
- Palpate for lymph node enlargement.
- Examine underlying structures such as mouth (gums and teeth), sinuses, muscles, and joints.
- When the affected skin overlies a joint, evaluate that joint for fluid and for range of motion to rule out septic arthritis (a surgical emergency).
- With facial involvement, evaluate (and document) extraocular movements to rule out orbital cellulitis.
- Remove the diaper to check for rashes, gluteal and perirectal abscesses, and inguinal adenopathy.

Tests for Consideration
- **Complete blood count (CBC) with differential** $116
- To follow response to therapy:
  - **C-reactive protein** $69
  - **Erythrocyte sedimentation rate** $85

- **Blood culture:** In ill-appearing patients $152
- **Wound Gram stain and culture:** To identify an organism and
  sensitivities $180
- **Electrolytes, blood urea nitrogen (BUN), and creatinine:**
  In sicker patients or if contrast will be administered $174
- **Purified protein derivative (PPD):** If concern for atypical
  mycobacterium $174

IMAGING CONSIDERATIONS

→ **Computed tomography (CT) of affected area with
  contrast:** To evaluate for abscess or deeper involvement
  - **CT neck** $150
  - **CT abdomen/pelvis** $1691
→ **CT of face and orbits with contrast:** If concern for
  orbital cellulitis $1875
→ **Ultrasound or magnetic resonance imaging (MRI) of
  affected joint:** To evaluate for septic arthritis
  - **Ultrasound hip** $675
  - **MRI hip** $1700
→ **MRI or bone scan:** If there is concern for osteomyelitis
  - **MRI leg** $1100
  - **Bone scan** $1512

Clinical Entities	Medical Knowledge

Cellulitis

Pφ ***Cellulitis*** is an acute infection of the skin. Inflammation of the
    dermis and subcutaneous tissues causes swelling, warmth,
    redness, and tenderness. Often a break in the skin is the portal
    of entry. The most common bacteria are *S. aureus* and
    Streptococcus species, especially group A. With soil or fresh
    water exposure, consider gram-negative organisms, specifically
    Aeromonas. In immunocompromised individuals, *Streptococcus
    pneumoniae* may cause rapidly progressing infection.

TP There is often a "bug bite," and the area of redness enlarges,
    becoming tender and warm. Some patients develop fever and
    signs of systemic illness.

Dx Diagnosis can be made with history and clinical findings.

Tx	Treatment consists of antibiotics and close follow-up to monitor for resolution. Knowledge of susceptibility patterns in your community and patient factors is critical. If the patient is systemically ill, immunocompromised, very young, if the affected area is on the face or overlies a joint, or if the patient has failed outpatient therapy, admission for intravenous antibiotics is indicated. For outpatient therapy, oral clindamycin (there is increasing *S. aureus* resistance in some areas) or sulfamethoxazole-trimethoprim (does not cover group A streptococcus [GAS] and can cause Stevens-Johnson syndrome) are good choices given the rise in community-acquired MRSA. For inpatient therapy, intravenous clindamycin is often used. Vancomycin should be considered for severe infections with systemic signs or joint involvement. For facial cellulitis, ceftriaxone or others that cover respiratory flora should be used. **See Nelson Essentials 98.**

Abscess

Pφ	An *abscess* is a discrete collection of pus in a cavity, which forms as a result of the body's immune response to infection or a foreign body. The bacteria (or foreign body) trigger the inflammatory response, increasing blood flow and white blood cell influx. The surrounding healthy tissue walls off the infected area to limit spread. Within the abscess capsule, bacteria may continue to grow, and antibiotic penetration into the abscess may be limited. The most common cause is *S. aureus*, although an abscess may be polymicrobial and include anaerobes.
TP	Patients present most commonly with a "bug bite," a "risin," or a boil that becomes progressively red, swollen, and tender, and may spontaneously drain pus.
Dx	Diagnosis is clinical. Imaging may be helpful. Gram stain and culture of pus are indicated to guide therapy.
Tx	Drainage is therapeutic and also allows obtaining a specimen for Gram stain and culture. Warm soaks and sitz baths may promote spontaneous drainage. Small, superficial abscesses may be opened with a needle. Larger abscesses require incision and drainage with possible packing. Antibiotics can be used in conjunction with drainage because there is often accompanying cellulitis. Prescribe antibiotics with good *Staphylococcus* coverage. **See Nelson Essentials 98.**

Necrotizing Fasciitis

Pφ   **Necrotizing fasciitis** infects the deeper layers of skin and subcutaneous tissues and spreads across fascial planes. Many bacteria can be responsible, including GAS, *Vibrio vulnificus*, *Clostridium perfringens*, and *Bacteroides fragilis*. The bacteria produce toxins or virulence factors that destroy soft tissue.

TP   This uncommon infection may begin at a site of trauma, a bite, or foreign body, and poor perfusion or local necrosis to the area may be a predisposing factor. If the infection is deep, there may be pain without visible signs. If more superficial, there will be warmth, redness, and swelling. The skin changes rapidly from red to purple with blisters and necrosis. The systemic inflammatory response often causes fever and vomiting.

Dx   Cultures of blood, pus, and tissue help identify causative bacteria. CT scan with contrast may help define extent of the infection.

Tx   Antibiotics should be started immediately. Vancomycin and clindamycin are often used. Early consultation with surgery is essential. Treatment includes aggressive debridement. Sometimes amputation is needed to stop the spread of infection. Hyperbaric oxygen therapy may be useful in select cases. **See Nelson Essentials 98.**

Pyomyositis

Pφ   **Pyomyositis** is a purulent infection of a muscle. The most common bacterial cause is *S. aureus*. Bacteria invade the muscle, and pus forms in the muscle.

TP   Patients often present with a history of minor trauma to the area followed by painful swelling. The area is usually swollen, warm, and tender. It may be very painful to move the affected muscle. The overlying skin may be affected, and some patients will be febrile.

Dx   CBC, CRP, and blood culture are usually indicated. Ultrasound, CT, or MRI may give useful information about whether there is drainable pus. Gram stain and culture of pus is sent to identify organism(s).

Tx   Intravenous antibiotics with good coverage of *S. aureus*, such as clindamycin or vancomycin, are typically used. Often surgical drainage is indicated.

Erysipelas	
Pφ	*Erysipelas* is an acute infection of the dermis, usually caused by GAS, resulting in inflammation that extends into underlying fat tissue. The bacteria enter the skin through an area of minor trauma such as eczema or insect bites. People with impaired lymph or venous drainage or immunodeficiencies are at higher risk.
TP	Patients typically present with a rapidly enlarging erythematous skin lesion with a sharply demarcated raised edge. It appears as a red, warm, tender, firm swollen area similar in consistency to an orange peel. Streaking erythema toward draining lymph nodes may be seen. Lymph nodes may be enlarged. The infection can occur anywhere on the body but most often on extremities. Systemic symptoms, including high fevers, shaking chills, fatigue, headaches, and vomiting, may occur. Spread to blood, joints, and heart valves is possible.
Dx	Erysipelas is diagnosed by the characteristic appearance of the rash. The antistreptolysin O (ASO) titer becomes elevated after approximately 10 days of illness.
Tx	Antibiotics with good *Streptococcus* coverage such as penicillin or clindamycin are effective. The route of administration (IV or PO) depends on the severity of the infection. **See Nelson Essentials 98.**

Superficial Thrombophlebitis	
Pφ	*Superficial thrombophlebitis* is inflammation of a superficial vein, usually accompanied by infection and thrombus. Common bacteria are *Staphylococcus* and *Streptococcus*.
TP	Pain and/or erythema may develop at an IV site. The area is red, warm, tender, and swollen.
Dx	Diagnosis can be made by history and physical examination. If possible, obtain a culture through the IV, and send the actual IV catheter for culture.
Tx	Remove any devices from the vein. Initiate antibiotics with good *Staphylococcus* and *Streptococcus* coverage. Nonsteroidal -antiinflammatory drugs (NSAIDs) can help control pain and inflammation. Elevation will help minimize swelling. If there is significant swelling, consider evaluating for more extensive thrombus and possible anticoagulation. **See Nelson Essentials 98.**

ZEBRA ZONE

a. **Immune deficiencies (Job, Wiskott-Aldrich, Omenn):** Often present with unusual rashes that do not respond to antibiotics or corticosteroids.

b. **Acute febrile neutrophilic dermatosis (Sweet syndrome):** Starts as a single plaque but then spreads. The rash and associated fevers do not respond to antibiotics.

c. **Scrofula:** Caused by atypical mycobacterium; presents as an enlarged lymph node with overlying erythema/discoloration.

Practice-Based Learning and Improvement

Title
Skin and soft-tissue infections caused by methicillin-resistant *Staphylococcus aureus*

Author
Daum RS

Reference
N Engl J Med 357(4):380-390, 2007

Problem
Review of management strategies for skin and soft tissue infections caused by MRSA

Comparison/control (quality of evidence)
Review article with cited references in peer-reviewed journal

Outcome/effect
Beta-lactams can no longer be considered reliable for community-acquired skin infections. Clindamycin is often effective against MRSA, but resistance (sometimes inducible) is rising. Trimethoprim-sulfamethoxazole and tetracyclines have good activity against MRSA, but not against GAS. Linezolid has excellent activity against MRSA and GAS but is expensive and there is concern about developing resistance with widespread use. Vancomycin is considered first-line treatment for hospitalized patients with invasive *S. aureus* infection until susceptibilities are determined.

Historical significance/comments
There has been a dramatic increase in the occurrence of community-acquired MRSA infections over the past decade. Older antibiotics such as clindamycin and trimethoprim-sulfamethoxazole are often used for empirical therapy, but increasing resistance is a major concern. There is a relative scarcity of newer agents, especially for children.

Interpersonal and Communication Skills

Document the Margins of Skin Lesions to Monitor Progression

It is essential that you clearly document the extent of the infection (erythema and swelling), as well as the time of your examination. This is often done in the medical record by drawing a diagram of a human body and shading the affected site. It is also wise to outline, on the patient's body, any area of erythema with pen or a marker and write the date and time next to the line. Using the diagram in the medical record and the line drawn around the erythema, your colleagues will later will be able to judge if the infection is improving or worsening—and how rapidly.

Professionalism

Respecting Patients, Maintaining Privacy

Skin issues can be painful and embarrassing. Keeping the patient covered except for the area being examined shows respect for patient privacy. The examination should be done with the door closed. Parents should be present during examinations of children. Ask older adolescents if they prefer the parent to stay or step out. To avoid questions of inappropriate touching, consider asking a staff member of the same sex as the patient to remain in the room during the examination.

Systems-Based Practice

Health-Care Economics: Claims, Coding, and Billing

Some of the top reasons insurance companies deny claims and do not reimburse for services are because of duplicated claims (two claims submitted for the same service)—48%; termination of coverage (patient is no longer covered by the insurance)—22%; and noncovered benefit (the service is not a covered benefit under the patient's plan)—20%.

Therefore it is important to ensure the following for all submitted claims: (1) they have the patient's demographic data and insurance ID, (2) the Current Procedural Terminology (CPT) and International Classification of Diseases, 9th edition (ICD-9) codes are correct and correlated to each other, (3) the date of service is marked, and (4) the physician has signed and dated the form. In addition, with each visit the office staff needs to confirm the patient's coverage before services are rendered.[1]

Reference

1. American Academy of Dermatology: Practice management. Available at http://www.aad.org.

Chapter 52
The Limping Child
(Case 21)

Christopher P. Raab MD

Case: Parents report their 3-year-old child has a new limp.

Differential Diagnosis

Trauma	Slipped capital femoral epiphysis (SCFE)	Child abuse
Acute osteomyelitis	Transient synovitis	Septic arthritis

Speaking Intelligently

My first step in evaluating a limping child is a comprehensive history and examination, including ascertaining if the limp is painful. Duration of symptoms allows distinction between congenital and acquired problems. For a febrile or ill-appearing child, I order blood work including complete blood count (CBC), sedimentation rate, and C-reactive protein (CRP) to check for evidence of infection or inflammation. For suspected trauma, a radiograph is obtained to assess for fracture, whereas bone scan or magnetic resonance imaging (MRI) may help localize a lesion of uncertain location. Well-appearing children with painful, nontraumatic limps are often difficult cases. Diagnoses such as transient synovitis can usually be suggested by history and examination alone.

PATIENT CARE

Clinical Thinking
• Do symptoms require immediate evaluation and treatment?
• Is **prompt surgical intervention** needed for possible SCFE, compound fracture, or septic joint?
• Is there concern for **physical abuse?**

History
- Is the limp **painful?**
- **Fever and limp** in an otherwise healthy child suggest an infection such as osteomyelitis or septic arthritis or possibly a rheumatic disease such as juvenile idiopathic arthritis (JIA)
- Inquire about **trauma** to suggest fracture, sprain, contusion, or SCFE.
- Inquire about recent **viral illness** to suggest transient synovitis.
- Inquire about additional systemic symptoms.
- Inquire about history of **tick bite.**
- Inquire about family history of rheumatologic disease.

Physical Examination
- Elevated heart rate and blood pressure may be secondary to pain.
- Although limp is generally of lower extremity origin, a complete examination is required.
- An older child may be able to pinpoint the site of pain with a single digit.
- Lower extremity pain can be referred from one joint to another (e.g., **knee pain may indicate hip pathology**).
- Each joint should be assessed for effusion and range of motion.
- Palpate all bony surfaces and prominences.
- Check for bruising, tenderness, or lesions. Some rashes are associated with specific disorders such as erythema migrans and Lyme disease.
- Muscle atrophy and/or weakness occur with neurologic processes.
- Abdominal pathology can present with limp.
- **Gait analysis** is done preferably over a long hallway. Gait has two major phases: stance and swing.
  - With an antalgic gait, the stance phase is shortened, signifying pain.
  - With a Trendelenburg gait, the pelvis drops during the swing phase signifying gluteal medius weakness or paralysis. It is associated with hip pathology such as Legg-Calvé-Perthes disease and developmental dysplasia of the hip (DDH).
  - With a stiff gait, there is decreased pelvic rotation and a rigid trunk, typically signifying spinal pathology.
  - With a spastic gait, there may be toe walking without heel strike caused by increased tone; increased adductor tone can result in a "scissor" gait.

Tests for Consideration
- **CBC:** Elevated white count in infection; anemia in systemic diseases such as malignancy or rheumatic disease; platelet elevation as an acute phase reactant — $116
- **Erythrocyte sedimentation rate (ESR):** For inflammation — $85
- **CRP:** For inflammation — $69
- **Lyme titers:** If joint effusion — $180
- **Parvovirus B19 titers:** If joint effusion — $437

- **Synovial fluid:**
  - Synovial fluid cell count, Gram stain $105
  - Synovial fluid Lyme titers $180
  - Synovial culture $152
- **Blood culture:** If ill appearing $152
- **Antinuclear antibodies (ANA):** If concern for rheumatic
  disorder $334
- **Lactate dehydrogenase (LDH) and alkaline phosphatase:**
  If concern for bone malignancy $140

IMAGING CONSIDERATIONS

→ **Plain radiographs:** These are obtained first. Radiologic
  evidence of fracture or osteomyelitis may lag behind the
  clinical picture. Plain films assess fractures, joint
  pathology, and benign or malignant bony lesions.
  Include one joint above and below suspected site,
  2 view AP and lateral (cost depending on
  anatomic location). $200-300
→ **Technetium-99 bone scintigraphy (bone anatomic
  location):** To assess inflammatory or infectious
  processes when lesion site is unknown.
  Cost varies by anatomical location. $1100 (leg)
→ **MRI:** The most specific tool to assess bony lesions.
  Cost varies by anatomical location. $1100 (leg)

Clinical Entities   Medical Knowledge

Trauma

Pφ   Pediatric traumatic lower extremity injuries are common. The
     growth plate is the weakest component of pediatric bone, and
     therefore growth plate injuries (Salter-Harris type I fracture)
     are more common than sprains in children. The Salter-Harris
     classification of fractures divides growth plate fractures into
     five categories depending on where the fracture is in
     relationship to the growth plate (see Chapter 53, Teaching
     Visual: Growth Plate Fracture Classification). Pain and limp also
     may be secondary to muscle contusion.

TP   Typically there is a painful limp and inability to bear weight.
     The patient and parents may be unaware of clinically significant
     trauma. Fractures and sprains both often present with edema,
     ecchymosis, and point tenderness at the involved site.

Dx   Diagnosis can be made by history and physical findings; however, confirmatory imaging is usually performed. Occult fractures can usually be seen on a radiograph. At least two views, usually anteroposterior (AP) and lateral, are required. Check pulses and capillary refill to assess perfusion. Assess neurovascular function by checking movement and sensation.

Tx   Displaced fractures are treated with orthopedic alignment under sedation. Simple aligned fractures typically require splinting and pain control. A fracture surrounding a joint will be casted for several weeks after initial edema has resolved. Simple sprains require rest, ice, compression with elastic bandages, and elevation (RICE). Pain control is often necessary. **See Nelson Essentials 198.**

Slipped Capital Femoral Epiphysis

Pφ   **SCFE** is displacement of the femoral head through the physis. During adolescence, the angle of the physis changes from horizontal to oblique. Rapid increase in body mass may cause shearing force on the physis, initially causing microfractures and eventually posterior and medial slippage of the femoral head from the physis.

TP   The typical patient is an obese male adolescent who may play sports. There is pain and limp with activity. The pain is usually located on the proximal anterior thigh but can be referred to the knee or even the ankle.

Dx   The history, physical examination, and radiologic findings together are diagnostic. There is loss of internal rotation of the hip, especially with the hip in flexion. AP and frog-leg lateral radiographs classically show displacement of the femoral head, often described as "ice cream slipping off the cone."

Tx   Immediate orthopedic consultation and cessation of weight bearing is mandatory for suspected SCFE. Ultimate treatment depends on degree of displacement and involves surgical stabilization with a percutaneous pin or screw. **See Nelson Essentials 199.**

Acute Osteomyelitis

Pφ Bacterial bone infection occurs through hematologic spread, after trauma, or via direct inoculation. The predominant organism is *S. aureus*. Other bacteria in special circumstances include group B streptococcus in neonates, *Salmonella* in patients with sickle cell disease, *Pseudomonas* in puncture wounds to the foot, or *Kingella kingae*.

TP Local tenderness and limp are typical early signs. Systemic signs such as fever and malaise may develop as the child begins to look ill, although some patients are quite well-appearing. Warmth, redness, swelling, and tenderness often occur with possible spasm of adjacent muscles.

Dx Diagnosis can be made with history and examination, along with laboratory and imaging studies. CBC may demonstrate leukocytosis and thrombocytosis. ESR and CRP are useful to monitor response to treatment. Blood culture is recommended, but the gold standard is Gram stain and culture of bone aspirate. Plain radiographs may be helpful but lag behind the clinical picture. Bone scan may be performed in early osteomyelitis, though MRI has greater specificity in distinguishing bone from joint inflammation.

Tx Intravenous antibiotics are started promptly for suspected osteomyelitis. Length of IV treatment is controversial; most practitioners treat with IV antibiotics for 3 to 4 weeks, followed by several weeks of oral antibiotics. **See Nelson Essentials 117.**

Transient Synovitis

Pφ ***Transient synovitis*** (formerly called "toxic" synovitis) is a self-resolving joint effusion, typically involving the hip. The underlying cause is unknown but is likely secondary to minor trauma or a viral infection.

TP A typical patient is a healthy male between 2 and 5 years of age who suddenly develops a limp or inability to bear weight. The child often will complain of pain in the proximal thigh or groin and will resist hip movement, but is otherwise well appearing. There may be recent upper respiratory symptoms. On examination, there is mildly restricted motion of the affected hip, and the patient will often lay with hips flexed and abducted.

Dx	Diagnosis is made clinically. Radiographs and laboratory tests are generally not necessary. Concern about chronic latent osteomyelitis should prompt AP and frogleg radiographs.
Tx	Treatment is supportive; with rest, recovery occurs within 3 to 14 days. **See Nelson Essentials 199.**

Child Abuse

See Chapter 96, Physical Abuse.

Septic Arthritis

Pφ	Joint infections may be caused by hematogenous spread, direct seeding from wounds, or direct extension of osteomyelitis. Lower extremity large joints are typically affected. The inflammatory response damages cartilage, sometimes irrevocably. *S. aureus* predominates across all age-groups, although other causes differ by age. In neonates, group B streptococcus, *Escherichia coli*, and other Gram-negative organisms are causative. In an adolescent, consider gonococcus.
TP	There is usually acute onset of pain with guarding of the affected joint. Initially pain may be poorly localized, but localization improves as symptoms progress. Children may limp or refuse to bear weight. The patient is typically ill appearing and febrile with the affected joint held in a position of comfort. A hip will be flexed, abducted, and externally rotated. A knee will be slightly flexed.
Dx	This is a medical emergency, and when suspected, the joint should be aspirated and fluid sent for Gram stain and culture. Blood culture may be negative. Plain radiographs and ultrasound, although not diagnostic, are useful to identify effusion.
Tx	Treatment includes IV antibiotics and joint drainage. Antibiotic coverage should be based on Gram stain and culture results. Treatment duration depends on the specific organism, but may be up to 6 weeks with a portion as IV therapy. A percutaneous intravenous central catheter (PICC) may be required for outpatient IV antibiotics. **See Nelson Essentials 118.**

ZEBRA ZONE

a. **Legg-Calvé-Perthes disease:** Osteonecrosis of the femoral head usually secondary to insufficient arterial blood flow.

b. **Reactive arthritis:** Autoimmune condition that develops in response to an infection in another part of the body.

c. **Malignant tumor:** Leukemia, Ewing sarcoma, osteosarcoma and rhabdomyosarcoma can all present with limp.

Practice-Based Learning and Improvement

Title:	
Imaging the child with a limp	
Authors:	
Myers MR, Thompson GH	
Reference:	
Pediatr Clin North Am 44:637-658, 1997	
Problem:	
Review of causes of limp and appropriate imaging studies	
Comparison/control (quality of evidence):	
Article presents an evidence-based approach in the use of diagnostic imaging in the evaluation of a child with a limp.	
Historical significance/comments:	
Evidence-based studies were compiled with standardization of the radiographic workup for limp.	

Interpersonal and Communication Skills

Begin With Open-Ended Questions to Obtain an Accurate History in a Limping Child

The differential diagnosis in the limping child is extensive. A careful history will often narrow the possibilities. Many parents assume their child is limping because of trauma. Even though the parent may begin the conversation focusing on some minor traumatic event, it is important to use open-ended questions to try to deduce the exact sequence of events and what other symptoms may be temporally associated. Establishing the presence or absence of fever can be helpful because it is unusual to have acute osteomyelitis or septic arthritis in the absence of fever outside the neonatal period (neonates sometimes do not mount good febrile responses to bacterial infections). Use open-ended questions to continue through the interview, including questions pertaining to family history of bone, joint, or rheumatologic disease, travel, animal exposure, and tick bites.

Professionalism

Reliability and Responsibility: Collaborate to Identify Systems Errors to Prevent Future Harm

In 1999 the Institute of Medicine issued a report entitled *To Err Is Human: Building a Safer Health System*. This report demonstrated that a large number of medical errors were occurring and that these errors resulted in significant patient morbidity and mortality. A chief area of interest was medication errors. In an effort to decrease medical errors, many health-care institutions have instituted changes in medication delivery systems. One example is medication bar coding. When a medication order is entered in the computer, a pharmacist receives the order and a bar-coded sticker. The pharmacist then checks the dosing per weight, and if correct, prepares the medication. The bar-coded sticker is placed on the medication. When the medication is delivered to the inpatient unit, the bar code is scanned and only that patient's medication drawer opens, to prevent misplacement of the medication. When the nurse administers the medication, he/she must first scan the patient's bar-coded bracelet, as well as the medication's bar code. This ensures that the correct patient is receiving the correct medication, correctly dosed, and at the correct time.

Systems-Based Practice

Risk Management: Make Appropriate Transition of Care to the Outpatient Setting

Physicians need to be aware of the medicolegal pitfalls associated with the diagnosis and transition of care of a limping child.

All patients with underlying malignancy or other conditions with potential for long-term morbidity should be set up with appropriate discharge instructions and follow-up with the primary care physician, appropriate specialist, radiologist, and laboratory. Failure to identify and address the transition of care gaps—either patient or health system–related—may lead to adverse clinical outcomes and physician liability.

Chapter 53
Teaching Visual: Growth Plate Fracture Classification

Nicole A. Green MD *and Robert LaTerra* MD

Objectives

- Recognize important differences in the growing skeleton that make child fractures unique.
- Diagram the different regions in a growing bone.
- Understand the Salter-Harris classification of growth plate injuries.
- Draw each fracture pattern according to the Salter-Harris classification for your patient.

MEDICAL KNOWLEDGE

The pediatric skeleton has unique features that allow for growth and contribute to patterns of injury different from those of an adult. The periosteum of a child is thicker and stronger and has greater osteogenic potential, leading to more rapid callus formation in the setting of fracture. The cortex of pediatric bone is more porous, making it more flexible and able to withstand a greater degree of deformation.[1] In addition, remodeling (correction of fractured bone alignment) is generally more predictable. For these reasons, children are generally less likely than their adult counterparts to require surgical management of uncomplicated fractures.[2] However, they are also susceptible to unique complications, including growth arrest.[3]

The immature long bone comprises different anatomic regions. Longitudinal bone growth occurs at the location of the physis, or growth plate. The physis separates the articular end (epiphysis) from the metaphysis, which is the subterminal, actively growing section of the long bone. Adjacent to the metaphysis on the side opposite the physis is the diaphysis.

The physis is composed of radiolucent cartilage that is weaker than bone and therefore more susceptible to fracture.[1,2] Although uncommon, growth disturbance can occur as a complication of physeal fracture and is related to a number of factors, including the location within the affected physis. Classification of physeal fractures is paramount to

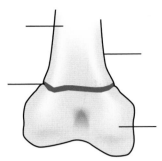

Choices

• Epiphysis
• Diaphysis
• Physis
• Metaphysis

Figure 53-1 The anatomic regions of the immature long bone, displaying the locations of the epiphysis, cartilaginous physis, metaphysis, and diaphysis.

guiding management, assessing risk, and predicting prognosis.[1] **In Figure 53-1, label the parts of the immature long bone as described in the text.**

Since its inception in 1963, the five-part Salter-Harris classification of physeal fractures remains the most commonly used system. Type I is a fracture through the physis, whereby the epiphysis is completely separated from the metaphysis. Radiographs of nondisplaced type I fractures appear normal with the exception of possible soft tissue swelling.[5] Diagnosis and proper management therefore depend on clinical suspicion.[1] Important clues on examination include the presence of swelling and point tenderness at the site of the growth plate. In type II, the fracture extends from the physis into the metaphysis at the opposite end of the fracture. The fragment includes the entirety of the epiphysis as well as a portion of the metaphysis (named the Thurston-Holland fragment).[3] Salter-Harris type III fractures extend through the articular surface of the epiphysis and across the physis to the periphery. This pattern is uncommon, usually occurring in a partially closed growth plate such as a distal tibia. Type IV fractures extend from the articular surface across the growth plate to the metaphysis.[1] Type V is a compression fracture through the physis from a severe crushing force.[6] Diagnosis of a type V fracture is often made retrospectively because radiographs may appear normal.[5]

Interpersonal and Communication Skills

It is important to understand the Salter-Harris classification system so that you can accurately describe injuries to patients and their families. In general, severity and risk for complication tend to increase with increasing Salter-Harris classification, although a number of exceptions exist. Parents may be relieved to know that

Using Figure 53-2 as a guide, trace the fracture patterns for each of the Salter-Harris types.

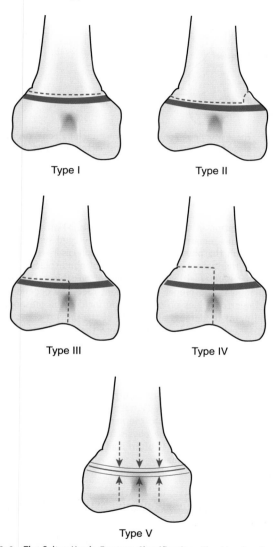

Type I

Type II

Type III

Type IV

Type V

Figure 53-2 The Salter-Harris Fracture Classification. The *blue bands* represent the locations of the physis. *Red dotted lines* depict the associated paths of fracture due to propagation. The *red arrows* (on the Salter-Harris type V image) indicate the direction of the compression forces acting on the affected portion of the physis.

most Salter-Harris fractures heal without complication. Although 30% of all Salter-Harris fractures may result in growth rate disturbance, less than 2% cause significant functional disturbance.[7] Types I and II fractures do not affect the articular surface, and with certain exceptions the management is straightforward and prognosis is excellent. Patients generally require closed reduction and casting for a 4- to 6-week period. Surgical intervention may be necessary for fracture types III and IV, and prognosis for growth disturbance is guarded. In type V fractures, prognosis is poor because growth arrest and angular deformity are common. You must warn parents of the possibility of growth arrest and angulation primarily in type III to V fractures. These complications can later be corrected by procedures such as osteotomy, epiphysiodesis, or limb-lengthening procedures. It is crucial that parents understand the importance of good orthopedic follow-up for all fracture types because some will require regular evaluations until the child's bones have stopped growing.[3]

References

1. Rang M, Wenger D: Children are not just small adults. In Wenger D, Pring M, editors: *Rang's Children's Fractures*, ed 3, Philadelphia, 2005, Lippincott.
2. Rab G: Pediatric orthopedic surgery. In Skinner H, editor: *Current Diagnosis and Treatment in Orthopedics*, ed 3, New York, 2003, Lange/McGraw-Hill.
3. Koval K, Zuckerman J: *Handbook of Fractures*, ed 3, Philadelphia, 2006, Lippincott Williams & Wilkins.
4. Salter R, Harris W: Injuries involving the epiphyseal plate. *J Bone Joint Surg* 45:587-622, 1963.
5. Rathjen K, Birch J: Physeal injuries and growth disturbances. In Beaty JH, Kasser JR, editors: *Rockwood and Wilkins' Fractures in Children*, ed 6, Philadelphia, 2006, Lippincott.
6. Thompson J: *Netter's Concise Atlas of Orthopaedic Anatomy*. Yardley, PA, 2002, Icon Learning Systems.
7. Shapiro F: Epiphyseal growth plate fracture-separations: a pathophysiologic approach. *Orthopedics* 5:720-736, 1982.

Professor's Pearls
Section III: The Inpatient Ward
John Carlton Gartner Jr. MD

Consider the following clinical problems and questions posed. Then refer to a discussion of these issues by John Carlton Gartner Jr. MD, Pediatrician-in-Chief, General Pediatrics/Diagnostic Referral Division, Nemours/Alfred I. duPont Hospital for Children, Wilmington, Delaware.

1. **Case:** An 8-year-old boy is admitted to the hospital for daily fever for more than 2 weeks. No diagnosis has been made despite several careful physical examinations as an outpatient and multiple negative cultures, including throat, blood, urine, and stool. The patient had had some initial abdominal pain and mild diarrhea, which resolved. Other routine laboratory work results includes an elevated sedimentation rate and C-reactive protein. What would be the most helpful part of your initial evaluation? What other tests should be done (e.g., computed tomography [CT], bone marrow examination)?

2. **Case:** A 10-year-old girl is sent to the hospital emergency department by her primary care physician because of the sudden onset of decreased movement of the left side of her face. She has been previously well and had a flulike illness with onset about 4 days ago. What conditions are associated with facial paralysis? Specifically, are there conditions that should be treated promptly? What other clues might be present on physical examination?

3. **Case:** A 15-year-old girl presents to your office for increasing headaches for the past 4 weeks and several episodes of morning vomiting. She has been followed closely in your office for the past year because of moderate weight gain. She has been well otherwise. Examination reveals an obese girl who is alert and cooperative, with normal vital signs. What part of the physical examination is most critical in this case? Is imaging of the brain necessary? What are the possible causes of her headache?

4. **Case:** A 14-month-old boy is sent for admission by his primary care physician because of swelling of his lower extremities and pallor. He has been a healthy infant with normal growth and development. Immunizations are up to date. Diet includes whole milk and some table food. Initial screening laboratory tests include the following: hemoglobin, 5 g/dL, and hematocrit (Hct), 17%, with normal white blood cell (WBC) and platelet count; comprehensive metabolic profile is normal except that the total protein is 3.5 g/dL and albumin 1.5 g/dL. What is the most likely cause of the swelling? What key laboratory tests should be done promptly? What additional history is critical?

5. **Case:** A 10-year-old girl is undergoing evaluation by an endocrinologist for short stature. She was normal at birth and grew at the 50th percentile for her first 18 months. She then had a slow decline in growth parameters and now is at the 10th percentile with only a 3 cm increase in the past year. She has been fairly healthy otherwise except for some irritability and poor weight gain in addition to decreased growth velocity. Parents and siblings are all of average height. What further questions might help make a diagnosis in this case? Could there be clues on examination? What screening laboratory test is important?

6. **Case:** A 9-year-old boy is brought to the office for ankle pain and swelling and some abdominal pain for 24 hours. He was previously well but developed mild crampy abdominal pain without emesis 1 day previously, and then this morning noted some swelling and pain in the left ankle. He has been afebrile but was given some acetaminophen for discomfort. What are key parts of the physical examination in this case? What condition must be considered first? What laboratory testing could be helpful?

Discussion by John Carlton Gartner Jr. MD, Pediatrician-in-Chief, General Pediatrics/Diagnostic Referral Division, Nemours/Alfred I. duPont Hospital for Children, Wilmington, Delaware

1. **Discussion:** Prolonged fever, or fever of unknown origin (FUO), is clearly defined in adults as 2 weeks of fever and no diagnosis after 1 week in the hospital. In pediatric patients it is generally accepted that more than 1 week of fever and no diagnosis from routine examination and laboratory results are sufficient. Time spent on history is often most revealing—with further testing not done randomly. For example, routine CT scan is helpful only if there are clues. Abdominal pain, change in bowel habits might warrant CT of the abdomen. In this case, further history was obtained. The patient had a new kitten for several months and had been licked and scratched. Examination also revealed several fading papules on the hands, and titers confirmed exposure to *Bartonella henselae,* the recognized cause of cat-scratch disease. CT scan was done before the return of the titers and revealed typical annular filling defects in the liver—likely granulomas from cat scratch disease.

2. **Discussion:** Peripheral facial palsy usually is associated with injury/inflammation of the seventh cranial nerve and is called Bell palsy. It is important to distinguish peripheral from central palsy—peripheral lesions affect the entire face, but central lesions usually spare the upper face because there are crossing fibers. Several infectious agents have been associated with peripheral facial palsy, including herpes simplex virus and *Borrelia burgdorferi*, the causative agent of Lyme disease. Our patient had a peripheral palsy and an otherwise normal neurologic examination. There was no known exposure to ticks, but she lived in an endemic area and careful search of her skin—done carefully with parents present but full skin exposure—revealed a 5-cm erythematous lesion with central clearing in her groin area. These are sufficient data to make a clinical diagnosis of Lyme disease and initiate treatment. Antibody titers may take several weeks to develop and should not delay antibiotic treatment in this case.

3. **Discussion:** This history is suggestive of increased intracranial pressure—headache is worsening over weeks and now associated with morning vomiting. Progressive headache should always be

distinguished from recurrent headache. Raised intracranial pressure should be your first concern, and a careful funduscopic examination is mandatory—and in this case reveals moderate papilledema. The differential diagnosis would include mass lesions, including tumors, bleeding from an aneurysm or trauma, and also primary increase in intracranial pressure, known as pseudotumor cerebri. This condition can be related to certain medications, such as tetracycline, but often is related to obesity. Imaging of the brain is important—CT or magnetic resonance imaging (MRI)—and was normal in this case, making pseudotumor the likely diagnosis. Lumbar puncture, done after a normal imaging study, can be done to confirm the increased pressure, which can often be managed with medication.

4. **Discussion:** The cause of swelling in this case is likely the low albumin level and consequent low oncotic pressure. Swelling often is in dependent areas, and this child is now walking. Critical initial laboratory testing is to find the most likely source of protein loss—in the urine. Failure of synthesis of albumin is extremely rare and related most often to severe hepatic insufficiency, which is highly unlikely with otherwise normal chemistries. Urinalysis in this case is normal, which suggests that another source of protein loss must be found—likely the gastrointestinal (GI) tract. The mean corpuscular volume (MCV) is also important and is quite low: 58 fL. Key additional history is that the child actually drinks almost exclusively whole milk from a bottle—8 ounces at least 6 times per day. Cow's milk protein is associated with iron deficiency and protein-losing enteropathy—likely related to an allergic reaction in the GI tract. Treatment involves not only iron therapy for months, but also reduction or elimination of the cow's milk from the diet, aided by cessation of bottle feeding.

5. **Discussion:** The growth curve in this case is somewhat unusual. The patient had normal growth until around 18 months, and parents are of average height. Most children with genetic short stature have small parents, and growth falls off in the first year. Children with constitutional delay (late puberty, eventual normal height) have a similar slowing in the first year and a family history of delay. Because our patient fell off later, one must consider an endocrine or other systemic disorder. Careful history reveals that the patient has a poor appetite and "bloating" after meals. Physical examination reveals diminished adipose tissue and some digital clubbing. Stool Hemoccult is negative, but stool fat stain is positive. There is mild anemia but normal sedimentation rate. Before starting detailed endocrine testing for growth hormone, the physician orders screening tests for celiac disease, which are strongly positive, and the patient is referred to a gastroenterologist. It is important to note that celiac disease is a more common cause of short stature than is growth hormone

deficiency but may be missed because symptoms related to the GI tract may be quite mild.

6. **Discussion:** One must always consider a surgical condition with abdominal pain, especially acute appendicitis. In this case, there is no fever and the patient also has ankle pain and swelling—not usually associated with appendicitis. Physical examination reveals a boy with mild abdominal discomfort but no guarding or rebound. The ankle is swollen, but range of movement is normal. Key in evaluation of acute joint swelling is to consider infectious/septic arthritis. The patient has no fever and good range of motion, making this much less of a consideration. The rest of the examination is normal, but stool Hemoccult is positive. Complete blood count (CBC) and urinalysis are normal. The experienced examiner decides to watch the patient at home carefully. The next day the patient develops a rash on his lower extremities that looks initially like insect bites but when evaluated in the office is clearly purpuric with scattered lesions on the lower extremities and buttocks. This is a good presentation for Henoch-Schönlein or anaphylactoid purpura (HSP). This is a type of vasculitis seen predominantly in children and usually has a good long-term outcome, unless there is serious renal involvement. Occasionally, intestinal involvement, including acute intussusception, is the major presentation.

Section IV
THE NEWBORN NURSERY

Section Editor

Jennifer R. Miller MD

Section Contents

Chapter 54
The Newborn Examination

Nilufer R. Goyal MD, FAAP

Speaking Intelligently

The first examination of the newborn takes place at the time of delivery, with the assignment of Apgar scores, which provide a quick assessment of transition to extrauterine life. In uncomplicated vaginal deliveries, this initial assessment is performed by the delivery room nurse. The newborn is monitored closely in the first several hours. The complete newborn physical examination in the normal newborn is performed by the pediatrician within the first 24 hours of life. Most infants in the term nursery are healthy and have a normal course. The goal of reviewing the prenatal history and performing a complete physical examination is to identify abnormalities and congenital anomalies that may require prompt attention. Many abnormalities are identified with prenatal testing.

Medical Knowledge and Patient Care

Evaluation of the neonate begins in the delivery room. The 1- and 5-minute Apgar scores provide assessment of the newborn's extrauterine transition. The vital signs, tone, color, perfusion, level of activity, and level of consciousness of the newborn are monitored closely during the first several hours after birth. In addition to performing daily physical examinations in the hospital, the pediatrician must be familiar with birth injuries and presentations of acute neonatal illnesses such as sepsis, pneumonia, and severe hyperbilirubinemia.

Basic Newborn Examination

General Observations: The first look will be a general assessment of wellness. Is the infant breathing comfortably? Is he/she alert, sleeping, or crying as if hungry or otherwise distressed? Are there any obvious anomalies? Look at the length, weight, and head circumference in relation to gestational age. These provide a general estimation of the in utero environment and nutrition. The order of the examination **proceeds from the least- to most-intrusive maneuver.** Many begin with cardiac auscultation of the calm infant.

Posture and Tone: Degree of flexion of extremities lends clues to the gestational age of the child as well as overall well-being. Sick infants may be limp and hold extremities more lax (hypotonia).

Head and Scalp Examination: The average head circumference for a term neonate is 35 cm. Molding resulting from overriding sutures may be prominent but resolves in the first few days. The anterior fontanelle is easy to palpate, whereas often the posterior fontanelle is not typically appreciated. Both should be soft and flat. Caput succedaneum is a boggy, indistinct swelling of the scalp, sometimes with bruising. As it recedes, there may be an underlying cephalohematoma. A cephalohematoma is a subperiosteal hematoma with clearly demarcated borders limited by suture lines. Observe for plagiocephaly, and check for an accompanying torticollis by assessing the sternocleidomastoid range of motion.

Face: Note the general features and position of the eyes and ears, and carefully observe the philtrum for clues to syndromic manifestations. To test for low-set ears, a line drawn from the inner canthus of the eye through the outer canthus should extend to intersect the ear. Abnormal formation of an ear pinna may be a clue to a urologic abnormality.

Eyes: Observe for a brief period of eye fixation, and check the red reflex by ophthalmoscope. A coloboma of the iris may be noted. Pressure during birth may cause a subconjunctival hemorrhage.

Oropharynx: Natal teeth are occasionally present. Epstein pearls are common benign fluid-filled nodules on the palate. A short lingual frenulum, or "tongue-tie," can limit upward tongue movement and cause difficulty with breastfeeding. A cleft lip or palate is often an isolated finding. Submucous clefts are easily missed without palatal palpation. Clefts frequently cause significant feeding difficulties with poor suck and nasal regurgitation.

Neck and Clavicle Examination: The neck should be checked for cystic hygromas. There should be full range of motion. Clavicle fracture is detected by palpation for crepitus or discontinuity.

Anterior Chest and Breast Examination: Observe the shape of the chest. Some newborns have transient pronounced breast development.

Lung and Cardiovascular Auscultation: Assess rate and effort of breathing. Grunting, flaring, or retractions indicate respiratory distress. The cardiovascular examination should be performed in a quiet room using a pediatric stethoscope. Assess heart rate, rhythm, and point of maximal impulse. For murmurs, note the intensity, timing in the cardiac cycle, and characteristics. Auscultate both axillae and the back. Palpate femoral pulses, and assess for brachiofemoral delay.

Abdominal Examination, Including Umbilical Cord: The abdomen is optimally examined with a calm newborn. Assessment of hepatosplenomegaly and abdominal mass may be facilitated by flexion of the knees. Single umbilical artery may be associated with a renal anomaly.

Hip Examination: Developmental dysplasia of the hip (DDH) is assessed by observation for gluteal asymmetry and performing of the Ortolani and Barlow maneuvers (see Chapter 17, Teaching Visual: Examination of the Infant Hip).

Genital Examination: In normal-appearing male genitalia, identify the urethral meatal opening, signs of hypospadias or epispadias (which may be relative contraindications to circumcision), and also bilaterally descended testes and absence of hernia or hydrocele. Differentiate retractile testes from cryptorchidism by milking the testicle toward the scrotum.

Externally normal female genitalia have prominent labia minora with the labia majora incompletely covering the minora. Transient white vaginal discharge or drops of blood are due to maternal hormone effect. If there is concern for clitoral enlargement, promptly consult endocrinology regarding ambiguous genitalia.

Often urate crystals are seen in the diaper. These appear as orange, sandy stains on the diaper and may at times be mistaken for blood. This otherwise benign finding may be an indicator of relative dehydration and can cause significant parental anxiety.

Back and Spine Examination: Note the presence of sacral pits, hemangiomas, or tufts of hair in the midline of the spine. Mongolian spots are benign skin markings, usually found in children of darker skin and are not associated with any illness.

Extremity Examination: Note polydactyly, syndactyly, or clinodactyly. Check the feet for deformity. Evaluate for brachial plexus injury by assessing asymmetry of upper extremity movement and symmetry of the Moro reflex.

Neurologic Examination: This includes observation of activity, tone, and primitive reflexes. In **the Moro reflex** the legs and head extend while the arms jerk up and out with the palms up and thumbs flexed. Shortly afterward the arms are brought together and the hands clench into fists, and the infant often cries. In **the rooting reflex,** newborns will turn their head toward anything that strokes their cheek or mouth, searching for the object by moving their heads in steadily decreasing arcs until the object is found. The rooting and suck reflexes are related. With rooting, the newborn infant will turn his/her head toward anything that strokes his/her cheek or mouth, and the **suck reflex** allows the child to instinctively suck at anything that touches the roof of the mouth. The **Babinski reflex** appears when the side of the foot is stroked, causing the toes to fan out and the great toe to extend. The reflex is caused by a lack of myelination in the corticospinal tract in young children. The Babinski reflex is a sign of neurologic abnormality in adults and older children.

Skin Examination: There are many neonatal rashes. Some common benign exanthems include erythema toxicum and milia. **Erythema toxicum neonatorum** consists of small erythematous papules and occasionally pustules surrounded by a distinctive blotchy erythematous halo. Individual lesions are transient, often disappearing within hours and then appearing elsewhere on the body. **Milia** are tiny white papules found on the face that are due to trapped sebaceous material in glands of the skin (see Chapter 16, The Newborn Well Visit).

Practice-Based Learning and Improvement

Common rashes and birthmarks, two important issues in diagnosis and management of newborn skin, are reviewed in the following articles, which include excellent photographs.

Title
Newborn skin. I. Common rashes

Authors
O'Connor NR, McLaughlin MR, Ham P

Reference
Am Fam Physician 77(1):47-52, 2008

Title
Newborn skin. II. Birthmarks

Authors
McLaughlin MR, O'Connor NR, Ham P

Reference
Am Fam Physician 2008;77(1):56-60

Interpersonal and Communication Skills

Maintain Complete and Legible Medical Records

The newborn examination is important because some potentially serious conditions have physical manifestations that if recognized early can be treated effectively, such as congenital hip dislocation. Physician documentation is usually in the form of notes that become a permanent part of the patient's medical and legal record. Attention to detail, including documentation of positive and negative findings of the physical examination, is an important part of the infant's medical record. Accuracy and legibility (for nonelectronic health records) in documentation should be the goal and responsibility of the physician.

Professionalism

Demonstrate Reliability and Responsibility: Time Your Nursery Rounds to Optimize Opportunity for Maternal-Infant Bonding

Most newborn nurseries having a "rooming-in" policy, whereby infants spend most of their time with the mother. This facilitates bonding and the initiation of breastfeeding. Physicians who work in the nursery need to be sensitive to the needs of the mothers and nursing staff caring for the mother-infant dyads. Timing rounds to cause as little disruption as possible, rounding at a consistent time, and informing the staff of a change in rounding time is not only courteous but also desirable.

Systems-Based Practice

Levels and Acuity of Nursery Care

The AAP Committee on Fetus and Newborn[1] classifies the facilities providing inpatient care for newborns into three levels. They are based on the following functional capabilities:

1. Level I (basic) is a hospital nursery able to evaluate and provide postnatal care of healthy newborn infants, stabilize and provide care for infants born at 35 to 37 weeks' gestation who remain physiologically stable, and stabilize newborn infants born at less than 35 weeks gestational age or ill until transfer to a higher-level facility.
2. Level II (specialty) is a hospital special care nursery able to provide care to infants born at more than 32 weeks gestation and weighing more than 1500 grams who have physiologic immaturity such as apnea of prematurity, inability to maintain body temperature, or inability to take oral feedings; or who are moderately ill with problems that are not anticipated to need subspecialty services on an urgent basis.
3. Level III (subspecialty) is a hospital neonatal intensive care unit (NICU) capable of providing continuous life support and comprehensive care for extremely high-risk newborn infants with birth weight of less than 1000 grams and gestational age of less than 28 weeks, and those with complex and critical illness.

Reference

1. American Academy of Pediatrics: Policy statement: organizational principles to guide and define the child health care system and/or improve the health of all children, committee on fetus and newborn, *Pediatrics* 114:1341-1347, 2004.

Chapter 55
Dysmorphology

Louis E. Bartoshesky MD, MPH

Speaking Intelligently

When I am asked to see an infant with dysmorphic features or a birth defect, I realize that most likely the parents are stressed. I explain that I will ask many questions to obtain a detailed history about the infant, the pregnancy, as well as family history in search of clues to help identify the problem. After performing a complete examination, I share my impressions and make recommendations for possible laboratory testing, imaging studies, or subspecialty consultation. In some cases, a diagnosis will be possible with history and examination; in others, a definitive diagnosis will take time to elucidate; and in many instances, no specific diagnosis is made. Despite this, therapy and ongoing care will be needed to maximize the child's health and development. Adequate time should be allotted at every step of the process for explanation of findings and answering family questions.

Medical Knowledge and Patient Care

Background and Definitions

A birth defect is an abnormality of structure, function, or metabolism present at birth. Major birth defects are those requiring medical or surgical intervention or affecting normal growth and development. Birth defects are the second leading cause of death in the first year of life and a leading cause of mortality, morbidity, and hospitalization throughout childhood. Three to five percent of newborns have a major birth defect.

Some children have a birth defect that is an isolated single anomaly; others have multiple congenital anomalies (MCA). A **malformation** is a primary structural birth defect arising from a local error in morphogenesis. A **deformation** is a structural birth defect resulting from some extrinsic effect on a developing organ or tissue with no intrinsic error in morphogenesis; for example, uterine crowding resulting in a clubfoot. **Disruptions** are structural defects resulting from destruction of a normally formed part, often resulting from interference with vascular supply to that structure. **Dysplasias** are localized or generalized abnormal organizations of cells with structural consequences. Hemangiomas can be considered to be localized dysplasias; skeletal dysplasias are generalized. A clubfoot, dislocated hips, neurogenic bladder, and Chiari type II anomaly all may result from a **single neural tube defect**—a lumbosacral meningomyelocele. An MCA syndrome, sometimes referred to as a **sequence,** is one in which there are developmental variants in more than one organ system and in which it is assumed (and sometimes proved) that there is common etiology for the multiple anomalies. An **association** is multiple anomalies occurring together more often than expected by chance but not with a single etiology.

Etiology

Isolated birth defects are usually argued to be **multifactorial traits,** that is, there are probably several variant genes along with environmental factors that are the causes for the anomaly. However, in some cases the defect may be the result of a mutation at a single gene locus. In many cases (probably 40% to 60%) the cause for multiple congenital anomalies is not clear. However, there are known **environmental and genetic causes of MCA.** Environmental factors that play a role in the etiology of birth defects include infectious agents (rubella, toxoplasmosis, syphilis, cytomegalovirus, varicella, and perhaps others); drugs (alcohol, certain anticonvulsants, warfarin sodium, probably cigarettes, and others); nutritional deficiencies (folic acid); radiation (but only at doses well above those of standard diagnostic studies); and maternal health (poorly controlled diabetes mellitus, maternal phenylketonuria).

MCA can be related to genetic factors. **Chromosome anomalies,** including aneuploidy (other than 46 chromosomes), deletions, duplications, unbalanced translocations, and inversions are all associated with MCA. Many **single-gene defects** are expressed as MCA. **Autosomal dominant traits** include many skeletal dysplasias (perhaps achondroplasia being the best known and most common), connective tissue disorders such as Marfan syndrome, neurocutaneous syndromes such as neurofibromatosis, tuberous sclerosis, von Hippel-Lindau, and others. **Autosomal recessive traits** presenting as MCA include lysosomal storage disorders (various categories such as mucopolysaccharidoses, oligosaccharidoses, sphingolipid disorders); peroxisomal disorders such as Zellweger syndrome; disorders of sterol metabolism such as Smith-Lemli-Opitz syndrome; disorders of metal metabolism; as well as some disorders of organic acid or amino acid metabolism and disorders of energy metabolism. Previously it had been taught that "metabolic disorders" were not associated with MCA, but it is now clear that a number of these disorders are associated with dysmorphic features and multiple anomalies. **X-linked MCA syndromes** include Hunter syndrome (mucopolysaccharidosis II), Menkes syndrome (disorder of copper metabolism), certain ectodermal dysplasias, and a number of syndromes associated with cognitive delay (such as fragile X syndrome). Some of the disorders of energy metabolism are related to mutations in the mitochondrial genome, and some of these present in infancy with dysmorphic features, hypotonia, hearing and vision disorders, seizures, and developmental delay. With improving chromosome technology and molecular genetic techniques made possible through the Human Genome Project, more and more causes for MCA are being determined.

Approach to the Child With Multiple Congenital Anomalies

History and Physical Examination

History includes determination of maternal risk factors such as maternal health, particularly diabetes control; maternal exposures in pregnancy—drugs, alcohol, and infections; maternal immunization status; history of maternal fever or exposure to known teratogenic infectious agents; and use of folic acid before conception. A careful three-generation family history is important with particular attention to infant and childhood death, infant and childhood disabilities, infertility, and consanguinity. Family history may be "negative," but it is never "noncontributory." Other pregnancy factors of possible importance to understanding a child with MCA include fetal activity (reduced in babies with certain neuromuscular disorders) and amniotic fluid quantities (elevated in certain syndromes such as Down or Turner syndromes and in the presence of fetal esophageal atresia, and reduced in cases of renal agenesis or obstructive uropathy). Reduced amniotic fluid (oligohydramnios) is a risk factor in fetal akinesia sequence—inhibited fetal movement resulting in joint contractures, flat face, flat ears, and pulmonary hypoplasia. Fetal growth is inhibited in congenital infection syndromes, in many chromosomal variant syndromes, and in many other syndromes of many different etiologies. Breech presentation may be associated with deformations such as clubfoot.

Careful examination starts with determination of length, weight, and head circumference. Measurements of interocular distances, palpebral fissure length, philtrum length, ear length, middle finger and total hand length, foot length, penile size, and testicular size are valuable in identifying a syndrome, and standards for these are available in several resources.

The presence of major anomalies is usually obvious. For example, cleft lip and palate, clubfoot, abdominal wall defects, heart malformations associated with persistent cyanosis or heart failure, tracheoesophageal fistula (TEF), diaphragmatic hernia, open neural tube defects, hypospadias, limb deficiencies, or imperforate anus are difficult to miss or at least become apparent after relatively simple evaluations—chest radiograph for diaphragmatic hernia, nasogastric tube passage for TEF and esophageal atresia, recognition of cardiac failure or cyanosis followed by echocardiography. However, major anomalies of renal structure, cataracts, deafness, and noncyanotic heart malformations require careful examination, alertness to subtle functional alterations, and awareness of important associations (such as the association of vertebral anomalies, cardiac malformations, and renal structural defects with TEF and/or anorectal anomalies—the **VATER association**—or of deafness, cardiac and renal anomalies with choanal atresia and iris and retinal colobomas—**CHARGE syndrome**).

Up to 50% of infants have a minor birth defect—one present in less than 5% of the population, but of little or no functional or cosmetic importance. However, **the presence of several such minor anomalies may suggest a specific syndrome** and indicate the need for further evaluation. Note should be made of color, distribution, and consistency of hair; number of hair whorls; and presence of a frontal upsweep. Size of palpebral fissures, the presence of epicanthal folds and slant or palpebral fissures, and the nature of brows and lashes may be helpful in identifying a syndrome. Ear position (low-set ears are those in which the top of the ear is below a line drawn from medial canthus of the eye) and structure, as well as presence of ear pits or preauricular tags, should be noted. Position of nose, integrity of alae nasi, and status of nasal bridge (depressed or prominent) and tip (upturned) may be helpful. Variations of length and markings of philtrum, condition of vermillion border of upper lip, symmetry of mouth movement, presence of lip pits, and defects at angle of mouth may give clues to an underlying syndrome. Cleft of soft palate may be missed on a cursory oral examination, whereas presence of a notch in the uvula or frank bifid uvula may indicate the presence of a submucus cleft.

Pits or tags on the face or neck are seen in certain oral-facial-digital syndromes. Short, broad neck or webbing is seen in children with Down syndrome, Turner syndrome, Noonan syndrome, and in the presence of cervical vertebral anomalies—including the Klippel-Feil anomaly. Inter-nipple distance is increased in Turner syndrome (a variation in chromosome number or structure) and Noonan syndrome (a disorder associated with a mutation at a single gene locus).

Hypospadias, sometimes subtle when at the corona; testicular maldescent; clitoromegaly; and labial hypoplasia or asymmetry are seen in various disorders of sexual development but also in more generalized MCA syndromes. Simple sacrococcygeal dimples are rarely of clinical importance, but when associated with a hairy patch, a hemangioma, or palpable bony defect they may indicate an underlying neural tube defect—a disorder of secondary neurulation.

Careful measurement of limb length and circumference, search for limb asymmetry, and measurement of fingers may give clues to the presence of a syndrome. Palmar and digital crease anomalies are seen in various syndromes—the transverse crease seen in children with Down syndrome being well known. The absence or underdevelopment of digital creases indicates reduced fetal movement in utero. Nail dysplasia or hypoplasia is seen in fetal alcohol and fetal phenytoin syndromes but also in ectodermal dysplasias and in other MCA syndromes. Any asymmetry of limb growth should be noted.

Hypopigmented or hyperpigmented areas of the skin may suggest a neurocutaneous disorder. There are a number of chromosomal disorders and other syndromes associated with hemangiomas and other cutaneous defects. Seborrhea-like changes and verrucous skin may be associated with certain syndromes.

Careful neurologic examination is, of course, essential in evaluating the child with MCA. Symmetry of movement, muscle tone, and deep tendon reflexes are to be observed and recorded.

Testing: A major anomaly, when isolated, does not require further laboratory study except in certain circumstances such as a child with a cleft lip and palate whose parent and grandparent also have clefts. Specific molecular DNA testing could be of value in such a child/family. A minor anomaly demands a careful search for minor anomalies. There is no specific number of minor anomalies the presence of which should suggest chromosome studies. Clinical judgment is required.

High-resolution chromosome studies will detect aneuploidies and many duplications, deletions, or complex rearrangements. Children with MCA who have normal high-resolution chromosome studies may be candidates for more specific studies. Certain syndromes, when suspected, can be confirmed with **specific fluorescent in situ hybridization (FISH) studies.** These include Williams, velocardiofacial/DiGeorge (22q11 microdeletion syndrome), Smith Magenis, Miller-Dieker, and trichorhinophalangeal syndromes. More are likely to be added as time goes on and technology improves. Prader-Willi and Angelman syndromes are included on this list but are best ruled out by determination of methylation pattern at the appropriate loci on chromosome 15.

Comparative genomic hybridization (CGH) using microarray and other new technologies is now available. Up to 10% of children with MCA and developmental delay may have a chromosome variant (deletions, duplications, inversions, complex rearrangements) detectable by CGH that could not be detected on high-resolution studies.

When a **congenital infection** (rubella, cytomegalovirus [CMV], toxoplasmosis, syphilis) is suspected, specific studies for that infection should be obtained. The term *TORCH* was a valuable reminder of some of the infectious agents that could be associated with birth defects. However, ordering "TORCH titers" is no longer logical. If congenital toxoplasmosis is suggested, serologic studies for antibodies are indicated. If CMV is suspected, urine for CMV should be collected. Congenital rubella is very rare now, although it should not be ignored as a possibility, particularly in populations in which there might be underimmunization. Herpes, the "H" in TORCH, is a rare cause of structural congenital anomalies, although it is an important cause of serious neonatal infection. There are no antibodies for "O."

Specialized studies are available for babies with MCA in whom lysosomal storage, peroxisomal disorders, sterol disorders, or disorders of metal metabolism are suspected. Such studies should only be obtained when there are suspicious clinical features. A "shotgun" approach of ordering everything in every baby is neither efficient nor cost effective.

Imaging studies and consultations (e.g., ophthalmology, cardiology, audiology, urology, nephrology) are ordered as indicated by information collected on history and physical examination.

In the evaluation, historical factors should be listed and major and minor anomalies described. References to texts (such as *Smith's Recognizable Patterns of Human Malformation*) or databases (e.g., London Dysmorphology Data Base) and consultation with appropriate specialists may be needed to determine what syndrome is possible. Up to half of children with MCA are not assigned a diagnosis, although that figure continues to shrink as technology advances.[1,2]

Practice-Based Learning and Improvement

The following websites are valuable resources for identifying birth defects:

http://www.cdc.gov/ncbddd (National Center for Birth Defects and Developmental Disabilities)
http://www.marchofdimes.com/pnhec
http://www.genetests.com
http://www.omim.org

Interpersonal and Communication Skills

Explain the Diagnostic Purpose for Specific Testing

During an evaluation of a child with congenital anomalies, it is important to be supportive and keep the family informed of the tests being done and the reasons for each test. It is a good idea to start off the explanation with: "Congratulations on the birth of your new baby," using the child's name if possible. Most families appreciate a detailed outline of the possible causes of the anomaly (anomalies) and an explanation of the proposed testing. Unless a specific genetic syndrome is suspected, the family should be told that in many cases no specific cause is determined.

Professionalism

Be Honest When Discussing Etiology and Potential Outcomes

Many people mistakenly believe that environmental agents are the cause of most birth defects and are looking for some exposure to explain their child's MCA. These beliefs should be dealt with honestly and with compassion. Parents are also concerned about developmental concerns of MCA: "Will my baby be delayed?" Honesty is most important, including admitting that cognitive outcome is uncertain in many cases.

Systems-Based Practice

Coordination and Case Management of Children With Complex Needs

Case management is a systematic process of assessment, planning, service coordination, and care delivery for patients with complex medical conditions or special social situations. It is an integrated approach through which the multiple service needs of these patients are met. Case management aims to achieve a controlled balance between cost and quality of patient care for special needs patients. All Medicaid and many commercial insurances offer case management services as a benefit to their members who meet the eligibility requirements. Children with congenital conditions and dysmorphic syndromes will meet such requirements, and physicians should promptly refer these patients.

References

1. Jones KL: *Smith's recognizable patterns of human malformation*, ed 6, Philadelphia, 2005, Elsevier.
2. Rimoin D, Connor JM, Pyeritz R, Korf B: *Principles and practice of medical genetics*, Philadelphia, 2007, Churchill Livingstone.

Chapter 56
Infant Feeding

Edelveis R. M. Clapp DO

Speaking Intelligently

As pediatricians we encourage mothers to breastfeed, and we provide support with counseling, weight checks, and recommendation of lactation consultants when needed. It is important to recognize that not all mothers will be willing or able to breastfeed. Successful breastfeeding is a learning curve for both mother and infant, and ultimately some parents may choose formula feeding. It is important to be supportive and encourage families to make the decision that best works for their lives, whether it be breastfeeding or formula feeding. As the pediatrician, you are the person who helps shape and guide the parents' view on infant nutrition, and they will look to you for advice. It is important to be well informed and to stay current with American Academy of Pediatrics (AAP) recommendations.

Medical Knowledge and Patient Care

Feeding an infant can be very confusing, especially for first-time parents. The AAP recommends exclusive breastfeeding for the first 6 months of life with continuation until 12 months, or as long as mother and child mutually desire.[1,2] For those who choose not to breastfeed, cow's milk–based formula is an acceptable alternative. At birth, 70% of infants are breastfed. By 6 months only one third are breastfed.[3] The pediatrician should be able to counsel about both breastfeeding and formula feeding, and guide parents to provide optimal nutrition.

Breast Milk Composition

Breast milk provides optimal infant nutrition. Its composition is 70% whey and 30% casein, compared with cow's milk, which is 18% whey and 82% casein.[1,2] Whey proteins are more easily digested in that they are more resistant to precipitation in stomach acid, and this promotes gastric emptying. Whey proteins such as lactoferrin, lysozyme, and secretory immunoglobulin A are involved in host defense.[1] Human milk also contains oligosaccharides, nucleotides, cellular components, and growth factors that enhance the newborn's immune system.

Lipids provide approximately 50% of the total calories, and human milk is high in essential fatty acids. Derivatives of these play important roles in neural and retinal function.

The major carbohydrate is lactose, which is hydrolyzed to glucose and galactose by lactase in the small intestine. Lactose that passes to the distal small intestine promotes proliferation of lactobacilli, which serves to suppress growth of more pathogenic bacteria and promote calcium and phosphorous absorption.[2]

Human milk contains many micronutrients, minerals and vitamins that promote optimal growth and development. However, there is little biologically active vitamin D in breast milk. Infants who are exclusively breastfed require 400 international units per day of vitamin D to be started soon after birth to prevent vitamin D deficiency and rickets.[4]

There are numerous advantages to breastfeeding:

- It is relatively low cost. Lactating mothers must optimize their caloric intake and eat a well-balanced varied diet that includes foods rich in calcium, zinc, magnesium, vitamin B_6, and folate.
- Breast milk is always available, requires no preparation, and is specifically tailored for human nutrition.
- Breastfeeding is associated with a lower incidence of allergies, otitis media, gastroenteritis, pneumonia, bacteremia, and meningitis during the first year of life.[3]
- Advantages to mother include faster weight loss because breastfeeding metabolizes an additional 500 calories per day. It also promotes involution of the uterus.

Contraindications to Breastfeeding

- Maternal infections are generally not a contraindication to breastfeeding. Two exceptions are infection with human immunodeficiency virus (HIV) in the United States and a maternal herpesvirus outbreak with lesions on the breast.[5]
- Drugs that are contraindicated in lactation include cimetidine, cyclophosphamide, ergotamine, and thiouracil.[6] In most cases, there is a reasonable substitute for these medications that is not contraindicated in breastfeeding.
- Some drugs (e.g., those used for radiology studies) require temporary cessation of breastfeeding.
- Some inborn errors of metabolism, such as galactosemia, are contraindications to breastfeeding.

Formula

Breast milk is the standard upon which infant formula composition is based. Infant formula must meet the minimum requirements of nutrients without exceeding the maximum recommended for each nutrient required for normal growth and development.[2]

Iron-fortified cow's milk–based formulas are an excellent feeding alternative. Nutritional studies comparing breastfed and formula-fed infants show little to no differences. Iron-fortified formula can be used:

- As a substitute for nonbreastfed infants
- As a supplement when mothers choose not to exclusively breastfeed
- As a supplement for breastfed infants with inadequate weight gain

Mothers who bottle feed can establish the same infant bonding as those who breastfeed. Feedings can last from 5 to 25 minutes, depending on the infant's efficiency.[5] Feeding time will shorten as the infant grows and develops a more mature suck and swallow. Emphasize to parents that the bottle should not be propped. It limits physical contact and bonding and is a risk for aspiration.

Feeding Guidelines

Feeding should be initiated as soon as possible after birth to promote maternal-infant bonding and maintain normal metabolism during extrauterine transition (see Chapter 67, Neonatal Hypoglycemia).

In general, breastfed infants want shorter intervals between feeds than formula-fed infants. Infants should be nursed on demand, with the goal of at least 8 to 12 times in a 24-hour period until lactation is well established.[5] Initially the interval between feeds should be no longer than 4 hours. Feeding times will vary. Infants may want to nurse anywhere from 5 minutes to 45 minutes. Breast milk is produced in a supply-and-demand fashion. The more the infant demands, the more breast milk will be produced. When lactation is being established, latching time should be unrestricted. An electric breast pump to promote complete emptying may help stimulate lactogenesis. Once the milk supply is established, latching longer than 30 minutes may suggest some degree of nonnutritive sucking. During early weeks, nursing sessions usually take more time. As the baby becomes more efficient with nursing, and effectively empties the breast, feeding time will decrease.

For formula-fed infants, a good rule of thumb is 1 ounce of formula per feed for every kilogram of weight, with an average total of 24 to 32 ounces per day. Intake should be adequate to maintain an average weight gain of 15 to 30 g/day during the first 2 months, 15 to 20 g/day during the next 3 months, and 10 to 15 g/day during months 6 through 12.[1-3]

In the first few days, infants usually lose weight, up to 10% of their birth weight, resulting from metabolism of subcutaneous water stores to prevent dehydration until lactation is established. Infants should be gaining weight by the end of the first week and be back to their birth weight by 14 days. If the infant is not waking to feed, parents should be instructed to wake the infants every 2 to 3 hours around-the-clock. Those who continue to lose weight will require supplementation with either pumped breast milk or formula. Emphasize that the infant should usually nurse followed by supplementation. Once birth weight is surpassed and daily weight gain is adequate (15 to 30 g/day), feeding can be on demand.

To assess hydration status and adequacy of intake, monitor wet diapers and the number and quality of stools. There should be at least one void and meconium stool within the first 24 hours. By day 3, the infant should have 3 or 4 wet diapers, and one to two transitional stools. With full feeds, there should be 6 wet diapers per day; stool frequency is variable, but often there is a bowel movement with each feed. Breastmilk stool is usually yellow and seedy.

Burping the infant will allow swallowed air to escape; this will decrease regurgitation and abdominal discomfort. Inform parents that all infants have some gastroesophageal reflux (GER) because of a relaxed lower esophageal sphincter. Overfed infants will spit more, as will those with significant GER. It is important for the physician to determine whether the reflux is pathologic in nature, caused by overfeeding, or within normal limits (physiologic GER). Any infant who is uncomfortable during feedings, is not gaining weight, has projectile emesis, or emesis that is bilious or bloody, requires further evaluation.

Some breastfed infants develop intolerance to cow's milk and soy protein through exposure in the maternal diet and may experience colitis with significant discomfort, poor weight gain, and Hemoccult-positive stools. In these cases, breastfeeding is often successful with a strict maternal elimination diet. Another option is feeding a protein hydrolysate formula.

Practice-Based Learning and Improvement

Title
Infant feeding

Authors
Hall RT, Carroll RE

Reference
Pediatr Rev 21(6):191-199, 2000

Historical significance/comments
Review article that outlines the benefits of infant nutrition with human milk along with satisfactory formula substitutes for healthy term and near-term infants. Specialized formulas, introduction of solids, and how to assess growth and nutritional status are reviewed.

Interpersonal and Communication Skills

Be Supportive of the Family's Feeding Choice

When a breastfed newborn is not gaining adequate weight, the pediatrician and parents become quickly engaged to turn things around. The utmost skill may be needed to gently convince a mom to offer supplemental formula temporarily. Empathic listening may help you understand that she may feel like a failure and does not understand that lactation may take a full week or more to be well established. Be encouraging and empathic, but not judgmental, should the parents opt for formula feeding. Although it is important to discuss the benefits of breastfeeding, it is also important to support the parents in their feeding decisions. Having both the support and understanding of their physician can give a mother confidence and reassurance, which can help to improve the feeding relationship the parents are establishing with their infant.

Professionalism

Advocate for Breastfeeding

Many hospitals give new mothers "gift packs" when they are discharged that include samples of infant formula as well as other products. As advocates for breastfeeding, physicians should be aware of the subtle message given to the breastfeeding mother by supplying her with a formula sample. Elimination of gift packs, and the implied endorsement of the products in the pack, should be discussed with hospital administration and other colleagues.

Systems-Based Practice

Comprehensive Nutrition Services for Financially Eligible Women, Infants, and Children

The Special Supplemental Nutrition Program for Women, Infants, and Children (WIC) provides federal grants to states for supplemental foods, health-care referrals, and nutrition education for patients who meet the following eligibility criteria:

- **Category**
  - □ Pregnant women
  - □ Women who are breastfeeding an infant (under 1 year of age)
  - □ Postpartum women to the sixth month after delivery
  - □ Children from birth to 5 years of age
- **Income**
  - □ Income eligibility requires that a household have gross a income at or below 185% of the federal poverty level.

- ■ **Nutrition risk**
  - □ Nutrition risk is any medical or health problem that can be corrected or lessened by proper amounts and types of food intake. Examples of nutrition risk are:
    - ● Iron deficiency
    - ● Inadequate growth (i.e., low weight for age, low weight for height)
    - ● Premature delivery
    - ● Inadequate dietary intake (types or amounts of food)

References

1. American Academy of Pediatrics: *Pediatric nutrition handbook*, 6th ed, Elk Grove Village, IL, 2009, American Academy of Pediatrics.
2. Hall RT, Carroll RE: Infant feeding. *Pediatr Rev* 21(6):191-199, 2000.
3. Behrman RE: *Nelson textbook of pediatrics*, 17th ed, Philadelphia, 2004, Saunders.
4. Wagner CL: Prevention of rickets and vitamin D deficiency in infants, children, and adolescents. *Pediatrics* 122(5):1142-1152, 2008.
5. Chandran L, Gelfer P: Breastfeeding: The essential principles. *Pediatr Rev* 27(11):409-417, 2006.
6. Lawrence RA: The pediatrician's role in infant feeding decision-making. *Pediatr Rev* 14(7):265-272, 1993.

Chapter 57
Newborn Screening

Louis E. Bartoshesky MD, MPH

Speaking Intelligently

Newborn screening (NBS) is of proven public health value. Although it is true that the disorders screened for are relatively uncommon (ranging from congenital hypothyroidism occurring about 1 per 4000 live births to some of the organic acidopathies or fatty acid oxidation disorders occurring less than 1 per 100,000), when taken together the disorders are common enough that screening is clearly cost-effective. About 1 in every 600 infants has a disorder identifiable by newborn screening. Newborn blood spot screening is a program, not just a laboratory test. The mission of NBS programs is to eliminate or reduce morbidity, mortality, and disability that result from disorders in the screening panel. To accomplish this, all affected newborns must receive early confirmatory diagnosis and optimal long-term management.

Medical Knowledge and Patient Care

The components of a newborn screening program are:

1. **Screening:** The laboratory testing
2. **Follow-up:** Rapid location and referral of potentially affected infants
3. **Diagnosis:** Confirmation or exclusion of the presumptive diagnosis
4. **Management:** Planning and implementation of long-term management, ideally coordinated in the child's medical home (see Chapter 25, The Special Needs Child)
5. **Evaluation** and quality assurance: Validation of testing material, assessment of efficiency of follow-up procedures, analysis of cost-benefit ratios, and assessment of benefit to patients, families, and the public
6. **Education** of health-care institutions and providers and the public

The NBS team includes the birth hospital where the specimen is obtained; the screening laboratory where testing is carried out; the follow-up team whose job is to communicate results and recommendations for follow-up with family, primary care provider, and referral center; the family; the public health infrastructure; specialty referral centers; and the primary care pediatrician whose job is to coordinate the often complex evaluation and follow-up of infants who test positive.[1]

Interpretation of an NBS result requires **an understanding of population screening** and appreciation of the **features of a good screening test:**[2]

- Reasonable sensitivity, specificity, and predictive value
- Reasonable prevalence rate of the disorder
- Cost-effectiveness
- Availability of an effective intervention
- Reproducible results and timely reports
- Public health and community resources to do adequate follow-up and management of detected disorders

Life-threatening disorders (e.g., congenital adrenal hyperplasia, galactosemia, maple syrup urine disease, propionic acidemia and other organic acidopathies, disorders of urea cycle) demand immediate response, and **others** are **associated with increasing disability with delay in intervention** (e.g., congenital hypothyroidism, phenylketonuria [PKU]). Some disorders do not require immediate attention (e.g., hemoglobinopathies, cystic fibrosis [CF]), but should be dealt with promptly by the NBS program and pediatrician.

Family history is important in evaluating a newborn with a suspicious newborn screening result. Previous infant deaths, relatives with metabolic, endocrinologic, and hematologic disorders are important to know about. The NBS program should know the birth weight and gestational age of babies screened. Interpretation of results on very low-birth-weight (VLBW) infants may be difficult. Amino acids may be elevated in infants receiving parenteral nutrition. VLBW infants may have low thyroxine (T_4) level with normal thyroid-stimulating hormone (TSH) level. Certain acyl carnitines detected by tandem mass spectroscopy (MS-MS) may appear elevated in babies on certain antibiotics. 17-Hydroxyprogesterone (the analyte elevated in infants with 21-hydroxylase deficiency congenital adrenal hyperplasia [CAH]) levels are higher in low-birth-weight infants and sometimes in more mature babies who are stressed (e.g., neonatal sepsis).

Some disorders, particularly organic acidopathies and amino acidopathies, may be characterized by poor feeding, irritability, and/or seizures, with onset before the NBS result is available.

The NBS specimen is usually collected on day 2 to 3 of life, but **the infant should be at least 24 hours old and fed at least twice at the time of specimen collection.** In some situations (e.g., a sick newborn being transferred to another hospital), an earlier specimen may be obtained, but early specimens (before 24 hours) must be followed by a repeat screen at a week or so. Some states have a mandatory second screen at 2 to 4 weeks of age. Some infants with congenital hypothyroidism, a few with CAH, and some with other disorders may be missed on first screen and detected on the second. Evidence of the value of a mandatory screen is anecdotal, although a collaborative study comparing one-screen and two-screen states is under way.

States that perform a single NBS may suggest a prompt repeat screen for a suspicious but not definitively abnormal initial NBS. For example, if the cutoff or "action level" at a given newborn screening laboratory for phenylalanine (the analyte elevated in PKU) is 121 µmole/L, but the level known to be associated with PKU is >150 µmole/L, the NBS program may suggest a prompt repeat screen for babies whose initial level is >120 but <150 µmole/L.

The point of newborn screening is to identify affected infants before symptoms develop, so physical examination is usually normal in the newborn nursery. However, certain features may give clues to a disorder in the NBS. Ambiguous genitalia and/or increased pigmentation may be seen in infants with 21-hydroxylase deficiency; children with certain organic or amino acidopathies may be irritable, hypertonic, or hypotonic; infants with glutaric aciduria I may have macrocephaly; infants with galactosemia may have detectable cataracts, direct hyperbilirubinemia, and/or clinical evidence of coagulopathy; infants with disorders of urea cycle may have tachypnea and irritability associated with hyperammonemia; infants with certain organic or amino acidopathies may have a characteristic smell such as the smell of maple syrup.

Each state decides for which disorders it wishes to screen. However, recently an expert panel convened by the American College of Medical Genetics with support from the federal Genetics Branch of the Maternal and Child Health Bureau recommended a panel of 28 disorders (29 including newborn hearing screening) as **the "core panel."** Another 25 or so disorders (the number may vary depending on how multiple possible hemoglobinopathies are counted) were recommended as "secondary targets" that a state may wish to include as part of its program. Some secondary targets are identified by the same analytes that identify core disorders (e.g., tyrosinemia types I, II, and III are all identified by elevated blood tyrosine level.). Recently, severe combined immunodeficiency (SCID) was approved to be included in the core panel.[3,4]

The 29 disorders on the core panel are:

Organic acidopathies: Isovaleric aciduria, glutaric aciduria I, 3-OH 3CH3 glutaric aciduria (HMG), multiple carboxylase deficiency, methylmalonic acidemia, 3-methylcrotonyl CoA carboxylase deficiency, cobalamine A, B disorders, propionic acidemia, β-ketothiolase deficiency.

Fatty acid oxidation disorders: Medium-chain acyl-CoA dehydrogenase (MCAD) deficiency, very-long-chain acyl-CoA dehydrogenase (VLCAD) deficiency, long-chain acyl-CoA dehydrogenase (LCHAD) deficiency, trifunctional protein deficiency, carnitine uptake defect.

Aminoacidopathies: PKU, maple syrup urine disease (MSUD), homocystinuria, citrullinemia, tyrosinemia type I, argininosuccinic acidemia. Of note, the most common urea cycle disorder, ornithine transcarbamylase (OTC) deficiency, is not detected on newborn screening.

Hemoglobinopathies: Variants of sickle cell disease, including Hb SS, Hb SC, Hb S/beta-thalassemia.

Others: Congenital hypothyroidism, congenital adrenal hyperplasia, biotinidase deficiency, galactosemia, cystic fibrosis, and hearing loss.

The amino acidopathies, organic acidopathies, and disorders of fatty acid oxidation (FAO) are detected by **tandem mass spectrometric (MS/MS) measurement** of amino acids and various acyl carnitines. Interpretation is complex and depends not only on the levels of the various analytes, but also on ratios of analytes.

Other methods are used for detection of congenital hypothyroidism, galactosemia, biotinidase deficiency, congenital adrenal hyperplasia,[5] hemoglobinopathies, and cystic fibrosis.

Further evaluation for children with abnormal or suspicious newborn screening depends on the disorder in question. Most newborn screening programs and the American College of Medical Genetics strongly recommend that all babies with abnormal newborn screens be seen urgently in many cases (PKU, organic acidopathies, amino acidopathies, fatty acid oxidation disorders, congenital hypothyroidism, congenital adrenal hyperplasia) and promptly in others (hemoglobinopathies, CF, biotinidase deficiency) at a specialized metabolic, endocrinologic, or hematologic referral center. These disorders are all complex and require specialized care.

Definitive diagnosis involves specific measurement of metabolites, sometimes molecular testing (DNA), sweat test, hemoglobin electrophoresis, or other specialized studies. **Management** of the metabolic disorders (organic acidopathies, amino acidopathies, disorders of fatty acid metabolism) is particularly complex and sometimes controversial. Although management of hemoglobinopathies and endocrine disorders may seem less complex, nevertheless there are complex aspects to these as well and **specialty referral is strongly recommended.**[6]

Practice-Based Learning and Improvement

Title
Expanded newborn screening for biochemical disorders: The effect of a false-positive result

Authors
Gurian EA, Kinnamon DD, Henry JH, Waisbren SE

Reference
Pediatrics 117(6):1915-1921, 2006

Historical significance/comments
NBS programs identify more than 50 disorders in some states. With increased biochemical disorders screened for by tandem mass spectroscopy (MS/MS), the number of false-positive results has increased. This inevitable result is due to the high sensitivity of a good screening test in detecting affected individuals while striving for a minimal false-negative rate. This study assessed the impact of a false-positive NBS result on parental stress, family relationships, and perceptions of the child's health by conducting interviews of parents who received a false-positive NBS screen result compared with parents whose infants had normal NBS results. All parents completed a parenting stress index. Findings suggest that false-positive screening results may adversely affect parental stress levels as well as the parent-child relationship.

Interpersonal and Communication Skills

Provide Verbal and Written Information on Newborn Screening

In almost all states newborn screening is mandatory. Nevertheless, every effort needs to be made to ensure that families are well informed about screening. Information should be provided by obstetricians and other prenatal care providers. Pediatricians should be prepared to inform families in the prenatal period about newborn screening and should be able to discuss, in at least a preliminary fashion, the screening results. Each state has brochures designed for families, and most states also have a detailed practitioner's manual. Written information about the testing is helpful because new parents may be overwhelmed or focused on getting answers to their own questions. Having some written communication that can be read at home later is helpful to reinforce the points made at the office visit. Pediatricians should have some mechanism in their offices to ensure that each baby they see has had an appropriate newborn screen.[7,8]

Professionalism

Communication and Collaboration: Explain the Process and Benefits of Newborn Screening Programs

Recently some observers have questioned whether it is appropriate for newborn screening to be mandatory. Perhaps there should be carefully obtained informed consent from parents before a specimen is obtained. Others say that it would be difficult, if not impossible, to obtain such consent during the stressful time of labor, childbirth, and the neonatal period. It is argued that there are proven benefits of newborn screening, and that if the baby were competent he/she would choose to have the heel stick and the possibility of a false-positive result with potential further pain and anxiety in order that a disorder that is responsive to intervention not be missed. The pediatrician should be prepared to discuss these issues with parents.[7,9]

Systems-Based Practice

Health-Care Economics: Cost-Benefits of Newborn Screening Programs

There are numerous cost-benefit ratio studies on screening for PKU, congenital hypothyroidism, and congenital adrenal hyperplasia in the United States and Europe. All have shown a favorable cost-benefit ratio. Cost-effectiveness studies of the entire 28-disorder panel are under way, but preliminary reports indicate that adoption of the expanded panel for newborn screening is cost-effective. However, physicians need to recognize the costs of false-positive findings, which include direct costs (e.g., necessary diagnostic workup), indirect costs (e.g., absence from work of parents), and intangible costs (e.g., anxiety and distress).[7,9,10]

References

1. Therrell B, Johnson A, Williams D: Status of newborn screening programs in the United States. *Pediatrics* 117:212-252, 2006.
2. Van Dyck P, Edwards ES: A look at newborn screening: Today and tomorrow. *Pediatrics* 117:S193, 2006.
3. American College of Medical Genetics Report: Newborn screening: Toward a uniform screening panel and system. *Genet Med* 8(suppl 1):S1-252S, 2006.
4. Calonge N, Green NS, Rinaldo P, et al: Method for evaluating conditions nominated for population-based screening of newborns. *Genet Med* 12:153-159, 2010.
5. Botkin J, Clayton E, Fost N, et al: Newborn screening technology: Proceed with caution. *Pediatrics* 117:1793-1797, 2006.
6. Puryear M, Tonniges T, van Dyck P, et al: American Academy of Pediatrics Newborn Screening Task Force recommendations: How far have we come? *Pediatrics* 117:S194, 2006.
7. Health Resources and Services Administration: These tests could save your baby's life. Available at http://www.genes-r-us.uthscsa.edu.
8. Perrin JM, Knapp AA, Browning MF, et al: An evidence based developmental process for newborn screening. *Genet Med* 12:131-134, 2010.
9. Pollitt RJ: Newborn blood spot screening: New opportunities, old problems. *J Inherit Metab Dis* 32:395, 2009.
10. Johnson K, Puryear M, Mann M, et al: Financing state newborn screening programs and uses of funds. *Pediatrics* 117:S270, 2006.

Chapter 58
Newborn Hearing Screen (Case 22)

Judith A. Turow MD

Medical Knowledge and Patient Care

Background

Before the implementation of formal screening programs, congenital hearing impairment was historically difficult to detect. Many children were well over 2 years of age before significant hearing loss was identified, and therefore intervention was lacking during the critical time for language development. The incidence of congenital deafness is estimated at 1 to 3:1000 among term well babies and 2 to 4:1000 among infants with neonatal intensive care unit (NICU) admission.[1-3] Identification of newborns with defective hearing and prompt intervention before 6 months of age has been shown to significantly improve both receptive and expressive language development.

Universal Newborn Hearing Screening (UNHS) was established in the 1990s, and was endorsed by the American Academy of Pediatrics (AAP) in 1999. The AAP 2007 position paper recommends initial screening by 1 month of age. For those with a positive screen, comprehensive audiologic evaluation should occur by 3 months of age, with appropriate intervention by age 6 months for those with confirmed hearing loss (HL). Ongoing surveillance to include addressing parental concerns, middle ear examination, development, and behavior assessment of hearing for all children is recommended during routine well child visits beginning at age 2 months.[4] Children at risk should be evaluated throughout childhood with repeat audiologic testing every 6 months until 3 years of age. Low-risk children should have routine surveillance and repeat hearing testing before kindergarten entry.[3] An infant with delayed speech or concern for hearing impairment should be evaluated, even if a prior hearing screen was passed.[4]

Categories of Hearing Loss

There are three types of HL: sensorineural, conductive, and mixed. **Sensorineural hearing loss (SNHL)** includes the inner ear, cochlea, semicircular canals and internal auditory canals, the auditory nerve, the brainstem, and auditory neural pathway to the auditory cortex. **Conductive hearing loss (CHL)** involves impedance of sound through the outer and/or middle ear. **Mixed HL** is a combination of both.[1,2]

The magnitude of HL is classified by decibels (dB) of HL as **mild, moderate, severe, or profound.** Mild HL ranges from 20 to 40 dB, moderate from 40 to 60 dB, severe from 60 to 80 dB, and profound greater than 80 dB.

Newborn nursery screening programs have been instituted to identify bilateral and unilateral sensorineural HL and permanent conductive HL. Infants admitted to the NICU are screened for sensorineural HL, which may include a cochlear abnormality or auditory neuropathy/dyssynchrony (AN).[4] AN is characterized by a normal response to sound (the cochlear hair cells are spared), but affected individuals are unable to process sounds (sound transmission in the eighth nerve is disordered); therefore the ability to understand speech and language is compromised.[5]

Screening Tests

Two screening tests for newborns are used: the **automated auditory brainstem response (AABR)** and the **transient evoked otoacoustic emissions (OAE).** They are noninvasive and record physiologic activity of normal auditory function. With OAE, an external ear probe (with a sensitive microphone) records cochlear outer hair cell responses to a series of soft clicks. Normal cochlear hairs respond to sound waves with echoes. The OAE measures response of these hair cells to the clicks, compares them to computerized standardized responses, and generates a pass or fail (i.e., refer). The status of the peripheral auditory system from the pinna to the cochlear outer hair cells is assessed. AABR measures action potentials in the auditory pathway from the peripheral hearing system, the eighth cranial nerve, and the brainstem to the level of the midbrain. Earphones emit a series of soft clicks. Three electrodes placed on the infant's forehead, mastoid, and nape of the neck measure electroencephalographic wave activity generated by the cochlea, eighth nerve, and the lower brainstem auditory pathway. Neural responses are compared with computerized standardized responses, and a pass or fail is generated. Infants who fail the initial screen are given a repeat screen by 4 weeks of age. If the repeat screen is not passed, complete audiologic evaluation with a diagnostic auditory brainstem response (ABR) is the next diagnostic step.[3,4] If an infant fails complete audiologic testing, evaluation by a team of professionals, including a pediatric otolaryngologist, geneticist, early intervention educator, speech pathologist, and pediatric ophthalmologist is indicated, with appropriate intervention instituted by 6 months of age.

Limitations of Screening

Screening has several limitations. Only moderate to severe hearing loss is detected. Some who initially pass will later be shown to have some degree of HL. This may reflect progressive degeneration, as in asymptomatic congenital cytomegalovirus infection, or the limited sensitivity of the screening tools to detect mild HL. Neural conduction disorders or auditory neuropathy/dyssynchrony are not detected with OAE. Adverse environmental conditions can affect screening results; testing is facilitated in a quiet environment. An abnormal screen is repeated by 4 weeks of age, and systems need to be in place for follow-up of abnormal results, including communication with the pediatrician.

A one-step screening procedure uses a single technology, either OAE or AABR, and has a higher false-positive detection rate.[4] A two-step program initially uses OAE, and retesting for those who do not pass is either a second attempt with OAE or an AABR. The two-step procedure is more expensive but has a lower false-positive rate; hence fewer infants are referred for unnecessary complete audiologic testing.[4] If an infant is tested twice using OAE, or initially with OAE and then with AABR and passes the second test, the infant is considered to pass.[4] If the initial AABR is not passed, the infant should not be rescreened using OAE, because there could be auditory neuropathy/dyssynchrony, which is undetected with OAE.

Infants who spend at least 5 days in the NICU are at risk for auditory neuropathy/dyssynchrony and should only be screened with AABR. All infants with a positive screen should be referred to audiology for diagnostic ABR. Both ears should be rescreened in those who refer in one ear. For an infant in the NICU with a risk factor such as hyperbilirubinemia requiring exchange transfusion or culture-positive sepsis, rescreening is recommended before discharge.

Differential Diagnosis

Nonsyndromic congenital hearing loss	Craniofacial anomaly–associated hearing loss
Congenital syndrome–associated hearing loss	Congenital infection–associated hearing loss

Introduction

When I evaluate an infant with a positive newborn hearing screen, I perform a comprehensive evaluation that begins with a history and physical examination. I inquire if the parents have a written copy of the results and whether a second screen was performed. I realize congenital hearing loss is often due to a single gene mutation, but check for other causes such as a primary maternal cytomegalovirus (CMV) infection.[1,4,6] Birth history is relevant if there was significant asphyxia requiring mechanical ventilation, severe hyperbilirubinemia, or admission to the neonatal intensive care unit (NICU).[1,6] The examination should focus on clues such as a craniofacial anomaly or dysmorphic features suggestive of a specific syndrome.[1,6] An infant with confirmed hearing loss is referred for comprehensive team evaluation for diagnosis of etiology and management, which may include hearing aid or eventual cochlear implant.[1,6] Definitive intervention by age 6 months of age will help maximize expressive and receptive language development.[1,6,7]

Clinical Entities	Medical Knowledge

Nonsyndromic Congenital Hearing Loss

Pφ	Over 60 genetic loci have been identified that cause isolated hearing loss, and at least 70% are autosomal recessive. Some are mutations in the gap junction proteins β2 and β6. For example, a mutation of GJβ2, which encodes the connexin protein 26 in the cochlea, results in moderate to severe bilateral hearing loss.
TP	Normal-appearing child with a normal physical examination.
Dx	A confirmed positive hearing screen is followed up with a diagnostic avditory brainstem response (ABR).
Tx	The multidisciplinary team approach is described in detail above. The goal is to implement amplification and early intervention services by 6 months of age and to bring appropriate candidates to a tertiary facility for evaluation for cochlear implantation. **See Nelson Essentials 10.**

Craniofacial Anomaly–Associated Hearing Loss

Pφ	There are a wide array of anomalies involving the auricle and external auditory canal associated with conductive hearing loss (CHL) and/or SNHL.
TP	There may be a malformed and/or misplaced pinna, atretic or absent external ear canal, and/or preauricular pits or appendages.
Dx	The evaluation at birth and beyond is diagnostic ABR, high-resolution imaging, and a skilled multidisciplinary team of professionals that includes audiology, otolaryngology, genetics, educators from early intervention, speech pathology, and ophthalmology, and perhaps plastic surgery. Specific imaging and genetic testing are determined on an individual basis.
Tx	Treatment is individualized based on the evaluation and may involve cochlear implant and/or reconstructive surgery. **See Nelson Essentials 50.**

Congenital Infection–Associated Hearing Loss

Pφ Several maternal infections can result in perinatal hearing loss.

CMV: Both primary and reactivation infections occur during pregnancy. Primary infections are more likely to be transmitted to the neonate than reactivation infection (40% versus 1%), and there is greater likelihood of symptoms at birth that may be isolated progressive hearing progressive loss or a full-blown syndrome affecting the brain, eyes, liver, and skin.

Toxoplasmosis: A primary infection in pregnancy with the protozoan *Toxoplasma gondii* can infect the fetus and either be asymptomatic or produce direct effects on the brain, eyes, liver, spleen, and skin.

Syphilis: A maternal infection with the spirochete *Treponema pallidum* can cause congenital syphilis, and the newborn may range from asymptomatic to the protean manifestations outlined below.

TP *CMV:* There may be asymptomatic infection with development of progressive SNHL or the full-blown syndrome with microcephaly, cranial periventricular calcifications, jaundice, hepatitis, petechiae and thrombocytopenia, seizures, abnormal muscle tone, and severe intellectual disability.

Toxoplasmosis: At birth, 70% to 90% of infected infants are asymptomatic and normal appearing. The classic triad in symptomatic infants is chorioretinitis, hydrocephalus, and intracranial calcifications. Findings at birth may include fever, maculopapular rash, hepatosplenomegaly, seizures, jaundice, thrombocytopenia, microcephaly, and rarely generalized lymphadenopathy.

Syphilis: Most with congenital infection are asymptomatic with a normal examination at birth. Fetal findings may include hydrops and stillbirth, with in utero death in up to 25% of cases. Early findings in the symptomatic newborn include rash on palms and soles, hepatosplenomegaly, jaundice, anemia, and "snuffles." There may be periostitis and metaphyseal dystrophy noted on radiographs.

Dx *CMV:* Urine CMV culture to be sent by 3 weeks of age to document congenital infection.

Toxoplasmosis: Specific maternal and infant titers.

Syphilis: Positive rapid plasma reagin (RPR) with a confirming specific treponemal test. A spinal tap is performed to exclude meningitis.

Tx   *CMV:* In the full clinical syndrome, ganciclovir has been used, in addition to supportive care to the extent needed, followed by early intervention for therapy and development tracking. The asymptomatic child with a confirmed case is monitored with hearing evaluations through age 6 years. Augmentative hearing-assist devices or cochlear implant may be indicated. *Toxoplasmosis:* There is no specific treatment, and supportive care and early intervention is provided as needed. Augmentative hearing-assist devices or cochlear implant may be indicated. *Syphilis:* Treatment is with parenteral penicillin. **See Nelson Essentials 66.**

Congenital Syndrome–Associated Hearing Loss

Approximately one third of hereditary hearing loss is syndromic. There are over 500 syndromes with associated hearing loss, and 80% of these are autosomal recessive (AR), 18% are autosomal dominant (AD), and 2% are X-linked recessive. Below is a list of several syndromes and their manifestations.[1,4]

AR inheritance of hearing loss includes syndromes such as Alport syndrome, Usher syndrome, Pendred syndrome, and Jervell and Lange-Nielsen syndrome.

- In Alport syndrome there is a defect in hearing in addition to renal disease. Hematuria is the usual presenting feature, with onset of hearing loss later, usually by late childhood or early adolescence, and generally before the onset of renal failure.
- Usher syndrome occurs in 3% to 6% of deaf children and perhaps another 3% to 6% of those who are hard of hearing. There is a combination of congenital hearing loss and retinitis pigmentosa. Hearing can range from normal to profound hearing loss at birth, as well as a loss of balance. Vision changes are noted between late school-age and young adult years.
- Pendred syndrome is an inherited disorder that accounts for as much as 10% of hereditary deafness and is associated with a malformation of the cochlea with congenital hearing loss and impaired balance, goiter, and intellectual disability.
- Jervell and Lange-Nielsen syndrome is a rare cause of profound congenital hearing loss associated with prolonged QT syndrome and cardiac arrhythmia.

AD inheritance of hearing loss includes Waardenburg syndrome, neurofibromatosis, and branchio-oto-renal (BOR) syndrome.

- Waardenburg syndrome is associated with piebaldism, heterochromia, and SNHL in 20% of cases.
- Neurofibromatosis is associated with tumors of the nerves, and in the case of neurofibromatosis II bilateral tumors of the eighth nerve, with hearing loss as early as adolesence, and possible tinnitus and poor balance.
- BOR syndrome affects the ear, kidneys and neck. There is an underdeveloped or absent kidney, preauricular pits or appendages, malformed or absent pinna and/or middle ear, and occasional fistula of the neck. People with BOR may have mild to profound hearing loss, which may be CHL, SNHL, or mixed

  Syndromes with deafness and associated craniofacial abnormalities: Treacher Collins, Goldenhar, Crouzon disease, and Apert

  Syndromes with deafness and associated visual loss: Usher, Alström, Cockayne, and Refsum. **See Nelson Essentials 48, 56, 163, and 186.**

Practice-Based Learning and Improvement

Title
Language of early and later identified children with hearing loss

Authors
Yoshinaga-Itano C, Sedey A, Coulter D, Mehl A

Reference
Pediatrics 102(5):1161-1171, 1998

Historical significance/comments
Despite intensive intervention services, improved hearing aid equipment, and improved educational services, children in the latter part of the twentieth century with congenital deafness had dismal educational statistics that had showed little improvement in 30 years. In this study, children whose HL was identified by 6 months of age had significantly greater expressive and receptive language abilities with language quotients >20 points above those identified later.

Practice-Based Learning and Improvement: Evidence-Based Pediatrics

Title
The evaluation of children with hearing loss

Authors
Greinwald JH, Hartnick C

Reference
Arch Otolaryngol Head Neck Surg 2002;128:84-87

Problem

As incidence of hearing loss from infection has fallen with better preventive care, the incidence of nonsyndromic hearing loss from genetic causes has risen.

Intervention

Single gene mutation *GJB2*, encoding connexin protein (Cx26), appears responsible for approximately 40% of severe to profound SNHL. Targeted genetic screening of this population allows families an opportunity for diagnosis and genetic counseling.

Historical significance/comments

A suggested approach to evaluation of hearing loss is provided along with discussion that most isolated congenital hearing loss is due to a single gene mutation.

Interpersonal and Communication Skills

Review Test Results and Explain Follow-Up Procedures

In preparation for discharge, it is important to review with the parents the results of tests done on the baby. Be sure to provide the results of the hearing screen and provide a few educational points to the parents. Discuss normal speech development depends upon the child having normal hearing. For infants who need a repeat hearing screen, explain that in most cases the result will be normal on rescreening, but identification of true hearing loss in the neonatal period is critically important for appropriate intervention. The parents should be given an appointment for outpatient follow-up as part of the discharge instructions.

Professionalism

Reliability and Responsibility: Follow Through the Diagnostic Process

All newborns should be screened before discharge. If needed, rescreening should occur by 1 month of age. Failure of the rescreening should trigger a comprehensive audiologic evaluation by 3 months of age. Professionals with expertise in congenital HL should initiate appropriate intervention by no later than 6 months of age. In addition, consultation may be needed with genetics, ophthalmology, neurology, and developmental pediatrics. Services for evaluation and treatment should be coordinated by the primary care professional within the medical home. The primary care physician must be reliable and responsible to ensure that this critical timeline in both evaluation and initiation of services is maintained for optimal speech and language development.

Systems-Based Practice

Mandated Newborn Hearing Screening

Forty-one states, including the District of Columbia, have mandated Universal Newborn Hearing Screening (UNHS), and approximately 95% of infants born in the United States have their hearing screened.[1,7] However, almost half who do not pass either fail to receive confirmatory audiologic evaluation or come to the attention of early intervention services. The essential components of a successful program are initial screening, and identification, evaluation, and tracking with follow-up and referrals coordination.[6] Screening involves systematic universal newborn screening and rescreening where appropriate. Identification and intervention involve successfully reaching and treating all newborns with significant HL. Evaluation involves reviewing the components of the entire program. Tracking and follow-up entail development of programs to monitor all referrals and missed referrals, and to communicate with the child's family and physicians.[6] For a positive screening, specialty referrals include audiology and otolaryngology, speech-language pathologists, special educators with specific training in hearing impairment, and other early intervention professionals, including a care coordinator.

References

1. Wrightson S: Universal Newborn Hearing Screening. *Am Fam Physician* 75(9):1349-1352, 2007.
2. Yoshinaga-Itano C, Coulter D, Thomson V: Infant hearing impairment and universal hearing screening. *J Perinatol* 20:S131-S136, 2000.
3. Firkser, Shyan Sun: Universal newborn hearing screenings: A three-year experience; NIH consensus statement: Early identification of hearing impairment in infants and young children. *Pediatrics* 99(6):e4, 1997. doi:10.1542/peds.99.6.e4.
4. Year 2007 position statement: Principles and guidelines for early hearing detection and intervention programs, Joint Commission on Infant Hearing. *Pediatrics* 120(4):898-921, 2007.
5. Rance G: Auditory neuropathy/dys-synchrony and its perceptual consequences. *Trends Amplif* 9(1):1-43, 2005. doi:10.1177/108471380500900102. Available at http://tia.sagepub.com/cgi/content/short/9/1/1
6. Gregg R, Wiorek S, Arvedson J: Pediatric audiology: A review. *Pediatr Rev* 25:224-234, 2004.
7. Yoshinaga-Itano C, Sedey A, Coulter D, Mehl A: Language of early and later identified children with hearing loss. *Pediatrics* 102(5):1161-1171, 1998.

Chapter 59
The Late-Preterm Infant

Marilee C. Allen MD

Speaking Intelligently

When caring for a late-preterm infant, I realize that although these newborns may look and seem identical to term newborns, they are a vulnerable group whose needs may be overlooked in the term nursery. They deserve careful monitoring because they as a group have a high rate of hospital readmission soon after discharge for hyperbilirubinemia, respiratory illnesses, sepsis, and feeding difficulties. In addition, they have increased neurodevelopmental disability compared with term neonates. Before discharge, I perform a complete assessment that includes adequacy of feeding, especially if breastfeeding, and ensure timely arrangement of the first office visit to monitor weight and assess for jaundice.

Medical Knowledge and Patient Care

Caring for the sickest and most immature preterm infants is complex and time consuming. In a busy neonatal intensive care unit (NICU), the less acute issues that arise when caring for larger preterm infants may get less attention. These issues are nonetheless important.

Increased Neonatal Complications

Many infants born after 34 weeks' gestation do not require intensive care and room-in with their mothers or are cared for in intermediate care units. Those that are admitted to the NICU for respiratory distress, temperature instability, hypoglycemia, infection, hyperbilirubinemia, or feeding problems tend to improve within days. Overlooking the vulnerability of larger preterm infants by failing to recognize their prematurity or failing to monitor and address their specific needs can be catastrophic. Claudine Amiel-Tison views these infants, whom she calls "macropremies," as "underprivileged newborns."[1] Whether we call them macropremies, near-term infants, or late-preterm infants, there is no doubt that their relative immaturity makes them vulnerable to complications; they have higher mortality, morbidity, and neurodevelopmental disability rates than do full-term neonates.[2]

Obstetric and neonatal intensive care advances have progressively lowered the limit of viability, but most (71%) preterm infants are born at gestational age (GA) 34 to 36 weeks and 13% are born at GA 32 to 33 weeks. In contrast, infants born before 28 weeks' gestation constitute only 2% of live births and 6% of preterm births.[3]

At each week of GA, there is individual variation in size and degree of maturity: just as a 10-year-old can be tall or short for age, a newborn can be large for gestational age (LGA) or small for gestational age (SGA) and more or less mature than other infants born at the same GA. A 35-week gestational age infant may be able to suck well, maintain his/her temperature with bundling, and go home with his/her mother. Another infant born at GA 35 weeks may develop **hypoglycemia, temperature instability, feeding problems, respiratory distress, hyperbilirubinemia, apnea, patent ductus arteriosus, or sepsis.** As a group, infants born at GA 33 to 36 weeks have three to four times the neonatal complication rate as full-term neonates. Hyperbilirubinemia is twice as common and often more prolonged in near-term infants than in full-term infants. Coordination of sucking, swallowing, and breathing improves with GA. Lower muscle tone and lower exercise tolerance in late-preterm infants contributes to poor feeding, which in turn may lead to dehydration and higher bilirubin levels.

As a result of these complications, population studies demonstrate higher mortality rates, longer mean hospital stays, and higher hospital costs in late-preterm infants than in full-term neonates. Most infants born before 35 weeks' gestation are admitted to a NICU, and NICU admission rates decrease from approximately 50% at GA 35 weeks to 2% to 3% after 37 weeks' gestation. Neonatal mortality rates (death before 28 days) and infant mortality rates (death before 1 year) are three to four times higher in late-preterm infants than in full-term infants. Infants born at GA 34 to 36 weeks have higher rates of rehospitalization soon after discharge than full-term neonates.[4]

Neurologic Complications

Exactly how preterm birth and its various complications contribute to brain injury is unknown. There is no doubt that vulnerability to insults during this critical period of brain growth and development leads to more neurologic complications and higher rates of cerebral palsy in late-preterm infants compared with full-term infants. Brain volume increases linearly with GA, gray matter volume increases threefold from 30 to 40 weeks' GA, and myelinated white matter volume increases dramatically between 35 and 40 weeks GA. Cerebral palsy rates are six to nine times higher in preterm infants born at GA 32 to 36 weeks or with birth weights (BW) 1500 to 2499 grams than infants born full-term or with normal birth weight.[5,6]

Despite the lack of focused longitudinal developmental follow-up studies, there are data to suggest higher rates of delayed infant milestones, cognitive impairments, academic difficulties, and behavioral problems in children born at GA 32 to 36 weeks than in children born at term. Biologic factors (low GA or BW, male gender, the presence of congenital anomalies), abnormalities on infant neurodevelopmental exams and neuroimaging studies, and environmental factors (socioeconomic status, parental education, maternal psychological distress or depression, infant enrichment and educational programs) are also important predictors of neurodevelopmental outcome.[7]

Practice-Based Learning and Improvement

Whenever possible, take the opportunity to carefully examine very preterm, late-preterm/near-term, and full-term infants. Learn how they differ with respect to physical and neurologic signs of maturity. Compare examination findings between preterm LGA infants and full-term appropriate-for-gestational-age (AGA) infants, and between preterm AGA infants and full-term SGA infants. Familiarize yourself with the various prenatal and postnatal methods of estimating gestational age, and know their limitations (i.e., postnatal estimates are not as accurate as early prenatal estimates of gestational age). While in the NICU, notice how infants of different sizes and maturity respond to cold stress, infection, metabolic derangements, and feedings.

Interpersonal and Communication Skills

Explore Family Beliefs, Concerns, and Expectations About Their Premature Newborn

Although physicians may find late-preterm infants to be commonplace, parents may be very distressed about having a premature delivery. Recognize parental anxiety and explore their concerns and understanding of the condition. Listen empathically. In understandable language, discuss and answer parents' questions about the potential problems the near-term infant faces, including difficulty with temperature regulation, transition from fetal to postnatal circulation patterns, breathing, glucose control, infection risk, coordination of feeding, and risk for hyperbilirubinemia.

If the baby is stable, cautiously reassure parents that the majority of late-preterm infants do well, but these infants do need close monitoring in the hospital and good pediatric follow-up. Just as children at a given age vary in size and maturity, infants at a given gestational age will vary in size and degree of maturity.

Professionalism

Communication and Collaboration: Identify and Communicate With the Primary Care Pediatrician

Before hospital discharge, communicate, in person if possible, with the infant's primary care provider about the infant's diagnoses, hospital course, and any concerns or recommendations for further care. A legible and comprehensive discharge summary should be given to the parents and also sent, by mail or electronically, to the physician/s who will be following the baby after discharge.

Systems-Based Practice

Care Coordination: Hospital Discharge Planning

The discharge planning coordinator plays a vital role in the successful discharge and transition of a premature infant from the NICU by arranging necessary follow-up appointments after hospital discharge and helping the families connect with special services and resources available in the community and through the insurance company. For example, specialized infant formula may be required that is not readily available in stores, and the discharge planner will be the liaison between family and supplier. If specialized equipment or a medical supply (e.g., nasogastric tubes or suction catheters) need to be obtained, then the discharge planner will coordinate the service with the insurance company.

References

1. Amiel-Tison C, Allen MC, Lebrun F, Rogowski J: Macropremies: Underprivileged newborns. *Ment Retard Dev Disabil Res Rev* 8:281-292, 2002.
2. Engle WA, Tomashek KM, Wallman C: "Late-preterm" infants: A population at risk. *Pediatrics* 120:281-292, 2007.
3. Institute of Medicine Committee on Understanding Premature Birth and Assuring Healthy Outcomes: In Behrman R, Stith Butler A, editors: *Preterm birth: Causes, consequences, and prevention*, Washington, DC, 2007, National Academies Press.
4. Jain L, Raju TNK, editors: Late preterm pregnancy and the newborn. *Clin Perinatol* 33:751-972, 2006.
5. Allen MC: Preterm development. In Accardo PJ, editor: *Capute and Accardo's neurodevelopmental disabilities in infancy and childhood*, vol 2, Baltimore, 2008, Paul H. Brookes Publishing Co, pp 29-45.
6. Allen MC: The neonatal neurodevelopmental examination. In Accardo PJ, editor: *Capute and Accardo's neurodevelopmental disabilities in infancy and childhood*, vol 1, Baltimore, 2008, Paul H. Brookes, pp 333-366.
7. Raju TN, Higgins RD, Stark AR, Leveno KJ: Optimizing care and outcome for late preterm (near-term) infants: A summary of the workshop sponsored by the National Institute of Child Health and Human Development. *Pediatrics* 118:1207-1214, 2006.

Chapter 60
Jaundice (Case 23)

Kathryn Rausch Crowell MD

Case: A 48-hour-old term infant has jaundice extending to the abdomen. He was delivered at 39 weeks gestation via spontaneous vaginal delivery. Maternal blood type is A positive. His birth weight was 3240 grams and he is breastfeeding every 4 hours. Today his weight is 2950 grams.

Differential Diagnosis

Physiologic jaundice	Sepsis	ABO hemolytic disease
Glucose-6-phosphate dehydrogenase (G6PD) deficiency	Jaundice associated with breastfeeding	

Speaking Intelligently

All newborns have an increase in serum bilirubin that usually peaks by 72 hours of age, and jaundice is a common finding. Although most jaundice is benign, infants must be monitored and carefully assessed to **identify those at risk for development of severe hyperbilirubinemia.** This includes review of risk factors, assessment of feeding adequacy, and possibly a measurement of bilirubin, either transcutaneous or a serum level. A nomogram that plots bilirubin according to age in hours helps stratify infants into risk groups and identify who needs close follow-up. When assessing a newborn before discharge, I note how well the baby is nursing. Successful establishment of lactation with frequent feeding and minimal weight loss helps minimize peak serum bilirubin levels. A previous child who required phototherapy, gestation of less than 38 weeks, bruising or a cephalohematoma, and maternal-infant ABO blood group incompatibility are some additional risk factors associated with possible development of significant hyperbilirubinemia. Risk increases with more than one risk factor. With early hospital discharge, it is key to assess risk and arrange for the first office visit within 24 to 48 hours of discharge.

At high serum levels, bilirubin can diffuse into the brain and is toxic to the neonatal central nervous system. In rare cases, severe hyperbilirubinemia may result in acute bilirubin-induced neurologic dysfunction (BIND). Kernicterus, a syndrome of neurologic damage with muscle tone abnormality, cognitive deficits, and hearing impairment, results when these changes are permanent.

PATIENT CARE

Clinical Thinking
- Review prenatal information.
- Assess **adequacy of feeding,** especially if breastfed.
- Because visual estimation of the degree of jaundice is inaccurate, it is wise to check a transcutaneous or serum **bilirubin level** on all infants with visible jaundice.
- Total bilirubin is assessed based on the age of the infant in hours and plotted on an **hour-specific nomogram** to identify **risk level as low, low intermediate, high intermediate, or high** (Figure 60-1).
- Review the history, and perform testing to determine the cause of jaundice. Is it "physiologic?" Is it worsened by feeding difficulty and/ or excessive weight loss? Is there hemolysis resulting from ABO incompatibility, G6PD deficiency, or other hemolytic disease?
- Determine whether phototherapy is necessary (Figure 60-2). In many cases without active hemolysis, home phototherapy is safe with daily monitoring of feeding, weight gain, and bilirubin levels.

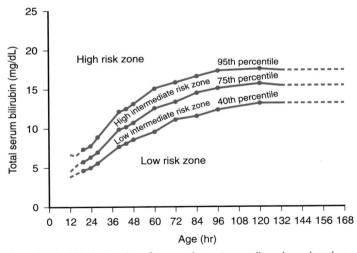

Figure 60-1 Risk designation of term and near-term well newborns based on their hour-specific bilirubin values. (Reproduced with permission from Bhutani VK, Johnson L, Sivieri EM: Predictive ability of a predischarge hour-specific bilirubin for subsequent significant hyperbilirubinemia in healthy term and near-term newborns. *Pediatrics*, 103:6-14, 1999, Fig. 2, Copyright © 1999 by the AAP.)

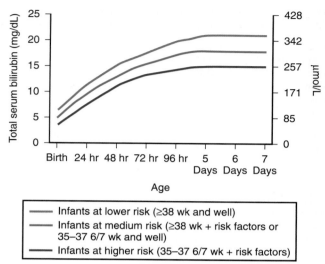

Figure 60-2 Guidelines for phototherapy in hospitalized infants of 35 or more weeks of gestation. (Reproduced with permission from AAP Clinical Practice Guideline. Subcommittee on Hyperbilirubinemia: Management of hyperbilirubinemia in the newborn infant 35 or more weeks of gestation. *Pediatrics* 114:297-316, 2004, Fig. 3, Copyright © 2004 by the AAP.)

History

- Consider **gestational age.** Late-preterm infants (35 to 37 weeks' gestation) need close monitoring and are at risk because of immaturity of the liver and blood-brain barrier (see Chapter 59, The Late-Preterm Infant).
- Consider **chronologic age.** Jaundice within the first 24 hours of life is pathologic. In addition, a rate of rise greater than 0.5 mg/dL/hr is concerning for active hemolysis.
- **Maternal blood type and antibody screen** should be documented. For maternal group O or Rh-negative mothers, infants should have a blood type and direct antibody (Coombs test) sent to determine if there is a "setup" for hemolysis.
- Consider **ethnicity.** Individuals of Mediterranean, Middle Eastern, Southeast Asian, and African descent may have G6PD deficiency causing hemolysis.
- Babies of Southeast Asian descent may have higher bilirubin levels independent of other factors.
- Has a **previous child** required phototherapy?
- Have any family members had splenectomy or cholecystectomy to suggest **hereditary spherocytosis?**

Physical Examination

- Jaundice develops in a **cephalocaudal** progression and is usually first seen in the face with progression to the trunk and extremities.
- Note icteric sclerae.
- Review vital signs, including head circumference, length, and weight. Note degree of **weight loss.**
- **Hepatomegaly** may indicate biliary atresia or congenital infection.
- Note bruising or a cephalohematoma.

Tests for Consideration

• **Transcutaneous (Tc) bilirubin level**	$85
• **Serum total and direct bilirubin level**	$194
• **Maternal blood group and antibody screen**	$650
• **Infant blood group**	$350
• **Direct antibody test (DAT) or direct Coombs:** To check presence of maternal anti-A and/or anti-B antibodies bound to infant red blood cells	$87
• **Complete blood count (CBC):** Hemoglobin as an indicator of degree of hemolysis; thrombocytopenia and elevated or depressed white cell count raise concern for sepsis	$116
• **Peripheral blood smear:** Note microspherocytes as evidence of hemolysis	$75
• **Reticulocyte count:** To evaluate response to hemolysis	$74
• **Quantitative G6PD:** Consider if appropriate ethnicity	$61
• **Blood culture:** If concern for sepsis	$152
• **Cerebrospinal fluid analysis and culture:** If concern for sepsis	$557
• **Newborn screen—thyroid-stimulating hormone (TSH) or thyroxine:** Congenital hypothyroidism is associated with prolonged jaundice. **Qualitative G6PD:** Is included in most newborn screens	$227

IMAGING CONSIDERATIONS

→ **Abdominal ultrasound:** If elevated direct bilirubin to identify biliary atresia or other hepatobiliary pathology	$846

ABO Hemolytic Disease

Pφ Infants who have blood group A or B born to a mother who is blood type O may have maternal anti-A or anti-B IgG antibodies attached to their red blood cells, and this is confirmed by a positive direct antiglobulin test (DAT or Coombs test). These antibodies occasionally trigger red cell hemolysis and increase the infant's bilirubin load, causing significant jaundice.

TP These babies are a "setup," and most who are affected present with significant elevation of total bilirubin and jaundice within the first 24 hours of life.

Dx Diagnosis is made with maternal blood group O, infant group A or B; positive DAT (Coombs test); jaundice appearing in the first 24 hours after birth; and microspherocytes on peripheral blood smear. Other factors such as difficulty with breastfeeding and excessive weight loss contribute to elevated levels of bilirubin.

Tx Phototherapy is indicated for significant bilirubin elevation, again assessed according to age in hours. The degree of ongoing hemolysis is monitored by following the hemoglobin and reticulocyte counts in addition to serum bilirubin. Transcutaneous bilirubin measurements are not accurate once phototherapy has been initiated. With an active hemolytic process, many pediatricians obtain a "rebound" total bilirubin within 12 to 24 hours after stopping phototherapy.[1,2] **See Nelson Essentials 62.**

Glucose-6-Phosphate Dehydrogenase Deficiency

Pφ G6PD is an enzyme that promotes red blood cell membrane stability. With *G6PD deficiency,* there may be excessive hemolysis and prolonged jaundice triggered by the stress of birth, or later in life due to oxidative stress induced by certain medications, foods, or infection. The *G6PD* gene is located on the X chromosome, so hemizygous males have the full enzyme deficiency. However, heterozygote females are also at increased risk. These neonates have increased heme turnover and an impaired ability to conjugate bilirubin.

TP G6PD deficiency occurs in those of Mediterranean, Middle Eastern, southeast Asian, and African decent and *should be suspected in jaundiced infants whose family history or ethnic background are suggestive or in infants with poor response to phototherapy.*

Dx	Quantitative G6PD level confirms the diagnosis. Qualitative screening is included in many newborn screens.
Tx	These infants are managed as described under ABO hemolytic disease. In addition, the family should be counseled about this condition and the need to avoid certain medications and foods (fava beans) that precipitate hemolysis (see Chapter 45, Anemia). **See Nelson Essentials 150.**

Sepsis

Pφ	*Sepsis* may cause an increase in red blood cell hemolysis and a decrease in the hepatic excretion of bilirubin, with elevation in indirect and/or direct bilirubin.
TP Dx Tx	Consider sepsis when a jaundiced infant presents with temperature instability, poor feeding, hypoglycemia, irritability, hypotonia, apnea, or respiratory difficulty (see Chapter 46, Neonatal Fever; Chapter 62, Early-Onset Group B Streptococcal Disease; Chapter 66, Transient Tachypnea of the Newborn; and Chapter 77, Neonatal Sepsis). **See Nelson Essentials 65.**

ZEBRA ZONE

a. **Biliary atresia:** Paucity of extrahepatic bile ducts leads to cholestasis and direct hyperbilirubinemia; surgical intervention with the Kasai procedure (hepatoportoenterostomy) by 6 weeks of age is associated with a better outcome.

b. **Galactose-1-phosphate uridyl transferase deficiency:** Classic galactosemia with complete enzyme deficiency—the inability to metabolize galactose-1-phosphate with toxicity to the kidneys, liver, and brain.

Practice-Based Learning and Improvement: Evidence-Based Pediatrics

Title
A primer on phototherapy for the jaundiced newborn

Author
Maisels MJ

Reference
Contemp Pediatr 22:38-57, 2005

Historical significance/comments
This tutorial on phototherapy, written by a thought leader in the field, provides an excellent understandable treatise on technical and historical aspects of phototherapy for the general practitioner.

Interpersonal and Communication Skills

Maintain Complete and Legible Medical Records

Successful identification and treatment of jaundiced newborns requires a team approach. Often nurses or midlevel providers are the first to recognize that an infant is jaundiced, and this must be communicated to the physician. Laboratory results from both the mother and infant are important to be communicated. In babies with extreme jaundice or jaundice that develops in the first 24 hours of life, evaluation of serial bilirubin levels is usually indicated. In some cases, phototherapy might be instituted. Infants who require phototherapy should be closely monitored by all staff. Appropriate evaluation of these infants and subsequent monitoring requires medical record documentation so that all members of the health-care team are aware of laboratory test results, changes, and new findings. At institutions without electronic medical records, legible handwriting is crucial.

Professionalism

Advocacy: Provide Opportunity for Maternal-Infant Bonding

Infants who require phototherapy are often separated from their mother for extended periods of time. Support for bonding and maintenance of breastfeeding is very important. Physicians should encourage their hospital to allow a mother to stay on the postpartum floor beyond the usual time of discharge to be with their infant who is under phototherapy. If this request is denied, transferring the infant to a pediatric ward where the mother can stay in the infant's room is another option.

Systems-Based Practice

Managed Care: Authorization for Home Phototherapy

Well established in safety and efficacy, phototherapy is the treatment of choice for hyperbilirubinemia. There are no standardized methods for the delivery of phototherapy, and there are numerous light sources available in the market approved by the U.S. Food and Drug Administration (FDA). If the total serum bilirubin (TSB) level meets criteria for home treatment as outlined in the American Academy of Pediatrics 2004 guideline, home phototherapy may be initiated as opposed to readmitting the child to the hospital. Coverage for home phototherapy devices is usually subject to the terms, conditions, and limitations of the applicable patient's insurance benefit plan and more specifically the durable medical equipment (DME) benefit. Under many benefit plans, coverage for DME is limited to the lowest-cost alternative. In addition, some DME items need to be authorized in advance by the insurance company before they are actually provided to the patient. Some insurance policies authorize a daily home visit during phototherapy for a feeding assessment, weight check, and obtaining a heelstick bilirubin level to monitor progression of therapy.

References

1. American Academy of Pediatrics, Subcommittee on Hyperbilirubinemia: Clinical practice guideline: management of hyperbilirubinemia in the newborn infant 35 or more weeks of gestation, *Pediatrics* 2004;114:297-316.
2. Maisels MJ: Neonatal hyperbilirubinemia. In Polin RA, Yoder MC, editors: *Workbook in practical neonatology*, Philadelphia, 2007, Elsevier, pp 53-71.

Chapter 61
Feeding Difficulty in the Newborn (Case 24)

Edelveis R. M. Clapp DO

Case: A 7-day-old term infant has lost 9% of her birth weight. She is breastfeeding every 3 hours and has four wet and two stool diapers per day. The prenatal and newborn nursery course were normal, and she is well appearing.

Differential Diagnosis

Inadequate caloric intake	Sepsis	Maternal depression

Speaking Intelligently

When I approach a newborn who is not gaining weight at a rate of 15 to 30 g/day, I first consider the most obvious cause. Malnutrition is the most common culprit, especially in a breastfed infant. An accurate history is key in sorting out the difficulty. Is the infant latching well? Is mother's milk in? How often is the infant feeding? Are there socioeconomic factors that could be affecting the well-being of the child? It is also important to rule out congenital abnormality or infection as the underlying cause of inadequate weight gain.

PATIENT CARE

Clinical Thinking
- Review the prenatal history, newborn course, and family history.
- Check vital signs—is the heart rate or respiratory rate elevated? Is the baby in distress and requiring stabilization with IV fluids or antibiotics?
- Is the infant **dehydrated? Jaundiced?** Is the skin turgor poor? Wetting diapers?
- A complete evaluation may be needed if there is concern for **sepsis.**
- What is the interaction between the mother and child? Are there concerns for **postpartum depression?** How does the mother feel about breastfeeding?

History
- Any problems in the nursery?
- How frequently is the infant feeding? How long do the feedings last? Does the infant **tire or sweat with feeds?** Is there **cyanosis?** Does the baby **spit up excessively or vomit?** Has mother's milk come in?
- Address hydration status by number of wet diapers, and stool frequency and quality.
- Check **mental status.** Is the baby alert and vigorous, or difficult to arouse? Is the infant irritable or in pain?
- Are there **signs or symptoms of infection?** Is there fever? Hypothermia?
- Has the infant had phototherapy?

Physical Examination
- Vital signs: Changes associated with dehydration include tachypnea, tachycardia, and weight loss. Hypotension is a late sign. Check for fever or hypothermia.
- Assess hydration status. Check the fontanelle, skin turgor, and mucous membranes.
- Check the tongue for **short frenulum.**

- Auscultate the heart for murmurs, abnormal rate and sounds.
- Palpate **femoral pulses,** and check capillary refill.
- Look for signs of **focal infection,** such as cellulitis.
- Watch the baby feed. Does he/she **latch well?** Is there milk transfer? Does the baby seem to swallow? Is the baby satisfied after a feed?

Tests for Consideration
- **Newborn metabolic screen:** Results may take up to 2 weeks. $227
- **Electrolytes:** If concern for dehydration. $174
- If the infant is lethargic, fontanelle is bulging, or infection is suspected:
  - **Complete blood count** $116
  - **Urinalysis** $95
  - **Urine culture** $148
  - **Blood culture** $152
  - **Cerebrospinal fluid (CSF) culture** $152
  - **CSF cell count** $150
  - **CSF Gram stain** $180
  - **CSF protein and glucose** $75
  - **Total bilirubin** $97
  - **Direct bilirubin** $97

IMAGING CONSIDERATIONS

→ **Abdominal radiographs:** If vomiting or delayed passage of meconium $219
→ **Echocardiogram:** Consider if murmur or diminished femoral pulses are noted $1630
→ If concern for abuse or focal neurologic findings:
  - **Head ultrasound** $361
  - **Head computed tomography** $1827

Clinical Entities	Medical Knowledge

Inadequate Caloric Intake

PF Underfeeding is the most common reason for failure to gain weight. The breastfed infant may have a poor latch or immature suck-swallow mechanism. The mother's milk supply may not be well established or inadequate; therefore, the infant may not be getting adequate calories. Inquire if there is audible gulping and swallowing, or if milk is seen in the baby's mouth. Check if breast engorgement has occurred, and if the mother experiences a let-down reflex. All of these support adequate caloric intake. Inquire precisely how formula is prepared.

TP	Typically newborns are at their lowest weight on day 3 or 4. Up to 10% of birth weight can be lost, but weight should be increasing by the end of the first week and past birth weight by 14 days.[1] A mother may report she does not feel her milk is in, or engorgement was not significant (there is typically significant discomfort with engorgement), or they are having difficulty latching the baby.
Dx	The mother should feel engorged when her breast milk is in and may begin leaking before the next feeding. For formula fed infants, it is important to ask how formula is prepared. Infants who are ingesting inadequate calories will either continue to lose weight, not gain weight, or gain inadequate weight. Check carefully for a short frenulum that may interfere with effective latching. Infants are expected to gain 15 to 30 g/day for the first 3 months.[1] A detailed history will help identify the underlying cause of poor weight gain.
Tx	Newborns should be fed every 2 to 3 hours around-the-clock. Lactation consultants can be helpful with latching technique, positioning for feeds, and suggesting methods to stimulate production, such as fenugreek. Re-enforce that once the milk supply is established, breastfeeding functions as a supply-and-demand operation, and more frequent feeds that empty the breast result in increased milk production. Use of a breast pump will facilitate complete emptying. If weight gain is still inadequate with breastfeeding alone, it is appropriate to supplement after nursing with either pumped breast milk or formula. Stress that in most instances the infant should nurse first and then be offered supplemental bottle feeding. Weight should be closely monitored until a good pattern of gain is established. **See Nelson Essentials 22 and 27.**

Sepsis

See Chapter 46, Neonatal Fever; Chapter 62, Early-Onset Group B Streptococcal Disease; Chapter 66, Transient Tachypnea of the Newborn; and Chapter 77, Neonatal Sepsis, for discussions on sepsis.

Maternal Depression

Pφ Maternal factors that play a role in inadequate infant weight gain are many fold, and encompass the following: There may be poor maternal-infant bonding as a result of postpartum depression, chronic depression, or another preexisting maternal medical condition.[5] Socioeconomic factors such as poverty and lack of paternal involvement may compound the impact of *maternal depression.* In addition, any of the concerns discussed above under inadequate caloric intake may be present.

TP A new mother may report the infant is very demanding or always crying. Some will even tell you that the baby doesn't like them, or rarely that they have thoughts of hurting their baby. Mothers with postpartum depression are often emotionally labile or have a flat affect. When there is poor infant-maternal bonding, the baby may be observed on the examination table while mom is sitting on the other side of the room. Inquire about involvement of the father or support available from family and/or friends.

Dx Every mother should be screened for postpartum depression at minimum for the first 6 weeks of the infant's life. Inquire about prior episodes of postpartum depression or major depression. Carefully assess the degree of maternal-infant bonding and the need for outside support. Determine if food insecurity and poverty is an issue. See Chapter 16, The Newborn Well Child Visit, for a discussion on screening for postpartum depression.

Tx The most important thing a physician can do for the parent is offer encouragement and support while monitoring the infant's progress, and refer a mother to her obstetrician for counseling and antidepressant therapy, especially if there have been previous episodes of postpartum depression or major depressive episodes. Recommend lactation support to maximize successful nursing, but there may be some instances in which breastfeeding is too stressful for the mother and encouragement to bottle-feed is indicated. For families who cannot afford formula or supplies for the infant, a social worker should be involved where possible. Some families may be eligible for the Special Supplemental Nutrition Program for Women, Infants, and Children (WIC) (see Chapter 56, Infant Feeding) or programs that provide formula at low cost.

ZEBRA ZONE

a. **Congenital heart disease:** Infants with lesions such as coarctation of the aorta or severe aortic stenosis are acyanotic with left-sided outflow tract obstruction. They may present with signs of congestive heart failure or poor feeding or sweating during feeds.

Practice-Based Learning and Improvement

Title
The pediatrician's role in infant feeding and decision-making

Author
Lawrence, RA

Reference
Pediatr Rev 14(7):265-272, 1993

Historical significance/outcome
Discussion of the role and influence of the pediatrician in the education and guidance for parental decisions about infant feeding and nutrition.

Interpersonal and Communication Skills

Demonstrate Appreciation of Assistance of Other Health-Care Professionals

The cause of feeding difficulties may range from simple to complex etiologies. In some cases the problem may require involvement and support from a variety of health-care team members, including lactation consultants, nutritionists, nurses, and social workers. It is important to maintain good working relationships with these important members of the comprehensive care team. Verbally thanking the consultant for seeing the patient or communicating thanks in your daily note is appreciated.

Professionalism

Indentify Parental Fears and Concerns

It is important to have good rapport with the family. Take some time, and use empathic listening skills to hear their concerns and fears. Often parents need only encouragement, positive reinforcement, and reassurance from their pediatrician to promote confidence for successful infant feeding.

Systems-Based Practice

Coordinate Resources to Achieve Optimal Feeding

Families of newborns with inadequate weight gain often need just support and reassurance. For those who require intervention, frequent outpatient weight checks, screens for postpartum depression, and judicious use of visiting nursing agencies and lactation consultants can all help prevent unnecessary emergency department visits and costly hospitalizations. Physicians must be knowledgeable about the standard services offered by the hospital lactation departments—monthly breastfeeding classes, lactation consultant visits, and breast pumps for purchase or rent. With more and more newborns discharged from the nursery early, primary care providers will need to become comfortable managing all inpatient and outpatient issues and coordinating the infant's care in the most efficient way.

References

1. American Academy of Pediatrics: *Pediatric nutrition handbook*, 6th ed, Elk Grove Village, IL, 2009, American Academy of Pediatrics.
2. Behrman RE: *Nelson textbook of pediatrics*, 18th ed, Philadelphia, 2004, Saunders.
3. Hay WW, Hayward AR, Levin MJ, et al: *Current pediatric diagnosis and treatment*, 16th ed, New York, 2003, Lange Medical Books, McGraw-Hill.
4. Lawrence RA: The pediatrician's role in infant feeding decision-making. *Pediatr Rev* 14(7):265-272, 1993.
5. Stellwagen L, Boles E: Care of the well newborn, *Pediatr Rev* 27(3):89-98, 2004.

Chapter 62
Early-Onset Group B Streptococcal Disease (Case 25)

Jennifer R. Miller MD

Case: A 37⅔-week infant with Apgar scores 8 and 9 presents at 1 hour of life with hypoxia, hypothermia, and tachypnea. Prenatal laboratory test results were normal except for unknown maternal group B streptococcus status. On examination, the infant is in moderate respiratory distress with tachypnea, flaring, retractions, grunting, and crackles at lung bases. There is a grade II/VI systolic murmur at the left midsternal border. Oxygen saturation is 88% on room air.

Differential Diagnosis

Early-onset group B streptococcal disease	Pneumothorax	Perinatal pneumonia
Transient tachypnea of the newborn	Non–group B streptococcal sepsis	

Speaking Intelligently

When I evaluate a newborn with respiratory distress, I first check the airway, breathing, and circulation (ABCs), position the airway, and provide supplemental oxygen if there is significant tachypnea and/or hypoxemia. I quickly review the course of labor and any risk factors for sepsis. I determine if antibiotics were administered during labor for prolonged rupture of membranes or a positive maternal group B streptococcus (GBS) screen and if prophylaxis was adequate. I send a complete blood count (CBC) as a sepsis screen. However, if the clinical condition warrants or suspicion is high, I obtain the CBC, along with a blood culture, and promptly begin antibiotics. I realize that transient tachypnea of the newborn (TTNB) is a diagnosis of exclusion and should be considered in the appropriate setting (i.e., a cesarean delivery or precipitous vaginal delivery without specific risk factors for sepsis).

Up to 30% of women of childbearing age have rectovaginal colonization with GBS, and there is a 50% rate of vertical transmission from a colonized mother to the fetus. Up to 2% of colonized neonates develop early-onset group B streptococcus (EOGBS) disease.[1-3] Before the adoption of protocols, there were up to 7500 cases annually in the United States. The 1996 Centers for Disease Control and Prevention (CDC) guideline for prevention of early-onset group B streptococcal disease specified identification of risk factors for invasive GBS disease, and specified administration of intrapartum antibiotic prophylaxis (IAP) during labor to those mothers with either a positive GBS culture or specific risk factors.[4] Since the 2002 CDC guideline recommended universal screening of pregnant women at 35 to 37 weeks gestation with administration of IAP to all who test positive, there has been a decline of over 70% in EOGBS disease. Despite the marked decline in incidence, GBS remains the chief cause of neonatal infectious disease. The 2010 revised CDC guideline maintains universal antenatal screening at 35 to 37 weeks gestation with IAP for GBS-positive mothers. In addition, women with an unknown GBS status and one or more risk factors: gestation less than 37 weeks, prolonged rupture of membranes (PROM), temperature of at least 100.4° F, GBS bacteriuria at any time during the pregnancy, and history of a previous infant with invasive GBS disease regardless of current maternal GBS status should continue to receive IAP. The new guideline introduces use of point-of-care nucleic acid amplification testing (NAAT), and clarifies criteria for prophylaxis in penicillin allergic mothers.[1,5]

PATIENT CARE

Clinical Thinking
- Assess and support the **ABCs.**
- Quickly review the prenatal laboratory test results and labor history, and note **risk factors for sepsis.**
- Place an IV line, obtain laboratory studies, and start antibiotics when indicated.
- Do not delay the start of antibiotics while considering a lumbar puncture (LP).
- LP is deferred if there is cardiorespiratory instability.
- If the infant is unstable or requires specific monitoring, consider transfer to a newborn intensive care unit.

History
- Was this a vaginal or cesarean delivery (with intact membranes)?

- Specific **risk factors for fetal GBS infection** include:
  - Maternal rectovaginal GBS colonization
  - Birth of a previous child with invasive GBS disease
  - GBS bacteriuria during pregnancy
  - Preterm delivery before GBS screening
  - Maternal fever and/or prolonged rupture of membranes (PROM, >18 hours) with unknown GBS status
- Was adequate IAP administered? Infants who received incomplete prophylaxis should be observed for 48 hours in the hospital with possible complete blood count (CBC) at 6 to 12 hours of life.
- EOGBS disease usually presents within 24 hours of life, but is possible through day 6.
- Additional **maternal risk factors for sepsis** are:
  - Premature prolonged rupture of membranes (PPROM) (i.e., prolonged rupture of membranes before start of labor)
  - Chorioamnionitis: Maternal fever >38° C and at least two of the following:
    - Fetal tachycardia
    - Maternal tachycardia
    - Uterine tenderness
    - Foul-smelling discharge
    - Maternal leukocytosis
- **Infant risk factors for sepsis** are low birth weight and prematurity.

Physical Examination
- Vital signs: Note tachypnea, tachycardia, temperature instability, or abnormal pulse oximetry.
- Perform a complete examination, and note general appearance: an infected infant may be asymptomatic or poorly responsive and hypotonic.
- Note signs of **respiratory distress:** tachypnea, retractions, grunting, flaring, inspiratory crackles, or decreased aeration.
- Note **neurologic signs of depression:** lethargy, poor feeding, decreased muscle tone.

Tests for Consideration
- **Glucose** $70
- **CBC with manual differential:** Depressed or elevated white blood cell count (WBC), an elevated immature: mature (I:T) ratio, or thrombocytopenia $116
- **Blood culture:** The diagnostic gold standard $152
- **C-reactive protein** $69
- **Cerebrospinal fluid (CSF) fluid analysis:** Gram stain, cell count, glucose, protein, and culture $557

IMAGING CONSIDERATIONS

→ **Chest radiograph:** For pneumonia, pleural effusion, cardiac silhouette, or pneumothorax $231

Clinical Entities	Medical Knowledge

Early-Onset Group B Streptococcal Disease

Pφ	Group B streptococcus (GBS, *Streptococcus agalactiae*), a gram-positive cocci, is transmitted to the fetus via ascension from maternal rectovaginal colonization, usually after labor has begun with ruptured membranes. The infected amniotic fluid may result in fetal colonization or infection. Heavy maternal colonization increases the risk for fetal transmission. Neonatal immunologic defenses are not well developed. Early-onset disease occurs as bacteremia, pneumonia, or meningitis. Since universal IAP during labor for GBS colonized women was instituted, the incidence has decreased by 80%.
TP	The Apgar scores may be depressed, or after an initial normal period the infant develops pallor, respiratory distress, temperature instability, lethargy, poor feeding, hypoglycemia, and/or abdominal distention with vomiting. Less than 10% present as meningitis with bulging fontanelle, irritability, and/or seizure.
Dx	The gold standard is blood culture. CSF culture is important to obtain if the infant is stable to tolerate the procedure, because meningitis may be present with a negative blood culture. Supporting data include elevated or depressed white blood count or elevated C-reactive protein.
Tx	Ampicillin and gentamicin are synergistic against GBS, or alternatively ampicillin and a third-generation cephalosporin is administered. Individualized supportive care to maintain adequate respiration and nutrition status is provided. Pneumonia and bacteremia are treated for 10 days, whereas uncomplicated meningitis is treated for 14 days.[3,6] **See Nelson Essentials 65.**

Other Early-Onset Sepsis

Pφ Neonatal sepsis is a systemic pathophysiologic response to microorganisms or their toxins in the first 28 days of life.[6] *Escherichia coli* is the most common organism other than GBS. Others include *Haemophilus influenzae, Klebsiella,* and *Enterococcus* species, *Staphylococcus aureus, Staphylococcus epidermidis,* and herpes simplex virus (HSV). *Listeria monocytogenes* is uncommon.

TP The presentation of bacterial sepsis may be identical to EOGBS disease. Disseminated herpes infection is unusual before day 4 of life and may present with the characteristic vesicular rash, respiratory distress, irritability, seizures, and possible jaundice.

Dx Identification of the pathogen depends on its ability to grow in culture; for bacteria, blood culture is the gold standard. Herpes is detected by polymerase chain reaction (PCR) and may also cause elevated liver function test results, as well as meningitis/encephalitis with red blood cells in the CSF. Lumbar puncture is done in many cases, but is deferred if there is cardiorespiratory instability.

Tx Initial treatment is broad-spectrum antibiotics as listed above with suspected GBS infection. Acyclovir is added if HSV is suspected. Therapy is tailored when specific results are available. Clinical judgment is key in determining duration of therapy in an ill-appearing infant with good clinical response to initiation of antibiotics with negative culture results. Individualized supportive care to maintain respiration and nutrition is provided. See Chapter 77, Neonatal Sepsis. **See Nelson Essentials 65.**

Perinatal Pneumonia

See Chapter 66, Transient Tachypnea of the Newborn, for discussion of pneumonia.

Transient Tachypnea of the Newborn

See Chapter 66, Transient Tachypnea of the Newborn.

Pneumothorax	
Pφ	Pneumothorax occurs in 1% to 2% of all newborns. Most pneumothoraces are asymptomatic, and they are more common in term or postterm males or in infants with underlying lung disease. Alveolar hyperinflation (either idiopathic or iatrogenic) is the most common cause.
TP	Asymptomatic affected infants are found by noting decreased breath sounds or hyperresonance on examination. Symptomatic infants will have tachypnea, respiratory distress, cyanosis, and irritability. The chest may be asymmetrical, and breath sounds diminished or unequal. With tension pneumothorax, there may be signs of shock.
Dx	Diagnosis is usually suspected clinically, with confirmation on chest radiograph. Mediastinal shift occurs with tension pneumothorax.
Tx	Asymptomatic pneumothorax will usually spontaneously resolve. Supplemental oxygen may hasten resorption of pleural air. Needle evacuation of air or chest tube placement is usually necessary with tension pneumothorax in an unstable infant. **See Nelson Essentials 61 and 138.**

ZEBRA ZONE

a. **Congenital anomalies of the airway such as choanal atresia or tracheoesophageal fistula:** May present with respiratory distress and hypoxemia

b. **Malformations of the lung such as congenital cystic adenomatoid malformation (CCAM) and diaphragmatic hernia:** Also may present with respiratory distress and hypoxemia (See Chapter 75 Tracheoesophageal Fistula.)

Practice-Based Learning and Improvement: Evidence-Based Pediatrics

Title
Changing patterns in neonatal *Escherichia coli* sepsis and ampicillin resistance in the era of intrapartum antibiotic prophylaxis

Authors
Bizzarro MJ, Dembry LM, Baltimore RS, Gallagher PG

Reference
Pediatrics 121:689-696, 2008

Historical significance/comments
This study reviews rates of neonatal *E. coli* sepsis in one institution during the era of intrapartum antibiotic prophylaxis for group B streptococcus. The rate of late-onset *E. coli* sepsis in term and preterm infants has increased, and early-onset *E. coli* sepsis in the very low-birth-weight preterm infant has increased, all in the face of marked decrease in early-onset group B streptococcal disease. This trend in *E. coli* sepsis will continue to be monitored along with the incidence of early-onset group B streptococcal disease.

Interpersonal and Communication Skills

Provide Person-to-Person Communication

The clinical status of a septic infant can change very quickly. The physician must be in constant communication with nursing staff, as well as with newborn intensivists if the situation necessitates. Parents need to be updated frequently on the status of the newborn as well as the status of the investigation. Because this situation may be potentially life threatening, a calm, honest discussion with parents is necessary, and appropriate ancillary staff to support the family is crucial.

Professionalism

Reliability and Responsibility: Accountability and Collaboration in the Search of System Errors to Prevent Future Harm

It is the pediatrician's responsibility to check maternal prenatal laboratory tests because, in the case of group B streptococcal infection, a positive test will affect the well-being and management of the newborn. If the values are unavailable, it is important to ascertain why and to collaborate with obstetric colleagues, nursing, and systems analysts to find workable solutions to prevent this from happening in the future.

Systems-Based Practice

Health-Care Economics: Cost Benefit of Prevention Guidelines

Cost-benefit analysis in health care is the analysis of health-care resource expenditures relative to possible medical benefit. This analysis may be helpful and necessary in setting priorities when choices must be made in the face of limited resources. This analysis is used in determining the degree of access to, or benefits of, health care to be provided.

Implementation of the GBS prevention guidelines has lead to improved clinical outcomes for mothers with GBS colonizations and their babies. A cost-benefit analysis completed by the CDC showed that the cost of delivering antibiotics is worthwhile and minimal given the benefit derived from decreased infant morbidity and mortality with successful prevention of early-onset group B streptococcal disease.[7]

References

1. Prevention of Perinatal Group B Streptococcal Disease: Revised Guidelines from CDC, 2010. *MMWR* 59(RR-10): 1-32, 2010.
2. Prevention of perinatal group B streptococcal disease: Revised guidelines from the CDC. *MMWR* 51(RR11):1-22, 2002.
3. Red book: 2009 Report of the Committee on Infectious Diseases. Elk Grove Village, IL, 2009, American Academy of Pediatrics.
4. Committee on Infectious Diseases and Committee on Fetus and Newborn: Revised guidelines for prevention of early-onset group B streptococcal (GBS) infection. *Pediatrics* 99:489-496, 1997.
5. Pulver LS, Hopfenbeck MM, Young GJ, et al: Continued early onset group B streptococcal infections in the era of intrapartum prophylaxis. *J Perinatol* 29:20-25, 2008.
6. Benitz W: Neonatal sepsis. In Polin R, Yoder M, editors: *Workbook in practical neonatology*, ed 4, Philadelphia, 2006, Saunders, pp 221-247.
7. CDC Policy Information Center. Available at http://aspe.hhs.gov/PIC/perfimp/2001/cdc.html.

Chapter 63
Delayed Meconium Passage (Case 26)

Jody Ross MD

Case: A full-term infant at 36 hours of age who has not yet passed meconium develops difficulty feeding and abdominal distention.

Differential Diagnosis

Meconium ileus/meconium plug syndrome	Hirschsprung disease
Small left colon syndrome	Intestinal/anal malformations

Speaking Intelligently

Almost 99% of healthy infants pass meconium within 24 hours after birth, and 100% of healthy infants pass meconium by 48 hours of age. Therefore meconium retention past 24 hours may signal intestinal obstruction and necessitates a prompt evaluation. The evaluation must include the infant's history and clinical examination as well as the maternal history, including drugs administered before and during labor. Radiographic studies, starting with plain abdominal radiographs, and consultation with a pediatric surgeon will usually be required.

PATIENT CARE

Clinical Thinking
- Review the prenatal, peripartum, and family history.
- Provide prompt **stabilization** for the distressed infant.
- Evaluate the infant for signs of **intestinal obstruction.**
- Place a nasogastric tube in the vomiting infant.
- Review the most likely differential diagnoses given the patient's history and physical examination.
- Consult with the pediatric surgeon, and systematically order radiographic studies.

History
- Review the infant's prenatal course, maternal history, and family history.
- Inquire about **drugs taken during pregnancy or labor,** because illicit drugs and magnesium sulfate can interfere with meconium passage.
- Review the infant's feeding history, especially the presence or absence of **bilious vomiting.**

Physical Examination
- Check vital signs: Tachycardia or bradycardia, weak pulses, and respiratory distress all indicate a distressed infant and the need for **possible emergency surgery.**
- Examine the infant with attention to the abdomen: Distention, visible dilated bowel loops, bowel sounds, position and patency of anus.
- Assess for **dysmorphic features:** 8% of patients with Hirschsprung disease have Down syndrome, and 70% of patients with anorectal malformations have other associated anomalies (**v**ertebral defects, **a**norectal anomalies, **c**ardiac defects, **t**racheoesophageal fistulas, **r**enal defects, and **r**adial upper **l**imb hypoplasia, the VACTRL association).

Tests for Consideration
- **Complete blood count (CBC):** If concern for sepsis $116
- **C-reactive protein:** If concern for sepsis $69
- **Blood culture:** Sepsis can complicate neonatal bowel obstruction and cause delayed meconium passage $152
- **Newborn screen for hypothyroidism and cystic fibrosis** $227
- **Electrolytes:** Hypercalcemia and hypokalemia can cause ileus and delayed meconium passage. Electrolyte derangement and acidosis may also signal a surgical emergency (e.g., malrotation with volvulus) $174
- **Anorectal manometry:** If considering Hirschsprung disease $555
- **Rectal suction biopsy:** Demonstrates lack of ganglion cells for diagnostic confirmation of Hirschsprung disease $606

IMAGING CONSIDERATIONS

→ **Plain abdominal radiographs:** A screen for obstruction—dilated loops, air fluid levels, stool retention $219
→ **Contrast enema:** To identify transition zone in Hirschsprung disease $530
→ **Ultrasound:** To delineate genitourinary anomalies associated with imperforate anus/anorectal atresia $563
→ **Magnetic resonance imaging (MRI):** Adjunct to evaluate spinal and genitourinary malformations associated with anorectal anomalies $1838

Clinical Entities	Medical Knowledge

Meconium Ileus/Meconium Plug Syndrome

Pφ **Meconium ileus** and **meconium plug syndrome** differ in location of the obstruction. Meconium plug syndrome is the mildest and most common form of distal obstruction in the newborn, involving the distal colon or rectum. The etiology of meconium plug syndrome is unclear, and after the initial plug is passed, bowel movements are normal. Meconium ileus may be simple or complicated when it is associated with volvulus, bowel perforation, or peritonitis. Meconium ileus occurs in up to 15% of patients with cystic fibrosis.

TP Both of these entities may present similarly with feeding difficulty, abdominal distention, and failure to pass meconium.

Dx Diagnosis can be made with the combination of plain radiographs and contrast enema.

Tx Treatment of meconium plug syndrome may be accomplished with digital rectal examination, other rectal stimulation, or the contrast enema. Simple meconium ileus may be treated by Gastrografin enema (water-soluble contrast) sometimes done serially. Complicated meconium ileus will require urgent surgical intervention. **See Nelson Essentials 137.**

Hirschsprung Disease

Pφ Congenital aganglionic megacolon, or **Hirschsprung disease,** is caused by failure of complete distal migration of neural crest cells, which results in an aganglionic segment of intestine. The internal anal sphincter is abnormally innervated as are variable lengths of other parts of the colon, most often the rectosigmoid colon. Hirschsprung disease accounts for up to one fourth of neonatal intestinal obstruction.

TP Infants present with failure to pass meconium, distended abdomen, and a tight anus. If the diagnosis is not recognized in the early newborn period, enterocolitis may develop, heralded by bleeding and diarrhea and possible sepsis.

Dx Diagnosis can be suspected based on physical examination, plain radiograph findings, and contrast enema results. The plain radiographs will show dilated bowel loops with gas and stool mixed in the colon or gas that is not seen past the pelvic rim. Contrast enema may show a transition zone between affected and unaffected bowel segments. Diagnosis is confirmed by rectal suction biopsy that demonstrates lack of ganglion cells.

Tx   Treatment is surgical resection of the aganglionic segment of colon. The trend is toward primary repair with a pull-through procedure. In cases involving extensive aganglionic segments, a colostomy is placed with future reanastomosis when possible. **See Nelson Essentials 126 and 129.**

Intestinal/Anal Malformations

Pφ   Failure of proper embryologic development of the gut leads to various atresias and stenoses. In "high" anal atresia, the rectum ends above the levator ani muscles and may involve a fistula with stool emptying into the vaginal vault in females or the urethra in males. "Low" anal atresia involves the rectum descending at least partially through the levator ani muscles and may have an associated perineal fistula.

TP   Newborns will either fail to pass any meconium or will have small ribbon-like stool passed through a stenotic anus or fistula.

Dx   Diagnosis is made with physical examination and various imaging modalities, including contrast enema and ultrasound. MRI may be used as well to further delineate the anatomy.

Tx   Treatment of anal stenosis can be accomplished with anal dilation. Anal atresia is treated with reconstructive surgery and possibly fistula dilation until definitive repair is done. Patients with high anal atresia will require colostomy. **See Nelson Essentials 129.**

Small Left Colon Syndrome

Pφ   This is a rare cause of neonatal intestinal obstruction. More than 50% of affected newborns are children of diabetic mothers. Transient dysmotility occurs because of unclear mechanisms. Other cases of *small left colon syndrome* have been reported in association with maternal psychotropic drug use, hypothyroidism, and hypermagnesemia. The affected bowel is normally innervated.

TP   Infants with small left colon syndrome usually develop functional obstruction after the initial passage of meconium.

Dx   Diagnosis is made based on appearance on plain abdominal
      radiographs and contrast enema—a small-caliber colon that
      lacks the usual tortuosity distal to the splenic flexure.

Tx   Treatment varies depending on severity of symptoms and may
      be accomplished with successive water-soluble enemas or
      temporary colostomy.

ZEBRA ZONE

a. **Hypoganglionosis:** A rare disorder with decreased innervation
   of the myenteric plexus presenting in a similar fashion to
   Hirschsprung disease. This is diagnosed on biopsy.

b. **Neuronal intestinal dysplasia types A, B:** Aberrant innervation
   of the gut, type A has ganglion cells present, distinguishing it
   from Hirschsprung disease. This is diagnosed on biopsy. Type B
   may coexist with Hirschsprung disease.

c. **Megacystis-microcolon–intestinal hypoperistalsis syndrome:**
   A rare condition characterized by lax abdominal musculature,
   incomplete intestinal rotation, abdominal distention, and
   deficient intestinal peristalsis. A large bladder and often
   vesicoureteral reflux are seen. Female neonates are typically
   affected; it is usually fatal in first year of life.

Practice-Based Learning and Improvement

Title
**Treatment of uncomplicated meconium ileus by Gastrografin
enema: A preliminary report**

Author
Noblett HR

Reference
J Pediatr Surg 1(2):190-197, 1969

Problem
Meconium ileus

Intervention
Gastrografin enema

Comparison/control (quality of evidence)
Case report

Outcome/effect
Successful nonsurgical treatment of meconium ileus

Historical significance/comments
As introduced in this important case report from 1969, gastrografin enema is now the standard of care for diagnosis and initial treatment of uncomplicated meconium ileus.

Interpersonal and Communication Skills

Provide Person-to-Person Communication to Consultants Whenever Feasible

When a newborn has a delay in passage of meconium, the infant is evaluated to determine the cause. Etiologies include intestinal obstruction (imperforate anus, Hirschsprung disease, meconium plug), hypothyroidism, or certain maternal drugs. The evaluation sometimes involves radiologists, surgeons, and other subspecialists. Clinical information must succinctly and thoroughly be presented to these consultants to ensure timely intervention and possible hospital transfer when needed for appropriate level of care. In most instances, a telephone call to the consultant is preferred to ensure timely care as opposed to simply leaving a note in the chart.

Professionalism

Communication: Informed Consent

Understanding this ethical and legal mandate is crucial because the infant with delayed meconium passage will require invasive testing and procedures. Always document conversations with consultants, as well as the informed consent process with the patient's family.

Systems-Based Practice

Risk Management in Newborns With Delayed Meconium Passage

The landmark 1999 Institute of Medicine (IOM) report To Err Is Human states that as many as 98,000 deaths in the United States each year result from medical errors. But the IOM also found that at least 90% of these deaths are the result of failed systems and procedures, not the negligence of physicians.

Medical-legal risk management of delayed meconium passage requires well-designed systems in place—standardized protocols/clinical pathways, standing physician orders, the availability of timely imaging resources, and open communication among the health-care providers and between providers and patients.

Chapter 64
Antenatal Hydronephrosis (Case 27)

David J. Sas DO, MPH

Case: A routine prenatal ultrasound of a 20–weeks'-gestation male fetus reveals bilateral hydronephrosis.

Differential Diagnosis

| Multicystic dysplastic kidneys (MCDK) |
| Vesicoureteral reflux (VUR) |
| Urinary tract obstruction |

Speaking Intelligently

When antenatal hydronephrosis is detected, I assess the degree of hydronephrosis and plan additional evaluation after birth. Although the definition of hydronephrosis is not universally agreed upon, most experts consider an anterior-posterior renal pelvis diameter of >5 mm in a second-trimester ultrasound abnormal. The degree of hydronephrosis predicts the likelihood of significant renal pathology. Patients with antenatal hydronephrosis not detected in utero often present postnatally with urinary tract infection, poor urinary stream, failure to thrive, dehydration, neonatal sepsis, or respiratory distress. It is important to determine the mechanism of hydronephrosis, because some are amenable to surgical intervention. As with all kidney disease, the goal is to protect residual renal function.

PATIENT CARE

Clinical Thinking
- The **degree** of prenatal hydronephrosis is an important predictor of renal pathology.
- Newborns with enlarged kidneys can have impaired respiratory function either through mass effect or pulmonary hypoplasia

secondary to oligohydramnios. ***Impaired respiratory function*** is the most important predictor of survival in babies born with renal insufficiency.
- After birth a thorough physical examination is performed, and urine output is carefully monitored.
- There may be excessive water and electrolyte loss, so hydration status is monitored carefully and electrolytes are checked as needed.

History
- Review the prenatal record, including laboratory investigations and ultrasound reports.
- A ***history of oligohydramnios*** increases the likelihood of significant postnatal renal impairment and potential respiratory problems at birth.
- A careful family history focusing on cystic kidneys, solitary kidney, or obstructive uropathy should be elicited.

Physical Examination
- The initial assessment should focus on vital signs, as well as ***respiratory effort*** and lung auscultation.
- Be particularly wary of masses and abnormal musculature on abdominal examination.
- Carefully note the presence or absence of descended testicles, anatomy of the penile/urethral meatus, and quality of the urinary stream.
- A complete physical examination is performed, looking for other anatomic anomalies that may suggest an associated syndrome.

Tests for Consideration
- **Serum electrolytes and measure of kidney function:** Should be monitored carefully because abnormalities may develop over time. Initial creatinine values reflect the mother's renal function rather than the baby's. This normally persists until about 5 to 7 days of life but varies in babies with renal insufficiency. $174
- **Urine culture:** Urinary tract abnormalities increase the risk for infection. $148

IMAGING CONSIDERATIONS

→ **Renal ultrasound:** If performed during the first 48 hours of life, renal ultrasound may falsely minimize hydronephrosis because of the normal oliguric state during the newborn period. By 2 to 4 weeks, the infant should be feeding well and gaining weight, and the renal ultrasound will provide accurate assessment of the degree of postnatal hydronephrosis. About one third of babies with mild prenatal hydronephrosis will have an abnormal postnatal ultrasound; the more severe the prenatal hydronephrosis, the more likely the postnatal scan will demonstrate persistence. If anterior-posterior renal pelvis diameter is >10 mm, start antimicrobial prophylaxis with amoxicillin 20 mg/kg once daily. $590

→ **Voiding cystourethrogram (VCUG): VCUG** is used for detection of vesicoureteral reflux. Start antimicrobial prophylaxis as above if the VCUG reveals grade 4 or 5 reflux; some start prophylaxis for lesser grades. However, the utility of prophylactic antibiotics in prevention of recurrent urinary tract infection (UTI) in infants with VUR is currently under investigation, and many expect it to be demonstrated that there is little utility in prophylaxis. $600

→ **Dimercaptosuccinic acid (DMSA) scan:** DMSA scan can evaluate renal function vis-à-vis proximal tubule uptake. This test is useful for patients suspected of having little functioning renal parenchyma. $1524

→ **Diuretic renography:** Like the DMSA, this study can also evaluate renal function but is most useful for evaluating for obstruction. $906

Clinical Entities	Medical Knowledge

Multicystic Dysplastic Kidneys

Pφ **MCDK** is the second most common cause of abdominal mass in neonates. The pathogenesis is not completely understood but is thought to be the result of abnormal coordination between the branching ureteric bud and developing metanephros. A number of different genes have been implicated and are under investigation. There is about a 50% risk for contralateral urologic abnormalities.

TP	MCDK usually presents with abdominal mass with or without respiratory impairment. Depending on the condition of the contralateral kidney, newborns with MCDK can present with signs and symptoms of renal failure.
Dx	Diagnosis is made primarily with a renal ultrasound. The classic findings are described as a "bunch of grapes" illustrating the noncommunicating cysts. There is usually no identifiable renal parenchyma on renal ultrasound, and DMSA confirms the lack of functioning kidney tissue.
Tx	Treatment is support for the degree of renal insufficiency. Nephrectomy may be indicated if the mass effect of the enlarged kidney is causing problems or if the patient has uncontrollable hypertension. **See Nelson Essentials 168.**

Urinary Tract Obstruction

Pφ	Kidney damage from a urinary tract obstruction is the result of pressure obliterating renal tubular and parenchymal tissue. An obstruction can be caused by an abnormal anatomic blockage anywhere along the urinary tract but is most commonly caused by posterior urethral valves (PUV) (in boys), ureteropelvic junction (UPJ) obstruction, ureterovesicle junction obstruction, or ureterocele.
TP	Newborns with a urinary tract obstruction can present with sepsis, renal failure, respiratory distress, oliguria, urinary tract infection, electrolyte disturbances, failure to thrive, or simply poor urinary stream (with obstruction distal to the bladder, as in PUV).
Dx	Renal ultrasound can often make the diagnosis and help to localize the obstruction, because dilatation will occur just proximal to the obstruction site with no dilatation distally. Though often not required, diuretic renography can confirm the presence of an obstruction.
Tx	Treatment is surgical correction of the obstruction. When possible, a transurethral catheter should be placed to reduce pressure. In more proximal obstructions, a nephrostomy tube may be placed to allow urine to drain from the kidney. **See Nelson Essentials 168.**

Vesicoureteral Reflux

Pφ **VUR** is the abnormal retrograde flow of urine from the bladder to the upper urinary tract. It can be caused by an anatomic obstruction or, more commonly, by a physiologically incompetent urinary tract causing the pressure proximally to be lower than the pressure distally, thus leading to urinary back flow. This physiologic impairment can be caused by abnormal innervation (neurogenic bladder), behavioral disorders ("dysfunctional elimination syndrome"), or abnormal compression of the distal ureters within the bladder wall during voiding.

TP Patients with VUR usually present with a urinary tract infection; although if undetected, severe VUR with recurrent urinary infections can present with chronic renal insufficiency or end-stage renal disease.

Dx VUR is diagnosed by VCUG and graded I to V according to the degree of retrograde filling and ureteral/pelvic dilatation (Figure 64-1).

Tx The treatment of VUR with surgical intervention and antimicrobial prophylaxis is controversial and under investigation. Traditionally, patients with more severe reflux (grades IV to V) are treated with an open surgical procedure. Newer endoscopic procedures that use a bulking agent to mechanically reduce reflux have been successful and are less invasive. Daily low-dose antibiotics are used for prophylaxis until the patient no longer has reflux on VCUG. For lower grades, traditional treatment has been with antibiotics until follow-up VCUG is negative for reflux. Studies of the natural history of VUR show that mild-to-moderate VUR will often resolve without intervention. However, VUR significant enough to cause antenatal hydronephrosis is likely to be pathologic. **See Nelson Essentials 167.**

ZEBRA ZONE

a. **Prune belly syndrome:** Triad of abnormal urologic anatomy, undescended testes, and absent abdominal musculature

b. **VACTERL association:** Variable combination of vertebral anomalies, anal atresia, cardiac lesions, tracheoesophageal fistula, renal/urologic anomalies, and limb defects

c. **Potter sequence:** Results from oligohydramnios from prenatal urinary tract obstruction leading to pulmonary hypoplasia, low-set ears, wide-set eyes, micrognathia, and orthopedic problems

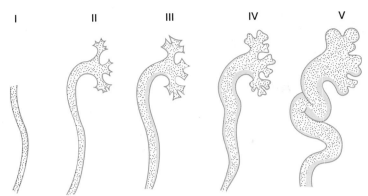

Figure 64-1 Classification of vesicoureteral reflux.

Practice-Based Learning and Improvement: Evidence for Postnatal Imaging

Title
Prospective study of outcome in antenatally diagnosed renal pelvis dilatation

Authors
Jaswon MS, Dibble L, Puri S, et al

Reference
Arch Dis Child Fetal Neonatal Ed 1999;80:F135-F138

Problem
Does follow-up postnatal imaging provide any added benefit to patients with hydronephrosis diagnosed prenatally?

Intervention
Postnatal renal ultrasound and VCUG in babies diagnosed prenatally with hydronephrosis

Comparison/control (quality of evidence)
Prospective clinical trial with cited references in peer-reviewed journal

Outcome/effect
Postnatal renal ultrasound does not adequately predict VUR; a VCUG should be performed in all infants diagnosed prenatally with hydronephrosis.

Historical significance/comments
Like many pediatric studies, the sample size is small and thus may not provide results that accurately reflect the entire population designated for study. Secondly, there is a larger question that remains to be answered: Does mild VUR (which does not cause hydronephrosis visible on renal ultrasound) require any intervention?

Interpersonal and Communication Skills

Encourage Questions and Make Yourself Available to Answer Future Ones

Abnormal findings on fetal ultrasound may be devastating to parents. The clinician should be sensitive to the emotional needs of the family and provide accurate information regarding the likely outcome and prospective morbidity. I always start with a plain description and simple illustration of the urinary tract and what the kidneys do before I go on to discuss any abnormalities. I encourage questions, recognizing that parents may have several now, and will certainly have more later as they begin to process the news I have delivered. They may worry that there are other yet undiagnosed problems or that their child has a genetic syndrome. Sometimes these questions cannot be definitively answered until after birth, and that should be acknowledged. I always ensure that the parents have access to a means of communicating with me because questions invariably arise later on. I specifically let them know that it will not be a bother for them to contact me later should the need to do so arise.

Professionalism

Acknowledge and Discuss Errors Openly

You are caring for a febrile 6-week-old boy admitted to the hospital with a urine culture positive for >100,000 CFU *Escherichia coli*. A renal ultrasound reveals bilateral moderate hydronephrosis. You learn that this patient was diagnosed with hydronephrosis on prenatal ultrasound but according to the parents, appropriate treatment and follow-up were not instituted. The parents ask if this current illness is related to the prenatal diagnosis of "big kidneys." You wish to avoid accusing other practitioners of wrongdoing, especially because you were not directly involved with the patient's care at the time. However, it is quite acceptable to explain to the parents what is usually done for newborns with this condition and be prepared to answer, in general terms, any further questions they may have.

Systems-Based Practice

The Patient-Centered Medical Home

The patient-centered medical home (PCMH) is now a frequently used term in the lexicon of medicine and medical economics. The general concept is an approach to providing comprehensive primary care that centralizes the often complex care patients require and facilitates partnerships between patients and their providers. It is thought that such "medical homes" might allow better access to health care and increase satisfaction with care, ultimately improving health. Prenatal diagnoses such as antenatal hydronephrosis, which presents a challenge of communicating across multiple subspecialties (including obstetrics/gynecology, pediatric urology, pediatric nephrology, neonatology, and general pediatrics), demonstrate how the concept of a "medical home" might facilitate the centralization and coordination of care. As it is likely that each of the aforementioned specialists will be involved in the care of these patients, it is imperative that each member of the care team be kept up to date regarding the postnatal plan. For now, before the "medical home" perhaps becomes the norm of practice, good communication with the general pediatrician from all subspecialists involved are the keys to ensuring that all of the child's health-care needs are met. See Chapter 25, The Special Needs Child.

Chapter 65
The Newborn With a Murmur (Case 28)

Elizabeth E. Adams DO

Case: During your initial evaluation of a 12-hour-old, term, appropriate-for-gestational-age male, you auscultate a grade II/VI continuous murmur below the left clavicle, which does not appear to radiate. The infant is otherwise doing well. Heart rate is 150 beats per minute, respiratory rate is 34 breaths per minute, and blood pressure is 76/50 mm Hg.

Differential Diagnosis

Patent ductus arteriosus (PDA)	Ventricular septal defect (VSD)	Coarctation of the aorta
Pulmonary valve stenosis	Peripheral pulmonary stenosis (PPS)	

Speaking Intelligently

Murmurs are commonly heard during the newborn period and can be heard in up to 50% of all term newborns during the first few weeks of life. Most murmurs heard within the first few days are from the normal transition from a fetal circulation to an extrauterine circulation, or they result from relatively benign conditions that are unlikely to cause hemodynamic collapse. **Beware: The absence of a murmur does not rule out a serious congenital heart defect!**

PATIENT CARE

Clinical Thinking
- Review the prenatal history, including ultrasounds.
- Check vital signs, including four extremity blood pressure readings and **oxygen saturation** in the right arm and at least one leg. An oxygen saturation that is dramatically different **preductus** (right arm) and **postductus** (other limbs) suggests a serious congenital heart defect (CHD). **Blood pressure** in the legs that is significantly lower than one taken in the arms strongly suggests coarctation of the aorta. Palpation of the **femoral pulses** is also important— pulses that are difficult or impossible to palpate should raise your suspicion for coarctation.
- If the murmur is heard consistently during the newborn's hospital stay, consultation with a pediatric cardiologist and an echocardiogram may be indicated before discharge. Close follow-up by a physician is imperative, and the infant should be seen within 1 week of hospital discharge.

History
- Elicit **family history of CHD,** especially in a parent or sibling. The baseline incidence of CHD across all populations is just under 1%. However, with an affected first-degree relative, the risk for CHD increases to 5% to 10% for the infant.
- Have any infants died shortly after birth? Any late miscarriages or children in the family with chromosome anomalies?
- Review any specific prenatal testing, including fetal echocardiograms.

Physical Examination
- Check vital signs (weight, height, head circumference, heart rate, respiratory rate, temperature, four extremity blood pressure readings, and oxygen saturation).
- Perform a complete examination. Focus on the cardiovascular system and any findings suggestive of genetic syndromes. Many **genetic syndromes** have associations with specific congenital heart defects, such as the correlation between Down syndrome and atrioventricular

(AV) canal defects, Turner syndrome and coarctation of the aorta, or Noonan syndrome and pulmonic stenosis.

- Inspect and palpate the precordium for chest wall deformities, cardiac thrills, and the point of maximal impulse. Determine where the murmur is heard best, its timing in the cardiac cycle (systole or diastole), any patterns of radiation, its intensity (1 to 6), and any other defining characteristics. Check pulses in both arms and legs. An infant with diminished or absent femoral pulses has coarctation of the aorta until proved otherwise.

Tests for Consideration
- **Electrocardiogram:** For cardiac rhythm, chamber enlargement, and QTc interval $217

IMAGING CONSIDERATIONS

→ **Chest radiograph:** To identify increased or decreased pulmonary blood flow, position of the aortic arch, cardiomegaly, or characteristic patterns such as the "egg on a string" pattern seen with transposition of the great vessels $231
→ **Echocardiogram:** To verify cardiac anatomy and blood flow pattern $1630

Clinical Entities	Medical Knowledge

Patent Ductus Arteriosus

Pφ   The ductus arteriosus, essential to fetal circulation, allows blood to bypass the unused lungs and flow directly from the pulmonary artery to the aorta. This muscular artery functionally closes after birth, usually within the first 24 hours, and should be completely closed by 2 to 3 weeks of age. When closure fails to occur, the ductus remains patent, maintaining a connection between the pulmonary artery and the aorta. With a large ductus there is significant shunting of blood from the aorta to the pulmonary artery because of the higher left-sided pressure. The persistent excessive pulmonary blood flow may lead to congestive heart failure (CHF).

TP   Every newborn has a PDA at birth. Many times ductus is audible while closing. This murmur is classically described as a "continuous machinery murmur"; however, it may be heard only in systole. A small persistent PDA is asymptomatic. With a large PDA, CHF may develop, and the infant will develop tachypnea, tachycardia, poor feeding, and failure to thrive.

Dx   Definitive diagnosis is made with echocardiogram; however, an experienced pediatrician or pediatric cardiologist can often make this diagnosis based on auscultation of the characteristic continuous machinery murmur heard below the left clavicle.

Tx   Treatment depends on the size of the ductus and age of the infant. In most term infants, "watchful waiting" is appropriate, because most PDAs will close spontaneously in the first several weeks. In extremely premature infants, PDAs may be surgically ligated or treated medically with indomethacin. PDAs may also be closed in the cardiac catheterization laboratory in older children. **See Nelson Essentials 61 and 143.**

Ventricular Septal Defect

Pφ   ***Ventricular septal defects*** are most commonly located in the membranous septum just below the aortic and pulmonic valves, or in the muscular septum, and result in left-to-right shunting and increased pulmonary blood flow. A small VSD produces turbulent blood flow, and frequently a loud murmur, but is rarely problematic. A large VSD may be asymptomatic with no murmur in the first few weeks of life until pulmonary vascular resistance drops and the pressure gradient from left ventricle to right increases, resulting in increased blood flow through the defect and an audible murmur. Over the first few months of life, the volume overload to the lungs with a large VSD will lead to CHF. VSDs constitute 20% of all CHD.

TP   A small VSD is asymptomatic but produces a harsh holosystolic murmur. With a large VSD, there is often development of CHF over the first few months of life with tachypnea, tachycardia, poor feeding, and inadequate weight gain, in addition to the characteristic murmur.

Dx   Diagnosis is made based on clinical findings and echocardiogram.

Tx   A small VSD will rarely require treatment, and many close over time. A large VSD with uncontrollable heart failure will require surgical repair. Infants are often treated preoperatively with furosemide and digitalis to improve the heart function and facilitate weight gain and nutritional status before definitive repair. Many defects get smaller with time and eventually close, so watchful waiting is often indicated in the absence of CHF. **See Nelson Essentials 143.**

Coarctation of the Aorta

Pφ	This obstructive lesion is caused by a narrowing in the aorta, most commonly located at the origin of the ductus arteriosus and involving varying segment lengths of the aorta. It is frequently associated with bicuspid aortic valve. There is diminished lower extremity (LE) blood flow, with decreased LE blood pressure and decreased or absent pulses in the legs with strong upper extremity pulses. In its extreme form there is complete interruption of the aorta, which is a life-threatening, ductal-dependent lesion.
TP	There is a systolic murmur along the left sternal border with a loud second heart sound. There are decreased or absent lower extremity pulses with strong upper extremity pulses. A neonate with severe coarctation will have lower extremity hypoperfusion and acidosis when the ductus closes. An infant with strong, easily palpable femoral pulses is unlikely to have coarctation of the aorta.
Dx	Diagnosis is made with clinical findings and echocardiogram.
Tx	Treatment depends on degree of narrowing. Close monitoring of perfusion and blood pressure is key. An acutely ill neonate requires a prostaglandin E_1 infusion to reopen the ductus arteriosus until the child has definitive surgical repair. **See Nelson Essentials 143.**

Pulmonary Valve Stenosis

Pφ	*Pulmonary valve stenosis* is caused by narrowing of the pulmonary valve orifice or thickening of the valve leaflets. The valve opens incompletely in systole resulting in right ventricular outflow obstruction in proportion to the degree of narrowing. There is increased right ventricular pressure, with eventual development of right ventricular hypertrophy.
TP	There are no symptoms with mild to moderate stenosis. On auscultation there is a harsh systolic ejection murmur heard best at the left upper sternal border and possibly an associated click.
Dx	Diagnosis is made with echocardiogram, along with a careful evaluation for rarely associated diagnoses such as Noonan syndrome.

Tx   A mild degree of pulmonary valve stenosis is generally well tolerated for many years; however, more severe forms may require early intervention. In its most severe form, pulmonary valve stenosis is a life-threatening, ductal-dependent lesion that requires prompt intervention in the first few days of life, often initially with balloon valvuloplasty. **See Nelson Essentials 143.**

Peripheral Pulmonary Stenosis

Pφ   ***Peripheral pulmonary stenosis* (PPS)** is due to the acute angle that the left and right pulmonary arteries form where they branch from the main pulmonary artery.

TP   There are no symptoms, and auscultation reveals a characteristic soft systolic murmur heard best at the left upper sternal border with radiation to both axillae.

Dx   Diagnosis is most often clinical, but definite diagnosis is with echocardiogram.

Tx   No treatment is required in most cases. This innocent murmur resolves as the infant grows. If a murmur thought to be from PPS persists beyond 6 months of age, cardiology referral should be considered. **See Nelson Essentials 143.**

ZEBRA ZONE

a. **Tetralogy of Fallot:** A combination of four entities: VSD, an aorta that is "overriding" the VSD, right ventricular hypertrophy, and pulmonary stenosis/right ventricular outflow obstruction. The pulmonary stenosis is usually at the level of the valve ring. The murmur heard is generally from the pulmonary stenosis; the VSD may or may not be audible.

Practice-Based Learning and Improvement

Title
Initial evaluation of heart murmurs: Are laboratory tests necessary?

Authors
Smythe JF, Teixeira O, Vlad P, et al

Reference
Pediatrics 86(4):497-500, 1990

Problem
Evaluation of innocent murmurs with advanced imaging techniques is costly and time consuming; this prospective study looked at predictive value of auscultation in determining the presence or absence of significant congenital heart disease.

Comparison/control (quality of evidence)
Clinical examination by a pediatric cardiologist had a sensitivity of 96% and specificity of 95% for diagnosing serious congenital heart defects.

Outcome/effect
Pediatric cardiologists can reliably identify innocent murmurs and pathologic murmurs based on examination findings.

Historical significance/comments
Clinical examination by a pediatric cardiologist has a high degree of accuracy, and additional testing may not always be required.

Interpersonal and Communication Skills

Share Information With Clarity and a Calm Demeanor

Effective communication with parents is a good way to prevent panic! Being told that their infant has a heart murmur is frightening for many parents. However, a good explanation of what a murmur is and what steps are needed to make a definitive diagnosis is usually reassuring. Avoid the pitfall of telling parents that everything will be fine when the infant may in fact have a serious heart problem.

Professionalism

Honesty and Integrity: Share Pertinent Examination Findings

Many infants in the newborn nursery have transient heart murmurs that resolve quickly. Should families be told that the infant has a heart murmur when the pediatrician is almost certain that the murmur is innocent and will likely resolve, or should discussion of the murmur only take place when the pediatrician decides that further evaluation is necessary? Most practitioners would agree that families should be informed of a clinically diagnosed innocent murmur at the time of discharge from the newborn nursery.

Systems-Based Practice

Coordination of Care for the Infant With a Complex Problem

Management of infants and children with congenital heart disease requires care coordination and expertise from multiple disciplines—primary care, cardiology, surgery, case management, home care, and social workers.

From the time a congenital heart defect is diagnosed—whether in utero or in the newborn period—communication and coordination is a must for success: the cardiologist completes a diagnostic evaluation and, if needed, will consult cardiothoracic surgery for surgical intervention. Case management and home care provide necessary services and support for discharge, again with frequent interaction with physicians for smooth transition and delivery of service. Ideally, the primary care physician remains aware and central to what is happening to child and the family.

Chapter 66
Transient Tachypnea
of the Newborn (Case 29)

Faizah N. Bhatti MD, MS

Case: A 37-weeks'-gestation infant delivered 3 hours ago by cesarean delivery for failure to progress has developed tachypnea and grunting after attempting his first feed. Apgar scores were 6 and 9, with initial cyanosis that resolved quickly with administration of blow-by oxygen.

Differential Diagnosis

Pneumonia	Respiratory distress syndrome (RDS)
Transient tachypnea of the newborn (TTNB)	Neonatal sepsis

Speaking Intelligently

Transient tachypnea of the newborn (TTNB) occurs in term and near-term infants, usually presenting as mild to moderate respiratory distress, often with hypoxemia. Because TTNB is a diagnosis of exclusion, I consider the dangerous entities in the differential. If there are risk factors for sepsis, or the tachypnea lasts more than 4 hours, I initiate a targeted workup, the extent of which will be determined by the baby's clinical status. Most important, supportive measures should be initiated promptly, and the neonatal intensive care unit (NICU) staff notified early for a potential transfer. The major goal is to ensure that a more serious diagnosis is not missed: TTNB can coexist with early sepsis or respiratory distress syndrome.

PATIENT CARE

Clinical Thinking
- Review the events of labor. Were there **fetal distress indicators** such as heart rate instability (poor beat-to-beat variability, bradycardia, late decelerations)? Was **meconium** passed in utero?
- Are there risk factors for **sepsis** such as prolonged rupture of membranes or inadequate intrapartum antibiotic prophylaxis (IAP) for group B streptococcus (GBS)? Maternal fever raises the possibility of **chorioamnionitis.**
- Check vital signs, oxygen saturation, blood glucose level, and temperature stability.
- Initiate supplemental oxygen if needed.
- Provide close monitoring with frequent reassessment.
- **Confer with NICU** regarding the potential for transfer.

History
- Review **maternal history.** Were prenatal ultrasounds normal? Were there risk factors such as preeclampsia or infection? What was mother's GBS status? If positive, was IAP administered?
- Was it a term gestation? If preterm, was a cause determined? Were antenatal corticosteroids administered? It can be difficult to distinguish TTNB from RDS, but RDS increases in frequency with degree of prematurity.
- Meconium aspiration is rare in infants less than 37 weeks gestation.
- Was it a precipitous vaginal or cesarean delivery? Was there a nuchal cord? What were the Apgar scores? Was resuscitation required in the delivery room?
- Has the infant **tolerated feeding?**

Physical Examination
- Check vital signs: heart rate, respiratory rate, temperature, weight, length, and head circumference.
- Perform a complete **physical examination,** with attention to respiratory effort, work of breathing (nasal flaring, intercostal and subcostal retractions), and aeration.
- Assess degree of alertness.

- Check pulse oximetry.
- Concerning signs for sepsis include temperature instability, hypoglycemia, tachypnea with hypoxemia, tachycardia, hypotonia, and/or lethargy.

Tests for Consideration

- **Complete blood count (CBC):** Neutropenia and/or an increased immature to total neutrophil (I:T) ratio and/or thrombocytopenia suggest infection $116
- **C-Reactive Protein (CRP):** Initial level with repeat at 12 and 24 hours may be helpful to exclude sepsis $69
- **Blood culture:** If concern for infection $152
- **Cerebrospinal fluid culture:** Is gold standard for meningitis diagnosis $152
- **Cerebrospinal fluid Gram stain, glucose, protein, cell count (red and white cell counts):** Provides quick assessment for meningitis $405
- **Blood glucose level** $70

IMAGING CONSIDERATIONS

→ **Chest radiograph:** To help differentiate TTNB from pneumonia or RDS or pneumothorax $231

Clinical Entities   Medical Knowledge

Transient Tachypnea of the Newborn

Pφ   Transient tachypnea of the newborn (TTNB) is caused by pulmonary edema secondary to delayed clearing of fetal lung fluid. It may be seen in cesarean deliveries without preceding onset of labor, perhaps due to the lack of surge in catecholamines that occurs naturally with the onset of labor. It has also been seen in conditions with ventricular dysfunction and increased central venous pressure. These babies are generally in mild respiratory distress and do not require aggressive management.

TP   TTNB occurs in term and near-term infants. There is tachypnea with respiratory rates of 60 to 80 breaths per minute, along with nasal flaring and retractions within a few minutes to a few hours of life. Grunting is more common with RDS, which can be difficult to distinguish from TTNB. On physical examination, there should be no abnormalities of other organ systems. Hypoxemia is generally corrected by no more than 40% inspired oxygen.

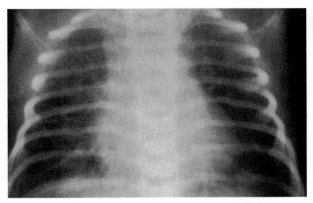

Figure 66-1   Radiograph of transient tachypnea of the newborn. Note prominent vascular markings.

Dx	Diagnosis can be made with an accurate maternal history that excludes risk factors for serious disease and the newborn physical examination. In addition, pulse oximetry and a chest radiograph may provide clues. The chest radiograph will generally show prominent vascular markings, fluid in the fissures, and possible pleural effusions (Figure 66-1). **Remember: This is a diagnosis of exclusion!**
Tx	Close observation and supportive care, including supplemental oxygen, are the mainstay. More-distressed babies may benefit from a short trial of nasal continuous positive airway pressure (CPAP). Clinical improvement occurs within a few hours to a few days, which helps to distinguish this from other clinical entities such as RDS, which may evolve as worsening respiratory distress. **See Nelson Essentials 61.**

Pneumonia

Pφ   The most important neonatal bacterial pathogens are group B
streptococcus, *Escherichia coli,* and *Listeria monocytogenes*,
followed by *Chlamydia trachomatis*. Transmission is perinatal.
Herpes simplex is the most important viral pathogen and often
occurs with disseminated herpes infection. **Pneumonia** may be
acquired in utero (true congenital pneumonia from aspiration of
infected amniotic fluid or maternal-fetal transmission across
placenta), intrapartum, or postnatally. It can be acquired via
hematogenous spread or via direct inoculation from the airways.
If sepsis is also present, this can result in lactate accumulation
in tissues, which triggers a hyperventilatory response. In
addition, the systemic release of cytokines directly damages
lung tissue, and there can be secondary persistent pulmonary
hypertension.

TP   In early-onset pneumonia, there is respiratory distress with
tachypnea, often with hypoxemia, or even apnea, which may
be present at birth or develop in the first few days of life.
On examination there is increased work of breathing with
retractions, nasal flaring, grunting, and/or cyanosis. The quality
of secretions may be altered, becoming thick yellow-green or
brown. With tachypnea there may be difficulty with oral
feeding, and nasogastric feeds or intravenous fluids may be
required. There may be temperature instability and/or
hypoglycemia.

Dx   Chest radiography is important for diagnosis and may show one
or more discrete infiltrates or a diffuse patchy infiltrative
pattern. It may be difficult to distinguish from RDS. A CBC and
CRP are obtained, and a blood culture may identify an
organism.

Tx   Broad-spectrum antibiotics such as ampicillin and gentamicin or
cefotaxime are initiated. If an organism is isolated in the blood
culture, therapy is tailored appropriately. Duration of therapy is
influenced by clinical response and the presence of other
diagnoses such as meningitis, but in most cases would be 7 to
10 days. **See Nelson Essentials 110.**

Neonatal Sepsis

See Chapter 62, Early-Onset Group B Streptococcal Disease, and
Chapter 77, Neonatal Sepsis.

Respiratory Distress Syndrome

See Chapter 73, Respiratory Distress Syndrome.

ZEBRA ZONE

a. **Persistent pulmonary hypertension:** There is failure of pulmonary vascular resistance to fall after birth, with a subsequent increase in right atrial pressure, leading to poor oxygenation and respiratory distress. Diagnosis is made with echocardiogram, and treatment is supportive.

b. **Air leak syndromes/pneumothorax:** Pneumothorax is not rare in newborns, although most cases are asymptomatic. Larger air leaks and those involving the mediastinum may lead to respiratory distress and hypoxemia. Small air leaks may spontaneously resorb, but larger air leaks may need evacuation with needle aspiration.

**Practice-Based Learning and Improvement:
Evidence-Based Pediatrics**

Title
Hypoxic respiratory failure in the late preterm infant

Authors
Dudell GG, Jain L

Reference
Clin Perinatol 33:803-830, 2006

Problem
Late-preterm infants (34 to 37 weeks gestation) have an increased incidence of respiratory distress and respiratory failure. They are usually in the well baby nursery, often similar appearing to the term infant. Hence their vulnerability can be underrecognized.

Comparison/control (quality of evidence)
Review article with cited references summarizing diagnosis and care for late-preterm infants with early-onset respiratory distress.

Historical significance/comments
Late-preterm infants are often passed along as term newborns, and their increased incidence of complications can be missed in the early newborn period, resulting in increased morbidities and hospital readmissions. (See Chapter 59, The Late-Preterm Infant.)

Interpersonal and Communication Skills

Acknowledge and Respond to the Family's Expressed Need for Information

Always communicate with the parents in a timely fashion about any clinical concern for the newborn's respiratory status. This includes that you have reviewed the maternal history and events of labor and have determined if there are risk factors for serious disease, and that their baby will be closely monitored and supported, and tests will be ordered as indicated, depending on the baby's progress in the first few hours of life. Answer all questions, and realize that the depth of answers required may vary depending on the educational and professional background of the parents. Become comfortable in providing emotional support as well as clinical information to parents regardless of their education and occupation. Parents who are themselves physicians compared with parents who lack a medical background are likely to have more in-depth questions and potentially greater fear as they may more readily realize the possibility of a serious diagnosis.

Professionalism

Reliability and Responsibility: The Importance of Effective Hand Washing

The critical importance of effective hand washing or use of hand sanitizer before and after hands-on patient care cannot be overestimated. About 2 million hospitalized patients per year acquire a nosocomial infection, and up to 90,000 of these patients die from their infection. Antibiotic resistance and the evolution of drug-resistant "superbugs," along with the lack of new antibiotic mechanisms in pharmaceutical pipelines, makes effective and consistent hand washing a professional imperative for all health-care providers.

Systems-Based Practice

Risk Management

Risk management is a planned and systematic process to reduce and/or eliminate the probability that losses will occur in a specific setting. It consists of three distinct yet interrelated areas: (1) risk identification and loss prevention, (2) loss reduction, and (3) risk financing. To be most effective in the hospital setting, risk management involves a multidisciplinary and proactive approach.

Physicians play a central role in the risk management of a common medical-legal pitfall—assuming that respiratory distress is solely transient tachypnea of the newborn (TTNB) and not a more serious disorder (e.g., sepsis, pneumonia, persistent pulmonary hypertension, or cyanotic congenital heart disease). The key to limiting missed diagnoses is to follow the basics: think broadly, carefully review the history for risk factors, monitor the infant closely, and reassess frequently. A judicious workup should be done if there is no improvement after 4 hours. Consult neonatology as needed, and fully document your clinical findings and plan. Always communicate with the parents, answer all questions, and provide updates on the newborn's status in a timely fashion.

Chapter 67
Neonatal Hypoglycemia (Case 30)

Jennifer R. Miller MD

Case: A full-term infant born 90 minutes ago has a blood glucose level of 38 mg/dL. The mother is a 33-year-old G1P0 who had normal laboratory findings except for an abnormal glucose tolerance test. Apgar scores were 9 at 1 and 5 minutes.

Differential Diagnosis

Infant of diabetic mother	Inappropriate-for-gestational-age infant	Sepsis

Speaking Intelligently

Hypoglycemia in the newborn is a common and potentially serious problem. Glucose is the key substrate for the brain, and significant or persistent hypoglycemia can result in permanent impairment in brain growth and development. At delivery there is an abrupt interruption of placental glucose transport, causing a decrease in the newborn's glucose level in the first 4 to 6 hours. Healthy newborns rebound well because they have enhanced glycogen stores that are mobilized by increased levels of catecholamines and glucagon. Insulin levels are also decreased in the first few days of life.[1] All newborns are observed carefully in the first several hours of life, and most nurseries have nurse-driven protocols in place for testing of those with specific risk factors, because hypoglycemia can be asymptomatic (chemical hypoglycemia) or symptomatic. There is increasing agreement that a glucose level below 50 mg/dL should be treated.[1,2] Oral feeds are attempted first, with either breast milk or formula. Gavage feeds or an intravenous bolus of dextrose is used if necessary. Follow-up testing is done to ensure adequate response. Problems with maintaining glucose homeostasis are related to increased utilization or decreased production of glucose, or increased production of insulin.[1] A complete evaluation is done promptly to determine the cause for hypoglycemia, and if not readily corrected, consultation with a neonatologist is indicated.

PATIENT CARE

Clinical Thinking

- Determine if the infant is **symptomatic.** Signs and symptoms of hypoglycemia include tremors/jitteriness, lethargy, irritability, hypotonia, tachypnea or respiratory distress, apnea, cyanosis, temperature instability, and/or seizures.
- Review prenatal and labor history. Note maternal health complications, such as glucose intolerance, and any risk factors for **sepsis** such as maternal fever, prolonged rupture of membranes, or group B streptococcus colonization.
- Check for **hypoglycemia risk factors:** maternal diabetes, certain maternal medications, small for gestational age (SGA) or large for gestational age (LGA), prematurity, asphyxia, or sepsis.
- Look for signs of dysmorphology.
- Check serum glucose: Whole blood Dextrostix level is about 10% lower than the plasma level due to the effects of red blood cell mass.[1]
- Treatment options include breastfeeding or bottle feeding, IV bolus of 2 mL/kg of D10W, or a continuous infusion of glucose to maintain glucose level above 50 g/dL.
- Repeat glucose testing after treatment to **ensure normalization.** Poor response to treatment may indicate a significant underlying problem and will require transfer to neonatology for stabilization, diagnosis, and management.

History

- Any history of **maternal medications** such as beta-blockers, terbutaline, systemic steroids, beta-agonists, oral hypoglycemic agents, salicylates, or alcohol?

- Review **maternal diabetes** history. Does the mother have type 1, 2, or gestational diabetes? How is glycemic control? Did she require insulin, or was the diabetes diet controlled?
- Review prenatal testing including ultrasounds. Was there concern for anomalies or a large-for-gestational-age infant?
- Review events in the **delivery room:** Low Apgar scores and cold stress are hypoglycemia risk factors.
- **SGA** infants have inadequate glycogen stores and may be poor feeders; they are more likely to have symptomatic hypoglycemia.[1]
- **Premature** infants are susceptible due to inadequate glycogen and fat stores and decreased response to glucagon.[1]
- Infants of diabetic mothers (IDM) and **LGA** infants have a relative hyperinsulin state.
- Infants with sepsis can have increased utilization of glucose and decreased gluconeogenesis.[1,2]

Physical Examination
- Check vital signs (weight, height, head circumference, heart rate, respiratory rate, temperature).
- Perform a thorough newborn examination.
- Note any congenital anomalies, dysmorphic features, or signs of hypoglycemia.
- Observe for signs/symptoms of hypocalcemia in the infant of a diabetic mother: jitteriness, myoclonic jerks, hypothermia, respiratory distress or apnea, cyanosis, somnolence, seizure.

Tests for Consideration
- **Heelstick glucose:** Both a glucometer reading and serum glucose level are useful. Glucometer readings are fast, but may not be as accurate. $70
- **Serum calcium** $85
- **Ionized calcium** $105
- If considering sepsis:
  - **Complete blood count** $116
  - **Cerebrospinal fluid (CSF) culture** $152
  - **CSF Gram stain, glucose, protein, cell count** $405

IMAGING CONSIDERATIONS

→ **Echocardiogram:** If concern for cardiac anomaly	$1630
→ **Chest radiograph:** If respiratory symptoms or considering sepsis	$231

Infant of Diabetic Mother

Pφ   Poorly controlled diabetes creates a teratogenic milieu early on for the developing fetus, and *infants of diabetic mothers (IDM)* have a higher incidence of congenital anomalies that include congenital heart disease, caudal regression syndrome, and small left colon syndrome. In addition, they are often macrosomic due to the anabolic effects of insulin and are at risk for hypoglycemia soon after delivery due to an increased insulin level and precipitous drop in serum glucose. Maternal glucose crosses the placenta, whereas insulin does not. During pregnancy, the fetal pancreas is stimulated to increase insulin production in response to elevated glucose levels. At delivery, there is a sudden decline in glucose supply, while the infant retains its endogenous high insulin level. Hence, the infant becomes hypoglycemic, usually within the first 3 hours after birth. Difficulty with glucose regulation may last several days.[1] However, a small portion of these infants are SGA, frequently a complication of maternal vascular insufficiency and hypertension affecting placental function in maternal type 1 diabetes mellitus. These infants are also at risk for hypocalcemia, hypomagnesemia, and hyperbilirubinemia.

TP   Infants are typically LGA. They are hypoglycemic within a few hours of birth and may be so for several days. They may be asymptomatic or irritable, jittery, or hypothermic. The SGA infant is more likely to have symptoms.[1] Infants may be somnolent and feed poorly, which further contributes to difficulty maintaining a normal glucose level. In addition, they may have respiratory distress syndrome, transient tachypnea of the newborn, and/or hyperbilirubinemia.

Dx   Diagnosis can be made with accurate maternal history, newborn physical examination, and measurement of newborn glucose level. In addition, there is careful monitoring for other problems in the IDM such as respiratory distress symptoms, hyperbilirubinemia, and hypocalcemia.

Tx   Treatment of hypoglycemia begins with either breastfeeding or
      bottle feeding a stable infant with mild hypoglycemia. A
      symptomatic infant can be given a 2 mL/kg bolus of $D_{10}W$,
      or if hypoglycemia persists, an infusion of IV glucose is given
      to maintain glucose level of >50 mg/dL. Recurrent bolus
      administration is avoided because a drop in glucose can occur
      following the insulin surge with bolus administration. For
      difficult-to-control cases, transfer to neonatology is usually
      indicated. **See Nelson Essentials 59.**

Inappropriate-for-Gestational-Age Infant

Pφ   SGA infants have very little glycogen and fat stores, and
      through the transition to oral feeding they may have
      inadequate fuel for gluconeogenesis.[1] Infants who are LGA are
      often hyperinsulinemic and after delivery experience mismatch
      of insulin and glucose levels, resulting in hypoglycemia.[1]

TP   These infants present with typical hypoglycemic symptoms with
      SGA infants more likely to have overt symptoms, whereas
      chemical hypoglycemia is common in the LGA infant.[1]

Dx   Diagnosis is made by measurements of newborn size and
      glucose level. An evaluation to determine cause of the
      abnormal growth pattern may reveal intrauterine growth
      restriction (IUGR) in the term SGA infant, and further testing
      may be indicated to elucidate the cause of IUGR.

Tx   Treatment is similar to that of the IDM. Support of bottle
      feeding or breastfeeding is offered. Intravenous bolus or
      continuous IV glucose may be necessary with repeat glucose
      testing to ensure normalization. **See Nelson Essentials 60.**

Sepsis

See Chapter 46, Neonatal Fever; Chapter 62, Early-Onset Group B
Streptococcal Disease; Chapter 66, Transient Tachypnea of the
Newborn; and Chapter 77, Neonatal Sepsis, for discussions on sepsis.

ZEBRA ZONE

a. **Congenital hyperinsulinism:** Genetic defect in pancreatic insulin secretion that presents in early infancy with severe persistent hypoglycemia and seizures that requires immediate aggressive management to prevent permanent neurologic sequelae

b. **Beckwith-Weidmann syndrome:** A genetic overgrowth syndrome resulting from abnormal insulin-like growth factor II (IGF-II) with macrosomia, abdominal wall defect, and macroglossia

Practice-Based Learning and Improvement: Evidence-Based Pediatrics

Title
Infants of diabetic mothers

Authors
Nold JL, Georgieff MK

Reference
Pediatr Clin North Am 51(3):619-637, 2004

Problem
Infants of diabetic mothers are subject to numerous complications and have an increased incidence of congenital malformations throughout gestation.

Comparison/control (quality of evidence)
Review article summarizing diagnosis and care of these newborns

Interpersonal and Communication Skills

Provide Information in an Efficient and Focused Manner

Neonatal hypoglycemia necessitates rapid intervention and therefore efficient and succinct communication between all members of the health-care team. If the infant is stable and is able to feed, he/she should be breastfed or bottle fed as soon as possible. If necessary, a nasogastric tube may be placed for feeding. If neither of these is feasible, an IV must be started. All of these actions will require communication between the physician, the nursing staff, and the parents. If hypoglycemia persists, consultation with the neonatal intensive care unit will likely be indicated.

Professionalism

Reliability and Responsibility

It is essential to have clear guidelines about which infants should be evaluated for hypoglycemia and an algorithm to follow about further glucose testing and when to transfer to a more-equipped nursery for more-intense monitoring and/or treatment. Physicians should ensure that appropriate guidelines and algorithms are developed and implemented at their hospital and that nursery staff is trained. It is of utmost importance that the physician perform an appropriate and timely evaluation of any infant at risk for hypoglycemia.

Systems-Based Practice

Medical Management: Hospital Clinical Pathways

Many newborn nurseries have protocols for checking glucose level in newborns who are small or large for gestational age, babies born to diabetic mothers, or babies who are premature at the time of birth. Current consensus is that hypoglycemia is blood glucose level less than 50 mg/dL in the newborn.[1,2] If less than 50 mg/dL, guidelines to either feed the infant by mouth (or by nasogastric tube) or deliver a small bolus of D10W intravenously are useful. Glucose levels should then be monitored and treated appropriately until stabilized. Development of such standard guidelines helps ensure that babies at risk are identified and treated in a timely manner. Early identification and treatment of hypoglycemia can prevent significant morbidity and possible mortality and aid in a timely discharge of the infant.

References

1. Simmons RA: Glucose metabolism in the newborn infant. In Polin RA, Yoder MA, editors: *Workbook in practical neonatology*, ed 4, Philadelphia, 2007, Elsevier Saunders, pp 45-51.
2. Kliegman RM, Behrman RE, Jenson HB, et al: *Nelson textbook of pediatrics*, ed 18, Philadelphia, 2007, Saunders.

Professor's Pearls
Section IV: The Newborn Nursery
Jennifer R. Miller MD

Consider the following clinical problems and questions posed. Then refer to a discussion of these issues by Jennifer R. Miller MD, Assistant Professor, Associate Program Director, Pediatric Residency Program, Division of General Pediatrics, Pennsylvania State Hershey Children's Hospital, Hershey, Pennsylvania.

1. **Case:** You are seeing a 3-day-old infant in the nursery. She was born vaginally at term to a 21-year-old G1P0. Prenatal testing results were normal. Maternal and infant blood type is O Rh-positive. The infant is breastfeeding. Her birth weight was 3500 g, and her current weight is down 10%. She appears jaundiced to the nipple line. Otherwise her physical examination is normal. She is scheduled for discharge today. How do you proceed?

2. **Case:** You are called to the newborn nursery to evaluate a ½-hour-old female infant with respiratory distress. She was born at 36-⅓ weeks' gestation, by cesarean delivery for breech presentation to a 36-year-old G3P2002. Mother presented in labor, and the infant was found to be breech. Membranes were ruptured for 6 hours. Maternal laboratory test results were normal except group B streptococcus was positive. Mother was treated with one dose of clindamycin IV before the cesarean delivery. Apgar scores were 7 and 8 at 1 and 5 minutes, respectively. Over the next 20 minutes the infant began to develop tachypnea, grunting, and retractions. At the time of your examination, temperature is 37.2°C heart rate, 150 beats per minute; respiratory rate, 75 breaths per minute. Pulse oximetry is 87% on room air. Her examination is significant for crackles bilaterally at the lung bases, as well as grunting, retractions, and nasal flaring. There are no murmurs. She is vigorous. What is your approach to this patient?

3. **Case:** You are evaluating a male newborn in the nursery. As you review the maternal record, you note that a fetal ultrasound at 21 weeks of age showed left-sided hydronephrosis, with anteroposterior the diameter of the right renal pelvis at 5 mm, and the left at 8 mm. The infant is clinically well. His physical examination including the abdominal and genitourinary examination is normal. He has yet to void or pass stool. You are about to speak with the family. What should you tell them regarding this ultrasound abnormality? What studies will you order, and when should they be done?

4. **Case:** You are called to evaluate a 36-hour-old female in the nursery. This infant was born to a 16-year-old mother who received no prenatal care. The mother admits to using marijuana during pregnancy. The infant has not passed stool since birth. She was bottle feeding about 1 ounce every 3 hours. In the last two

feedings, however, her mother has struggled to get her to take $\frac{1}{2}$ ounce. She has voided four times in the last 36 hours. Her birth weight was 2875 grams, and her weight now is 2600 grams, down 6% from birth weight. Her vital signs are stable. She is jaundiced to the neck and mildly icteric. She is fussy and has a mildly distended abdomen. Otherwise her examination is normal. How will you evaluate this patient?

5. **Case:** A female newborn is being discharged from the nursery. Her mother was on selective serotonin reuptake inhibitor (SSRI) antidepressant therapy during pregnancy. Otherwise the prenatal and newborn nursery course has been uneventful. She has not passed her otoacoustic emissions (OAE) hearing screen. The nurses have attempted it three times, to no avail. What information and support can you offer to the family? What follow-up does this child require?

6. **Case:** You are called to a scheduled cesarean delivery. The infant is delivered at 37 weeks for suspected macrosomia. Maternal gestational diabetes has been diet controlled. Otherwise, prenatal labs and testing results were normal. The infant weighs 4000 g at birth. Apgar scores are 6 and 9 at 1 and 5 minutes, respectively. On examination, you note the macrosomia, and a grade II/VI systolic murmur at the left middle sternal border. There is no cyanosis or respiratory distress. The infant's pulses are full. How do you proceed?

Discussion by Jennifer R. Miller MD, Assistant Professor, Associate Program Director, Pediatric Residency Program, Division of General Pediatrics, Pennsylvania State Hershey Children's Hospital, Hershey, Pennsylvania.

1. **Discussion:** This infant is likely not feeding effectively. A young, first-time mother will usually require much guidance with breastfeeding. You may consider a lactation consultation to help with positioning, hold, timing of breastfeeding, and overall bonding with the newborn. Attempts at breastfeeding should be made every 2 to 3 hours around the clock. A breast pump to use after nursing may help stimulate the mother's milk production. This infant should be supplemented with either pumped breast milk or commercial formula after every breastfeeding attempt.

   This infant is jaundiced, and therefore a transcutaneous bilirubin or a total and direct serum bilirubin measurement is appropriate. The American Academy of Pediatrics offers guidelines on what levels require phototherapy, and what levels predict a high risk for needing phototherapy in the coming days.

   Close follow-up will be necessary, and the baby should be seen by a medical provider within 1 to 2 days of discharge depending on the bilirubin level. This can be accomplished with a trusted visiting nurse agency or with the patient's primary care provider.

2. **Discussion:** There are two major possibilities: transient tachypnea of the newborn (TTNB), and pneumonia/sepsis. Note that this infant is at risk for early-onset group B streptococcus (EOGBS) disease because the mother is GBS positive and had ruptured membranes with incomplete intrapartum antibiotic prophylaxis (IAP) because the drug used was clindamycin. Only penicillin, ampicillin, or cefazolin given at least 4 hours before delivery are considered adequate IAP. So one must be particularly careful in the evaluation of this newborn. After assessing the airway, breathing, and circulation (ABCs), oxygen should be placed on the infant. This may be accomplished by nasal cannula, face mask, or hood. A chest radiograph should be obtained. TTNB will often show a reticular hazy appearance, with increased interstitial fluid and fluid in the right horizontal fissure. Pneumonia will appear as a patchy infiltrate, usually without excess fluid. In addition, a complete blood count (CBC) and a blood culture should be obtained. If the radiographic findings are consistent with TTNB and the CBC is reassuring, the infant can be carefully monitored without antibiotics. Oxygen can be weaned as tolerated. IV fluids may be required, because a tachypneic infant may be at risk for aspiration with feeds. If the radiographic findings or CBC are not reassuring, a complete sepsis workup may be completed and IV antibiotics begun.

3. **Discussion:** This infant has unilateral hydronephrosis. Careful family history is important, looking for any kidney disorders (solitary kidney, dysplastic kidney). With a negative family history and normal physical examination, this baby is still at risk for renal pathology, unilateral urinary obstruction, and/or vesicoureteral reflux. He needs to be monitored carefully for presence of urination and if possible, strength of urinary stream. He should have a renal ultrasound and voiding cystourethrogram scheduled for about 1 t 2 weeks of life, once his normal fluid status is reestablished after the initial weight loss at birth. The decision to place him on prophylactic antibiotics is controversial. Ongoing studies are addressing the need for this measure. A consultation with a pediatric urologist may be considered, depending on the results of the postnatal ultrasound.

4. **Discussion:** Because this infant has not passed stool in the first 24 hours of life, she is at risk for an intestinal obstruction. She is not vomiting, so it is more likely to be a lower intestinal obstruction. The first step is to perform an inspection of the rectum and attempt a digital rectal examination. If there is a small meconium plug, this may eliminate the problem. If that is not successful, temporarily stop feeding the infant, administer IV fluids, and order a stat plain film of the abdomen. She may suffer from meconium ileus, more proximal meconium plug, Hirschsprung disease, or a small/malformed colon. Plain radiography may not delineate these, and barium enema may be necessary. Consultation

with the neonatal intensive care unit and a pediatric surgeon early in the workup is necessary, because the clinical status of the infant may change very quickly.

5. **Discussion:** Many newborns fail to pass (refer) their newborn hearing screens. Vernix in the ear canals, ambient noise in the nursery, fussy newborns, all contribute to false-positive (referred) results. In fact up to 10% of newborns may fail newborn hearing screen. There is good evidence that 80% who refer are subsequently found to have normal hearing thresholds.

This child requires a follow-up repeat hearing screen. This is usually accomplished with automated auditory brainstem response (AABR) testing. Rescreening should occur within the first month of life. Many hospitals have procedures in place to order rescreenings, so that infants at risk are sure to have follow-up scheduled. Information regarding the failure to pass the screen should also be forwarded to the child's primary care provider.

Finally, because this mother was on antidepressant therapy during her pregnancy, she will likely be at high risk for postpartum depression. Although no parent wants to hear that there is an abnormality with their child, the mother at risk for postpartum depression may react differently than most. Although it is important to be factual and honest while discussing any newborn concern, the physician must temper that with compassion and hope. If necessary, consultation with the obstetricians for formal depression evaluation may be appropriate.

6. **Discussion:** This is an infant of a diabetic mother (IDM) who requires close monitoring of glucose levels. It is appropriate to check a heelstick glucose with the routine initial assessment of such an infant. If the infant is stable, as in this case, and the glucose level is 50 mg/dL or less, most pediatricians would encourage the infant to feed by bottle or by breast if possible. This is often not possible because the mother is usually still recovering from the cesarean delivery. Most newborn nurseries have a specific protocol for glucose monitoring in these babies. For example, glucose could be checked every hour for four measurements. If all glucose measurements are over 50 mg/dL, the glucose level could be checked every 2 hours for two measurements, and if all are over 50 mg/dL, it could be checked progressively less often according to protocol.

Because of maternal gestational diabetes, this infant has increased risk for congenital abnormalities. Careful assessment of the infant's murmur is appropriate. The timing and the description of this murmur are consistent with a patent ductus arteriosus. If, however, this murmur is persistent through the nursery stay, or if the infant becomes cyanotic, tachypneic, or distressed, evaluation with four extremity blood pressures, chest radiography, and echocardiography would be appropriate.

Section V
THE NEONATAL
INTENSIVE CARE UNIT

Section Editor

Helen M. Towers MD

Section Contents

Chapter 68
Delivery Room Management of the Newborn Infant

Jane S. Lee MD, MPH

Medical Knowledge and Patient Care

Over 4 million infants are born each year in the United States. Approximately 10% of these newly born infants require active intervention in the delivery room, and approximately 1% require extensive resuscitation to sustain life. National guidelines have been developed to provide health-care workers with the necessary training for competency and uniformity in neonatal resuscitation.[1-3] They address a sequential increase in assistance based on the physiologic response of the infant to each intervention along an algorithm.

Initial Assessment: At least one appropriately trained medical person should be present to perform a rapid assessment of an infant after delivery. This assessment determines the infant's overall maturity, presence of meconium, quality of respirations, and degree of muscle tone. If transition to extrauterine life is uneventful, the infant receives routine care that comprises drying, warming, positioning, and possibly suctioning to clear the airway. In the event that extrauterine transition is delayed or inadequate, resuscitation is begun. Further intervention is administered based on an "evaluation-decision-action" assessment of the infant's respirations, heart rate, and color at 30-second intervals. An Apgar score is assigned to the infant at 1 minute and 5 minutes after birth. The Apgar score is a mechanism by which one can assess and summarize the condition of the newborn after childbirth and allows caregivers to understand the condition of the infant after birth. The Apgar score comprises five components: skin color, heart rate, reflex irritability, muscle tone, and respirations. Each component can be scored from 0 to 2 points, allowing the cumulative score to be between 0 and 10 points total.

Assisted Ventilation: Effective ventilation is the most crucial step in any resuscitation. Free-flow oxygen is administered to any infant who appears cyanotic but otherwise has adequate respiratory effort and heart rate. Supplemental oxygen may be gradually removed as the cyanosis resolves. However, if the cyanosis persists despite the administration of 100% oxygen, a trial of positive-pressure ventilation may be administered with bag and mask. Positive-pressure ventilation is also indicated for infants with persistent apnea or gasping respirations, despite brief tactile stimulation and for bradycardic infants whose heart rate is less than 100 beats per minute. The initial positive-pressure breaths often require higher inflation pressures to establish functional residual capacity. Subsequent breaths are delivered so that the infant receives the lowest inflation pressures necessary to produce adequate chest rise. Signs of effective ventilation are good chest movement, audible breath sounds, and rapid improvement in heart rate and color. Once positive-pressure ventilation is initiated, resuscitation should proceed with the use of 100% oxygen. A notable exception is the premature infant, for whom use of variable oxygen concentration between 21% and 100% may be used to maintain adequate oxygen saturation. If no appreciable improvement is observed within 90 seconds of initiating resuscitation with room air, supplemental oxygen should be provided.

Endotracheal Intubation: Endotracheal intubation is indicated when positive-pressure ventilation with bag and mask is ineffective or required for prolonged duration. Other indications include tracheal suctioning for meconium, continued chest compressions, endotracheal administration of medications, and special situations such as congenital diaphragmatic hernia and extreme prematurity. The infant should receive free-flow oxygen throughout the intubation in order to minimize hypoxia, and each attempt should be limited to less than 20 seconds duration. The best indication of successful endotracheal intubation is a prompt improvement in vital signs. Endotracheal placement should be confirmed by exhaled carbon dioxide (CO_2) detection. The most commonly used CO_2 detector is a colorimetric device that confirms placement by demonstrating a rapid change in detector color from violet to yellow. A false-negative result may occur in infants with decreased pulmonary blood flow or low cardiac output. Other clinical indicators such as condensed humidified gas within the endotracheal tube during exhalation and equal breath sounds on auscultation may be helpful but are not as reliable alone.

Meconium-Stained Amniotic Fluid: Meconium-stained amniotic fluid (MSAF) occurs in approximately 10% to 15% of all deliveries with increasing incidence as pregnancies extend beyond 42 weeks gestation. Of those infants born through MSAF, only 3% to 12% exhibit respiratory distress consistent with meconium aspiration syndrome (MAS). Up to 50% of infants who develop MAS will require intubation and mechanical ventilation. Evidence from multicenter, randomized controlled studies altered long-standing obstetric and neonatal practices, and now **routine intrapartum oropharyngeal and nasopharyngeal suctioning of the hypopharynx before delivery of the infant's shoulders is no longer advised** because these practices did not reduce the incidence of MAS. Endotracheal intubation and direct tracheal suctioning of meconium is still recommended in the infant who appears depressed at birth or who subsequently develops respiratory distress after initial assessment. Visible meconium is removed by bulb suction or large-bore catheter suction. If endotracheal intubation is indicated, continuous suctioning by means of a meconium aspirator should be applied as the tube is gradually removed. Repeat intubation and suctioning is recommended until no further meconium is recovered or until "significant bradycardia" indicates that resuscitation must proceed.

Chest Compressions: Chest compressions are indicated in any infant whose heart rate remains less than 60 beats per minute despite a minimum of 30 seconds of adequate ventilation. The lower third of the sternum is compressed a relative depth of approximately one-third of the anterior-posterior diameter of the chest with two-thumb encircling hand technique. Alternatively, a two-finger technique may be preferable during attempts at umbilical catheterization for intravenous access. Chest compressions are coordinated with assisted ventilation in a 3:1 ratio so that the infant receives 90 compressions for every 30 breaths. The heart rate is periodically reassessed by either palpating pulsations at the base of the umbilical cord or by auscultation of the infant's precordium. Once the heart rate exceeds 60 beats per minute, chest compressions may be discontinued. Positive-pressure ventilation then continues at a faster rate of 40 to 60 breaths per minute until the infant's heart rate exceeds 100 beats per minute and spontaneous respirations occur. If the heart rate remains less than 60 beats per minute despite coordinated ventilation–chest compression, administration of epinephrine is indicated.

Resuscitative Medications: Only a small minority of infants require resuscitative medications. The medications available for use in the delivery room are epinephrine, volume expanders, naloxone, and sodium bicarbonate. Although the intratracheal route is the most accessible route, intravenous administration via the umbilical vein is the preferred route of drug administration. Alternatively, peripheral venous cannulation may be attempted. If intravenous access cannot be obtained, intraosseous administration is an acceptable alternative.

Epinephrine should be administered if the infant's heart rate remains less than 60 beats per minute despite adequate coordinated ventilation and chest compressions of at least 30 seconds' duration. The recommended dose is 0.01 to 0.03 mg/kg of a 1:10,000 solution infused intravenously as quickly as possible followed by a 0.5 to 1 mL flush of normal saline. A larger dose (0.05 to 0.1 mg/kg) may be given via the intratracheal route while intravenous access is attempted. Repeat doses of epinephrine should be administered intravenously as necessary on a 3- to 5-minute interval.

In the setting of acute blood loss or shock, isotonic crystalloid solution (i.e., normal saline or Ringer's lactate) is indicated for volume expansion. Albumin should not be used as a volume expander because equally efficacious alternatives are available.

The recommended dose is 10 mL/kg infused intravenously or intraosseously over 5 to 10 minutes duration. However, rapid infusions of volume expanders should be avoided in premature infants given its association with intraventricular hemorrhage. Additional doses may be necessary depending on degree of suspected blood loss. If large blood loss is anticipated, O Rh-negative packed red blood cells may also be considered.

Rarely, other medications such as a narcotic antagonist, buffer, or vasopressor may be useful following initial resuscitation. However, these medications are not recommended for use in the delivery room.

Practice-Based Learning and Improvement

Title
A proposal for a new method of evaluation of the newborn infant

Author
Apgar V

Reference
Curr Res Anesth Analg 32:260-267, 1953

Problem
Need to develop a method to rapidly assess a newborn infant

Intervention
Chart review of 1760 infants born at a single institution over 1 year

Outcome/effect
Development of a scoring system to summarize newborn well-being

Historical significance/comments
Note that the Apgar score was developed from a retrospective study in 1953, arising from a need for an accurate and replicable method for evaluating and reporting on the newborn infant. The Apgar score is now used worldwide as a means of communicating the health of a newborn at 1- and 5-minute intervals after birth. It forms the basis of comparing populations when performing neonatal research and is an invaluable communication tool.

Interpersonal and Communication Skills

Reach Agreement on Problems and Plan: Explain Choices in Light of Family Goal and Values

If resuscitation is anticipated because of perinatal circumstances, the parents should meet with both the obstetric and neonatal providers before delivery so that they may receive relevant and accurate information on the expected survival, the spectrum of possible outcomes and treatment options, and the potential risks associated with the available therapies. Once the resuscitation commences, the family should be kept informed periodically as to what is happening. As the resuscitation progresses, it is critical that ongoing discussions occur between the medical team and the parents so that they may participate in the decision making concerning the care of their infant.

Professionalism

Self-Improvement: Commit to Lifelong Learning and Education

The acquisition and maintenance of knowledge and skills is an important part of medical training and practice. Certification in neonatal resuscitation is available and should be updated regularly. Individuals who work in the delivery room must be certified, and certification is recommended for health-care personnel who work in the emergency department, where deliveries occur quite frequently. A competent and efficient resuscitation of a neonate and its consequent outcomes depend on the presence of a team of health-care providers who are familiar with and practice neonatal resuscitation in accordance with the national guidelines.

Systems-Based Practice

Quality Improvement: The Joint Commission and Sentinel Event Policy

A sentinel event is considered a significant adverse unexpected event that occurs to a patient. The Joint Commission (formerly known as JCAHO) reviews sentinel events in order to identify important systems issues that may have contributed to the event occurrence. The Joint Commission defines what cases must be reported for review under its sentinel event policy. For the delivery room, the types of cases considered reviewable under the sentinel event policy are "any perinatal death or major permanent loss of function unrelated to a congenital condition in an infant having a birth weight greater than 2,500 grams." Based upon reviews of these events, The Joint Commission publishes root causes, risk reduction strategies, and recommendations for improvement in order to reduce the likelihood of similar events occurring at other institutions. These findings can be seen at The Joint Commission website.[4]

References

1. Perman JM, Wyllie J, Kattwinkel J, et al, Neonatal Resuscitation Chapter Collaborators: Part 11: Neonatal Resuscitation: 2010 International Consensus on Cardiopulmonary Resuscitation and Emergency Cardiovascular Care Science With Treatment Recommendations. *Circulation* 122(16 Suppl 2):S516-S538, 2010.
2. Kattwinkel J, Perlman JM, Aziz K, et al: Part 15: Neonatal Resuscitation: 2010 American Heart Association Guidelines for Cardiopulmonary Resuscitation and Emergency Cardiovascular Care. *Circulation* 122(18 Suppl 3):S909-S919, 2010.
3. Kattwinkel J, editor: *Textbook of Neonatal Resuscitation*, ed 5. Elk Grove Village, IL, 2006, American Academy of Pediatrics/American Heart Association.
4. Joint Commission. Sentinel event alert. Available at: http://www.jointcommission.org/SentinelEvents/SentinelEventAlert/sea_30.htm.

Chapter 69
The Preterm Infant

Christiana R. Farkouh MD, MPH

Patient Care and Medical Knowledge

A preterm birth refers to any baby born before the thirty-seventh week of pregnancy. Infants born prematurely can be further classified into three categories based on birth weight. Low-birth-weight (LBW) infants are those with a birth weight below 2500 grams. A very low-birth-weight (VLBW) infant weighs less than 1500 grams, and an extremely low-birth-weight (ELBW) infant weighs less than 1000 grams. Although an infant born at 25 weeks' and one born at 35 weeks' gestation are both considered premature, the medical concerns and care required to support each differ considerably in terms of required resources, and the infants may have vastly different outcomes.

Major concerns relating to prematurity include stabilization in the delivery room and evaluation of the degree of immaturity of vital organ systems. Following initial stabilization, attention is closely paid to ongoing cardiorespiratory needs, hemodynamic status, fluid administration, electrolyte monitoring, neurologic status, temperature stability, likely infectious complications, and ultimately feeding tolerance and readiness for discharge. It is these factors that will ultimately determine the duration of the infant's neonatal intensive care unit (NICU) stay. A systems approach is best in identifying and providing overall medical needs of the infant:

Cardiovascular: Hemodynamic stability is an important consideration requiring ongoing monitoring, with indwelling catheters required in the smallest and sickest of patients. Fluctuations in blood pressure may affect the pressure passive cerebral circulation. The effect of a large patent ductus arteriosus may impact the respiratory, cardiac, and renal systems and pose a risk to blood supply to the gastrointestinal (GI) tract.

Infectious Disease: Perinatal and postnatal infection, in the face of an immature immune system, can pose a tremendous challenge, affecting the infant's respiratory status, hemodynamic stability, fluid and electrolyte balance, and ultimate neurodevelopmental outcome.

Neurologic: Early serial evaluations for intraventricular/intracranial hemorrhage and periventricular leukomalacia play a vital role in counseling families about possible long-term neurodevelopmental concerns, but extreme caution must be maintained in making predictions of long-term neurodevelopmental outcome based on ultrasound findings.

Developmental immaturity of the respiratory control centers can result in apnea of prematurity. For some preterm infants the resultant apnea, bradycardia, and desaturation events may be few and self-limiting; however, for others, these events can be quite frequent, requiring significant stimulation. Medical therapy with caffeine has been used. Intubation is occasionally necessary.

Pulmonary: Respiratory distress syndrome (RDS) (see Chapter 73, Respiratory Distress Syndrome), resulting from an immaturity in lung surfactant development, carries a risk for development of air leaks, including pneumothorax and pulmonary interstitial emphysema. The respiratory system is often the focus of care during the initial hours, days, and possibly weeks of a premature infant's life. The most preterm infants, those less than 26 completed weeks' gestation, are most susceptible to respiratory complications as a result of both an immature pulmonary surfactant system and also an arrest of alveolar development. Most infants below 28 weeks' gestation will require intubation and mechanical ventilation with surfactant administration and supplemental oxygen as needed to adequately support oxygenation. Efforts are made to avoid hyperoxia in preterm infants under 32 to 34 weeks due to concerns of free radical production and its impact on lung tissue injury as well as on the developing retinal vasculature, leading to retinopathy of prematurity (ROP). Many NICUs have adopted target oxygen saturation levels that range from 88% to 92% for infants on increased ambient oxygen as an effort to prevent the deleterious effects of hyperoxia.

Gastrointestinal: Intravenous access via either an umbilical catheter or peripheral intravenous line is needed to ensure adequate fluid administration, caloric intake, and hemodynamic stability. A central venous catheter (i.e., percutaneous central venous line (PCVL), peripherally inserted central catheter [PICC]) may be required to ensure maximal caloric intake that favors optimal growth. When on sufficient parenteral caloric support, fluid requirements of 120 to 140 mL/kg/day can provide sufficient caloric support of 120 kcal/kg/day for a growing preterm infant. Infants under 750 g may require even higher fluid amounts as a result of significant insensible fluid losses through their immature skin. Because urine output is not a reliable marker of fluid status in the first 24 to 48 hours of life, monitoring serum electrolytes at a regular interval will assist in assessing overall fluid status. Frequent blood monitoring carries the high likelihood of need for blood transfusion, and efforts should be made to minimize exposure to multiple donors.

Early initiation of enteral nutrition, otherwise called "trophic feeds" of volume ≤10 mL/kg/day, via a nasogastric or orogastric tube in hemodynamically stable preterm infants is encouraged. Trophic feedings aid in priming the immature gut, encourage normal gastrointestinal hormonal release, and have not been associated with increased incidence of necrotizing enterocolitis, which is a significant pathologic condition in preterm infants (see Chapter 72, Necrotizing Enterocolitis).

All mothers of preterm infants should be encouraged to provide breast milk feedings for their infants because the immunologic benefits of breast milk have yet to be matched by specially designed preterm infant formulas. Once feeds are tolerated, they can be advanced by ≤20mL/kg/day. Fortification of breast milk is usually necessary to provide the appropriate caloric intake as well as calcium and phosphorus requirements for a growing preterm infant. As the preterm infant approaches 33 to 34 weeks and demonstrates a coordinated suck-swallow-breathing mechanism, the advancement to oral bottle feeding or breastfeeding may begin.

Ophthalmologic: Retinopathy of prematurity (ROP) screening protocols exist in most NICUs to follow retinal vascular development and identify those at high risk for ROP requiring intervention with laser therapy. Current standards are to screen all infants under 1500 g or less than 28 weeks or those with an unstable clinical course felt to be at high risk by the attending caregiver.

The Late-Preterm Infant

Recently, attention has been paid to the late preterm infant. These infants are born prematurely between 34 and 36 5/7 weeks gestation. Although many of these infants may be the size of a full-term infant and may also be cared for in the well baby nursery, they do carry some of the risks seen in the preterm population. In addition, they experience prolonged hospitalizations and rehospitalization at greater rates than their full term counterparts. (See Chapter 59, The Late-Preterm Infant.)

Practice-Based Learning and Improvement

Title
Early surfactant administration with brief ventilation vs. selective surfactant and continued mechanical ventilation for preterm infants with or at risk for respiratory distress syndrome

Authors
Stevens TP, Harrington EW, Blennow M, Soll RF

Reference
Cochrane Neonatal Group, *Cochrane Database Syst* Rev 4, 2007

Problem
Should surfactant be given early to all premature infants with signs of RDS?

Intervention
Studies of early surfactant administration

Comparison/control
Studies of later selective surfactant administration

Quality of evidence
Systematic review of randomized controlled trials

Outcome/effect
In early surfactant administration, there is lower incidence of mechanical ventilation, air leak syndromes, and bronchopulmonary dysplasia (BPD).

Historical significance/comments
This is the basis for the current strategy of surfactant administration use in premature infants.

Interpersonal and Communication Skills

Establish Rapport and Encourage Partnership Between Physician and Family

If the situation allows, meeting the parent before the delivery can be a valuable step in the process of caring for a preterm infant. This early meeting allows the parents to meet the physician who will be caring for their infant and gives the physician the opportunity to begin to develop a relationship with the family. Important information regarding a health-care plan can be shared at this meeting. This conversation is often the parents' first time to become aware of the multiple medical conditions their infant may be at risk for, and the information may be tailored depending on the degree of prematurity and presence of other complicating factors. Such an introduction lays the framework for ongoing discussions regarding the infant's clinical status. It is also the vital first step to development of a strong partnership between the physician and the family.

Professionalism

Advocacy for Parents in the Neonatal Intensive Care Unit

Parents are often over whelmed by the NICU and often do not feel they can "parent" their child in this setting. Allowing the parents to have as much interaction with their infant as possible, including physical handling, will facilitate bonding and increase their self-efficacy and confidence as parents. Parents should not only be offered assistance by the medical staff but also by social workers, psychologists, and chaplains to help them adjust to their altered parenting role while coping with the stress, anxiety, and uncertainty of having a premature infant.

Systems-Based Practice

Care Coordination for Neonatal Intensive Care Unit "Graduates"

Pediatricians should be aware of the short- and long-term needs of premature infants. Neonatal follow-up clinics are primarily for the surveillance of the babies' progress in terms of their growth and development. In general, visits to such a clinic are scheduled at 4, 8, 12, 18, and 24 months corrected age. Extremely premature babies and babies who endured more serious complications may need to be followed more frequently and for a longer duration.

About 25% of the youngest and smallest babies who "graduate" from NICU care live with long-term health problems, including cerebral palsy, blindness, and chronic conditions.[1] Children born prematurely are at greater risk for lower cognitive test scores, learning difficulties, and behavioral problems when compared with full-term children.[2]

References

1. Hack M, Flannery DJ, Schluchter M, et al: Outcomes in young adulthood for very-low-birth-weight infants. *N Engl J Med* 346:149-157, 2002.
2. Bhutta AT, Cleves MA, Casey PH, et al: Cognitive and behavioral outcomes of school-aged children who were born preterm. *JAMA* 288:728-737, 2002.

Chapter 70
The Growth-Restricted Infant

Christiana R. Farkouh MD, MPH

Medical Knowledge and Patient Care

Background and Definition

Intrauterine growth restriction (IUGR) represents a deviation and reduction in the expected fetal growth pattern. Fetal growth restriction complicates 5% to 8% of all pregnancies. IUGR is associated with a higher incidence of pregnancy complications, including stillbirth, prematurity, and perinatal morbidity and mortality. Often the terms *small for gestational age (SGA)* and *IUGR* are used interchangeably, but incorrectly. The critical distinction in the difference between SGA and IUGR is in the fetal growth potential. An SGA infant is one whose birth weight is below the 10th percentile, whereas an IUGR infant has failed to meet his or her growth potential or has shown a deceleration in the growth pattern during gestation.

The multiple causes of IUGR can be divided into three major categories of origin: **fetal, placental,** and **maternal.** Approximately 40% of cases of IUGR have no identifiable cause. Traditionally IUGR has been divided into symmetric or asymmetric growth restriction. The distinction between the two may relate to the timing of an intrauterine insult, as well as the possible cause and indeed even the severity of any inciting factor, but it is unclear if this distinction alone is tied to ultimate outcome.

Symmetric IUGR refers to any infant with a decrease in all parameters of weight, length, and head circumference. It is generally considered to be due to an event or process that occurs early in the pregnancy. Infants with **asymmetric IUGR** have decreased weight and length but demonstrate a relative head sparing; this event or process is believed to occur later in pregnancy.

Fetal Factors

Fetal factors that can impact in utero growth include chromosomal abnormalities such as trisomy 21, 18, or 13 or Turner syndrome. Genetic syndromes, including Russell-Silver and Cornelia de Lange as well as congenital malformations, multiple gestations, and congenital infection, have been associated with intrauterine growth restriction. The viral infections associated with IUGR have been given the acronym TORCH: toxoplasmosis, other (syphilis and other viruses), rubella, cytomegalovirus (CMV), and herpes.

Placental Factors

Placental factors that are associated with an increased risk for development of IUGR include abnormal placental implantation (velamentous cord insertions, previa, abruption), abnormal morphology, placental lesions, placental infarction, and placental infection.

Maternal Factors

Maternal factors that can impact fetal growth include chronic medical conditions such as diabetes, vascular diseases, auto immune diseases, hemoglobinopathy, hypertension, and preeclampsia. These chronic medical conditions can affect uterine blood flow as well as placental development and function. Factors related to maternal constitutional factors such as prepregnancy weight as well as weight gain during pregnancy correlate with fetal growth. Maternal cigarette, alcohol, drug (cocaine, heroin), and certain medications (warfarin, tretinoin [Retin-A]) use have all been associated with poor fetal growth both by the direct impact that these exposures have on placental function and also as a correlate of maternal nutrition. In addition, a prior history of a pregnancy complicated by IUGR, stillbirth, and/or spontaneous abortion is associated with an increased incidence of IUGR in a subsequent pregnancy.

Both **term and preterm infants** may manifest intrauterine growth restriction. The ultimate long-term outcome relates not only to the gestational age at birth but also the etiology, as well as the degree of the growth restriction. The incidence of perinatal morbidities correlates with the severity of the growth restriction. Morbidities such as respiratory distress syndrome, perinatal asphyxia, hyperviscosity-polycythemia syndrome, immunodeficiency, and metabolic derangements such as hypoglycemia, hypothermia, and hypocalcemia all occur at greater frequency in infants with IUGR compared with their appropriate-for-gestational-age (AGA) counterparts. The potential **neurodevelopmental long-term outcomes** associated with IUGR infants manifest as motor issues such as cerebral palsy, as well as learning and behavioral problems and altered postnatal growth.

Epidemiologic studies have demonstrated that **altered fetal growth may be associated with the development of adult diseases** such as insulin resistance, type 2 diabetes mellitus, obesity, hypertension, and cardiovascular disease. It has been hypothesized that the developmental adaptations that occur as a result of the altered fetal growth permanently alters postnatal physiology. This period of fetal development represents a period of rapid cell division, during which an insult or stressor may have long-lasting consequences on the tissue or organ function. This hypothesis is referred to the Barker hypothesis or the fetal origins hypothesis.

Practice-Based Improvement: Evidence-Based Medicine

Title
Neonatal management and long-term sequelae

Authors
Halliday H

Reference
Best Pract Res Clin Obstet Gynaecol 23:871-880, 2009

Problem
This is a full review of the definition and terminology used in IUGR, including a discussion of all possible etiologies. Neonatal outcomes, implications for the newborn infant, and long-term sequelae are discussed.

Interpersonal and Communication Skills

Identify Resources and Support When Preterm Delivery Is Anticipated

If a preterm delivery is anticipated, the mother should be counseled regarding the short- and long-term morbidities that a preterm, growth-restricted infant is at higher risk for developing. As in any delivery of a preterm infant, this discussion often serves as the initial introduction that the mother and her family may have to neonatal intensive care and all the stresses entailed in admission to an intensive care unit. Most mothers need support during this difficult time. Identifying family support, as well as discussing hospital support systems, may reassure the parents that there will be systems in place to help them through this process. Hospital support systems that may be appropriate depending on the circumstances include nutritionists, social workers, geneticists (if a genetic syndrome is suspected), and maternal support groups. Confirming understanding, and being available for follow-up questions will be the foundation of developing a good relationship between the family and the health-care team.

Professionalism

Responsibility and Self-Improvement: Remain Current on Assessment Tools for Gestational Age

Accurate assessment of gestational age is required before infant growth parameters can be plotted on the standard newborn growth curves and a determination of symmetric or asymmetric IUGR made. Optimal management of newborns depends on whether they are classified as AGA, SGA, or LGA. This classification is made using the Ballard (formerly Dubowitz) gestational age assessment tool, which includes a series of physical and neurologic maturity items that are scored. Physicians who care for newborns must not only be familiar with this gestational age assessment tool but also skilled in administering it and willing to take the time to perform the assessment.

Systems-Based Practice

Health-Care Economics: Claims, Coding, and Billing

In 1983 Medicare established what is called the Prospective Payment System (PPS). Under this system, a patient is classified into a Diagnosis-Related Group (DRG). This grouping is based upon the clinical condition(s) of the patient, including the diagnosis, comorbidities, procedures, and discharge disposition as well as patient demographics such as age and gender. PPS then pays a flat rate for any given DRG. With a flat rate payment system, there is incentive for the health-care provider to provide efficient health-care delivery because the provider will receive that flat rate regardless of the duration or type of care they provide.

To receive the highest reimbursement, hospital personnel must thoroughly document the above information. This documentation allows each important billable service to be "coded." This code is known as the ICD-9-CM or ICD-9. This is a coding system with thousands of diagnoses and procedures, each of which receives an assigned number within the code. It is this coding that ultimately determines the DRG for that patient. In some systems the physicians themselves assign the ICD-9 codes for the patient; however, many hospitals employ trained coders who are experienced in determining all of the possible ICD-9 codes that can be applied to the patient. This model is often used because trained coders are excellent at assigning ICD-9 codes that physicians often do not consider. This then leads to a better-paying DRG assignment and a higher rate of reimbursement. Ultimately though, without supporting documentation in the medical record in the form of clear and concise notes, these codes cannot be applied and in some cases may be considered fraudulent.[1]

Reference

1. American Hospital Directory: Available at http://www.ahd.com/pps.html.

Chapter 71
Follow-Up Care of the Premature Infant

Jane S. Lee MD, MPH

Medical Knowledge and Patient Care

Technologic advances in perinatal care have led to an improvement in survival of infants born prematurely. Currently, an estimated 13% of all newly born infants in the United States are born preterm (defined as birth before 37 weeks gestation). Although the total number of survivors has increased, these infants continue to remain vulnerable to a variety of medical and developmental morbidities associated with their underlying immaturity. The importance of the role of the family as partners in providing care for their infant before and after discharge from a neonatal intensive care unit (NICU) cannot be underestimated.

Preparation for Discharge from the NICU: In 1998 the American Academy of Pediatrics (AAP) proposed guidelines on hospital discharge of high-risk neonates. The essential physiologic competencies that must be achieved before discharge include **temperature regulation,** maintenance of **stable cardiorespiratory function,** and the **ability to nipple an adequate volume of feeding** to sustain an acceptable pattern of growth. Although interrelated, each of these competencies may not be necessarily accomplished by the same postnatal age because the maturation of these processes is influenced by the infant's birth weight (BW), gestational age (GA), and severity of associated medical illnesses. The majority of preterm infants typically attain these competencies between 34 and 36 weeks postmenstrual age (PMA).

Concurrently, the **parents must also demonstrate an ability to care for their infant.** As early as possible, at least two family members should participate in the infant's care to ensure ample time for education in acquiring the skills and judgment required to provide appropriate care.

Common Medical Issues

Immunization is a critical component of preventive care. The timing and dosing of routine primary immunization for diphtheria, tetanus, pertussis, *Haemophilus influenzae* type b, poliomyelitis, pneumococcal disease, and influenza should be based on chronologic age and not on adjusted age. Because of increased risk for hospitalization from viral gastroenteritis, the AAP supports rotavirus immunization in medically stable preterm infants between 6 and 12 weeks of age at the time of discharge or after the infant has been discharged home.

Infants less than 2 kg born to mothers who are hepatitis B surface antigen (HBsAg) negative should receive the initial dose of hepatitis B vaccine (HBV) at 30 days (chronologic) or at hospital discharge, whichever occurs earliest. If maternal HBsAg status is unknown, HBV and hepatitis B immune globulin should be administered within the first 12 hours of age, because preterm and low-birth-weight infants may have a less predictable response to HBV. Infants born to HBsAg-positive mothers should receive HBV and hepatitis B immune globulin (HBIG) within 12 hours after birth as well as a series of three additional doses starting at 1 month of age.

Immunoprophylaxis with palivizumab has been shown to decrease the rate of hospital-associated respiratory syncytial virus (RSV). Prophylaxis is recommended for preterm infants and children younger than 2 years of age with chronic lung disease who require medical therapy (i.e., supplemental oxygen, bronchodilator, diuretic, or corticosteroid therapy) within 6 months before the anticipated start of the RSV season. Other groups for whom RSV prophylaxis is recommended include infants born ≤28 weeks' gestation during the first 12 months, infants born between 29 and 31 weeks' gestation during the first 6 months, and infants born between 32 and 35 weeks gestation who are less than 6 months, chronologic age, with at least two risk factors (i.e., child care attendance, school-age siblings, congenital abnormalities of the airway, or severe neuromuscular disease). Once prophylaxis is initiated, a total of up to five consecutive monthly doses should be administered to provide sufficient protection for the entire RSV season, except for those with neuromuscular disease, who need prophylaxis until 90 days of age. Even after a documented RSV infection, prophylaxis should continue because various strains of RSV may cocirculate.

Apnea of prematurity (AOP) is defined as a cessation of breathing of at least 20 seconds duration or a cessation of breathing associated with bradycardia or oxygen desaturation. In hospitalized infants, episodes may be treated with methylxanthine therapy and/or continuous positive airway pressure. Although AOP typically resolves by 37 weeks PMA, episodes may persist until approximately 43 weeks PMA. Before discharge, infants are typically observed for a preset observation period during which the infant should remain event-free. For infants with an unusually prolonged course of recurrent severe AOP, home cardiorespiratory monitoring may be prescribed until approximately 43 weeks PMA or after the cessation of extreme episodes, whichever comes last. Evidence-based review of the literature suggests **there is no evidence that home monitoring will reduce apparent life-threatening events or deaths from sudden infant death syndrome.**

Bronchopulmonary disease (BPD) represents an evolving process of lung injury of multifactorial origin related to underlying lung immaturity, abnormal lung development, inflammatory mediated injury, and inadequate repair response. The incidence of BPD is inversely proportional to birth weight, and the overwhelming majority of affected infants weigh less than 1250 grams at birth. Diagnosis of BPD is based on the requirement for supplemental oxygen or continuous positive airway pressure support after 28 days of age and/or after 36 weeks PMA. Following NICU discharge, BPD remains a significant cause of long-term morbidity. In those infants with a history of prolonged or multiple intubations, airway problems include subglottic stenosis, tracheal or bronchial granulomas, and acquired tracheobronchomalacia. Infants with BPD are more susceptible to pulmonary infections and reactive airway disease. Serious long-term sequelae include cor pulmonale and pulmonary hypertension. Affected infants often continue to require high caloric intake secondary to the increased energy expenditure associated with increased work of breathing. Ongoing treatment of BPD may include bronchodilators, fluid restriction, diuretics, electrolyte supplementation, and antibiotics.

Nutrition: The overwhelming majority of very low-birth-weight infants exhibit poor postnatal growth. To sustain weight gain, these infants often require between 110 and 130 kcal/kg/day. Serial measurements of the infant's weight, length, and head circumference are necessary to assess overall growth pattern. The infant's adjusted age is typically used to plot these measurements until 18 months of age or catch-up growth has been achieved.

Human breast milk is the recommended source of nutrition for all infants. However, for many preterm infants, formulas are the major nutrition source upon discharge. Even preterm infants who are receiving breast milk may need to be supplemented with several feedings per day of preterm discharge formula, which typically provides 22 kcal/oz and is enriched with additional protein, minerals, vitamins, and trace elements. The AAP recommends continued use of postdischarge formula until 9 months postnatal age. Alternatively, the higher- calorie formula may be discontinued once catch-up growth is achieved. Introduction of solid foods is based on the infant's oral-motor readiness, which typically occurs between an adjusted age of 4 and 6 months. Similarly, transitioning to cow's milk should be avoided until 12 months adjusted age.

Additional vitamin and iron supplementation may be necessary. A vitamin D supplement of 400 International Units/day is recommended until 12 months of age in breastfed infants and formula-fed infants ingesting less than 500 mL/day of vitamin-D fortified formula. Iron supplementation is required through the first year of life. An oral supplement of 2 mg/kg/day should be given to all breastfed infants until 12 months of age. Formulas typically provide approximately 2 mg/kg/day of iron for the average premature infant consuming 150 mL/kg/day of formula. Depending on the degree of prematurity, an additional 1 mg/kg/day may be beneficial.

Gastroesophageal reflux disease (GERD) is a frequent problem in the preterm infant. The primary mechanism is believed to be related to a transient and inappropriate relaxation of the lower esophageal sphincter. GERD is often successfully managed with conservative measures such as flat prone/upright positioning, more-frequent smaller-volume feedings, formula thickening with cereal, and/or a trial of hypoallergenic formula. Medical therapy consisting of acid suppression with either an H_2 antagonist or a proton pump inhibitor is reserved for those infants with persistent moderate-to-severe symptoms. A prokinetic agent may also be considered in difficult to manage cases. In severe disease, transpyloric feeding or Nissen fundoplication may be indicated.

Neurodevelopmental Disabilities: Premature infants continue to face significant challenges into childhood. They are at risk for a variety of neurodevelopmental disabilities secondary to injury to the developing brain. Disabilities range from major disabilities such as cerebral palsy and intellectual deficits to subtle impairments of sensory integration, learning differences, and problems with behavior and temperament. A fundamental aspect of routine care is developmental surveillance. Using a standardized screening tool such as the Denver Developmental Screening test, the pediatrician may identify infants who require a more comprehensive evaluation. For the first 2 years of life, developmental milestones should be adjusted to account for the infant's prematurity. Once a delay is diagnosed, referral for early intervention services is recommended for infants and children less than 3 years of age with special developmental and educational needs. (See Chapter 25, The Special Needs Child.)

A subset of premature infants, typically the smallest and most premature, are also monitored through NICU-affiliated neonatal follow-up programs. These programs may not provide primary care but work in a consultative mode to monitor medical care by serial evaluation of health and neurodevelopmental outcomes. Detailed assessments typically include evaluation of alertness, posture, passive and active muscle tone, deep tendon reflexes, primitive reflexes, postural reactions, and formal testing of functional abilities using measures such as the Bayley Scales of Infant Development.

Retinopathy of prematurity (ROP) is a serious vasoproliferative disorder that may result in severe visual impairment or blindness in preterm infants. The AAP recommends ROP screening for preterm infants with BW ≤1500 grams or gestation age ≤30 weeks and for clinically unstable preterm infants with BW between 1500 and 2000 g or gestational age older than 30 weeks who are considered to be at high risk based on their medical course. Serial retinal examinations should be performed by an experienced ophthalmologist who has sufficient knowledge and experience to enable accurate identification of the location and sequential retinal changes of ROP. Treatment with laser therapy, when indicated, has been shown to decrease the incidence of retinal detachment and blindness. Upon discharge, it is imperative that ophthalmologic follow-up be documented and reviewed with the parents because infants with a history of ROP are at risk for subsequent ophthalmologic complications such as strabismus, significant refractive error, amblyopia, cataract formation, and impaired visual acuity. Careful monitoring and follow-up can minimize risk for long-term visual impairments.

Hearing Loss: Universal newborn hearing screening is recommended for all newborns. Acceptable methodologies for screening include auditory brainstem response and evoked otoacoustic emissions. Approximately 2% to 4% of preterm infants born at less than 32 weeks gestation will develop some degree of hearing loss. Additional evaluations are warranted if there are concerns about speech and hearing because hearing deficits may present after discharge. Early recognition of hearing impairment, appropriate hearing amplification, and early intervention services are critical for optimal language development. Prognosis depends largely on the degree of hearing impairment as well as the timing of diagnosis and treatment.

Practice-Based Learning and Improvement: Evidence-Based Medicine

Title
Hospital discharge of the high-risk neonate proposed guidelines

Authors
Committee on Fetus and Newborn

Reference
Pediatrics 102:411-417, 1998

Quality of evidence
Consensus statement

Historical significance/comments
The first formal statement of the American Academy of Pediatrics on the issue of hospital discharge of the high-risk neonate

Interpersonal and Communication Skills

Encourage Family to Participate in Decisions

Once parents have acclimated to the hospital environment and have had some time to process all of the initial information they have received, many parents want to actively participate in decisions regarding the health-care plan. Some decisions will be appropriate for discussion of alternatives and others will not be. However, involvement of the family to the extent possible serves to encourage bonding with the infant and development of a partnership between the family and the physician.

Professionalism

Advocacy for Improving Services for Disabled Children

Advocacy plays a significant role in the care of the premature infant. Many of these infants will benefit from special services in their community in order to enhance their future development. Advocating for improved services for disabled children in the community at local or national levels is a way in which physicians can live up to the principles of professionalism in their practice. The American Academy of Pediatrics (AAP) serves as an important partner at the national and state levels for advocating for these children.

Systems-Based Practice

Medical Management: Care Coordination Regarding Hospital Discharge

The 2008 AAP Guidelines on Hospital Discharge has indicated six critical components of the discharge-planning process:

1. Parental education
2. Completion of appropriate elements of primary care in the hospital
3. Development of management plan for unresolved medical problems
4. Development of a comprehensive home care plan
5. Identification and involvement of support services
6. Determination and designation of follow-up care

   The ability of the primary caregiver and other family support members to deliver care to the premature baby must be assessed before discharge. In-home evaluations regarding the availability of supplies, medications, complicated technologies, and nutritional support must also be started before discharge. Arrangements for follow-up appointments are usually made locally; however, this is not always possible. Some level II nurseries may be in relatively rural areas, and the infant will need to return to the tertiary center for certain services (e.g., ophthalmologic examinations, hearing assessments, developmental follow-up). In rural areas, home services may also be limited, which means that the primary care physician has additional responsibility in evaluating the transition to home care.

Chapter 72
Necrotizing Enterocolitis (Case 31)

Jane S. Lee MD, MPH

Case: A 14-day-old, 750-g, 27-weeks' gestation infant receiving enteral feedings of standard preterm formula develops bilious gastric aspirates and abdominal distention.

Differential Diagnosis

Necrotizing enterocolitis (NEC)	Spontaneous intestinal perforation (SIP)	Intestinal malrotation with midgut volvulus
Hirschsprung disease	Meconium obstruction of prematurity	Sepsis with ileus

Speaking Intelligently

Bilious gastric aspirate with abdominal distention suggests an intestinal obstruction distal to the ampulla of Vater. When a premature infant presents with these findings, I obtain baseline abdominal radiographs, including anteroposterior and left lateral decubitus views, to evaluate the bowel gas pattern and assess for pneumoperitoneum. If the infant appears hemodynamically stable and initial radiographs show nonspecific intestinal abnormalities, I closely monitor the infant for further evidence of feeding intolerance, ischemia, and infection. During this observation period, I typically discontinue enteral feeds, place a large-bore nasogastric tube to low intermittent wall suction to achieve intestinal decompression, perform a sepsis evaluation, and start broad-spectrum antibiotics empirically. I continue to obtain sequential laboratory studies and radiographs to assist me in narrowing my differential diagnosis. A surgical consultation is recommended if the workup reveals signs of intestinal ischemia, perforation, or continued clinical deterioration.

PATIENT CARE

Clinical Thinking
- **Radiographic** evaluation of the abdomen requires **two views** (anteroposterior and left lateral decubitus or cross table lateral) to evaluate bowel gas pattern and presence of intraperitoneal air. A prone view may be helpful in assessing for air-fluid levels.
- Surgical emergencies should be excluded.
- Medical therapy for NEC typically consists of bowel rest, intestinal decompression, and broad-spectrum antibiotic therapy.
- The cardinal principle of surgical management for NEC is resection of grossly necrotic bowel and preservation of as much bowel length as possible.

History
- Evaluate the **maternal risk factors:** Antenatal history of decreased placental perfusion, intrauterine growth restriction, maternal diabetes, hypermagnesemia, and administration of dexamethasone.

- Evaluate the **neonatal risk factors:** Degree of prematurity, postnatal age, comorbid conditions that might compromise intestinal perfusion or overall hemodynamic status (i.e., resuscitation at birth, patent ductus arteriosus, gastrointestinal malformation), and feeding regimen.
- Assess for symptoms of **feeding intolerance:** Evidence of delayed gastric emptying such as increased gastric residuals, abdominal distention, and evidence of occult or grossly bloody stools.
- Determine the risk factors for neonatal **sepsis:** Previous antibiotics for suspected or documented infection, presence of indwelling catheters in place type of respiratory support, and use of acid suppressive therapy.

Physical Examination
- **Vital signs:** Monitor for apnea, bradycardia, temperature instability, or hypotension.
- **Signs of intestinal ileus:** Abdominal distention, decreased bowel sounds, and palpable bowel loops.
- **Signs of peritonitis:** Abdominal distention, tenderness, palpable mass, and erythema or discoloration of the abdominal wall.
- **Signs of shock:** Lethargy, pallor, mottling, delayed capillary perfusion, weak peripheral pulses, and bleeding diathesis.

Tests for Consideration
- **Arterial blood gas (ABG):** To evaluate for metabolic acidosis $45
- **Complete blood count (CBC) with differential:** To assess for leukopenia, leukocytosis, neutropenia, and thrombocytopenia $110
- **Coagulation profile, including prothrombin time, activated partial thromboplastin time, fibrinogen, and fibrin split products:** To monitor for a consumptive coagulopathy $300
- **Electrolytes, glucose, and calcium** $115
- **Cultures of the blood, urine, and cerebrospinal fluid (CSF):** To document bacterial infection $135 each
- **Examination of the stool:**
  For occult blood $15
  Reducing substance $45
  Bacterial culture $135

IMAGING CONSIDERATIONS

→ **Serial abdominal radiograph, including anteroposterior, left lateral decubitus, and prone views** $120 each
→ **Abdominal ultrasound:** To detect ascites or abscess formation. It will also document the position of superior mesenteric blood vessels $450
→ **Upper gastrointestinal (GI) series:** To evaluate gastrointestinal anatomy and gastric emptying. This procedure should not be performed for suspected NEC or intestinal perforation $630
→ **24-Hour pH probe:** To detect gastroesophageal reflux disease (GERD) $1175
→ **Nuclear technetium scintigraphy:** To assess GERD, gastric emptying and aspiration $745

Clinical Entities	Medical Knowledge

Necrotizing Enterocolitis

Pφ   **NEC** is a severe inflammatory disease of the gastrointestinal tract that predominantly affects premature infants and has multifactorial pathogenesis. It results from a complex interaction of factors related to abnormal bacterial colonization, intestinal ischemia, reperfusion injury with activation of a proinflammatory cascade, and intestinal mucosal immaturity. The majority of cases are sporadic, but outbreaks may occur in nurseries. The incidence varies inversely with birth weight and gestational age, and infants less than 1000 grams at birth and less than 28 weeks' gestation appear to be the most susceptible. The average age of onset is inversely related to gestational age. At the time of presentation, infants typically are advancing on enteral feedings or may have achieved full-volume feedings.

TP   Infants can present with increased gastric residuals, emesis, mild abdominal distention, decreased bowel sounds, or hematochezia, as well as systemic signs such as apnea, bradycardia, temperature instability, or lethargy. Physical examination may reveal increasing abdominal girth, visible intestinal loops, abdominal tenderness, palpable mass in the right lower quadrant, abdominal wall erythema secondary to necrotic loops adjacent to the abdominal wall, or abdominal discoloration from intraperitoneal meconium visible through the abdominal wall. Major systemic signs such as worsening respiratory failure, acidosis, decreased peripheral perfusion, shock, cardiovascular collapse, and bleeding diathesis can occur.

Dx   Radiographic imaging that includes two views is essential for diagnosing NEC and should be performed every 6 to 8 hours during the first 48 to 72 hours of disease to evaluate for pneumatosis intestinalis and pneumoperitoneum. Portal venous gas may be visible as thin, linear branching areas of radiolucency overlying the liver. The greatest risk for perforation is in the first 24 to 48 hours. A fixed dilated bowel loop that remains unchanged over serial radiographs may be a sign of intestinal ischemia or infarction. Metabolic derangements, including hyponatremia from fluid shifts, glucose instability, and metabolic acidosis, are commonly seen. Either leukocytosis or leucopenia as well as thrombocytopenia are often present.

Tx   The typical approach consists of bowel rest, intestinal decompression, systemic antibiotics, and parenteral nutrition. Broad-spectrum antibiotic coverage consisting of vancomycin, gentamicin, and metronidazole can be used. However, antimicrobial choices should be guided by local resistance patterns. Correction of electrolyte abnormalities, metabolic acidosis, and coagulopathy can be necessary. Arterial blood gas monitoring, ventilatory support necessitating intubation and fluid resuscitation with normal saline or colloid and pressor support may also be required. If surgical intervention is required, exploratory laparotomy usually involves resection of necrotic bowel and exteriorization of viable ends as an enterostomy and mucous fistula to allow for continued bowel decompression. Alternatively, primary peritoneal drainage can be considered in cases of perforated NEC in unstable or very low-birth-weight infants. **See Nelson Essentials 63.**

Meconium Obstruction of Prematurity

See Chapter 63, Delayed Meconium Passage.

Sepsis with Ileus

See Chapter 77, Neonatal Sepsis.

Spontaneous Intestinal Perforation

Pφ	SIP is a spontaneous, focal intestinal perforation may arise from regional ischemia to the mucosa that spreads into the deeper layers of the affected intestine eventually resulting in transmural involvement. Perforations are sharply demarcated lesions without gross necrosis and localized to the antimesenteric side of the terminal ileum. In comparison with NEC, SIP occurs more frequently in extremely premature infants and typically presents during the first 2 weeks following birth.
TP	Affected infants appear clinically well despite a sudden onset of abdominal distention. A bluish discoloration of the abdominal wall suggests the presence of an intestinal perforation.
Dx	Abdominal radiographs may initially show a normal bowel gas pattern or transient bowel distension. Subsequent radiographs may demonstrate a paucity of bowel gas or a gasless abdomen. Pneumatosis intestinalis is not typically observed. Once intestinal perforation occurs, a pneumoperitoneum may be observed. Laboratory studies are often not helpful in differentiating this disease from NEC.
Tx	Supportive measures including bowel rest, intestinal decompression, and broad-spectrum antibiotic therapy. Surgical management consists of primary peritoneal drainage or laparotomy. **See Nelson Essentials 63.**

Intestinal Malrotation With Midgut Volvulus

Pφ	Malrotation results from a failure of the gastrointestinal tract to complete its normal rotation as it returns to the abdominal cavity at 8 to 10 weeks gestation. Normal mesenteric attachments are absent, so the midgut is attached to the posterior abdominal wall only at the duodenum and at the proximal colon. Abnormal peritoneal bands called Ladd bands form between the colon and the duodenum, which can lead to duodenal obstruction. In addition, unfixed bowel may twist around its mesentery, resulting in ischemia of the bowel supplied by the superior mesenteric artery.
TP	Infants present with symptoms of a high intestinal obstruction such as sudden onset of bilious vomiting, abdominal distention, and hematochezia. As the obstruction progresses, the abdomen becomes more distended, firm, and tender, consistent with developing peritonitis.
Dx	Upper gastrointestinal series is the definitive study to document position of the duodenojejunal junction and assess for evidence of volvulus. **Malrotation** is present if the duodenojejunal junction is displaced to the right of midline or inferior to the level of the pylorus. **Midgut volvulus** is present if the duodenum appears dilated and fluid filled with a "corkscrew" appearance of the distal duodenum and proximal jejunum as it spirals downward into the right or mid-upper abdomen. Contrast enema may demonstrate an abnormal position of cecum to the right or upper abdomen but may not be helpful because the cecal position is highly variable. Ultrasonography may reveal a "whirlpool sign" of bowel twisting around its mesentery.
Tx	Volvulus is a gastrointestinal emergency that requires immediate surgical intervention. The Ladd procedure is performed, which consists of volvulus reduction, resection of grossly necrotic bowel followed by primary anastomosis or enterostomy, lysis of peritoneal bands, replacement of the bowel in a malrotated position, and appendectomy. In cases of extreme necrosis, a second-look laparotomy may be performed 12 to 36 hours after the initial surgery to assess intestinal viability. **See Nelson Essentials 129.**

Hirschsprung Disease

Pφ	Intestinal dysmotility and functional distal intestinal obstruction occurs as a result of congenital agenesis of ganglion cells in the myenteric and submucosal plexuses secondary to a failure of neural crest cell migration. The aganglionic segment causes a lack of propagation of peristalsis and absent relaxation of the internal anal sphincter. The length of affected bowel influences the severity of observed dysmotility.
TP	Infants present with a history of delay in meconium passage within the first 48 hours of life. Other symptoms include infrequent passage of stool, feeding intolerance, bilious vomiting, and abdominal distention. Presentation may be delayed in the preterm infant whose enteral feeds are initiated beyond the immediate neonatal period.
Dx	Abdominal radiograph typically shows dilated intestinal loops with air-fluid levels in the colon. Contrast enema characteristically demonstrates a funnel-shaped transition zone between the narrowed aganglionic distal bowel and the markedly dilated normally ganglionated, proximal bowel. However, a distinct transition zone may not always be readily apparent. In cases of total aganglionosis, the enema shows reduced caliber of the entire colon, no clear transition zone, and contrast refluxed into the distended ileum. Retention of contrast in the colon for more than 24 hours following the procedure is also suggestive of disease. Definitive diagnosis is established by rectal biopsy that reveals an absence of ganglion cells in the submucosal layer and acetylcholinesterase staining of the submucosa, which identifies abnormal nerve hypertrophy. A suction biopsy of the rectal mucosa and submucosa is typically performed at bedside.
Tx	Initial management consists of gastric decompression by placement of a Replogle tube and repeated rectal irrigation. The definitive surgical intervention is resection of aganglionic segment with pull-through of the normal innervated bowel down to the anus. (See Chapter 35, Constipation.) **See Nelson Essentials 126.**

ZEBRA ZONE

a. **Pneumatosis coli:** Isolated colonic pneumatosis intestinalis represents a benign form of NEC in which less severe inflammatory bowel changes occur.

b. **Intestinal neuronal dysplasia:** A rare, inherited form of intestinal obstruction secondary to hyperganglionosis of submucosal and myenteric plexuses with increased acetylcholinesterase activity.

c. **Metabolic disease:** Metabolic diseases such as hypothyroidism are rare causes of chronic, nonobstructive intestinal ileus that results in a functional bowel obstruction.

Practice-Based Learning and Improvement: Evidence-Based Medicine

Title
Laparotomy versus peritoneal drainage for necrotizing enterocolitis and perforation

Authors
Moss RL, Dimmitt RA, Barnhart DC, et al

Institution
Multiple NICUs in the United States and Canada (14 U.S. NICUs, 1 international)

Reference
N Engl J Med 354:2225-2234, 2006

Problem
To compare survival of very low-birth-weight preterm infants with perforated necrotizing enterocolitis following primary peritoneal drainage versus laparotomy and bowel resection.

Intervention
A total of 117 preterm infants with birth weight less than 1500 g and perforated necrotizing enterocolitis were enrolled from 15 participating centers. Infants were randomly assigned to receive peritoneal drainage (n = 55) or laparotomy (n = 62).

Quality of evidence
Level I evidence

Outcome/effect
There was no statistical difference in 3-month survival following primary peritoneal drainage and laparotomy with bowel resection. There was also no differences in dependence on parenteral nutrition 90 days postoperatively and duration of hospitalization.

Historical significance/comments
This multicenter, randomized clinical trial showed that primary peritoneal drainage was as efficacious as traditional laparotomy with bowel resection for surgical management of perforated necrotizing enterocolitis in the very low-birth-weight infant.

Interpersonal and Communication Skills

Listen and Consider What Others Have to Say About Relevant Issues

Although most cases of NEC can be medically managed, a pediatric surgeon should be consulted whenever NEC is strongly suspected or definitively diagnosed so that rapid mobilization for surgery may occur if surgical intervention is necessary. Close monitoring by both the medical and surgical services for signs of disease progression and good communication of clinical change is critical in providing optimal care.

Professionalism

Commitment to Life-Long Learning and Education

The study by Moss et al (cited previously in the Practice-Based Learning and Improvement competency) was a multicenter, randomized trial comparing the efficacy of primary peritoneal drainage with traditional laparotomy and bowel resection. It showed quite vividly that the former treatment is just as effective as the latter. This study illustrates how keeping up with the literature and the practice of evidence based medicine (EBM) improves quality of care and clinical outcomes. EBM is an essential component of professional behavior and requires you to ask focused clinical questions related to patients under your care, to research the answers, and to apply your findings in your practice.

Systems-Based Practice

Health-Care Economics: The Financial Impact of Preterm Birth

In 2005 the annual societal economic cost (medical, educational, and lost productivity) associated with preterm birth in the United States was around **$51,600** per infant born preterm.

There are three major factors that contribute to these costs. First, premature infants require longer hospitalizations (approximately 24.2 days average for children having a principal diagnosis of prematurity versus 2 days for a normal term newborn). Second is the loss of productivity for the caregivers of preterm infants. These infants have significantly more doctor's visits in their first year of life. These costs and the loss of work for parents leads to longer periods of short-term disability. Finally, these infants require on average many more early intervention and special education services than term newborns.[1,2]

References

1. Institute of Medicine: *Preterm birth: Causes, consequences, and prevention,* Washington, DC, 2006, National Academy Press.
2. March of Dimes Foundation: *The cost of saving babies.* Available at http://www.marchofdimes.com/hbhb/index.asp.

Chapter 73
Respiratory Distress Syndrome (Case 32)

Tara M. Randis MD

Case: A male infant delivered via stat cesarean delivery to a 36-year-old mother secondary to maternal hypertension at 35 weeks' gestation is brought to the neonatal intensive care unit (NICU) for evaluation and management of respiratory distress.

Differential Diagnosis		
Respiratory distress syndrome (RDS)	Aspiration	Infection/pneumonia
Pneumothorax	Transient tachypnea of the newborn (TTN)	

Speaking Intelligently

When an infant presents with respiratory distress, urgent assessment and intervention is required. I first clear the airway of secretions and then position the infant properly ("sniffing position"). If cyanosis is present, I administer supplemental oxygen immediately. Nasal continuous positive airway pressure (CPAP) may help expand the lungs, improving both oxygenation and ventilation, and avoiding the need for subsequent intubation. If there is little or no respiratory effort, I proceed with positive pressure ventilation followed by intubation and mechanical ventilation. A chest radiograph should be obtained for both diagnostic purposes and if necessary, endotracheal tube positioning. While caring for the infant I try to develop a differential diagnosis based upon prenatal history, birth history, initial clinical presentation, and examination.

PATIENT CARE

Clinical Thinking
- Support airway and spontaneous breathing effort, providing supplemental oxygen and ventilatory support as needed.
- Is there a reversible cause of distress that can be quickly relieved such as a **pneumothorax?**
- If this is respiratory distress syndrome (RDS), then prompt **surfactant** administration may be appropriate.

History
- What is the **gestational age** of this infant?
- Has the mother received antenatal corticosteroids?
- Are there risk factors for infection, such as maternal fever, untreated maternal group B streptococcus (GBS) colonization, prolonged rupture of membranes, and signs of fetal distress?
- Was meconium-stained amniotic fluid present? Were there signs of fetal hypoxemia or stress in utero (abnormal fetal heart tracings, abnormal umbilical artery blood gas levels)?
- Did the mother experience labor before delivery?

Physical Examination
- Vital signs: Abnormal respiratory pattern or effort may be present. Pulse oximetry may reveal hemoglobin desaturation. Bradycardia is commonly seen in the presence of hypoxia. Hypothermia itself may lead to respiratory distress. Tension pneumothorax results in hypotension.
- Signs of respiratory distress such a nasal flaring, grunting, or intercostal or subcostal retractions are often present.

- Hypotonia is often seen in sepsis, severe hypoxia, neurologic disorders, or exposure to maternal medications/drug use.
- A cardiac murmur, enlarged liver, or poor peripheral pulses are present in **some** congenital heart defects.
- Passage of meconium in utero often leads to staining of the finger nails or umbilical cord and meconium at or below the vocal cords.
- Pallor or even hydrops may be present in infants with severe anemia.

Tests for Consideration
- **Arterial blood gas (ABG)** $156
- **Complete blood count (CBC) with differential** $53
- **Blood culture** $100

IMAGING CONSIDERATIONS

→ **Chest radiograph** $75
→ **Echocardiogram:** If congenital heart disease or vascular abnormalities are suspected $325

Clinical Entities   Medical Knowledge

Respiratory Distress Syndrome

Pφ   *RDS* results from a deficiency of pulmonary surfactant. Surfactant, composed of phospholipids and proteins, reduces alveolar surface tension. Surfactant production by type 2 pneumocytes is generally sufficient by 34 to 35 weeks' of gestation. Inadequate surfactant production often leads to alveolar collapse. Primarily a disease of preterm infants, RDS may present in term infants with delayed lung maturity or decreased surfactant production (infants of diabetic mothers, perinatal asphyxia), or when surfactant is inactivated (meconium aspiration). Antenatal administration of glucocorticoids to mothers at risk for preterm delivery also accelerates lung maturity and has been proven to reduce the risk for RDS.

TP   Symptoms include nasal flaring, tachypnea, cyanosis, retractions, and expiratory grunting. Infants present with distress within the first 6 hours of life. The clinical course is characterized by progressive worsening of symptoms with a peak severity at 48 to 72 hours.

Dx   The diagnosis of RDS is based upon the combination of history, clinical features, and characteristic chest radiographs. Decreased breath sounds may be present. Chest films typically reveal a homogeneous "ground glass" or reticulogranular appearance secondary to diffuse atelectasis throughout the lung fields, and air bronchograms. ABG reveals hypoxemia, hypercarbia, and mixed acidosis.

Tx   Surfactant replacement therapy is either given prophylactically in the delivery room to at-risk infants or as a rescue therapy after clinical decompensation. Nasal CPAP helps to maintain functional residual capacity (FRC) and prevent alveolar collapse. Some infants require intubation and mechanical ventilation. **See Nelson Essentials 61.**

Transient Tachypnea of the Newborn

Pφ   This respiratory distress is caused by transient pulmonary edema secondary to delayed reabsorption of fetal lung fluid. Early in gestation, the pulmonary epithelium contributes to lung development and alveolar formation by secreting chloride into the alveolar space, creating an osmotic gradient that induces the flow of liquid in the air spaces. As the fetus matures, the pulmonary epithelium develops the capacity to reabsorb sodium. The surge of endogenous steroids and circulating catecholamines during labor and delivery further stimulates these epithelial cells to reabsorb sodium, pumping it into the interstitial space. Fetal lung fluid follows. Furthermore, prostaglandin secretion during labor leads to lymphatic dilatation, which aids in the clearance of fluid from the interstitium.

TP   Nasal flaring, retractions, grunting, tachypnea and cyanosis are often seen in the first few hours of life. When mild, TTN may last 12 to 24 hours. More severe cases may last 72 hours or longer.

Dx   TTN is a diagnosis of exclusion. Chest radiographs often reveal prominent perihilar streaking as a result of the engorgement of the lymphatic system and may have visible fluid in the fissures. ABG may reveal hypoxemia.

| Tx | This is a self-limiting disease, and treatment is supportive. Supplemental oxygen or nasal CPAP is the mainstay of therapy. Infants may require IV fluids and gavage feeding until symptoms resolve. (See Chapter 66, Transient Tachypnea of the Newborn.) **See Nelson Essentials 61.** |

Infection/Pneumonia

Pφ	Respiratory distress is often the first sign of **infection** in the neonate, and the lungs represent a common site for the establishment of sepsis in the newborn. Infections in the newborn may be bacterial or viral and may be acquired prenatally, during delivery, or early in the postnatal course. Most common causative agents are GBS, *Escherichia coli*, *Listeria monocytogenes*, and nontypable *Haemophilus influenzae*. Risk factors include prolonged rupture of membranes, chorioamnionitis, and fetal gasping due to asphyxia, which leads to increased risk for aspiration.
TP	These infants are typically lethargic and have some degree of respiratory distress. They may have trouble maintaining their body temperature. Eventually these infants demonstrate hypotension and poor perfusion as a sign of shock.
Dx	Chest radiographs often reveal patchy infiltrates, but they may also look similar to those seen in RDS, especially in the case of GBS pneumonia. White blood cell count, differential, platelet count, blood cultures, and Gram stain may be helpful. A spinal tap is necessary if the clinical suspicion for sepsis if high. Tracheal cultures should be interpreted with caution because it may not be possible to differentiate between true infection and early bacterial colonization.
Tx	Empiric use of intravenous antibiotics at the onset of distress to cover the most common pathogens and respiratory support are the mainstay of therapy. **See Nelson Essentials 110.**

Pneumothorax

| Pφ | **Pneumothorax** is accumulation of free air from ruptured alveoli between the parietal pleural lining of the chest wall and the visceral pleura of the lung. A tension pneumothorax occurs when the trapped air impedes venous return to the heart, leading to decreased cardiac output and hemodynamic instability. |

TP	An air leak should be suspected in any infant who has a sudden onset of respiratory distress or whose condition suddenly deteriorates. Infants often present with grunting, increased pallor or cyanosis, and retractions.
Dx	If there is a unilateral pneumothorax, breath sounds may be decreased on the affected side. Transillumination of the chest wall with a fiberoptic light source may be extraordinarily helpful, because intervention may be necessary before a chest film is obtained. Chest radiographs typically reveal a sharply demarcated, hyperlucent area without pulmonary parenchymal markings (Figure 73-1). Lateral decubitus films, in which the affected side is positioned up, are quite helpful. Hypoxemia on ABG and sudden drop in oxygen saturations on pulse oximetry are characteristic findings.
Tx	No specific treatment is necessary for an asymptomatic pneumothorax. Urgent chest tube insertion into the pleural space, anterior to the lung, is the definitive treatment for symptomatic infants. **See Nelson Essentials 138.**

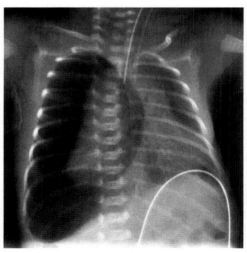

Figure 73-1 Right pneumothorax.

Aspiration	
Pφ	***Aspiration*** of meconium, blood, or amniotic fluid may lead to respiratory distress. The fetus may gasp in response to stress or hypoxemia in utero. Passage of meconium may also occur under these circumstances. Aspiration of these substances can occur before, during, or after delivery. Respiratory distress results from a variety of mechanisms, including physical obstruction of air passages, development of a chemical pneumonitis, and inactivation of lung surfactant. Superimposed bacterial infection may occur.
TP	Infants present with varying degrees of respiratory distress. After meconium aspiration, infants may have a "barrel chest" with audible rales or rhonchi on examination.
Dx	In addition to the clinical signs mentioned above, the chest radiograph may show patchy areas of atelectasis, hyperinflation, or even pneumothorax, which is seen in 10% to 20% of infants with meconium aspiration. ABG may reveal hypoxemia and acidosis.
Tx	Again, supportive care is the mainstay of therapy. If the infant is depressed with poor respiratory effort, direct visualization of the trachea should be performed followed by endotracheal suctioning. **See Nelson Essentials 61.**

ZEBRA ZONE

a. Congenital heart disease: See Chapter 79, Cyanotic Newborn.

b. Neurologic disorders: Physical examination findings such as hypotonia and poor respiratory effort are suggestive of neurologic disorders (hypoxic-ischemic encephalopathy, birth trauma, or neuromuscular diseases). Maternal medications such as magnesium sulfate, narcotics, or general anesthesia may present similarly, but their effects should not be sustained.

c. Anatomic abnormalities: Anatomic malformations, including congenital cystic adenomatoid malformation, congenital lobar emphysema, mediastinal tumors/masses, and congenital diaphragmatic hernia.

d. Severe anemia: Due to hypoxemia, subsequent metabolic acidosis with a compensatory tachypnea may occur.

Practice-Based Learning and Improvement: Evidence-Based Medicine

Title
Synthetic surfactant for respiratory distress syndrome in preterm infants

Author
Soll R

Reference
Cochrane Database Syst Rev 1998;(3)CD00149

Problem
Effectiveness of intratracheal administration of synthetic surfactant in premature newborns with established respiratory distress syndrome

Intervention
Surfactant administration to premature infants with respiratory distress

Comparison/control
Routine supportive therapy

Quality of evidence
Meta-analysis of randomized controlled trials

Historical significance/ comments
Promotes widespread use of exogenous surfactant among NICU populations

Interpersonal and Communication Skills

Establish Rapport and Maintain Personal Connection

Although initial assessment of infants with respiratory distress often occurs in the delivery room, further evaluation and management will likely take place in a neonatal intensive care unit or transitional nursery. Taking the infant from the delivery room will no doubt leave the parents feeling helpless and anxious. Because the primary physician caring for the infant is often unable to leave the bedside, it may be helpful to designate another member of the medical team to support the parents and maintain a connection by keeping them informed of the infant's status and new developments. This person should be skilled in presenting information that encourages the family to ask questions about the care. Because of the complex nature of the information, frequent checks for understanding should occur during the discussion. This can be accomplished simply by asking the parent(s) to summarize the things that were just told to them.

Professionalism

Respect: Maintain Patient Confidentiality

Extended family members often flock to the hospital upon hearing of an infant's birth. Frequent communication with the parents of the newborn is critical; however, it is inappropriate to discuss the infant's condition, diagnosis, and plan of care in front of visitors, including family members, unless the parents of the infant have given consent to share information.

Systems-Based Practice

Discharge Planning for High-Risk Neonates

The discharge planning of high-risk neonates should involve at minimum the following team of professionals: a neonatologist, a discharge planner or case manager, a social worker, patient's nurse, pediatric subspecialists depending on the clinical needs, and case manager or outreach worker from the patient's insurance plan.

The primary care physician should be identified, and he or she should be given periodic reports on the progress of the patient.

The 2008 American Academy of Pediatrics Guidelines on Hospital Discharge[1] has indicated six elements of the discharge planning process:
1. Parental education
2. Completion of appropriate elements of primary care in the hospital
3. Development of management plan for unresolved medical problems
4. Development of a comprehensive home care plan
5. Identification and involvement of support services
6. Determination and designation of follow-up care

Reference

1. Hospital discharge of the high-risk neonate. *Pediatrics* 122(5):1119-1126, 2008.

Chapter 74
Congenital Diaphragmatic Hernia (Case 33)

Christiana R. Farkouh MD, MPH

Case: A newborn term infant presents with cyanosis and respiratory distress at birth. Initial chest radiograph demonstrates translucencies of various sizes in the left hemithorax, and the cardiac silhouette is deviated into the right hemithorax.

Differential Diagnosis

Congenital diaphragmatic hernia (CDH)	Congenital cystic adenomatoid malformation (CCAM)	Bronchopulmonary sequestration (BPS)

Speaking Intelligently

If the diagnosis is known before birth, a thorough prenatal evaluation should ensue to determine if other congenital abnormalities are present that may represent a known genetic defect/ chromosomal anomaly or syndrome. Subsequently, these infants should be delivered in institutions that can provide maximal cardiorespiratory support in the form of extracorporeal membrane oxygenation (ECMO) because these infants can exhibit severe cardiorespiratory instability and pulmonary hypertension. Immediately after birth I intubate the airway and place a Replogle tube into the stomach with continuous suction to minimize gastric and intestinal distention with air. These interventions serve to secure lung expansion and minimize intestinal distention. Because the diagnosis is not always known before birth, I strongly recommend obtaining a chest radiograph immediately when a newborn infant presents with respiratory distress. Because of the clinical finding of diminished breath sounds on the side of the thorax where abdominal organs have herniated, the possibility of a pneumothorax exists and may subsequently lead to placement of a chest tube or needle thoracotomy before obtaining radiographic evidence of a pneumothorax. Such an intervention will not only be of no clinical benefit, but may be more injurious if any of the abdominal viscera are punctured.

PATIENT CARE

Clinical Thinking

- Once the infant is born, immediately **intubate the trachea** and place a **Replogle catheter into the stomach** with continuous low wall suction.
- Proper positioning of the infant with the affected side down also serves to support full expansion of the contralateral lung.
- Intravenous and arterial access is then obtained typically via umbilical vessels. However, umbilical venous catheters may be difficult to position, especially if the liver is also herniated into the chest.
- CDH is *not* a surgical emergency. **Stabilizing the infant's respiratory status** with either mechanical ventilation or with the use of ECMO is the priority.
- If ECMO appears likely given the degree of lung disease, serious discussions with the family are warranted, given the risks of ECMO itself and the concern for prolonged respiratory difficulties after repair is accomplished.
- In addition to the structural defect in the diaphragm that results in migration of abdominal contents into the chest, which impedes lung development on the affected side, the contralateral lung tissue is affected as well because of the shift in the mediastinal structures into the opposite chest.
- Some patients may also suffer from some degree of **pulmonary hypoplasia** on both sides of the lung as a result of interference in the normal growth and development of the lung.
- Because of the possible need for ECMO, these infants should all receive a head ultrasound, and echocardiogram should also be performed to visualize the cardiac structure, exclude any congenital heart defect, and ascertain overall cardiac function.

History

- Because CDH is readily identifiable on prenatal ultrasound, the majority of these infants are identified prenatally.
- History may be limited to the pregnancy history, prenatal ultrasounds, and even possibly prenatal magnetic resonance imaging (MRI).
- When not identified prenatally, these infants suffer respiratory distress immediately after birth, at which time the defect is identified on routine CXR.
- CXR demonstrates abdominal contents (stomach, bowel, and/or liver) in the thorax.

Physical Examination

- Vital signs: Tachypnea, respiratory distress, and hypoxia (cyanosis).
- The hallmark finding in infants with CDH is a scaphoid abdomen due to the abdominal contents being in the chest.
- Diminished breath sounds on the affected side and heart sounds may be better auscultated in the midline or more laterally depending on

the side of the defect. A left CDH may have better heart sounds in the midline or right side of the sternum.

- The actual size of the defect in the diaphragm cannot be ascertained until in the operating room.
- **Identify** if **other congenital anomalies** are apparent on examination.

Tests for Consideration
- **Arterial blood gas** $156
- **Electrolytes** $29
- **Karyotype with high-resolution chromosomes** $150

IMAGING CONSIDERATIONS

→ **Chest radiograph:** Anteroposterior views $75
→ **Echocardiogram** $325
→ **Head ultrasound** $550
→ **Renal ultrasound** $250

Clinical Entities   Medical Knowledge

Congenital Diaphragmatic Hernia

Pφ **Congential diaphragmatic hernia** results from herniation of the intestinal tract through a defect in the diaphragm. It results from the failure of closure of the pleuroperitoneal canal during the eighth week of fetal life.

The defect most frequently occurs at the foramen of Bochdalek. The defect can vary from several centimeters to complete absence of the involved hemidiaphragm.

In 85% of the cases the defect is of the left hemidiaphragm; less than 1% is bilateral.

TP After delivery, infants present with respiratory distress, cyanosis, and scaphoid abdomen.

Dx CDHs are often diagnosed prenatally with a prenatal ultrasound demonstrating the intra-abdominal contents in either the left or right hemithorax with a shift of the mediastinal structures into the opposite side of the thorax. Prenatal measurements of the lung to head ratio (LHR) are often calculated between 24 and 26 weeks gestation. If not diagnosed, a chest radiograph in the postnatal period may demonstrate presence of abdominal contents (stomach, liver, intestine) in the thorax.

Tx   Immediate tracheal intubation and placement of a nasogastric tube are undertaken to prevent gaseous distention of the herniated intestine. Treatment with nitric oxide was initially a mainstay of therapy, but recent studies may show that it provides no benefit. ECMO may be necessary in the more severe cases. The timing of surgical repair is based on the infant's respiratory status. Most centers delay repair of the diaphragm for a number of days to allow time for the pulmonary vasoreactivity to diminish. **See Nelson Essentials 58 and 61.**

Congenital Cystic Adenomatoid Malformation
Pφ   *Congenital cystic adenomatoid malformation (CCAM)* originates as an adenomatous growth in the terminal bronchioles early in gestation. Most CCAMs connect with the tracheobronchial tree, and as a result they can increase in size. Typically only one lobe of the lung is involved.
TP   Clinical symptoms may be few to none to severe respiratory distress. A cystic mass is noted on radiograph on the affected side.
Dx   Classically CCAMs are divided into microcystic, macrocystic, or mixed lesions (macrocystic and microcystic). Mediastinal shift, polyhydramnios, pulmonary hypoplasia, and hydrops fetalis may all be present or develop. Prenatal diagnosis may be difficult to discern between CCAM and BPS. In BPS fetal Doppler studies can demonstrate the systemic blood supply from the aorta.
Tx   Some fetal CCAMs will regress spontaneously; in others treatment is based on clinical symptomatology. Fetal therapy, including fetal lung resection for microcystic lesion or thoracoamniotic shunt for macrocystic lesions, has been performed in immature fetuses exhibiting signs of hydrops. In the postnatal period, infants with respiratory distress may require lobectomy in the neonatal period. Even in infants who are asymptomatic, elective removal of the affected lobe is recommended because of the concern regarding recurrent pulmonary infections and the possibility of malignant transformation.

Bronchopulmonary Sequestration

Pψ   The etiology is an accessory lung bud that originates lower down in the primitive foregut. ***Bronchopulmonary sequestration*** is characterized by the presence of nonfunctioning lung tissue that does not communicate with the tracheobronchial tree and derives its blood supply from the aorta. The affected lung is abnormal with areas of atelectasis intermixed with fluid-filled cysts. It can have associated malformations (i.e., CDH, congenital heart defect, rib or vertebral anomalies).

TP   Most newborns with BPS are asymptomatic; however, if the sequestered area is large, the infant may present with cyanosis and respiratory distress with or without pulmonary hypoplasia.

Dx   Antenatal ultrasound can demonstrate a solid, echogenic chest mass with the systemic blood supply visualized by color Doppler. Prenatal MRI is superior to ultrasound. The classic findings seen on chest radiograph after birth are a triangular or oval basal lung mass on one side of the chest. Ultrasound or Computed tomography (CT) examinations are also helpful in confirming the presence of a thoracic mass. Doppler studies or contrast studies delineating the feeding vessels to the sequestration are definitive.

Tx   In the postnatal period, infants with respiratory distress may require surgical resection of the mass in the neonatal period. Surgical excision of the mass in infants who are asymptomatic is debatable, but elective removal of the mass may be recommended because of the concern regarding recurrent pulmonary infections. However, spontaneous regressions both in the prenatal and postnatal period have been reported. In addition, embolization of the systemic feeding vessels may play a role in therapy.

ZEBRA ZONE

a. **Fryns syndrome:** Major diagnostic criteria include abnormal facies, small thorax, widely spaced hypoplastic nipples, distal limb and nail hypoplasia, and diaphragmatic hernia with pulmonary hypoplasia.

b. **Pentalogy of Cantrell:** Consists of a cleft sternum, anterior midline diaphragmatic defects, a pericardial defect, congenital cardiac abnormalities including ectopic cordis, and an upper abdominal omphalocele.

Practice-Based Learning and Improvement

Title
A randomized trial of fetal endoscopic occlusion for severe fetal congenital diaphragmatic hernia

Authors
Harrison M, Keller R, Hawgood S, et al

Reference
N Engl J Med 349:1916-1924, 2003

Problem
Does fetal endoscopic tracheal occlusion improve survival (measured to 90 days of life) in human fetuses with severe congenital left-sided diaphragmatic hernia?

Intervention
Fetal endoscopic tracheal occlusion or routine postnatal care

Comparison/control
A randomized controlled trial comparing fetal tracheal occlusion with standard postnatal care, institutional review board (IRB) approved

Outcome/effect
Tracheal occlusion did not improve survival or morbidity rates in this cohort of fetuses with left-sided congenital diaphragmatic hernia.

Historical significance/comments
This controversial study subjected pregnant women and their unborn babies to the risks for premature rupture and possible preterm delivery and infection. Before this randomized trial, data suggested that fetal endoscopic tracheal occlusion to induce lung growth may improve the outcome of severe CDH. This study was concluded before enrollment was complete because of the unexpectedly high survival rate of 77% in the group receiving standard care compared with 73% survival rate in the tracheal occlusion group.

Interpersonal Skills/Communication

The Value of Prenatal and Postnatal Multidisciplinary Collaboration

In the era of accurate prenatal diagnosis, multidisciplinary involvement before birth is almost routine and includes high-risk obstetricians, neonatologists, and pediatric surgeons. Because of the inability to accurately predict the clinical severity of this diagnosis before birth, coordinating the mode and timing of delivery among these services is needed to optimize the infant's care. Assessing the infant's cardiorespiratory status, possible need for ECMO, and timing of surgery requires frequent communication between surgery and neonatology in the postnatal period. The quality of these interactions is enhanced when a thorough history and physical examination are performed and an understanding of the clinical course and infant's response to certain interventions are demonstrated.

Professionalism

Prepare Families With Appropriate Prenatal Consultations

Most prenatal care includes an ultrasound to look for congenital anatomic defects. When conditions such as CDH are discovered, the obstetrician should refer the family, before the infant's delivery, for a consultation with the appropriate pediatric specialist and, if it is anticipated that NICU care will be required, the neonatologist. The meetings serve to educate and prepare the parents for their child's birth and medical management and the possibility of a critically ill infant. Discussion regarding the role and indication for high-technology interventions such as ECMO and morbidity and mortality risks are initiated at the meeting. The prenatal consultants should be available to the parents as further questions arise during the remainder of the pregnancy. The content of the discussions must be documented and communicated with the consultant's partners who might be on service or on call when the infant is born.

Systems-Based Practice

Hospital Clinical Pathways

The care of infants with CDH can become quite complex, and the patient may need the expertise from multiple medical and surgical specialties. This care must be coordinated well, and desired actions must be communicated without fail. To facilitate both the appropriate care and communication, many hospitals have developed clinical pathways for complex disease states. **A clinical pathway is designed after a thorough analysis of the medical literature to ensure the highest, evidence-based level of care.** The institutional experts, once the literature is reviewed, design a pathway that works well within the institution's working structure. The pathway is used for each patient with the specific diagnosis and is familiar to all the participating team members.

Chapter 75
Tracheoesophageal Fistula (Case 34)

Veniamin Ratner MD

Case: An apparently healthy term newborn with an unremarkable prenatal course is delivered. Prenatal ultrasound was significant only for mild polyhydramnios and a small stomach. Within the first few hours after birth, the infant develops copious oral secretions and is unable to tolerate oral feedings. Attempts at passing a feeding tube fail. Eventually, an increased respiratory rate and respiratory distress develop.

Differential Diagnosis

Esophageal atresia	VACTERL	CHARGE
Tracheoesophageal fistula (TEF)	**V**ertebral anomalies **A**nal atresia **C**ardiac anomaly **T**racheo- **E**sophageal fistula or atresia **R**enal and **L**imb abnormalities	**C**oloboma **H**eartdefects, choanal **A**tresia **R**etardation of growth and development **G**enital and **E**ar anomalies

Speaking Intelligently

When I suspect a patient has a tracheoesophageal fistula, my first thought is to quickly verify my suspicion by attempting to pass a nasogastric tube to the stomach and confirm its position by chest radiography. Once the diagnosis of esophageal atresia has been established, my next step is to provide continuous suction of the proximal esophageal pouch to minimize the degree of lung aspiration-related injury. Next, I position the infant with its head elevated to minimize reflux of gastric secretions into the lungs. Early involvement of the pediatric surgical team is necessary. If there is rapid progression of respiratory distress, I intubate the patient and provide mechanical ventilatory support. If there is a fistula between the trachea and the distal portion of the esophagus, the patient may develop marked abdominal distention, requiring urgent surgical intervention. When the patient's condition is stable, I evaluate for possible associated congenital defects (VACTERL, CHARGE). Laboratory work is rarely a priority; however, echocardiography is essential for identifying aortic arch anatomy and position to determine the appropriate surgical approach.

PATIENT CARE

Clinical Thinking
- Provide **continuous suction** of the secretions from the esophageal pouch and mouth to prevent significant aspiration lung injury.
- Spontaneous breathing is preferable, but if respiratory support is necessary, avoid nasal canula or continuous positive airway pressure.
- Early evaluation for possible associated **congenital anomalies** is essential for comprehensive appropriate management.

History
- Polyhydramnios and an absent or small stomach bubble on prenatal ultrasound should raise suspicion of esophageal atresia.
- A history of inability to swallow oral secretions and excessive drooling must be followed with an attempt to pass a tube into the stomach. Failure to pass the tube is considered diagnostic for esophageal atresia.
- Inability to tolerate feeding due to development of respiratory distress or cyanosis since the first day of life should prompt evaluation for tracheoesophageal fistula.

Physical Examination
- **Vital signs:** Increased respiratory rate may be the first sign of the development of lung injury. Intermittent oxygen desaturation early in the disease may progress to significant constant oxygen desaturation with clinically obvious cyanosis.
- Classically, the neonate with esophageal atresia has copious, white, frothy bubbles of mucus in the mouth and sometimes the nose.
- The infant may have **noisy breathing** and episodes of coughing and cyanosis. These episodes may be exaggerated during feeding if a fistula between the esophagus and the trachea is present.
- Abdominal distention develops as air builds up in the stomach. The abdomen will be scaphoid in the absence of a fistula.

Tests for Consideration
- **Chest and abdomen radiography with orogastric tube in place:** To visualize the position of the esophageal pouch, degree of lung involvement, and degree of stomach distention   **$75 and $45**
- **Serum electrolytes:** The infant might have an associated renal abnormality   **$29**
- **Arterial blood gas (ABG):** For the patient with respiratory distress or on mechanical respiratory support   **$156**

IMAGING CONSIDERATIONS

→ **Echocardiography:** To identify aortic arch anatomy and possible cardiac anomalies	$325
→ **Renal ultrasound:** If urine output is inadequate for age or electrolytes abnormalities are present	$250

Clinical Entities	Medical Knowledge

Esophageal Atresia and Tracheoesophageal Fistula

Pφ	***Esophageal atresia*** is characterized by incomplete formation of the esophagus and is frequently associated with a fistula between the trachea and the esophagus. Many anatomic variations of esophageal atresia with or without ***tracheoesophageal fistula*** have been described (Figure 75-1).
TP	Maternal polyhydramnios may be the first sign of esophageal atresia in the fetus. The inability to identify the fetal stomach bubble on a prenatal ultrasonogram in a mother with polyhydramnios makes the diagnosis of esophageal atresia more likely.
	Classically, the neonate with esophageal atresia has copious, white, frothy bubbles of mucus in the mouth and sometimes the nose. These secretions may clear with aggressive suctioning but eventually return. The infant may experience episodes of coughing, choking, and cyanosis, especially during feeding. Abdominal distention may be prominent if a fistula between the distal esophagus and the trachea is present. The abdomen will be scaphoid if no fistula exists.
Dx	Diagnosis can be made by failure to pass a feeding tube into the stomach; however, it needs to be confirmed by radiographic study of the chest and abdomen with the feeding tube in place. An infant with esophageal atresia should have an echocardiogram before surgery to define any structural anomaly of the heart or great blood vessels, and identify the side where the aortic arch lies.

Tx   Once a diagnosis of esophageal atresia is established, preparations should be made for surgical correction. A suction catheter (Replogle catheter, No. 8 to 10 French gauge) is placed in the upper esophageal pouch to suction secretions. An infant with respiratory distress requires endotracheal intubation and mechanical ventilation.

   The operative correction of an esophageal atresia is not regarded as an emergency procedure. The one exception is the preterm infant with severe respiratory distress syndrome requiring ventilatory support. There is the risk for gastric overdistention and rupture of the stomach due to escape of air down through the distal fistula into the stomach. **See Nelson Essentials 128.**

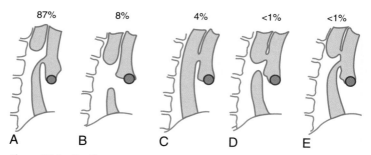

87%   8%   4%   <1%   <1%

A   B   C   D   E

Figure 75-1   The five most common forms of esophageal atresia and tracheoesophageal fistula, in order of frequency.

CHARGE

Pφ   CHARGE is an acronym for a cluster of anomalies that includes **C**oloboma, **H**eart defects, choanal **A**tresia, **R**etardation of growth and development, and **G**enital and **E**ar anomalies. Other associated features may include tracheoesophageal anomalies, urinary tract abnormalities, deafness, and characteristic facial and hand abnormalities. It is an autosomal dominant condition with genotypic heterogeneity. Most cases are due to mutations of the CHD7 gene, but other genetic mutations, including 22q11.2 deletions and single gene mutations, can occur.

TP   The presentation can be related to one or multiple organ systems. Cyanosis may occur secondary to heart disease or respiratory compromise. Other physical stigmata are found on physical examination and imaging studies.

Dx	The cluster of three cardinal signs or two cardinal signs and three minor anomalies usually is sufficient for the diagnosis. Fluorescence in situ hybridization (FISH) for DiGeorge syndrome and high-resolution karyotyping may be required. Echocardiography confirms the cardiac findings. Chest radiograph and abdominal ultrasound may exclude other midline defects. Skeletal survey will exclude skeletal abnormalities. Cranial ultrasound and head computed tomography (CT)/ magnetic resonance imaging (MRI) should be performed to exclude cerebral and ear abnormalities and to determine the level of choanal stenosis.
Tx	Multiple surgeries are expected for those infants who survive the neonatal period. Multiple specialty follow-up and specialized support services may be required. **See Nelson Essentials 79.**

VACTERL	
Pφ	VACTERL is an acronym for a cluster of abnormalities consisting of **V**ertebral anomalies, **A**nal atresia, **C**ardiac anomaly, **T**racheo**E**sophageal fistula or atresia, **R**enal and **L**imb (typically radius) abnormalities. The patient also may have associated growth deficiency. Occasionally, the acronym has an **S** at the end for association with single umbilical artery.
TP	Severity at birth is related to the presenting organ system. Further imaging reveals the nonrandom associated findings. No chromosomal abnormality or other etiology has been identified.
Dx	Skeletal survey, chest radiograph, echocardiography, and abdominal ultrasound may be required for confirmation of findings.
Tx	Treatment is based on surgical correction of esophageal and cardiac anomalies and long-term follow-up for growth deficiency. Multiple specialty follow-up and specialized support services may be required **See Nelson Essentials 128.**

ZEBRA ZONE

a. **Esophageal duplication cyst:** Cystic mass lined by intestinal epithelium that attaches to the esophagus

b. **Laryngotracheoesophageal clefts:** Common channel defect between the pharyngoesophagus and laryngotracheal lumens

Practice-Based Learning and Improvement: Evidence-Based Medicine

Title
Oesophageal atresia

Author
Spitz L

Reference
Orphanet J Rare Dis 2007; 2:24

Problem
Review of embryology, pathophysiology, and therapeutic surgical interventions for the repair of esophageal atresia

Comparison/control (quality of evidence)
Review article with cited references in peer-reviewed journal

Historical significance/comments
Robust review of historical references, pathophysiology, and treatment of TEF

Interpersonal and Communication Skills

Take Time to Understand Parents' Perspectives

The finding of tracheoesophageal fistula is often associated with a variety of other congenital defects, and families are faced with a newborn that is often not what they originally idealized. They may also be faced with multiple surgical interventions in order to correct defects in their new baby. It is important to listen well when discussing such distressing findings with parents. It is often difficult to know which problem the family finds most distressing. The child may have a serious heart defect that requires extensive surgical repair; however, the family may be more distressed by the facial abnormalities that have no significant effect other than cosmetic. Try to listen for and understand all of the family's concerns. This will help you ease their discomfort and communicate more effectively.

Professionalism

Altruism: Provision of Care for the Uninsured

Infants with multiple congenital abnormalities may require multiple surgical interventions and have a prolonged and protracted course. Infants with multiple congenital anomalies whose families have no health insurance can be treated pro bono. They should be referred to individuals or agencies that can assist the family in obtaining insurance as well as Supplemental Security Income (SSI), if warranted by the specifics of the diagnosis.

Systems-Based Practice

Inpatient Quality Indicators

Inpatient Quality Indicators (IQIs) are a set of measures defined by the Agency for Healthcare Research and Quality (AHRQ) that provide a perspective of hospital quality of care using hospital administrative data. Surgical quality of care, for example, includes average 30-day mortality and morbidity rates (postsurgical infections and readmission rates), average length of stay (LOS), and patient satisfaction. These indicators are used to help hospitals identify areas that may need quality improvement.

Chapter 76
Meconium Aspiration Syndrome (Case 35)

Jane S. Lee MD, MPH

Case: A term infant is delivered emergently by cesarean delivery because of a nonreassuring fetal heart tracing. The infant is covered in thick particulate meconium and following resuscitation develops severe respiratory distress.

Differential Diagnosis

Meconium aspiration syndrome (MAS)	Persistent pulmonary hypertension of the newborn (PPHN)	Infection/pneumonia
Transient tachypnea of the newborn (TTN)	Respiratory distress syndrome (RDS)	

Speaking Intelligently

In the setting of meconium-stained amniotic fluid, I rapidly assess if the infant is vigorous following delivery. Vigor is defined as the presence of spontaneous respirations, reasonable tone, and sustained heart rate above 100 beats per minute. If an infant is crying, he or she is vigorous. If the infant appears depressed at birth, immediate intervention is required. Additional personnel should be summoned at this time so that subsequent resuscitative measures may be performed simultaneously. Using either a bulb syringe or large-bore suction catheter, I clear any visible meconium from the infant's mouth and nose. It is important to suction the mouth first because nasopharyngeal suctioning may induce gasping and further aspiration of meconium. I then place the infant in the "sniffing" position so that the airway is as unobstructed as possible. While another member of the delivery room team administers free-flow oxygen to the infant, I perform endotracheal intubation and tracheal suctioning of meconium. This process is repeated until no meconium is recovered.

PATIENT CARE

Clinical Thinking

- Initiate neonatal resuscitation if the infant appears depressed at birth or develops respiratory distress shortly after birth.
- Remember **the ABCs** of resuscitation: airway, breathing, and circulation.
- If the infant remains cyanotic despite adequate ventilation, evaluate the infant for an acute, superimposing cause for the hypoxia such as air leak.
- When did the aspiration occur—in utero or following delivery? Is there evidence of **chronic hypoxia?** Consider an echocardiogram to evaluate for evidence of pulmonary hypertension.
- If no meconium is obtained upon tracheal suctioning, consider other diagnoses because meconium aspiration is less likely.

History

- Is there **antenatal history** of maternal diabetes, hypertension, preeclampsia, or maternal drug abuse?
- Did prenatal ultrasonography reveal evidence of congenital anomalies or abnormalities in amniotic fluid volume or uteroplacental blood flow?
- Were there **signs of fetal hypoxia** such as a nonreassuring fetal heart pattern, abnormal biophysical profile, oligohydramnios, intrauterine growth restriction, or metabolic acidosis on umbilical artery blood gas sampling?

- Evaluate **intrapartum risk factors.** Was the infant born by cesarean delivery without labor or a precipitous vaginal delivery? Is the pregnancy postterm? Are there other reasons for respiratory depression such as magnesium prophylaxis for preeclampsia or maternal narcotic administration within 4 hours before delivery?
- Are there risk factors for neonatal sepsis such as rupture of membranes of greater than 18 hours duration, maternal fever, chorioamnionitis, group B streptococcal vaginal colonization, presence of urinary tract infection or history of recurrent urinary tract infections in the mother, birth of previous infant with neonatal infection, or fetal tachycardia?

Physical Examination
- Vital signs: Bradycardia, tachypnea, oxygen desaturation.
- Overall condition: Determine the infant's vigorousness, alertness, tone.
- Symptoms of respiratory distress: Varying degree of tachypnea, nasal flaring, grunting, retractions, and cyanosis may be present. Central cyanosis is assessed by examining the face, trunk, and mucous membranes.
- Signs of **postmaturity:** Inspect for weight loss, loose skin folds, peeling of the skin, long fingernails, and yellowish staining of the skin, finger nails, and umbilical cord.
- Signs of shock: Evaluate for pallor, delayed capillary perfusion, and peripheral pulses that are not easily palpable.
- Cardiac examination: Assess for cardiac murmur or signs of congestive heart failure.

Tests for Consideration
- **Arterial blood gas (ABG)** $156
- **Complete blood count (CBC) with differential** $53
- **Electrolytes, including glucose and calcium** $29
- **Blood culture** $100

IMAGING CONSIDERATIONS

→ **Chest radiograph** $75
→ **Echocardiogram:** To evaluate for pulmonary hypertension, ventricular filling, cardiac contractility, and structural cardiac anomalies $325

Clinical Entities	Medical Knowledge

Meconium Aspiration Syndrome

Pφ   Passage of meconium is associated with up to 15% of deliveries and may represent a normal physiologic event associated with gastrointestinal maturation; it is rare before 37 weeks gestation. In utero aspiration of meconium-stained amniotic fluid occurs as in response to stress such as hypoxia, acidemia, or infection. Respiratory distress develops as a result of a variety of mechanisms. As the aspirated meconium moves into the distal airway, a partial or complete mechanical obstruction occurs. A partial "ball-valve" obstruction leads to air trapping and potential for air leak, whereas complete obstruction results in atelectasis. Over the first few hours of age, a chemical pneumonitis develops secondary to induction of an inflammatory response. Meconium inactivates the endogenous surfactant, which leads to a loss of alveolar stabilization, resulting in collapse of the lung or atelectasis and intrapulmonary shunting.

TP   The infant typically presents in severe respiratory distress with grunting, tachypnea, and retractions. There may be evidence of meconium staining of the skin, umbilical cord, and finger and toe nails, indicating exposure to meconium for some hours before delivery.

Dx   Evidence of meconium passage at delivery should be present. Chest radiograph typically reveals hyperinflation with flattened diaphragm and diffuse, asymmetric patchy infiltrates. Pleural effusion and cardiomegaly may also be present.

Tx   Tracheal suctioning of meconium should be performed immediately in all depressed infants. Once the meconium is cleared, the infant should receive supportive care as needed. In severe cases complicated by pulmonary hypertension, inhaled nitric oxide should be started. Replacement therapy with surfactant may also be administered. If severe hypoxemia persists despite other therapies, extracorporeal membrane oxygenation (ECMO) should be considered. **See Nelson Essentials 61.**

Persistent Pulmonary Hypertension of the Newborn

Pφ When pulmonary vascular resistance and pulmonary arterial pressures remain elevated after birth, inadequate gas exchange occurs secondary to shunting of blood away from the lungs through a patent ductus arteriosus. Pulmonary vasoconstriction may be further exacerbated by hypoxia, acidosis, and hypercapnia.

TP Symptoms include tachypnea, nasal flaring, grunting, tachycardia, and cyanosis. The examination may be notable for a systolic murmur of tricuspid regurgitation, hepatomegaly secondary to right ventricular failure, and poor peripheral perfusion as evidenced by delayed capillary refill and weak pulses.

Dx A chest radiograph is necessary to assess underlying lung disease and assess for cardiomegaly. The chest radiograph typically demonstrates poorly perfused lungs. An echocardiogram is indicated to exclude structural cardiac anomalies, assess myocardial function, and confirm the presence and severity of pulmonary hypertension. ABG will reveal severe hypoxemia and acidosis. Comparison of preductal and postductal oxygen saturation values will also reveal an oxygen gradient (>10% difference) and will help differentiate PPHN from structural heart disease.

Tx The goal of treatment is to lower pulmonary vascular resistance, which may be achieved by a regimen of minimal stimulation, intravenous fluid and nutritional support, correction of acidosis, and maintenance of adequate oxygenation and systemic blood pressure. Mechanical ventilation may be necessary. Administration of inhaled nitric oxide will selectively relax pulmonary vasculature, thereby permitting more blood flow to the lungs. If hypoxemia is refractory to other therapies, ECMO may be required. **See Nelson Essentials 61.**

Transient Tachypnea of the Newborn

See Chapter 66, Transient Tachypnea of the Newborn.

Infection/Pneumonia

See Chapter 77, Neonatal Sepsis.

Respiratory Distress Syndrome (RDS)

See Chapter 73, Respiratory Distress Syndrome.

ZEBRA ZONE

a. **Surfactant protein B deficiency:** A rare autosomal recessive congenital deficiency of surfactant protein B, which results in abnormal alveolar accumulation of other surfactant proteins. Affected infants present with severe respiratory distress unresponsive to exogenous surfactant therapy and ventilator management.

b. **Alveolar capillary dysplasia:** A rare cause of progressive fatal PPHN that arises from a failure of formation and growth of alveolar capillaries, hypertrophy of medial muscles of the pulmonary arteries, and abnormal alignment of pulmonary veins.

c. **Congenital lung abnormalities:** Severity of respiratory distress is related to the degree of pulmonary hypoplasia that arises from the underlying developmental abnormality. Examples include congenital diaphragmatic hernia, congenital cystic adenomatoid malformation, and pulmonary sequestration.

d. **Congenital heart disease:** See Chapter 79, Cyanotic Newborn.

Practice-Based Learning and Improvement: Evidence-Based Medicine

Title
Delivery room management of the apparently vigorous meconium-stained neonate: Results of the multicenter, international collaborative trial

Authors
Wiswell TE, Gannon CM, Jacob J, et al

Reference
Pediatrics 105:359-381, 2000

Problem
To compare endotracheal intubation and suctioning with expectant management of apparently vigorous meconium-stained term infants in reducing the incidence of MAS.

Intervention
A total of 2094 infants enrolled from 12 participating centers were randomly assigned to intubation and intratracheal suctioning (n = 1051) or to expectant management (n = 1043).

Comparison/control (quality of evidence)
Level I evidence

Outcome/effect
There was no statistical difference in the occurrence of MAS or other respiratory disorders between infants who received intubation and

intratracheal suctioning versus expectant management. There was a 3.8% intubation-related complication rate observed in this study.

Historical significance/comments
This multicenter, randomized clinical trial showed that expectant management was as efficacious as routine endotracheal intubation and suctioning in preventing MAS in vigorous term meconium-stained infants. The findings of this study led to a revision of national resuscitation guidelines on neonatal resuscitation of this subset of infants.

Interpersonal and Communication Skills

Reach Agreement With Family on Problems and Plans

Once a diagnosis has been established in the case of a severely compromised neonate, an ongoing dialogue must be established between the medical team and the infant's family. This will hopefully allow the family to understand the underlying etiology of the disease and enable them to be active participants in the decision-making process. When dealing with respiratory distress in the newborn period, the differential diagnosis may require inclusion of progressive or lethal disease and discussions with the families may include such sensitive issues as death. If death appears inevitable, the medical provider needs to discuss end-of-life issues such as do not resuscitate (DNR) orders and palliative care with the family.

Professionalism

Compassion: Designate a Liason to Family Whenever Necessary

Infants with meconium staining must have an individual skilled at neonatal intubation present at the delivery. If the infant requires intervention, that individual must focus on stabilizing the infant and will have no time to speak to the parents. It is distressing for parents to see activity at the infant warmer and sense the concern of the physicians and have no idea what problem/s their infant is experiencing.

Compassionate care includes designating a qualified individual to speak to and stay with the parents until the physician in charge of the resuscitation is able to give them more information.

Systems-Based Practice

Patient Safety: Three-Way Repeat-Back May Enhance Safety of Communication

Multiple factors contribute to medical error. In the delivery room, a team of individuals must work together in sometimes frantic situations while being vigilant to maintain patient safety. Poor communication in this setting can be a major contributing factor to medical error. Reports of neonatal death or injury as a result of mishaps and mistakes in neonatal resuscitation listed poor communication and coordination among the patient care team as a contributing factor in 72% of cases reviewed.[1]

The "three-way repeat-back" is thought to be a helpful error prevention technique when multiple tasks are being requested and recorded.

Leader: "Give atropine 0.1 mg!"
Follower: "That's atropine 0.1 mg."
Leader (confirming): "That's correct."

Reference

1. The Joint Commission: Preventing infant death and injury: Sentinel Event Alert (30), 2004.

Chapter 77
Neonatal Sepsis (Case 36)

Christiana R. Farkouh MD, MPH

Case: A 32-weeks-gestation female infant is born to a 29-year-old G2P1 mother whose serologic test results are:

Blood type A Rh-positive, antibody negative, rapid plasma reagin (RPR) NR, rubella immune, hepatitis B surface antigen (HBsAg) negative, GC/*Chlamydia* negative, human immunodeficiency virus (HIV) negative, group B streptococcus (GBS) unknown.

Delivery was via an emergency cesarean section due to a nonreassuring fetal heart tracing. The mother was admitted 48 hours before delivery with preterm rupture of membranes and received two doses of betamethasone and antibiotics. Her prenatal history was notable only for antibiotic therapy for an *Escherichia coli* urinary tract infection (UTI) 1 month before delivery. At 9 hours of life, there is temperature instability, tachypnea, and hypoglycemia.

Differential Diagnosis

Neonatal sepsis	Apnea of prematurity (AOP)
Necrotizing enterocolitis (NEC)	Neonatal herpes simplex virus (HSV)

Speaking Intelligently

When an infant is admitted after birth with prenatal/perinatal risk factors, or at any time develops clinical symptoms such as fever, hypothermia, glucose intolerance, alterations in respirations , feeding intolerance, or temperature irregularity, I perform a blood culture, complete blood count (CBC) with differential, and C-reactive protein (CRP). I start empiric antibiotic therapy after the blood culture is drawn because the symptoms of neonatal sepsis can be quite subtle and nonspecific, and delay in treatment may be fatal. The CBC, differential, and CRP are repeated at 24 hours. Treatment continues for at least 48 hours despite negative blood culture results. At delivery, however, particularly if mothers have been treated with antibiotics, blood culture results can be unreliable. The initial clinical presentation, response to therapy, presence of risk factors, and laboratory results will all play a role in determining the decision to continue antibiotics beyond the initial 48 hours of evaluation to rule out sepsis.

PATIENT CARE

Clinical Thinking
- Are there maternal or perinatal risk factors?
- What is the infant's presenting sign(s) or symptom(s)?
- Are there risk factors for sepsis, such as prolonged rupture of membranes, GBS colonization, maternal fever (temperature >38° C [100.4° F])?
- Does the infant have a central line?
- Is there concern for feeding intolerance?
- Has this infant been treated for sepsis previously?

History
- Consider **maternal factors** such as GBS colonization, maternal GBS UTI, prior children with GBS infection/sepsis.

- Consider **perinatal issues** such as prolonged rupture of membranes (>16 hours), maternal temperature >38° C (100.4° F), amniotic fluid characteristics, obstetric concern regarding chorioamnionitis.
- Consider **neonatal factors** such as prematurity, change in baseline clinical status, alterations in respiratory requirements, feeding intolerance, presence of a central line.
- Fever greater than 100.4° F in newborns is unusual and should immediately initiate a full infectious workup including blood, urine, and cerebrospinal fluid (CSF) studies.

Physical Examination
- Vital signs: Hypotension, tachycardia, increased frequency of apnea, increase in desaturation episodes or need for increased respiratory support, fluctuations in body temperature (especially hypothermia in preterm infants) not related to incubator environment.
- Initial assessment should focus on airway, breathing, and circulation (ABCs).
- Abdominal examination: Distention, assessment of bowel sounds, change in residual feed volumes.
- Overall tone and level of activity can be helpful, especially if changed from baseline.

Tests for Consideration
- **CBC with differential:** Determine ANC, determine the immature to total neutrophil ratio (I:T ratio). Serial levels at 12 and 24 hours may help. $116
- **CRP:** Serial levels at 12 and 24 hours may help. $69
- **Blood culture (both peripheral and from central catheter, if present)** $152
- **Urine culture and analysis** $148
- **CSF analysis Gram stain, cell count, for white blood cells (WBCs), red blood cells (RBCs), protein, glucose, and culture** $557
- **CSF HSV polymerase chain reaction (PCR)** $300
- **Coagulation studies: Prothrombin time and partial thromboplastin** if concern for coagulopathy in disseminated disease $105

IMAGING CONSIDERATIONS

→ **Chest radiograph**	$75
→ **Abdominal ultrasound (evaluate liver texture and size)**	$225
→ **Brain magnetic resonance imaging (MRI)**	$900
→ **Head computed tomography (CT) scan**	$750

Neonatal Sepsis

Pφ **Neonatal sepsis** can present as early-onset sepsis (EOS), occurring in the first 7 days of life, or late-onset sepsis (LOS), occurring between 7 days and 3 months of life. EOS is usually associated with *intrapartum* complications such as GBS colonization, *perinatal* risk factors such as prolonged rupture of membranes, chorioamnionitis, maternal fever, use of scalp electrodes, and *neonatal* risk factors, such as low birth weight and prematurity. The organisms associated with EOS are typically **transmitted vertically** from the maternal genital tract to the infant and include group B streptococcus *E. coli* enterococci, *Listeria monocytogenes,* and other gram-negative organisms. In contrast, LOS in preterm infants is usually caused by coagulase-negative staphylococcus, a gram-positive organism, and is associated with the use of central venous catheters. Other **nosocomial infections** may be acquired in association with reduced vigilance and low hand-washing rates.

TP Many infants with sepsis have signs of respiratory distress, and other nonspecific signs include feeding intolerance and lethargy.

Dx When a sepsis evaluation occurs after the initial delivery process, evaluation of blood, CSF, and urine is indicated. In older preterm infants who present with low-risk symptoms without focal signs of meningitis, it may be reasonable to obtain blood cultures from both peripheral and central sites, a urine culture by suprapubic catheterization or urethral catheterization, CBC with differential, and CRP before initiating therapy, performing CSF studies to ascertain meningitis and duration of antibiotic therapy only if the blood culture results are positive. However, approximately 15% of infants with meningitis will have negative blood cultures.

Tx Therapy for EOS consists of intravenous ampicillin and gentamicin. Ampicillin is the antibiotic of choice for treatment of GBS, *L. monocytogenes,* and most enterococci, and gentamicin provides coverage for possible gram-negative organisms. Cefotaxime, a third-generation cephalosporin, may be considered if meningitis due to gram-negative organisms is suspected. For infants undergoing evaluation for LOS, treatment with vancomycin and gentamicin may be preferred because many of these infants have central lines in situ, placing them at high risk for sepsis. See Chapter 62, Early-Onset Group B Streptococcal Disease. **See Nelson Essentials 65.**

Apnea of Prematurity

Pφ   The term *apnea* refers to the absence of both airflow and breathing movement. ***Apnea of prematurity*** can be defined as the cessation of breathing for >20 seconds or cessation of breathing <20 seconds accompanied by a bradycardia 20% below baseline heart rate or desaturation <80%. Apnea can be classified as **central, obstructive,** or **mixed,** based on the presence or absence of airflow and breathing movements. Roughly 40% of apnea is central in nature, approximately 10% is obstructive, and roughly 50% is mixed apnea (both central and obstructive). Apnea of prematurity typically resolves by 37 weeks post conception; however, it can persist until 45 weeks post conception.

TP   Apnea must be differentiated from periodic breathing, which is a normal breathing pattern in preterm and term newborns characterized by regular breathing for 10 to 15 seconds followed by a brief pause in breathing for <10 seconds without change in heart rate and oxygen saturation.

Dx   Only after other possible causes of apnea have been excluded (sepsis, pneumonia, neurologic disorders, hypothermia, hypoglycemia, and gastroesophageal reflux) can one make a diagnosis of apnea of prematurity. Most neonatologists consider apnea in the first 24 hours of life indicative of infection or neurologic abnormalities. As a result, **AOP is not considered in the differential diagnosis of apnea in the first 24 hours of life in any newborn regardless of the degree of prematurity.**

Tx   In mild forms, the apnea may resolve spontaneously or may need some mild stimulation to restore a regular breathing pattern. For more moderate or severe forms of apnea of prematurity, two main treatments exist: providing respiratory support, which can be in the form of nasal cannula, continuous positive airway pressure (CPAP), or intubation and mechanical ventilation. For difficult to control cases, another approach is medical therapy with methylxanthines (such as caffeine). **See Nelson Essentials 61 and 134.**

Herpes Simplex Virus

Pφ   ***Herpes simplex virus*** is a double-stranded DNA virus belonging to the family Herpesviridae, a virus characterized by the ability to invade the nervous system, replicate, remain latent, and reactivate at later stages in response to a variety of stressors.

TP	Presentation of HSV infection in newborns can occur in three forms: (1) disseminated infection involving the viscera, particularly the liver and lung; (2) central nervous system (CNS) disease; or (3) skin, eyes, and/or mouth (SEM) disease. Cutaneous vesicular lesions are often thought to be the hallmark of HSV disease; however, about 20% of infants with disseminated HSV do not develop these findings during their illness. The majority of neonates with HSV infection are born to asymptomatic mothers who developed a primary HSV infection during the pregnancy. In fact, it is the woman with a primary genital HSV infection who is at highest risk for transmitting the virus to her baby. Approximately 50% to 60% of infants delivered to women with a first-episode primary infection developed neonatal HSV disease compared with 2% of babies delivered to women with recurrent HSV disease.
Dx	Definitive testing includes early markers such as HSV PCR detection in CSF, blood/serum, and/or peripheral mononuclear cells. If there are vesicular skin lesions, unroof a lesion to send a swab for HSV monoclonal antibodies, which is diagnostic; results can be available in 1 hour. In addition, this testing can also distinguish between type 1 and type 2 disease. Cutaneous vesicular lesions are often thought to be the hallmark of HSV disease; however, about 20% of infants with disseminated HSV do not develop cutaneous findings. Liver function testing can also be a sensitive early marker of HSV infection and can aid in diagnosis.
Tx	After initiating antiviral therapy with acyclovir, supportive interventions are administered as needed. Because coagulopathy is a manifestation of disseminated disease, checking coagulation studies and measuring platelet levels is necessary. **See Nelson Essentials 66.**

Necrotizing Enterocolitis

See Chapter 72, Necrotizing Enterocolitis.

ZEBRA ZONE

a. **Congenital central hypoventilation syndrome:** Congenital central hypoventilation syndrome (CCHS), or Ondine's curse, is a life-threatening disorder involving an impaired ventilatory response to hypercarbia and hypoxemia. CCHS presents on the first day of life with prolonged apneas, elevated carbon dioxide levels, and small tidal volumes during sleep with more normal infant breathing patterns when awake.

b. **Galactosemia:** This is an autosomal recessive disease caused by deficient activity of galactose-1-phosphate uridyltransferase (GALT) as a result of a mutation at the GALT gene on chromosome 17q. Classic features in newborns are vomiting, diarrhea, hyperbilirubinemia, hepatomegaly, and *E. coli* sepsis a few days after starting cow milk formula or breast milk.

Practice-Based Learning and Improvement: Evidence-Based Medicine

Title
Neonatal herpes simplex infection

Authors
Kimberlin DW

Reference
Clin Microbiol Rev 17(1):1-13, 2004

Problem
Full review of the pathophysiology and recent developments of neonatal HSV

Comparison/control (quality of evidence)
Review article with cited references in peer-reviewed journal

Historical significance/comments
Excellent review of the current management of HSV infection in the newborn

Interpersonal and Communication Skills

Structure, Clarify, and Summarize Information

When sepsis is suspected, it is important to discuss your concerns with the family and keep them informed about the baby's condition and relevant data. Usually families will want to know why you suspect infection, what tests have been done, and what medicines have been started. Patients with sepsis may have multiple organ failure, and in some cases, this may be the most crucial and therapeutically complex issue to manage. Sharing the medical plan with the parents can reassure them that careful thought and consideration of their child's needs and best interest are being maintained. Keeping them apprised embraces them as integral members of the health-care team.

Professionalism

Respecting the Expertise of Nursing Colleagues

The initial signs of sepsis in neonates can be quite subtle and can rapidly progress to irreversible shock and death. The bedside nurse is often the first to raise concerns regarding change in an infant's baseline status. As for all clinical matters, it is essential to respect the clinical expertise of the nursing staff and respond immediately when a nurse raises concerns about the deteriorating clinical status of a patient. Besides being a core value of professionalism, such respect and regard may save a patient's life.

Systems-Based Practice

Quality Improvement: Process, Structure, Effectiveness, and Efficiency

Reducing practice variation in clinically complex patient populations is one of the biggest challenges in medicine. Variation often leads to less-than-optimal outcomes for newborns and unnecessary costs to the health-care system.

Treatment of neonates with suspected sepsis appears to be influenced by considerations other than maternal risk factors or the infant's clinical condition beyond the first day of life. There appears to be a great deal of practice variation among neonatologists confronted by patients with suspected sepsis. Awareness of this unnecessary variation may be of great value in reducing the duration of antibiotic therapy in the neonatal intensive care unit and shortening the length of stay.[1]

Reference

1. Spitzer AR, Kirkby S, Kornhauser M: Practice variation in suspected neonatal sepsis: A costly problem in neonatal intensive care. *J Perinatol* 25(4):265-269, 2005.

Chapter 78
Intraventricular Hemorrhage (Case 37)

Helen M. Towers MD

Case: An infant is born at 26 weeks gestation, weighing 740 grams, following placental abruption. He develops low blood pressure requiring pressor support. His hematocrit is 28% the following morning, requiring a packed red blood cell transfusion. On the second day of life, a head ultrasound reveals bilateral intraventricular hemorrhage with distension of the left ventricle and extension into the parenchyma.

Differential Diagnosis

Intraventricular hemorrhage (IVH)	Cerebellar hemorrhage	Epidural hemorrhage
Subdural hemorrhage	Subarachnoid hemorrhage	

Speaking Intelligently

When I suspect an infant has IVH, I assess the clinical presentation of the infant. I evaluate gestational age and the presence of other complications of prematurity, such as severe respiratory distress. I palpate the anterior fontanel for evidence of bulging secondary to increased intracranial pressure. A severe bleed may lead to acute altered hemodynamic status, requiring an increase in ventilator or pressor support. Imaging by head ultrasound determines the size, location, and extent of the bleeding. Laboratory tests include hemoglobin and platelet levels, as well as serum electrolytes, acid-base balance, and glucose levels. Coagulation studies can be of some help in term infants. Prompt discussion of the findings with the parents may guide further supportive measures, particularly if there is extensive bleeding present.

General support measures consist of blood transfusion, evaluation of acid-base balance, electrolyte balance, and serial ultrasounds for evidence of obstructive hydrocephalus over time.

PATIENT CARE

Clinical Thinking
- Infants less than 31 weeks gestation and <1500 grams have an approximately 30% risk for IVH.
- A requirement for intubation or for resuscitation in the delivery room indicates a sicker infant who may be more predisposed to IVH.
- Fluctuations in blood pressure and oxygenation may predispose to IVH.
- **Bulging fontanel** or **abnormal movements,** including posturing or seizure activity, may indicate presence of IVH.
- Evaluations of arterial blood gas (ABG) will provide information on oxygenation as well as acid-base balance.
- Serial head ultrasound evaluation provides valuable information to be shared with the parents.
- The parents need sufficient information that is provided in an unbiased manner and adequate emotional support to make decisions regarding life-sustaining efforts.

History
- **Prematurity** is the most common association with IVH with increasing likelihood of bleeding occurring in the most immature infants.
- Antenatal history of maternal sepsis and nontreatment with corticosteroids has been associated with IVH.
- In the postnatal period, the requirement for intubation shortly after delivery, as well the presence of pneumothorax, has been associated with IVH.
- Most IVH occurs within the first 72 hours of life.

Physical Examination
- Vital signs associated with the acute onset of IVH include hypotension, bradycardia, and apnea.
- A bulging anterior fontanel may be felt but is not a consistent finding.
- Seizures may be seen.
- Hyperglycemia may occur.

Tests for Consideration
- **Complete blood count (CBC)** $53
- **Serum electrolyte levels** $29
- **Blood glucose level** $25
- **Arterial blood gas (ABG)** $156
- **Coagulation studies, including prothrombin time (PT) and partial thromboplastin time (PTT)** $75

IMAGING CONSIDERATIONS

→ Head ultrasound (serial over time)	$550
→ Magnetic resonance imaging (MRI) of the brain	$900

Clinical Entities   **Medical Knowledge**

Intraventricular Hemorrhage

Pφ   ***Intraventricular-periventricular hemorrhage*** is the end result of bleeding from capillaries within the subependymal germinal matrix, a vascular network that lies in the periventricular region of the brain and is the source of cortical neurons and glial cells.

TP   Presentation generally occurs within the first 72 hours of life, and earlier in premature infants <750 grams. Most cases are silent and are found on surveillance ultrasound. Others may be associated with clinical changes such as metabolic acidosis, drop in hematocrit, glucose instability, and pulmonary hemorrhage.

Dx   Diagnosis is made by cranial ultrasound, computed tomography (CT), or MRI imaging. Grading is classically into four stages. Grade 1 is hemorrhage confined to the germinal matrix. Grade 2 has extension and filling of <50% of the lateral ventricle on sagittal view. Grade 3 has >50% ventricular filling with distension of the lateral ventricle. Grade 4 is associated with parenchymal extension of the hemorrhage. Extension of the bleed into the parenchyma of the brain predisposes to the development of porencephalic cyst formation and may have associated periventricular leukomalacia, which carries a worse neurodevelopmental prognosis.

Tx   There is no treatment currently available. Therapy is directed at prevention of further neurologic damage that may result from the development of obstructive hydrocephalus. Approximately 50% of hemorrhages will lead to hydrocephalus, and approximately 50% of these will resolve spontaneously. For those infants who develop increasing ventricles, serial lumbar puncture with removal of 10 to 15 mL/kg per tap is occasionally performed, usually to attempt to decompress before shunt placement in smaller infants. Some infants ultimately may require placement of a ventriculoperitoneal shunt when the infant approaches 1800 g. **See Nelson Essentials 64.**

Cerebellar Hemorrhage

Pφ **Cerebellar hemorrhage** is a potentially underrecognized problem of bleeding into the posterior fossa. It may occur independently or associated with severe intraventricular hemorrhage. It has been described in 10% to 25% of autopsies of low-birth-weight infants and occurs more frequently in surviving extremely low-birth-weight infants.

TP The presentation may be clinically silent, or it may occur in conjunction with a supratentorial bleed and be associated with alterations in blood pressure, glucose control, and metabolic acidosis. Perinatal risk factors include an abnormal fetal heart rate, delivery by emergent caesarian delivery, and lower Apgar scores, and postnatal risk factors include high-frequency ventilation, requirement for volume expanders or pressor support, as well as the presence of a patent ductus arteriosus (PDA) or pulmonary hemorrhage.

Dx Because the cerebellar vermis and tentorium are more echogenic, it is more difficult to diagnose a cerebellar bleed by head ultrasound. Performing imaging via the posterolateral or mastoid fontanel, at the junction of the squamosal, lamboidal, and occipital sutures allows for better visualization. CT imaging may provide better visualization when the infant is stable enough for transport.

Tx Management of a posterior fossa bleed involves serial evaluation. There is no treatment offered. Longer neurodevelopmental follow-up of infants suggests a worse outcome may be associated with the presence of a cerebellar bleed. **See Nelson Essentials 64.**

Epidural Hemorrhage

Pφ Epidural bleeds are caused by rupture of branches of the middle meningeal artery or bleeding from major veins or venous sinuses. It is a rare lesion in the newborn and may be associated with a skull fracture.

TP Bleeding into the epidural space may follow a traumatic or instrumented delivery and should be suspected in any infant who demonstrates signs of raised intracranial pressure with bulging fontanel, decreased tone, and increasing stupor in the first day of life. Seizures may occur. A unilateral fixed dilated pupil may indicate uncal herniation. Progressive scalp swelling may occur.

Dx	An emergency CT or MRI should be performed to identify the site and size of the hemorrhage. Ultrasound is not a reliable modality to identify an epidural bleed.
Tx	Surgical evacuation of the clot or needle aspiration may be performed. **See Nelson Essentials 184.**

Subdural Hemorrhage

Pφ	Subdural bleeding occurs as a result of laceration or injury to the veins and sinuses of the brain. It may occur in the subdural space over the cerebral convexity, in the posterior fossa, or along the longitudinal cerebral fissure. Bleeding results from trauma, usually rotational movements of the brain within the skull. Posterior fossa bleeds result from rupture of the transverse or straight sinuses or the vein of Galen.
TP	Acute neurologic changes may be present with hemiparesis or impaired oculomotor motion. Seizures can also occur.
Dx	CT or MRI imaging is required to confirm the location and size of the bleed.
Tx	Occasionally neurosurgical evacuation is required. Approximately 80% of infants who undergo evacuation of the hematoma have normal or minor developmental deficits on follow-up. **See Nelson Essentials 184.**

Subarachnoid Hemorrhage

Pφ	Blood may be found in the subarachnoid space by extension from subdural, intraventricular, or intracerebellar hemorrhage. Blood may be found over the cerebral convexities, especially posteriorly, as well as in the posterior fossa. It is thought to originate from bleeding between small vascular channels derived from anastomoses between leptomeningeal arteries or from bridging veins.
TP	Significant increase in intracranial pressure is rare. Hydrocephalus may develop secondary to adhesion formation, which may obstruct the flow of cerebrospinal fluid. It may be associated with hypoxic events and occurs more commonly in the term infant. It may be asymptomatic or may present with onset of seizures. More rarely, with massive subarachnoid hemorrhage, clinical deterioration is rapid and irreversible.

Dx	A bloody lumbar puncture with elevated protein count may be the first sign. Ultrasound is not the best modality to visualize a subarachnoid bleed because there is normally some increased echogenicity around the brain. CT is considered the best means of imaging the subarachnoid space and differentiating hemorrhage there from other intracerebral bleeds.
Tx	Close monitoring of the clinical presentation is the most usual course of action. There is no specific treatment. The outcome is generally favorable for infants who develop subarachnoid hemorrhage. Almost 90% of those infants who develop seizures will have normal follow-up. Hydrocephalus is a rare and late-occurring complication. **See Nelson Essentials 184.**

ZEBRA ZONE

Bleeding disorders: Intraventricular hemorrhage may be a rare complication of bleeding disorders such as **factor XIII deficiency** and **Glanzmann thrombasthenia,** a rare platelet abnormality caused by absent or dysfunctional platelet fibrinogen receptor. Late-onset neonatal bleeding with IVH may be seen in **vitamin K deficiency. Neonatal alloimmune thrombocytopenia (NAIT)** is a maternal-fetal platelet antigen incompatibility disorder diagnosed serologically by demonstrating parental platelet antigen incompatibility and the presence of maternal platelet antibodies.

Practice-Based Learning and Improvement: Evidence-Based Medicine

Title
Low-dose indomethacin and prevention of intraventricular hemorrhage: A multicenter randomized trial

Authors
Ment LR, Ehrenkranz RA, Duncan CC, et al

Reference
Pediatrics 93(4):543-550, 1994

Problem
Prophylactic use of indomethacin to reduce incidence of IVH in preterm infants <1250 grams

Intervention
Administration of 0.1 mg/kg indomethacin at 6 and 12 hours of age then once daily for next 2 days

Comparison/control
Placebo

Quality of evidence
Prospective, randomized, placebo-controlled multicenter trial

Outcome/effect
Reduction in incidence and severity of intraventricular hemorrhage, especially grade 4 IVH, noted as well as associated reduction in incidence of patent ductus arteriosus

Historical significance/comments
This is the first study to show reduction in severe intraventricular hemorrhage. Because grade 4 bleeds are associated with the worst neurologic outcomes, this therapy might be considered in those units that have higher-than-average incidence of severe grade 4 hemorrhage.

Interpersonal and Communication Skills

Communicate Sensitively When Families Face Life-Altering Consequences

The finding of a high-grade intraventricular hemorrhage in the first few days of a premature infant's life may have life-altering consequences. Great sensitivity is required in explaining the findings to the family. It is preferably done by a senior provider who has already met the family or intends to continue to provide care to them. A frank discussion of the potential neurodevelopmental outcomes should occur with referral for neurologic consultation as required. Social support, psychologic services, and chaplain services should be offered when available.

Professionalism

Altruism: Be Unselfish and Devoted to the Welfare of Others

Families may not be able to come in to the neonatal intensive care unit at the convenience of the physician. It is important to make oneself available after normal working hours to meet with parents. Even though it is acceptable to update parents by telephone, there is no substitute for a face-to-face meeting.

**Quality Improvement: Physician Compliance
With Clinical Practice Guidelines**

Physicians should not recommend or perform treatments and tests for which the value of expected benefit is less than expected cost. Following clinical practice guidelines (CPGs) and national practice standards is a critical factor in the quality- and value-based approach in health care.

One such guideline is the Practice Parameter: Neuroimaging of the Neonate: Report of the Quality Standards Subcommittee of the American Academy of Neurology and the Practice Committee of the Child Neurology Society from 2002.[1] It addresses the following questions regarding brain imaging of preterm infants:

- Which preterm infants should undergo routine screening ultrasonography (U/S)?
- When should these studies be performed?
- Do abnormalities on neonatal U/S require follow-up MRI?
- What is the ability of ultrasonography to accurately predict long-term neurodevelopmental outcome in this patient population?

Reference

1. Ment LR: Practice parameter: Neuroimaging of the neonate: Report of the Quality Standards Subcommittee of the American Academy of Neurology and the Practice Committee of the Child Neurology Society. *Neurology* 58(12):1726-1738, 2002.

Chapter 79
Cyanotic Newborn
(Case 38)

Ganga Krishnamurthy MD

Case: A newborn infant is noted to be cyanotic soon after birth.

Differential Diagnosis

Cyanotic congenital heart defect	Primary pulmonary disease
Neuromuscular condition associated with cyanosis	Persistent pulmonary hypertension of the newborn (PPHN)

Speaking Intelligently

The first step in evaluating a cyanotic infant is to distinguish between central cyanosis and peripheral cyanosis. Cyanosis is defined as a bluish discoloration of the skin and mucous membranes and is indicative of the presence of at least 3 to 5 g/dL of reduced hemoglobin in the circulation. A newborn infant often appears blue at birth. However, as the lungs assume the responsibility of becoming the organ of gas exchange following delivery, newborn infants who have undergone a normal transition will rapidly become pink. Although peripheral cyanosis occurs as a result of peripheral vasoconstriction and sluggish blood flow, central cyanosis is more ominous. If cyanosis is present without apparent respiratory distress, the likelihood of underlying cardiac disease is high on the differential and should lead to a prompt assessment of preductal and postductal saturation evaluations, four-extremity blood pressure measurement, chest radiograph study, electrocardiogram (ECG), arterial blood gas estimation, and echocardiography, all of which should guide the practitioner to an accurate diagnosis. Prostaglandin therapy may need to be started promptly if a ductal-dependent lesion is suspected.

PATIENT CARE

Clinical Thinking

- It is important to note if cyanosis resolves or improves with oxygen supplementation.
- Adequacy of airway, breathing, and circulation are primary considerations.
- If there is strong suspicion of a ductal-dependent congenital heart defect, rapid initiation of prostaglandins (prostaglandin E_1 [PGE_1]) is crucial to maintain ductal patency.
- Unstable infants or those on prostaglandin therapy may need to be placed on mechanical ventilation.
- The next step is to clinically determine the most likely anatomic etiology that is leading to cyanosis of the newborn.

History

- The mode of delivery, Apgar score, degree of resuscitation required after birth, and whether or not color improved with oxygen administration should be noted.
- Maternal history of fever, positive group B streptococcus (GBS) status, or prolonged rupture of membranes may suggest sepsis in the newborn.
- A history of meconium-stained amniotic fluid and a nonreassuring fetal tracing may be indicative of meconium aspiration syndrome.

Physical Examination

- Vital signs, including temperature, heart rate, respiratory rate, and four-extremity blood pressure recordings should be taken. Infants with serious underlying congenital heart defects often have a normal heart rate and blood pressure.
- Preductal (right arm) and postductal (leg) oxygen saturation indicate arterial supply before and after the ductus arteriosus, respectively. Hence, a pulse-oximetry probe placed on the right hand will indicate the saturation of blood flowing through the arterial distribution of the right subclavian artery, a preductal blood vessel. A differential greater than 15% between preductal and postductal saturation may indicate persistent pulmonary hypertension.
- Physical examination should distinguish central from peripheral cyanosis. Infants with a good cardiac output status will be warm and well perfused with good distal pulses and warm extremities. A polycythemic infant may appear "ruddy" and may have peripheral cyanosis because of sluggish peripheral blood flow.
- The presence of any phenotypic abnormalities suggestive of an underlying genetic disorder should be noted.
- Infants with an underlying pulmonary cause will have an increase in work of breathing.

- Precordial activity, heart sounds and the presence of a murmur should be noted. A normal precordial and auscultatory examination does not exclude serious underlying heart disease.

Tests for Consideration

- Hyperoxia test is used to distinguish central from peripheral cyanosis An arterial blood gas (ABG) is obtained before and after administration of 100% oxygen. PaO_2 values below 150 mm Hg despite administration of 100% oxygen are strongly suggestive of a cyanotic congenital heart defect.
- **Complete blood count (CBC)** $35
- **Blood culture** $100
- **Arterial blood gas (ABG)** $156
- **Arterial lactate** $25
- **ECG** $150

IMAGING CONSIDERATIONS

→ **Chest radiograph** $75
→ **Echocardiogram** $325

Clinical Entities   Medical Knowledge

Cyanotic Congenital Heart Defect

Pφ Cyanosis in the clinical setting of congenital heart disease is due to admixture of desaturated and saturated blood or, alternatively, decreased pulmonary blood flow. Examples of *cyanotic congenital heart defects* include truncus arteriosus, transposition of the great arteries, tetralogy of Fallot with pulmonary stenosis, critical pulmonary stenosis, pulmonary atresia with intact ventricular septum, tricuspid atresia, and total anomalous pulmonary venous connection.

TP Cyanosis associated with congenital heart disease is not usually accompanied by increase in the work of breathing, an important distinguishing characteristic from respiratory causes. For those lesions in which pulmonary blood flow is dependent on the patent ductus arteriosus, cyanosis may only become evident or worsen as the ductus arteriosus closes and pulmonary blood flow becomes compromised.

Dx	Accurate diagnosis may follow careful clinical examination, interpretation of the hyperoxia test, EKG, and chest radiograph and is generally confirmed by echocardiography. Infants with a cyanotic heart defect will have an abnormal hyperoxia test (i.e., the PaO_2 does not increase significantly after administration of 100% oxygen) because the hypoxia is due to right-to-left shunting and not to abnormal oxygenation in the lungs. The presence of cyanosis, an ejection systolic murmur in the pulmonary area, oligemic lung fields, and normal rightward axis on ECG leads to the likely diagnosis of critical pulmonary stenosis. The typical presentation of transposition of the great arteries is a cyanotic infant without a murmur, with a postductal saturation that is much higher than the preductal saturation, and a narrow superior mediastinal shadow on radiography.
Tx	Urgent consultation with a pediatric cardiologist is the first step. Most lesions, including transposition of the great arteries and total anomalous pulmonary venous return, will need surgical intervention in the newborn period. Transcatheter intervention is the first line of treatment in infants with critical pulmonary stenosis. Some lesions such as tetralogy of Fallot without significant obstruction to pulmonary blood flow may not need surgery in the newborn period but will require surgical intervention later on in infancy. **See Nelson Essentials 144.**

Primary Pulmonary Disease

Pφ	Newborn infants with *primary pulmonary disease* such as GBS pneumonia, meconium aspiration syndrome, respiratory distress syndrome, intrapleural collection of air or fluid, or airway anomalies may present with cyanosis. Cyanosis is due to defective oxygenation secondary to primary lung disease.
TP	Cyanosis secondary to a pulmonary etiology is usually accompanied by an increase in work of breathing. Auscultation may reveal abnormal air entry and adventitious sounds.
Dx	Diagnosis can be made by careful review of maternal and infant history, physical examination, and chest radiograph. CBC may reveal leukocytosis and bandemia in infants with pneumonia. ABG with significant hypoxia and hypercarbia suggests significant impairment of oxygenation and minute ventilation.

Tx   Defects in oxygenation or minute ventilation may be ameliorated or corrected by respiratory interventions, including oxygen, noninvasive ventilation (continuous positive airway pressure [CPAP]), or endotracheal intubation and mechanical ventilation. Antibiotic therapy is often needed. Surfactant replacement is required if the underlying defect is associated with surfactant deficiency. **See Nelson Essentials 136.**

Persistent Pulmonary Hypertension of the Newborn

Pφ   Pulmonary vascular resistance is high during fetal life and rapidly decreases after birth. Failure to follow this normal transition is called *persistent pulmonary hypertension of the newborn (PPHN).* It is anatomically described as persistence of fetal circulation due to failure of the closure of the foramen ovale and persistence of the patent ductus arteriosus.

TP   The manifesting features may be reflective of the underlying etiology of PPHN. These infants have differential cyanosis with postductal arterial saturations significantly lower than the preductal saturation.

Dx   Chest radiograph, history, and physical examination may help in differentiating the etiology of PPHN. Echocardiography provides evidence to support and quantify the degree of pulmonary hypertension.

Tx   Defects in oxygenation and minute ventilation may be corrected by respiratory interventions. These include placement on conventional or high-frequency oscillatory mechanical ventilation to provide oxygen as well as adjunctive therapy such as inhaled nitric oxide. Both oxygen and nitric oxide are pulmonary vasodilators. Antibiotic therapy is often needed. Placement on extracorporeal membrane oxygenation (ECMO) may be required if adequate oxygenation cannot be achieved with conventional therapy. **See Nelson Essentials 61.**

Neuromuscular Condition Associated With Cyanosis

Pφ   Infants who fail to achieve adequate ventilation will present with cyanosis. Infants with neuromuscular abnormalities such as spinal muscular atrophy type I or nemaline myopathy may present in the newborn period. The cyanosis is secondary to **inadequate respiratory effort** as a result of profound hypotonia.

TP	Severe neurologic or neuromuscular lesions may manifest in the newborn period with hypotonia. There may be an antecedent maternal history of poor fetal movements, persistent breech presentation, or polyhydramnios.
Dx	Additional testing is required to elucidate the etiology. Tests include serum creatine phosphokinase (CPK), serum and cerebrospinal fluid lactate and pyruvate, electromyography, nerve conduction velocity tests, and muscle biopsy. Genetic tests for triplet repeat sequence, fragile X, and other inherited abnormalities may be indicated. Neurologic examination of the mother may assist in the diagnosis of muscular dystrophy.
Tx	Attention must first be placed on securing the airway if needed and monitoring the adequacy of breathing. Endotracheal intubation and placement on mechanical ventilation may be needed. Further treatment is based on the underlying diagnosis and in many cases may be only supportive. **See Nelson Essentials 182.**

ZEBRA ZONE

Methemoglobinemia: Methemoglobinemia is an unusual condition in which the ferrous iron in the hemoglobin is reduced to the ferric state, producing methemoglobin. This compound is not capable of transporting oxygen, resulting in hypoxia. Infants may present with cyanosis and with few respiratory symptoms. Treatment with methylene blue is indicated in certain cases.

Practice-Based Learning and Improvement: Evidence-Based Medicine

Title
The surgical treatment of malformations of the heart in which there is pulmonary stenosis or pulmonary atresia

Authors
Blalock A, Taussig HB

Reference
JAMA 128(3):189-202, 1945

Problem
Before this point there was no reasonable treatment for pulmonary stenosis or atresia.

Intervention
Case series of three patients with systemic to pulmonary artery shunts for the treatment of cyanotic heart disease resulting in pulmonary artery obstruction with patent ductus arteriosus

Comparison/control
No surgical intervention

Outcome/effect
Demonstration of significant reduction of cyanosis

Historical significance/comments
Before this important work by Blalock and Taussig in 1945, pulmonary stenosis and pulmonary atresia were not considered surgically repairable. This study demonstrated the safe use of either the subclavian or innominate artery in reducing cyanosis without significant complications when anastomosed to the pulmonary artery. This led to significant advancement in the surgical treatment of cyanotic heart disease. It also described the safe use of anesthesia in these fragile infants.

Interpersonal and Communication Skills

Gather Information: Structure, Clarify, and Summarize Information

A cyanotic newborn requires urgent attention and intervention. Parents are often not prepared for the unexpected activity surrounding the need for prompt evaluation and diagnosis. A calm explanation of the need for further attention must be relayed with an assurance of full disclosure of information as it becomes available. The information that must be transmitted is often highly complex and emotionally charged, so structuring and summarizing the information, as well as clarifying and checking for understanding of that information, will improve the quality of communication.

Professionalism

Self-Awareness/Knowledge of Limits: Ask for Consultation or Assistance When Needed

The diagnosis of cyanotic congenital heart disease is one of the most complex in medicine. As in all cases when the medical needs of the patient are urgent, the amount of time to perform a clinical evaluation and synthesize information is limited. The physician "on the spot" needs immediate additional expertise from consultants and may need to call, often at off hours, physicians whose clinical care ultimately will not be needed. This can be met with resentment or even anger. Fear of this response should not limit consultation, because your primary responsibility is to provide the best care to your patient.

Systems-Based Practice

Health-Care Economics: Assessing Cost of Complex Health Care

Congenital heart disease surgeries are associated with high-cost admissions because of prolonged length of stay and extensive resource utilization. In a review of "Predictors of high cost admissions for congenital heart surgery"[1] the authors report that patients with greater disease complexity, younger age, prematurity, other anomalies, or Medicaid, and those admitted during a weekend are the cases most likely to result in high cost. Institutions of various types did not differ in frequency of high-cost admissions, regardless of whether they were designated as a children's hospital or held teaching status. Also, an institution's bed size, teaching status, hospital ownership, and hospital volume of cardiac cases are not independently associated with greater numbers of high-cost admissions.

Using hospital billing data as a surrogate for cost is considered useful to health-care providers, institutions, payers, and policy makers when formulating interventions and policies to allocate resources for complex congenital heart surgery.

Reference

1. Connor J, Gauvreau K, Jenkins K: Predictors of high cost admissions for congenital heart surgery. *Abstr Academy Health Meet* 21:abstract no. 1120, 2004.

Chapter 80
Teaching Visual: Fetal Circulation

Matthew Zinn DO *and Robert Palermo* DO

Objectives

- Describe the normal fetal circulatory pattern and the transition to neonatal circulation.
- Discuss the physiology and potential complications of a patent ductus arteriosus (PDA).
- Diagram a ductus arteriosus and the reason for its repair for the parents of your patient.

MEDICAL KNOWLEDGE

A patent ductus arteriosus is a remnant from fetal circulation that provides a connection between the pulmonary circulation and the systemic circulation at the level of the thoracic aorta to bypass the lungs in utero. To understand the impact of a PDA on a newborn, one must first comprehend the transitional pathway from the fetal circulation to the circulation in the postnatal period.

In the fetus, gas and nutrient exchange is provided via the placenta. The oxygenated blood is carried to the fetus via the umbilical vein. Most of the blood flows through the ductus venosus to the inferior vena cava (IVC), and the remainder perfuses the liver. As the blood enters the right atrium, the higher-velocity flow from the IVC is pushed across the foramen ovale and is ejected by the left ventricle into the aorta to perfuse the body. The blood flow entering the right atrium via the superior vena cava enters the pulmonary artery via the right ventricle. The ductus arteriosus allows the pulmonary artery blood flow to join the systemic circulation at the aorta, thus bypassing the lungs with the majority of the right ventricular output. *The location of the ductus arteriosus distal to the left subclavian artery allows the head and coronary vessels to receive blood with a relatively higher oxygen saturation compared with the rest of the body.*

Figure 80-1 illustrates the fetal circulation. As you trace the path of blood, start with the umbilical vein which sends oxygenated blood from the placenta to the fetal heart.

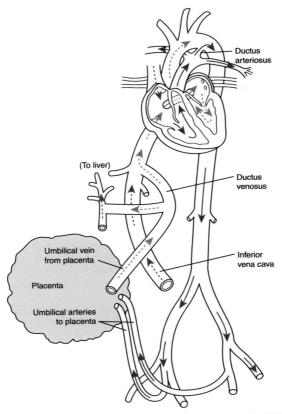

Figure 80-1 Fetal circulation. Connect the dots using red and blue pencils to trace the fetal circulation. (Note purple lines already drawn to denote the mixing of blood.)

Be sure to note the following progressions:

1. Umbilical vein → IVC → right atrium → thru the foramen ovale → left atrium → left ventricle → aorta → body
   MEANWHILE
2. Deoxygenated blood from SVC mixes with oxygenated blood from IVC → right ventricle → pulmonary artery → ductus arteriosus → aorta

Intrauterine lungs are filled with fluid and therefore have a higher pressure and vascular resistance than the systemic circulation. At birth, three things change that reverse this pressure differential: (1) the low-pressure placenta is removed from the circulatory system, thus increasing the systemic vascular resistance; (2) inhaled oxygen promotes pulmonary arterial vasodilation; and (3) alveolar fluid is eliminated. *These circulatory alterations increase the left atrial pressure compared with the right, leading to closure of the foramen ovale.* An increase in plasma oxygen tension and a decrease in prostaglandin E2 production cause the PDA to close.

The PDA functionally closes within 10 to 15 hours of life and then completely involutes after 2 to 3 weeks, becoming the ligamentum arteriosum. The ductus arteriosus fails to close in about 0.03% to 0.08% of infants. Failure to close is more prevalent in premature infants and those exposed to first-trimester perinatal rubella infection. If the ductus arteriosus remains patent, the flow reverses to a left-to-right shunt as the systemic vascular resistance increases during the neonatal transition. This shunt causes increased pulmonary blood flow and can eventually lead to left-sided volume overload of the heart and congestive heart failure if the shunt is severe. Signs of a PDA include (1) a continuous "machinery"-like murmur (heard best infraclavicularly on the left), (2) widened pulse pressure, (3) bounding peripheral pulses, and (4) a palpable thrill. Diagnosis is confirmed by an echocardiogram with Doppler color flow that demonstrates continuous turbulent flow between the aorta and the main pulmonary artery.

Congestive heart failure, pulmonary hypertension, and an increased risk for infective endocarditis are the main complications of a severe PDA. To prevent these complications, most cardiologists recommend closure of every PDA, unless it is found incidentally on an imaging study. Closure of a PDA in premature infants is initially attempted with medical management aimed at decreasing prostaglandin synthesis with indomethacin or ibuprofen. Nonsteroidal antiinflammatory drugs (NSAIDs) have been shown to be ineffective in term infants and older children; thus closure of the PDA requires occlusion via cardiac catheterization with an occluder device or coil. As a last resort, thoracotomy can be performed with surgical ligation or clip occlusion of the PDA.

Interpersonal and Communication Skills

A patent ductus arteriosus can be a difficult concept to explain to families. Consider Figure 80-2. To achieve success, we as physicians must completely understand the changing physiology and then convey this knowledge in a simple and concise manner.

1. I start the conversation by illustrating the normal fetal and neonatal anatomy outlined in the first section of this chapter. This provides the parents with a reference during the conversation. The extent to which I explain details depends upon the sophistication of the family.

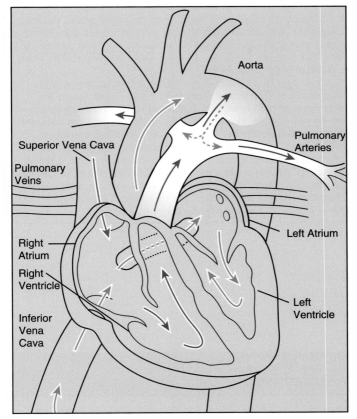

Figure 80-2 Fetal circulation. *Blue arrows,* Deoxygenated blood; *red arrows,* oxygenated blood; *purple arrows,* mixed blood.

2. The metaphor I find most beneficial when describing a PDA is that of a detour in a construction zone (see Figure 80-2). In normal neonatal physiology, blood leaves the right heart via the pulmonary artery and directly enters the aorta through the ductus arteriosus, effectively bypassing the lungs. I emphasize that the lungs are not used before birth. (If parents are left wondering how the blood receives oxygen when it never travels through the lungs, I explain that before birth oxygenated blood from the mother enters the baby through the placenta. Because there is no need for the baby to send already oxygenated blood to the lungs, nature has put a "detour" in place that bypasses the lungs, allowing maternally oxygenated blood to travel directly to the body.)

3. I explain that closure of the ductus arteriosus begins with the first breath. The sudden increase in blood oxygen results in constriction of the vessel, with functional closure occurring in the first 24 hours of life. However, as I point out, this process does not always proceed as planned. I explain that sometimes the ductus remains open, but now that the aortic pressures are higher than the pulmonary pressures, pulmonary overcirculation may result. I tell the parents that fortunately we can complete the process of closing the ductus by providing medicine that causes vasoconstriction or by surgically removing the "detour." (At this point, I draw a clip on the PDA of Figure 80-2 and the family is usually satisfied!)

Professor's Pearls
Section V: The Neonatal Intensive Care Unit
Linda M. Sacks MD

Consider the following clinical problems and questions posed. Then refer to a discussion of these issues by Linda M. Sacks MD, Mercer University School of Medicine, Macon, Georgia.

1. **Case:** A 1400-gram former 28-week preterm infant is now 31 weeks postconceptional age (PCA). She had mild respiratory distress syndrome (RDS) requiring <24 hours of ventilation and one dose of surfactant. She never received antibiotics and had no central lines of any kind. For the last 2 weeks she has been stable on a low-flow nasal cannula at Fio_2 24% in an isolette, tolerating

gavage feedings of fortified breast milk. On caffeine daily for apnea, she has two to four apneic episodes per day, all responsive to brief tactile stimulation. This morning the infant has a 10-mL bile-stained residual and moderate abdominal distention. Her apnea is now constant and requires vigorous stimulation. The last episode required positive pressure ventilation (PPV) with bag and mask. The nurse has increased her oxygen to 2 L/min at FiO$_2$ 40% to maintain saturation in the 88% to 90% range. On your examination, you find the infant's perfusion to be barely adequate, with capillary refill of 4 seconds. Her blood pressure (BP) is 45/25 mm Hg with a mean arterial pressure (MAP) of 32. What are the diagnostic possibilities, and how do you work them up and treat the infant?

2. **Case:** This infant was born by vaginal delivery after 10 hours of rupture of membranes (ROM) at 37 weeks to a 40-year-old mother with no prenatal care in a community hospital 60 miles from your center. The obstetrician noted polyhydramnios. The newborn "choked" on his first feeding and turned blue transiently. Helicopter transport to your neonatal intensive care unit (NICU) has been requested. What questions do you have for the referring physician? What stabilization should be done before the transport team arrives? What diagnosis do you suspect? How will you prove your diagnosis?

3. **Case:** A 3.5-kg white male infant was born by elective cesarean delivery at 38 weeks at maternal request. He develops grunting, retractions, and an oxygen requirement soon after birth. The infant is placed in a 30% oxyhood, but within 2 hours he requires 50% oxygen to maintain saturation above 92%. Chest radiographic study shows poor expansion and a ground glass appearance to the lungs. The infant is placed on nasal continuous positive airway pressure (CPAP) +6 cm, and an umbilical artery catheter (UAC) is placed. Blood gas determination shows pH of 7.26, PaCO$_2$ of 52 mm Hg and PaO$_2$ of 55 mm Hg. About 20 minutes after this gas level is obtained, the infant's oxygen requirement goes up to 90%, his heart rate (HR) rises to 180 beats per minute, and his blood pressure falls from a MAP of 50 to 30. He has an ashen appearance. What do you think has happened, and what should you do?

4. **Case:** An infant was born by spontaneous vaginal delivery (SVD) at 41⅔ weeks to a G2P1 32-year-old mother with negative laboratory test results, including group B streptococcus (GBS) (done at 36 weeks). Chromosomes and ultrasound at 22 weeks were normal. There was thick meconium in the amniotic fluid, but the infant was vigorous at birth, with Apgar scores of 7 and 9 at 1 and 5 minutes. Shortly after admission to the nursery she was noted to be cyanotic. Her respiratory rate is 70 breaths per minute, her HR is 145 beats per minute, and she is not distressed. Blood pressure

is normal and equal in all four extremities. She is transferred to the NICU. What are the diagnostic possibilities? What studies should you order?

5. **Case:** A term male infant is now 28 hours old. His mother is anxious to go home after her uncomplicated vaginal delivery. The infant has been breastfeeding well, has passed stool twice, and is voiding adequately. When you do his discharge examination, you note that he has just vomited a large amount of bile-stained colostrum. His abdomen is firm and possibly tender; it is hard to tell because he will not stop crying. Can this infant go home? What diagnostic possibilities must be ruled out?

Discussion by Linda M. Sacks MD, Mercer University School of Medicine, Macon, Georgia

1. **Discussion:** This infant's major symptoms are acute onset of increased apnea, feeding intolerance, abdominal distention, poor perfusion, and an increased oxygen requirement. Although each symptom alone may have a benign etiology, taken together they suggest serious bacterial infection or necrotizing enterocolitis (NEC). The first task is stabilization of the infant's physiology. This may require a high-flow nasal cannula, CPAP, or even intubation. A blood gas measurement will help determine which modality is most appropriate. The infant should also be made NPO so as not to stress her digestive tract, and a fluid bolus of saline should be given for her hypoperfused state. Initial blood work should include a complete blood count (CBC) (check for anemia and evidence of infection: left shift, neutropenia or elevated white blood cell count and thrombocytopenia). Obtain a blood culture and C-reactive protein (CRP) level. Order supine and decubitus films of the abdomen, looking for an ileus and/or signs of NEC (pneumatosis, portal air, thickened bowel wall, perforation with free air). If NEC is suspected or free air seen, surgical consultation should be obtained. Broad-spectrum antibiotic coverage for both gram-positive and gram-negative organisms should be started without waiting for test results. The coverage must be selected on the basis of sensitivities of the most common infections specific to your unit. A typical combination would include vancomycin, an aminoglycoside, and perhaps clindamycin. This infant's presentation is typical for both NEC and nosocomial infection. Suspected organisms might be *Staphylococcus aureus*, gram-negative rods, and late-onset GBS. Fungus is less likely in this situation of a larger infant with no antecedent antibiotics or central lines. A lumbar puncture (LP) should be performed when the infant's clinical condition permits. Although *Staphylococcus epidermolysis* sepsis is the most common nosocomial infection in many NICUs, it rarely presents in such a life-threatening manner.

2. **Discussion:** Clues to this infant's diagnosis are as follows: (1) Vaginal delivery with ROM for 10 hours and unknown GBS may suggest infection. (2) Advanced maternal age may suggest that the infant has trisomy 13, 18, or 21, in which case congenital anomalies may be expected. (3) Polyhydramnios implies that the infant did not swallow in utero (neurologic problem) or has a high gastrointestinal (GI) obstruction. (4) Choking suggests incoordination or esophageal obstruction with or without a tracheoesophageal fistula (TEF). Questions to ask the referring physician: (1) Are there any signs of chorioamnionitis in the mother? Did she receive antibiotics intrapartum? (2) Does the infant have any stigmata of trisomy 13, 18, or 21? (3) Has an orogastric (OG) tube been passed into the stomach to rule out esophageal atresia? Stabilization should include oxygen if needed and an OG tube. If the tube does not pass easily into the stomach, a film should be taken with the OG tube in place. With esophageal atresia the tube will coil in the blind proximal pouch, making the diagnosis. If there is air in the bowel in the presence of esophageal atresia, there is also a TEF. If there is no air, the baby has isolated esophageal atresia. Under no circumstances should a contrast study be done! Aspiration of contrast into the lungs is the usual result. The infant should be placed with his head elevated at least 15 degrees, and an IV started for fluid management. The OG tube can be placed to low intermittent suction as well. Although transfer to a surgical NICU is definitely indicated, ground transport is safer for both the baby and the transport team. There is nothing to be gained by a more expensive and dangerous helicopter ride in this situation of a stable infant.

3. **Discussion:** This infant has most likely developed a spontaneous tension pneumothorax. Before the days of surfactant, up to 40% of infants with RDS requiring CPAP or mechanical ventilation developed pneumothoraces. Increased HR, increased oxygen requirement, and hypotension all point to a tension pneumothorax rather than simple worsening of his RDS. One may hear decreased breath sounds on the side of the pneumothorax. Tracheal deviation and transillumination of the chest may be positive as well, although in large infants it is harder to demonstrate. A chest radiograph will show free air and deviation of mediastinal structures to the contralateral side of the pneumothorax. If the infant is stable, turn his oxygen up to 100% and wait for a chest radiograph before acting on the suspected pneumothorax. If he is unstable, or the chest radiograph will be delayed, attempt needle aspiration of the free air. Appropriate locations for needle placement are midclavicular line, second or third intercostal space, or fourth or fifth intercostal space along the anterior axillary line. The needle should be guided just over the rib to avoid the vessels

that run under the rib. Needle thoracentesis is followed by chest tube placement in most cases of tension pneumothorax. This infant should also receive surfactant. Babies born by elective cesarean delivery before 39 weeks are at risk for respiratory problems, including RDS, transient tachypnea of the newborn (TTNB), and pulmonary hypertension. Therefore the American College of Obstetricians and Gynecologists (ACOG) recommends that elective cesarean delivery not be performed before 39 weeks in the absence of proof of pulmonary maturity or a true maternal indication.

4. **Discussion:** Diagnostic possibilities for this infant include sepsis, meconium aspiration (MAS), pulmonary hypertension, and cyanotic congenital heart disease (CHD). The fact that the infant is not distressed points more toward CHD or pulmonary hypertension than to MAS or sepsis. A normal second-trimester ultrasound rules out hypoplastic left heart syndrome, but does not rule out several types of cyanotic congenital heart disease, such as transposition. Place the infant in 100% oxygen, and obtain a determination of blood gas levels. If her saturation remains <90%, she needs an echocardiogram to look for cyanotic CHD or pulmonary hypertension. Regardless of her response to 100% oxygen, she needs a septic workup and a chest radiograph. MAS will be visible on the chest radiograph, as will pneumonia. The heart may have an unusual configuration, and you will also be able to evaluate if pulmonary blood flow is increased or decreased. If cyanotic heart disease is suspected, transfer to a cardiac center is essential. In the interim, start the infant on antibiotics and a prostaglandin infusion. Watch for apnea, fever, and/or seizures with prostaglandin.

5. **Discussion:** Bile-stained emesis in the newborn infant should be considered pathologic until proven otherwise. This infant has passed stool, so a low obstruction is unlikely. Infants with Hirschsprung disease usually take longer than 28 hours to become obstructed to the point of bilious vomiting. Duodenal obstruction presents earlier than 28 hours. The abdomen in jejunal and ileal atresia is not tense or tender this early. The entities that are most worrisome are necrotizing enterocolitis and malrotation with volvulus. NEC would be unusual this early in an otherwise low-risk infant. Ruling out sepsis and malrotation would be high on my differential list. A kidney, ureter, and bladder (KUB) radiograph with volvulus would show an obstructive pattern, with the number of dilated loops dependent upon the site of the malrotation. Diagnosis can be made with an upper GI study looking for the position of the ligament of Treitz, or via a barium enema looking for malposition of the cecum.

Section VI
THE PEDIATRIC INTENSIVE CARE UNIT

Section Editor

Sharon Calaman MD

Section Contents

Chapter 81
Raised Intracranial Pressure (Case 39)

Glenn R. Stryjewski MD, MPH

Case: A 4-year-old child is brought to the emergency department with vomiting and severe headache. He has an elevated blood pressure and slow irregular heart rate. A CT scan of the head shows signs of raised intracranial pressure.

Differential Diagnosis

Hydrocephalus	Tumor/mass and edema
Infection	Intracranial hemorrhage

Speaking Intelligently

When I suspect a patient has raised intracranial pressure (ICP), I assess the patient's clinical status, simultaneously trying to determine the etiology. Knowing the underlying cause helps determine the likely time course of progression and facilitates decisions about possible therapies. Critical patients will require not only treatment of their intracranial pressure but also immediate support of their cardiorespiratory systems. After addressing the airway, breathing, and circulation (ABCs), I position the child with the head elevated to 45 degrees with the neck in midline and with neck stabilization if it appears to be a case of trauma. Next I administer osmotherapy with 3% saline, typically 3 mL/kg as an initial bolus. Mannitol is another option. At the same time I begin marshalling necessary resources such as the CT scan and the neurosurgeon, recognizing that both may require time to become available. If clinical progression of symptoms is rapid, I suspect some type of intracranial hemorrhage. Slower development usually implies hydrocephalus, tumor, or infection. Laboratory work is rarely a priority, but when an intracranial bleed is suspected, it is important to know the patient's hemoglobin, platelets, and PT/PTT values promptly. Serum electrolyte levels should also be obtained, because disorders of sodium can be both a cause and a consequence of raised ICP.

PATIENT CARE

Clinical Thinking
- Support the ABCs. ICP will worsen if the airway, breathing, and circulation are not supported.
- Is there an obvious problem you can do something about, such as a malfunctioning ventricular drain?

History
- Consider **underlying conditions** because these are often the contributing etiology, such as *hydrocephalus* or a *mass.*
- Fever in an otherwise healthy child with these symptoms may suggest an **infectious** cause such as *meningitis* or *encephalitis.*
- Recent trauma and rapid progression of symptoms is suggestive of *intraparenchymal, epidural, subdural, or subarachnoid* **hemorrhages.**
- Consider underlying conditions such as **hydrocephalus** or **mass** as possible etiologies.

Physical Examination
- Vital signs: Classic changes associated with a significant rise in ICP are hypertension, bradycardia, and an abnormal respiratory pattern. Early on, however, hypertension with tachycardia may be present. Realize that the normal range for heart rate, blood pressure, and respiratory rate varies with age.
- The first assessment should focus on airway, breathing, and circulation.
- Fontanelle size and character in infants can be helpful but are inconsistent findings.
- Papilledema is a more reliable finding to confirm your suspicions.
- **Focal findings** such as weakness or paralysis can help localize a lesion.
- Obtundation, posturing, or fixed and dilated pupil examination (unilateral or bilateral) implies impending herniation.

Tests for Consideration
- **Complete blood count (CBC):** May be useful if hemorrhage is suspected, especially in a young infant; platelet count may be helpful. $110
- **Electrolytes:** Screening for sodium disorders. $115
- **Arterial blood gas (ABG):** Checking that respiratory status is adequate. $45
- **PT:** Both PT and PTT are useful if hemorrhage is suspected because coagulopathy will need to be corrected. $75
- **PTT** $75

IMAGING CONSIDERATIONS

→ **Head CT:** Provides a rapid assessment for bleeding and hydrocephalus and may detect some masses if normal structures in the brain are displaced — $450

→ **Shunt series:** If a ventriculoperitoneal shunt is in place — $275

→ **Head ultrasound:** Would be appropriate in an infant 6 months or younger with an adequately open anterior fontanelle — $350

→ **Magnetic resonance imaging (MRI):** May be necessary to further delineate lesions; not generally necessary acutely — $1800

Clinical Entities	Medical Knowledge

Hydrocephalus

Pφ **Hydrocephalus** is the result of excessive cerebrospinal fluid (CSF) accumulation. This is usually due to inadequate reabsorption of CSF by the arachnoid villi. Obstruction of CSF flow through the ventricles and around the brain may also occur as a result of a new mass lesion or clotted blood. CSF is produced by the choroid plexus at an average of 400 to 500 mL/day, and the volume available within the brain is approximately 120 mL.

TP As CSF accumulates, the cerebral ventricles dilate. In infants this will be noticed as an enlarging head circumference and widening of the sutures. Eventually irritability, vomiting, and a restriction of upward gaze ("sunsetting") develop. In an older child the most common initial complaint is headache usually followed by vomiting. Lethargy and somnolence also develop. Papilledema is often present on examination.

Dx Diagnosis can be made with the clinical findings and history given above; however, confirmatory imaging is often performed.

Tx Treatment consists of elevation of the head and ensuring adequate ventilation, oxygenation, and perfusion. Acetazolamide can be used to reduce CSF production. A surgical shunt or drain may need to be placed. **See Nelson Essentials 184.**

Tumor/Mass and Edema

Pφ	An enlarging **mass** within the skull exerts direct pressure locally, and potentially throughout the brain. According to the Monro-Kellie doctrine,[1] the intracranial compartment contains three elements: blood, brain, and CSF. An increase in any one of these will cause a rise in pressure within the enclosed cranial vault.
TP	Constitutional findings such as headache and vomiting (especially in the early morning) are often present. Increased head circumference and widening of the sutures can be seen in the infant. Fundoscopic examination may reveal papilledema. There may be new-onset seizures. Other symptoms typically relate to local effects based on the location of the growing mass. A slowly growing mass may enlarge significantly without clinical signs or symptoms until late in the course.
Dx	Diagnosis can be made with the clinical findings and history given above; however, confirmatory imaging is often performed.
Tx	Treatment of the mass effect is similar to that of hydrocephalus discussed above. With edema surrounding the mass, there is a role for corticosteroid administration to reduce inflammation and edema. **See Nelson Essentials 184.**

Infection

Pφ	Bacteria, viruses, and fungi can all be responsible for **infections** of the central nervous system (CNS). Pathophysiology is either direct injury or inflammation of the supportive structures of the neurons, or the neurons themselves. We divide these infections into meningitis or encephalitis based on the area of the brain primarily infected. Raised intracranial pressure may develop related to inflammation from the infection itself and/or inflammation produced as a result of cell death.
TP	Patients will typically have fever. An altered level of consciousness, headaches, vomiting, bulging fontanelle, widened sutures, neck pain, and papilledema may all be present.

Dx	For meningitis, a lumbar puncture is usually diagnostic. In encephalitis, a lumbar puncture may or may not confirm the diagnosis. MRI may be helpful in better defining changes consistent with meningitis. In some cases only characteristic findings such as paroxysmal lateralizing electrical discharges (PLEDs) associated with herpes infections or a brain biopsy will yield the diagnosis.
Tx	Treatment is both correct antimicrobial therapy and supportive care to maintain oxygenation and perfusion of the brain. **See Nelson Essentials 100.**

Intracranial Hemorrhage

Pφ	An *intracranial hemorrhage* can occur in the epidural, subdural, or subarachnoid space, and/or in the parenchyma of the brain itself. Epidural bleeding occurs with injury to an arterial vessel above the dura. Subdural bleeding occurs with injury to the bridging veins between the dura and the surface of the brain. Subarachnoid and intraparenchymal bleeding can occur from a variety of sources. These events in children are often traumatic; however, they can also develop secondary to severe dehydration, anatomic abnormalities, and inherited metabolic disturbances.
TP	These events tend to be abrupt and dramatic in nature with the child having an altered level of consciousness and focal neurologic findings. It is of critical importance to determine if there has been a history of trauma.
Dx	With a good history, a specific diagnosis is almost always suspected. CT imaging of the head is the best modality to determine the presence of blood in the CNS.
Tx	With epidural and subdural bleeding a neurosurgical intervention to drain the clot is almost always necessary. Because these events develop quickly, the risk for impending herniation is very high. Immediate medical management includes the following: respiratory and hemodynamic support, head of bed (HOB) elevation with the neck midline, osmotherapy with 3% saline or mannitol, and adequate sedation and pain control. Hyperthermia should be avoided, and any seizure activity should be aggressively treated. If hypertension, bradycardia, and other signs of herniation are present, then hyperventilation is appropriate. **See Nelson Essentials 184.**

ZEBRA ZONE

a. **Pseudotumor cerebri:** Uncommon in children; presents with all the signs of increased ICP described (headache, papilledema) but without an apparent etiology

Practice-Based Learning and Improvement

Title
Critical Pathway for the Treatment of Established Intracranial Hypertension in Pediatric Traumatic Brain Injury

Author
Carney N, Chestnut R, Kochanek P

Reference
Pediatr Crit Care Med 4(suppl 3):S65-S67, 2003

Problem
How to provide consistent, evidence-based therapy to children with increased intracranial pressure resulting from traumatic brain injury.

Comparison/control (quality of evidence)
Evidence-based literature review with consensus guidelines established.

Outcome/effect
The development of treatment pathway utilizing an evidence-based medicine review as developed by experts in the field of pediatric traumatic brain injury.

Historical significance/ comments
This particular article developed the treatment algorithm by which raised intracranial pressure in children with traumatic brain injury is now managed. The entire supplement in this edition of Pediatric *Critical Care Medicine* is an outstanding resource not only for the clinical pathway as stated above, but for an evidence-based review of many aspects of raised ICP in traumatic brain injury.

Interpersonal and Communication Skills

Provide Information in an Efficient and Focused Manner

Raised ICP will often require rapid evaluation and intervention. However, this must be balanced with raising alarms unnecessarily. This balance can be difficult to achieve. However, due to the potential significance of increased intracranial pressure, it is appropriate to err on the side of caution. Early consultation with a neurosurgeon is appropriate. The quality of this interaction is enhanced when a thorough history and physical examination are performed in advance, so that an accurate and complete picture can be described for the physician who is not at the bedside.

Professionalism

Respect Others by Regarding Their Opinions Seriously

The clinical findings of raised ICP may be subtle; however, an astute clinician will often detect early changes—and early intervention will result in improved patient outcomes. Your examination findings may be benign despite the insistence of others (both clinicians and parents) that there is a problem. This will happen repeatedly in your career. Respect for other clinicians' findings and for the observations of parents is essential, even if they are not in agreement with your own.

Systems-Based Practice

CT Imaging of the Head: Practicing Cost-Effective Health Care Without Compromising Quality

Although one must learn to use expensive studies appropriately, we all recognize that the decision to obtain an imaging study of the head may have significant benefit. Here are my caveats for good systems-based practice in this regard:

1. Given a patient's history and physical examination, therapy may (and often *should*) be instituted without radiologic imaging.
2. In this day of digital imaging and transfer, be wary of repeating a CT scan unnecessarily simply because a patient is transferred from one institution to another.
3. Although serial imaging may have a role for monitoring some intracranial problems, be sure to conduct a thorough review of the literature in this matter in the context of your particular patient. This will assist you in deciding on the added value of such studies.

Reference

1. Wilkinson HA: Intracranial pressure. In Youmans JR, editor: *Neurological surgery*, Philadelphia, 1990, WB Saunders.

Chapter 82
Arrhythmia (Case 40)

Cara Garofalo MD

Case: An 8-year-old child presents with dizziness and an abnormal electrocardiogram

Differential Diagnosis

Sinus tachycardia and bradycardia	Supraventricular tachycardia (SVT)
Heart block	Ventricular tachycardia

Speaking Intelligently

When a child presents with an abnormal heart rhythm, I immediately assess the child's hemodynamic stability and identify the type of arrhythmia. In the unstable patient, with evidence of diminished cardiac output, assessment and support of airway, breathing, and circulation is performed rapidly. I place the child on a continuous cardiac monitor and obtain a 12-lead electrocardiogram (ECG). Identifying the type of arrhythmia begins with determining rate (fast or slow), regularity or irregularity, QRS morphology (narrow complex or wide complex), presence or absence of P waves, and relationship of P waves to QRS complexes. Whether or not the child is tolerating the arrhythmia hemodynamically determines my sequence of interventions, including attempts at pharmacologic or electric cardioversion. Algorithms for stable and unstable arrhythmias in the guidelines provided by the American Heart Association's PALS (Pediatric Advanced Life Support) should be followed. Initial laboratory work should include electrolytes (including calcium, magnesium, and potassium) and a complete blood count (CBC) to look for anemia in the patient with sinus tachycardia. I quickly consult a pediatric cardiologist.

PATIENT CARE

Clinical Thinking
- Support airway, breathing, and circulation.
- Identify the arrhythmia.
- Are there precipitating factors like abnormal electrolytes or medications?

History
- Is there a known history of **arrhythmia, cardiomyopathy,** or **congenital heart disease?**
- Onset and duration of arrhythmia should be elicited to determine potential for secondary sequelae (myocardial dysfunction, thromboembolism).
- A history of recent viral symptoms should raise concern for **myocarditis** as the cause of arrhythmia.
- A history of the patient's medications as well as **medications in the household** should be taken to elicit possible etiologies.

Physical Examination
- Initial assessment should focus on airway, breathing, circulation, and mental status.
- Heart rate, especially for narrow complex tachycardias, can provide a clue to the etiology of the arrhythmia. Reentrant SVTs are generally faster than sinus tachycardia or ectopic atrial tachycardias (EATs).
- Blood pressure, pulses, and overall perfusion should be monitored closely to assess adequacy of cardiac output. An irregularly irregular pulse is the hallmark of atrial fibrillation.
- Respiratory rate and effort may be increased if pulmonary edema develops as a result of poor cardiac output.
- Cardiac auscultation should focus on the regularity or irregularity of the rhythm and presence of adventitious sounds (murmur, gallop, rub).
- Hepatomegaly and peripheral edema are signs of congestive heart failure.
- Mental status is important as a marker for perfusion and cardiac output.

Tests for Consideration
- **Electrocardiogram (ECG)** — $150
- **Electrolytes (focusing on potassium, calcium, magnesium)** — $35
- **Arterial blood gas (ABG)** — $45
- **Thyroid function studies:** Hyperthyroidism associated with tachycardia — $45
- **CBC, erythrocyte sedimentation rate (ESR), and C-reactive protein (CRP):** In the child with possible myocarditis — $30

IMAGING CONSIDERATIONS

→ **Chest radiograph:** To identify cardiomegaly in the patient
  with possible myocarditis or cardiomyopathy $120
→ **Echocardiogram:** To identify any structural cause for
  arrhythmia and to assess ventricular function $275

Clinical Entities	Medical Knowledge

Sinus Tachycardia and Bradycardia

Pφ ***Sinus tachycardia*** and ***bradycardia*** originate from the sinoatrial
     node, and maintain normal conduction through the heart. Sinus
     bradycardia can be a manifestation of increased vagal tone,
     hypothermia, increased intracranial pressure, meningitis,
     hypothyroidism, anorexia, obstructive jaundice, and
     medications. Sinus tachycardia may occur in the setting of
     anemia, dehydration, pain, fever, infection, hypoxia,
     hypotension, anxiety, myocarditis or cardiomyopathy,
     hyperthyroidism, ingestion of certain medications, and
     pheochromocytoma.

TP   The child with sinus tachycardia or bradycardia often remains
     asymptomatic but may experience palpitations, light-
     headedness, and possibly syncope.

Dx   Diagnosis can be made on ECG by identification of P waves
     preceding each QRS complex and by orientation of the
     P-wave axis. In sinus rhythm P waves are upright in leads I,
     II, and aVF.

Tx   Treatment is directed by identifying and treating the cause.
     Medications (atropine, epinephrine) may be needed if
     bradycardia is severe enough. Very rarely, temporary or
     permanent cardiac pacing is required if medication fails to
     adequately improve perfusion. **See Nelson Essentials 142.**

Supraventricular Tachycardia

Pφ   **SVT** originating in the atria comprises a large family of arrhythmias. Reentrant tachycardias are perpetuated through accessory bypass tracts that circumvent the atrioventricular node. Ectopic atrial tachycardia (EAT) originates from an atrial focus away from the sinus node and is generally faster than sinus rhythm but slower than SVT. Atrial flutter and fibrillation are rare in children, except those with some forms of acquired heart disease or congenital heart disease. Junctional ectopic tachycardia (JET), a narrow complex tachycardia originating in the atrioventricular (AV) junction, occurs most commonly in postoperative cardiac surgery patients.

TP   Children with SVT often experience palpitations and may have chest pain and a fluttering feeling in the neck. Some children experience abdominal pain and nausea or vomiting. Dizziness may precede syncope or near-syncope. If the rate is fast enough, the child may have poor perfusion, delayed capillary refill, and hypotension.

Dx   Diagnosis can be made on 12-lead ECG. SVT rates in infants generally range from 220 to 320 beats per minute, and 150 to 250 beats per minute in older children. The ECG demonstrates narrow complex tachycardia. Ectopic atrial tachycardia is marked by P wave morphology, axis, and PR interval that differ from findings on normal sinus ECG. Atrial flutter can be identified by a "sawtooth" pattern of the P waves. In atrial fibrillation, flutter waves may be seen intermittently; however, atrial rate is very irregular.

Tx   Treatment is determined by the specific arrhythmia and the patient's stability or instability. In the stable patient with reentrant tachycardia, one can try vagal maneuvers, such as ice to the face or blowing through an occluded straw. Adenosine can be given if the SVT persists. Synchronized cardioversion should be performed in the hemodynamically unstable patient. The hemodynamically stable patient with atrial flutter or fibrillation should receive anticoagulation and rate control before cardioversion. Medications most commonly given for rate control include calcium channel blockers, beta-blockers, and digoxin (alone or in combination). Treatment of ectopic atrial tachycardia generally begins with beta-blockade. **See Nelson Essentials 142.**

Ventricular Tachycardia

Pφ **Ventricular tachycardia** can be idiopathic in children but also occurs in children with (1) congenital heart disease, (2) cardiomyopathy or myocarditis, (3) tumors or cardiac infiltrates, (4) primary arrhythmias (long QT syndrome, familial ventricular tachycardia), (5) electrolyte abnormalities, (6) medications and toxins (general anesthetics, catecholamines, tricyclic antidepressants, cocaine, and digoxin toxicity), and (7) blunt chest trauma.

TP Palpitations, dyspnea, chest or abdominal pain, dizziness, and syncope or near-syncope are most common in children with rates greater than 150 beats per minute. Sustained arrhythmia can produce signs of congestive heart failure.

Dx ECG features of ventricular tachycardia include wide QRS complexes with either left or right bundle branch block pattern and AV dissociation. Rates of ventricular tachycardia range from 120 to 300 beats per minute in children.

Tx Treatment is determined by the patient's hemodynamic status. In the stable patient with an identifiable cause that can be corrected, the underlying abnormality should be corrected. If the rhythm persists, patients should be given lidocaine or amiodarone. Patients with cardiac compromise require immediate synchronized cardioversion. Treatment of pulseless ventricular tachycardia follows the same PALS algorithm as ventricular fibrillation. **See Nelson Essentials 142.**

Heart Block

Pφ **Heart block** occurs when conduction of the cardiac impulse from the sinus node to the atrioventricular node, or from the atrioventricular node to the ventricles, is impaired. First-degree AV block, occurs with digoxin toxicity; with inflammatory conditions such as rheumatic heart disease, myocarditis, or Kawasaki disease; with some cardiac malformations; or after cardiac surgery. Second-degree AV block can occur in situations similar to first-degree AV block. Third-degree (complete) heart block is either congenital or acquired. The acquired form results from conditions similar to those causing first-degree AV block and infectious etiologies (Lyme). Maternal connective tissue disease is associated with congenital complete heart block. This can also occur in the setting of L- transposition of the great arteries and heterotaxy syndrome.

TP	First- and second-degree AV block are usually asymptomatic. Complete heart block often has hypotension and poor perfusion. Older children can experience exercise intolerance, easy fatigability, syncope, or near-syncope.
Dx	Diagnosis of heart block is made by 12-lead ECG. First-degree AV block is identified by prolonged PR interval. Second-degree type I (Wenckebach or Mobitz I) demonstrates progressive prolongation of the PR interval with eventual dropping of a QRS complex. In second-degree type II (Mobitz II), QRS complexes are dropped suddenly, without progressive prolongation of the PR interval. Complete heart block is marked by complete disassociation of P waves and QRS complexes, with the atrial rate faster than the ventricular rate.
Tx	Treatment of heart block is similar to that for symptomatic bradycardia (see above). **See Nelson Essentials 142.**

ZEBRA ZONE

a. **Wolf-Parkinson-White syndrome:** An abnormal conduction pathway in the myocardium that predisposes to SVT

Practice-Based Learning and Improvement: Evidence-Based Medicine

Title
Pediatric dysrhythmias

Authors
Doniger SJ, Sharieff GQ

Reference
Pediatr Clin North Am 53:85-105, 2006

Problem
Diagnosis and management of rhythm disturbances in children

Comparison/control (quality of evidence)
Review article in peer-reviewed journal

Historical significance/comments
Excellent review of rhythm disturbances and their management

Interpersonal and Communication Skills

Structure, Clarify, and Summarize Information

In order to gain effective assistance from an outside consultant, the physician should be able to describe the rhythm disturbance systematically, addressing **rate, morphology (narrow or wide), regularity, presence or absence of P waves, and association of P waves to QRS complexes, as well as the clinical appearance of the patient.** An awareness of the patient's medical problems and medications is also essential. Summarizing this information in a concise manner for the cardiologist will facilitate the consultant's ability to make recommendations.

Professionalism

Commit to Lifelong Learning and Education: Involve Yourself in Appropriate CME Activities

Although the rhythm disturbances themselves have not changed over time, the best medications and algorithms for the treatment and management have changed. If you routinely come in contact with children with potential rhythm disturbances, it is important to attend regular continuing medical education (CME) activities that address these conditions. Pediatric Advanced Life Support (PALS) is an excellent CME activity to help the practitioner remain up to date on appropriate therapy.

Systems-Based Practice

Primary Care Emergency Preparedness

Arrhythmia management is a medical emergency that is likely to happen quite rarely in pediatrics. However, these emergent situations may present to a primary care office instead of a more acute setting. Primary care settings need to balance the likelihood of such events with the level of training of staff as well as the cost of equipment available. To assist with these decisions the American Academy of Pediatrics[1] developed a policy statement identifying the best approaches for pediatric primary care providers to provide emergency care for pediatric patients:

Considerations for optimizing office preparedness of pediatric primary care providers for emergencies include the unique aspects of each office practice, the types of patients and emergencies likely to be encountered, on-site resources, and those of the larger emergency care system encompassing the pediatric primary care provider's office.

Reference

1. Committee on Pediatric Emergency Medicine: Preparation for emergencies in the offices of pediatricians and pediatric primary care providers. *Pediatrics* 120:200-212, 2007.

Chapter 83
Acute Respiratory Failure (Case 41)

Christine M. Schlichting MD

Case: A 2-year-old with tachypnea and increased work of breathing

Differential Diagnosis

Pneumonia	Bronchiolitis
Croup	Status asthmaticus
Pediatric acute respiratory distress syndrome (ARDS)	

Speaking Intelligently

When presented with an infant or child in respiratory distress, I think of the respiratory system and its components, why each component may fail, and how this presents clinically: central control of breathing, blockage in the upper airway, lower airways dysfunction, alveolar disease, and neuromuscular failure or "bellows dysfunction." It is important to note that respiratory failure may also occur in a patient who presents with multiple organ failure, such as septic shock, and this respiratory failure may involve many levels of the respiratory system all at once. Thinking through the cause of the distress helps me with my next interventions, which may involve taking control of the child's work of breathing with an artificial airway or supporting the child with oxygen and medications.

The end result of respiratory failure is ventilatory failure (hypercarbia or elevation of Pco_2) and/or hypoxemia (decrease in Po_2), both of which can be life threatening.

PATIENT CARE

Clinical Thinking
- It is helpful to take a stepwise approach to support of a patient in respiratory distress:

- **Oxygen** should be administered while an evaluation is in progress. Oxygenation improves with the delivery of supplemental oxygen or with the delivery of positive pressure, which recruits closed/ collapsed airways and alveoli and in so doing decreases $\dot{V}/\dot{Q}$ **mismatch.** Oxygen can be delivered by nasal cannula (delivers up to 32%), simple face mask (maximum delivery 35%), and a nonrebreather mask (maximum 60%). Because of poor mask fit and room air entrainment oxygen delivery by these simple devices may not approach these levels. Improvement of ventilation can be accomplished by improving the $\dot{V}/\dot{Q}$ match so positive pressure systems such as continuous positive airway pressure (CPAP) or bilevel positive airway pressure (BiPAP) are beneficial. Finally, patients may need the support that can only be delivered via tracheal intubation and use of mechanical ventilation.
- Although it is tempting to treat the symptomatic patient reactively, **it is essential, whenever possible, to gather full information, including history and appropriate tests, before interventions.**
- Support of a patient in severe respiratory failure will necessitate tracheal intubation and ventilator support. The guiding principle is support with the least morbidity. **Ventilators damage lungs** and should be used with settings that are as low as can deliver the desired level of support. Mean airway pressures below 20 cm H_2O reduce pressure injury to the alveoli (barotrauma). Permissive hypercapnia (allowing increased carbon dioxide) and subsequent respiratory acidosis is safer (if pH >7.25) than using higher airway pressures. Positive end-expiratory pressure (PEEP) should be set at a level that maintains open airways and effectively recruits collapsed lung units without decreasing cardiac output. Oxygen exposure should also be minimized: in general, inspired oxygen less than 60% is considered "safe."

History
- What are the presenting symptoms?
  - **Cough** indicates irritation in the airways with or without increased mucous (sputum) production. Where the secretions seem to originate is also helpful: copious nasal secretions in young children almost always indicate a viral illness, and a primary bacterial pneumonia usually has a cough producing sputum. The quality of the cough may also suggest a diagnosis
  - **Fever** is usually a sign of infection.
  - **Anxiety** or "air hunger" is not uncommon in patients with hypoxemia.
  - **Agitation** occurs in both hypoxemia and in patients with hypercarbia before the onset of lethargy and coma.
  - **Lethargy** demands careful evaluation because it can occur in many clinical scenarios of respiratory failure possibly suggesting hypercarbia.

- What is the time course of the illness? Was it sudden in onset, or had it been going on for some time and gradually worsened?
- Did the caretakers notice rapid breathing, retractions, or increased work of breathing?
- Does the patient have pertinent past medical history?

Physical Examination
- Evaluation of signs:
  - **Tachycardia** is not a specific sign; but it may indicate hypercarbia.
  - **Increased respiratory rate** may indicate the degree of respiratory failure, although it may be a sign of increased respiratory demand (e.g., the patient who is acidotic or with fever).
  - **Decreased respiratory rate** may indicate failure of central control that occurs in central nervous system diseases, metabolic diseases, and drug effects, but also occurs in severe status asthmaticus and hypothermia.
  - **Prolonged exhalation** usually indicates lower airways obstruction such as asthma but can be present in congestive heart failure (CHF) as well.
  - **Use of accessory muscles**, nasal flaring, and retractions (suprasternal, intercostal, subcostal, and sternal) is an indication of increased respiratory effort.
- **Breath sounds:**
  - **Rales** or **crackles** are indicative of air fluid interface in the alveoli.
  - **Rhonchi** are typical of mucus or other substance in the large airways.
  - **Wheezing** occurs in conditions that partially obstruct the small airways.
  - **Vocal resonance** occurs when auscultated spoken words sound similarly over both the lung and trachea. In the setting of diminished breath sounds it indicates the lung under the stethoscope is consolidated.
  - **Diminished breath sounds** also occur with pleural effusions, but vocal resonance is absent except at the top of the effusion, where the vocal resonance is distorted.
  - **Postural preference:** If the parents confirm that the patient has insisted on maintaining an upright position, the patient may have either intrathoracic airway obstruction or cardiac/vascular compression that is minimized in the upright position. Forcing the patient to lay supine may lead to cardiorespiratory arrest.

Tests for Consideration
- **Arterial blood gas (ABG):** Should be done in the patient whom you suspect will need intervention guided by the results. $45
- **Complete blood count (CBC) with differential:** The white blood cell (WBC) count and differential are useful in determining an infectious etiology. $110

- **Electrolytes:** Should be done in any patient with respiratory failure because there may be excess antidiuretic hormone circulating. $115
- **Sputum Gram stain and culture and nasal wash for viral studies** $130

IMAGING CONSIDERATIONS

→ **Chest radiograph:** Identifies infiltrates, atelectasis, pneumothorax, pneumomediastinum, pulmonary edema, pleural effusion, and other conditions $120
→ **Chest computed tomography (CT):** Identifies intraparenchymal lesions and delineates effusions $800

Clinical Entities	Medical Knowledge

Pneumonia

Pφ	***Pneumonia*** is an infection involving any or all parts of the lung. It can be caused by many infectious agents, including bacteria, viruses, and fungi.
TP	Presentation varies depending upon the patient's age and the etiology of the pneumonia. A typical bacterial pneumonia presents with acute onset of fever, malaise, and cough with variable respiratory distress and degrees of hypoxemia.
Dx	The chest radiograph is the key to making the diagnosis. There can be lobar, multilobar, or diffuse infiltrates. Specific diagnosis of an etiologic organism involves testing scrapings of the nasal mucosa for viruses, culturing those scrapings for virus, and staining and culturing sputum from the tracheobronchial tree (Figure 84-1).
Tx	Treatment involves directing specific antimicrobial agents toward the infectious etiology and supportive care as outlined above. **See Nelson Essentials 110.**

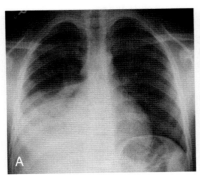 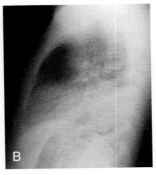

Figure 83-1   Radiographs of chest showing pneumonia.

Bronchiolitis	
Pφ	**Bronchiolitis** is a viral infection of the respiratory tract. It starts in the upper airway but progresses to the lower airways typically over a 3 to 5-day period. It is caused by a number of common viruses and occurs sporadically and in epidemics, especially during the winter months.
TP	It is typically a problem for young infants and for children with serious chronic diseases. Mucous production and inflammation leads to obstruction in the lower airways with wheezing. In small children who are obligate nose breathers, the initial coryza may also lead to significant nasal obstruction and respiratory distress. In neonates, the first symptom may be apnea, which then progresses to the more typical upper respiratory symptoms.
Dx	Diagnosis is by clinical presentation. Diagnosis of etiology is done by "nasal wash" with determination of viral antigen or fluorescent staining of nasal secretions or viral culture.
Tx	Treatment of bronchiolitis is largely supportive. Nasal suctioning and chest physiotherapy if tolerated are commonly ordered. Racemic epinephrine and albuterol aerosolized treatments may also be effective. Corticosteroids have not been shown to have beneficial effects in bronchiolitis and should only be considered in patients with known reactive airway disease. **See Nelson Essentials 109.**

Croup

Pφ	Laryngotracheitis, or *croup,* is an inflammatory process targeting the larynx and trachea, usually caused by infection. This impinges upon the radius of the airway, resulting in partial obstruction.
Tp	Viral croup most commonly occurs in children younger than 4 years of age. There is usually a short history of an upper respiratory infection. Fever, when it occurs, tends to be <38.3° C (101° F). The hallmarks are inspiratory stridor and a barky cough, described as "seal-like."
Dx	Diagnosis is made by clinical presentation.
Tx	Treatment for croup is supportive and primarily aimed at decreasing the inflammation. Cool mist is sometimes helpful. Aerosolized racemic epinephrine treatments and intravenous or intramuscular dexamethasone reduce airway edema. Patients who continue to exhibit unacceptable symptoms of upper airway obstruction may benefit from heliox (helium/oxygen gas mixture). **See Nelson Essentials 107.**

Pediatric Acute Respiratory Distress Syndrome

Pφ	*ARDS* presents at the end of a spectrum of lung pathology that starts with acute lung injury (ALI). This spectrum of pulmonary disease is caused by an acute inflammatory response leading to denaturation of surfactant and fluid extravasation into the alveolus. Later a reparative phase consists of fibroproliferation and organization of lung tissue. Finally, collagen is formed, leading to scarring and fibrosis.
Tp	The presentation of the patient with ARDS may be variable, depending upon the underlying etiology or trigger.
Dx	ALI is defined as a syndrome of acute and persistent lung inflammation with increased vascular permeability. ALI is characterized by three clinical features: (1) bilateral radiographic infiltrates, (2) a ratio of the partial pressure of arterial oxygen to the fraction of inspired oxygen (PaO_2/FiO_2) between 201 and 300 mm Hg, (3) no clinical evidence for an elevated left atrial pressure.
	The criteria for ARDS are the same as acute lung injury except that the hypoxemia is worse, requiring a PaO_2/FiO_2 ratio of ≤200 mm Hg.

Tx   Therapy is focused on identifying and treating the inciting cause if known and treatable. Supportive care is delivered as indicated clinically. **See Nelson Essentials 39.**

Status Asthmaticus

See Chapter 87, Status Asthmaticus.

ZEBRA ZONE

a. **Foreign body aspiration** can present much like croup or asthma. Prevalence is higher in toddlers.

b. **Severe metabolic acidosis** may present with respiratory distress. Diabetic ketoacidosis is a common diagnosis that may present this way.

c. **Pulmonary diagnoses** that present with respiratory distress and are uncommon include:
- Pulmonary hemosiderosis
- Pulmonary interstitial pneumonitis
- Acute chest syndrome, common in sickle cell disease
- **Mediastinal masses** can present with severe respiratory distress, and this underscores the need for careful evaluation of patients before interventions.

Practice-Based Learning and Improvement: Evidence-Based Medicine

Title
Ventilation with lower tidal volumes compared with traditional volumes for acute lung injury and the acute respiratory distress syndrome

Authors
The Acute Respiratory Distress Syndrome Network

Reference
N Engl J Med 342(18):1301-1308, 2000

Problem
Traditional lung volumes used in mechanical ventilation are associated with barotrauma.

Comparison/control (quality of evidence)
Well-powered and well-controlled multicenter study

Outcome/effect
Demonstrates improved survival with small tidal volumes used in management of ARDS

Historical significance/comments
This is a landmark adult study that was well powered and demonstrated a clear 9% improvement in mortality in patients managed with "low" 6 to 8 mL/kg tidal volumes versus 10 to 15 mL/kg.

Interpersonal and Communication Skills

Use Language the Patient and Family Can Understand

Communicating "bad" information to parents, and in some cases patients, is difficult. Use common language when speaking about the situation. For example, talk about the need for a **"breathing tube"** not an endotracheal (ET) tube. Describe the tube placement as being **"through the voice box into the wind pipe,"** not "through the larynx into the trachea." Watch the face and body language of family members closely while speaking to them. This helps give you feedback on many issues, including when to stop talking, whether there is an understanding of what you are trying to communicate, or when you may need to repeat something you have said.

Professionalism

Accountability to Patients and Their Families

Children with respiratory failure will frequently be admitted to a tertiary care hospital that is also a "teaching" hospital. Should only the most experienced staff (physicians, nurses, respiratory therapists) do procedures and care for these patients? If so, how will future generations learn these skills?

Reconciliation of this dilemma can take different tacks:
1. Use simulation and simulation laboratories to teach a procedure first before the trainee attempts the procedure on a real patient.
2. The supervising physician is present "at the elbow" of the trainee during the procedure.
3. The supervising physician may "take over" the procedure from the trainee when appropriate
4. The patient and family are never misled about who will do a procedure or care for their child.

Systems-Based Practice

Quality Improvement: The Joint Commission and VAPs

Ventilator-associated pneumonia (VAP) is a major cause of morbidity, mortality, and increased hospital stay (increased health-care cost). Recognized as a national problem, hospital accreditation from The Joint Commission (formerly known as JCAHO) now requires that programs implementing evidenced-based practice be established for use in intubated patients to decrease the risk for VAP. Such practices include using suction systems dedicated to the artificial airway, frequent mouth care, sterile suctioning techniques, and routine elevation of the head of the bed.

Chapter 84
Shock (Case 42)

Arun Chopra MD

Case: A previously healthy 4-year-old child presents to the emergency department with fever and listlessness. The patient has a heart rate of 190 beats per minute and is hypotensive with a blood pressure of 75/25 mm Hg. The respiratory rate is 35 breaths per minute with mildly increased work of breathing; the oxygen saturation is 100%. The parents say that their child has not eaten well in the last 24 hours and has had no urine output in the last 12 hours. The patient has been vomiting and has had some diarrhea for the last 24 hours.

Differential Diagnosis

Distributive shock—septic	Distributive shock—anaphylactic	Neurogenic shock
Hemorrhagic shock	Cardiogenic shock	
Obstructive shock	Hypovolemic shock	

Speaking Intelligently

When I admit a patient with shock, the first thing I do is assess the airway, breathing, and circulation (ABCs). It is crucial to ensure adequate oxygen delivery to the tissues because shock, regardless of etiology, is a state of *oxygen delivery inadequate to meet the demands of the tissues.* Oxygen delivery is a product of cardiac output and oxygen content of the blood. Therefore, the oxygen delivery to the body can be determined by the following equation:

$$CO \times Oxygen\ content\ of\ blood$$

$$[HR \times SV] \times [(1.36 \times Hgb \times Sa_{O_2}) + (0.003 \times Pa_{O_2})]$$

where
HR = Heart rate
SV = Stroke volume
Hgb = Hemoglobin in g/dL
Sa_{O_2} = Oxygen saturation
Pa_{O_2} = Partial pressure of arterial O_2

Bearing this in mind, one needs to provide oxygen to a patient in shock and have a low threshold for intubating the patient and taking over the patient's work of breathing. As I assess the child, I keep in mind that although many perceive hypotension as the hallmark of shock, in pediatrics this can be a late sign because *the ability of young patients to compensate with tachycardia to maintain cardiac output* can be significant. Therefore a significant tachycardia even with a normal blood pressure is very concerning. Volume resuscitation with fluid boluses of 20 mL/kg given quickly is the next priority. Basic lab work, most importantly a determination of blood gas levels, can help determine the severity of the situation by revealing the acid-base status. Some institutions can quickly obtain a "critical care" panel or i-STAT that will also provide electrolyte and lactate levels. History and a careful physical are important to determine the specific etiology of the shock state and to allow for tailoring of therapy.

PATIENT CARE

Clinical Thinking
- Always support the *ABCs.*
- *Volume resuscitation* is an essential part of the management of the majority of cases. While using volume resuscitation one needs to assess the response to volume and watch for signs of pulmonary edema.
- While resuscitating, look for *underlying illnesses* that may cause or contribute to the illness or modify how the patient responds.

- An early determination of whether the underlying cause is heart failure is mandatory because the early management is very different.
- Is there any chronic underlying illness?

History

- A history of fluid intake and output is vital to assessing both current fluid status and the possibility of dehydration as the cause of shock.
- *Infection* should be aggressively ruled out because sepsis is often a cause of shock in the pediatric population.
- A detailed recent past medical history should be obtained to evaluate for any *immunosuppression,* recent corticosteroid use, or malignancy because these can affect initial management and increase the risk for septic shock.
- Any history of *heart murmur* or cardiac anomaly should raise suspicion of cardiogenic shock.
- A history of recent *trauma* may suggest hemorrhage or spinal cord injury as the source of shock.

Physical Examination

- Vital signs: Tachycardia is usually the first sign of shock, followed by tachypnea and hypotension. Remember that neurogenic shock and late septic shock may present with bradycardia.
- *Extremity perfusion* should be noted, specifically capillary refill >2 seconds is concerning. Take note of whether the extremities are cooler than normal or warmer than normal (an indication of peripheral perfusion and systemic vascular resistance).
- Note should be taken of skin turgor, production of *tears while crying,* mucous membranes, and if applicable whether or not the fontanelle is sunken as markers of fluid status.
- If there is concern for spinal injury, lack of movement of extremities and rectal tone should be noted.
- *Rashes* can help identify underlying causes of infection or give a clue to coagulation defects that can be associated with severe shock.
- Open wounds or ongoing *blood loss* or other signs of trauma may suggest hemorrhagic or neurogenic shock.
- Increase in liver size, *cardiac gallop,* or displaced point of maximal impulse can suggest cardiogenic shock.
- Note should be made of an enlarged spleen because this could indicate sequestration or splenic injury leading to hemorrhagic shock.

Tests for Consideration

- **Complete blood count (CBC) with differential** $110
- **Electrolytes, blood urea nitrogen (BUN), and creatinine level** $115
- **Arterial blood gas (ABG) levels** $45
- **Electrocardiogram (ECG)** if suspected cardiogenic shock $217
- **Prothrombin time (PT) and partial thromboplastin time (PTT)** $75

- **Cortisol level** $25
- **Lactate level** $25

IMAGING CONSIDERATIONS

→ **Chest and abdominal anteroposterior (AP) films** $120
→ If suspected spinal cord injury
  - **Cervical spine (C-spine) and thoracic spine (T-spine) series:** $120 each
  - **Spinal magnetic resonance imaging (MRI):** $1100
→ **Echocardiography:** If suspected cardiogenic shock $1630

Clinical Entities	Medical Knowledge

Distributive Shock States: Septic Shock

Pφ	**Distributive shock** is the disruption of cardiac output by *distributing* the circulatory volume into a larger space by either vasodilation or vascular leak (septic shock is a specific type of distributive shock). **Septic shock** occurs when a high burden of infective particles—usually bacteria, but viral and fungal sepsis can occur—causes a cascade of inflammation that leads to vascular dysfunction, dilation, and increased vascular leak. Many infective particles also have a myocardial depressant effect. Furthermore, in profound sepsis there is also thought to be difficulty in extraction of oxygen at the tissue level.
TP	The classic presentation in septic shock is fever, tachycardia, hypotension, and vasodilation (warm extremities with poor capillary refill). Patients will often be confused or sleepy; young children sometimes present as irritable and inconsolable. Urine output is frequently decreased.
Dx	Signs of the **systemic inflammatory response syndrome (SIRS)**—high or low temperature, tachycardia, tachypnea, abnormal leukocyte count, and cardiovascular dysfunction—that is, hemodynamic compromise in the setting of a suspected or proved infection.

Tx Broad-spectrum antibiotics are the mainstay of early treatment. Treatment of the hemodynamic compromise includes fluid resuscitation of up to 60 mL/kg or more in the first hour followed by vasoactive drugs such as dopamine, epinephrine, and norepinephrine as continuous infusions to maintain cardiac output. If there is evidence of adrenal suppression (low or normal cortisol in the face of stress and hemodynamic compromise), consider hydrocortisone. **See Nelson Essentials 40.**

Distributive Shock States: Anaphylactic Shock

Pψ *Anaphylactic shock* is another form of distributive shock mediated by systemic inflammation and histamine release. Anaphylaxis occurs in individuals who are exposed to an allergen to which they have been previously sensitized.

TP The classic presentation in anaphylactic shock is tachycardia, hypotension, vasodilation, swelling, hives, bronchospasm, and airway compromise. Patients will often be irritable, complain of itching or swelling, and have increased secretions.

Dx This is usually a clinical diagnosis, when the patient presents in shock with a history of allergies and exposure to an allergen.

Tx The ABCs in anaphylactic shock are paramount. The swelling and increased secretions can rapidly lead to airway compromise, and early securing of the airway should be considered. Fluid resuscitation can help in reestablishing the circulating volume and maintaining cardiac output. Epinephrine subcutaneously or as an infusion can be used to treat the vasodilation and help decrease some of the airway symptoms, while antihistamines (both H_1- and H_2-blockers) and corticosteroids are used to treat ongoing inflammation. **See Nelson Essentials 81.**

Hemorrhagic Shock

Pψ *Hemorrhagic shock* is the disruption of oxygen-carrying capacity of the blood by anemia as well as hemodynamic compromise due to hypovolemia. (Remember, oxygen content is approximately $1.36 \times Hgb \times Sao_2$.)

TP Hypotension and tachycardia in the face of significant blood loss are usually associated with traumatic injury.

Dx	Anemia and hypovolemia as demonstrated by blood count and physical examination findings are the hallmarks of diagnosis for hemorrhagic shock. However, *be mindful that patients with acute blood loss may have a normal Hgb in the early phase of blood loss and shock.*
Tx	Volume resuscitation blood should be undertaken in an urgent or emergent fashion, often using type-specific noncrossmatched blood to restore the body's oxygen-carrying capacity. In significant anemia, 100% inspired oxygen can greatly increase the total oxygen delivery and should be started while giving blood. **See Nelson Essentials 148.**

Cardiogenic Shock

Pψ	*Cardiogenic shock* is the disruption of the cardiovascular system by failure of the myocardial pump. The stroke volume is decreased because the heart is not pumping effectively. The heart often becomes dilated, and therefore the myocytes do not effectively cross-link, resulting in decreased myocardial contractility.
TP	Tachycardia with cold extremities and an enlarged liver are typical. Children may present with abdominal symptoms due to decreased intestinal perfusion. In some patients, there may be signs of pulmonary edema.
Dx	The typical cases have an enlarged failing heart, and the initial clue will be found on a chest radiograph, which typically demonstrates cardiomegaly and, at times, dilated pulmonary vasculature and/or pleural effusion. Echocardiogram evaluates cardiac function (ejection fraction), and a cardiac biopsy may define the etiology. An ECG may demonstrate signs of inflammation, chamber enlargement, or specific ischemic patterns.
Tx	Always remember the ABCs. Fluid resuscitation is judiciously administered to optimize the intravascular volume, being careful to avoid fluid overload. Vasoactive agents to increase contractility and cardiac output and decrease systemic vascular resistance are indicated. Specifically, dobutamine and milrinone drips are the mainstays of pharmacologic therapy. Other drugs administered include digoxin (to increase contractility), diuretics (to remove excess fluid), and afterload-reducing drugs (such as captopril or enalapril to promote cardiac output by decreasing peripheral vascular resistance). **See Nelson Essentials 148.**

Hypovolemic Shock

Pψ | *Hypovolemic shock* is disruption of cardiac output due to severe depletion of the circulating blood volume. Increasing heart rate is a principal means of compensation to maintain cardiac output. Once the blood volume is decreased below the body's ability to compensate, there is decreased venous return to the right atrium, and it becomes difficult to maintain adequate cardiac output. Therefore oxygen delivery to the tissues is compromised.

TP | There is tachycardia and hypotension with a history of either decreased fluid intake or significant fluid loss through diarrhea, vomiting, or less commonly, fever and tachypnea accompanied by inadequate intake, diabetes, or third-space losses (pancreatitis, liver failure).

Dx | The typical cases manifest evidence of significant volume loss, which can be detected by a well-taken history and an accurate physical examination. Laboratory data that can supplement the diagnosis include blood urea nitrogen >20 times the creatinine level, suggesting "prerenal" disease or intravascular depletion.

Tx | Hypovolemic shock is treated by replacing volume intravenously, or by oral rehydration with a careful monitoring of electrolyte balance and ongoing fluid losses. **See Nelson Essentials 40.**

Obstructive Shock

Pψ | *Obstructive shock* is disruption of cardiac output by inhibiting blood flow into or out of the heart with a space-occupying lesion in the thorax such as tamponade, tension pneumothorax, or a coarctation of the aorta.

TP | The typical presentation is acute onset of hemodynamic collapse, often in the face of another illness that predisposes the patient to one of the common forms of obstruction.

Dx | Clinical findings such as decreased breath sounds on one side (pneumothorax) or radiographic studies will aid in diagnosis.

Tx | The fundamental treatment for all of the forms of obstructive shock is to remove the obstruction. If this cannot be done quickly, then the patient should be maintained with fluid resuscitation and potentially vasoactive medications, with the goal of keeping the heart "full and fast." **See Nelson Essentials 40.**

Neurogenic Shock

Pψ	*Neurogenic shock* occurs when there is disruption of the autonomic nervous system's ability to maintain a normal degree of sympathetic tone in the vasulature, resulting in vascular dilation and a relative bradycardia.
TP	The most common etiology of neurogenic shock is in the setting of trauma leading to a high spinal cord injury. Other causes include spinal tumors and spinal infections.
Dx	The combination of bradycardia or normal heart rate, hypotension, and increased vasodilation with a clinical history of spinal cord disruption should make the diagnosis. Physical examination findings such as decreased rectal tone, paralysis, or paresis will also help make the diagnosis.
Tx	Depending on the spinal injury, intubation to secure the airway and breathing is often needed. Fluid resuscitation is instituted early, followed quickly by administration medications to increase vascular tone, such as norepinephrine or phenylephrine drips. In addition, high-dose corticosteroids are often administered. **See Nelson Essentials 40.**

ZEBRA ZONE

a. **Acute onset hemolytic anemia due to glucose-6-phosphate dehydrogenase (G6PD):** Severe anemic state precipitated by a stressor such as infection or certain medications with inadequate stores of this enzyme in the red blood cell membrane. (See Chapter 45, Anemia.)

b. **Carbon monoxide poisoning:** Prevents oxygen binding to hemoglobin and hence there is inadequate oxygen delivery at the tissue level

c. **Splenic sequestration crisis in sickle cell disease:** There is inadequate venous return due to sequestration of blood volume within the spleen, in addition to the baseline anemia.

d. **Heat stroke:** A medical emergency with high body temperature that affects multiple body systems. There is profound peripheral vasodilation and volume depletion, due to a combination of distributive and hypovolemic states

Practice-Based Learning and Improvement: Evidence-Based Medicine

Title
Clinical practice parameters for hemodynamic support of pediatric and neonatal patients in septic shock

Authors
Carcillo JA, Fields AI, Task Force Committee Members

Reference
Crit Care Med 30(6):1365-1378, 2002

Comparison/control
Review article examining levels of evidence of practice with expert consensus on management guidelines

Quality of evidence
Level II evidence

Outcome/effect
Guidelines for management of pediatric and neonatal sepsis

Historical significance/comments
The first well-evaluated evidence-based algorithm to follow in treating pediatric septic shock

Interpersonal and Communication Skills

Perils of Intensive Care Unit Machinery: Dealing With Anxiety Provoked by Technology

It is important to remember that family members are quite unaccustomed to the technology used in the modern pediatric intensive care unit. Such bewilderment produces anxiety, which can often be alleviated by simple discussions explaining the function of each device and its role in the care of their child.[1]

Professionalism

Maintain Patient Confidentiality: The Temptation of the Electronic Medical Record

Health-care staff may know the family of or have a child who is friends with a child who is hospitalized where they work. Whereas it is natural to be concerned about the child's clinical status, individuals who are not part of the care team are not permitted to access the child's electronic medical record (EMR). To access a patient's record when you are not part of the care team is illegal and a serious breach of both confidentiality and protocol. Hospitals have software to monitor who has logged onto a patient's EMR. These programs are frequently used if a VIP or celebrity is hospitalized. If an individual who is not part of the legitimate caretaking team has logged onto a medical record (even if done out of innocent curiosity), very significant penalties may be imposed.

Systems-Based Practice

Acute Care Level of Service: Consider Cost-Effective, Quality Options

Acute inpatient care for the *recovered* shock patient may not be appropriate. There are alternate levels of care, such as subacute care facilities or home care. Evaluate other services or levels of care that may be appropriate to adequately address the patient's current medical condition, social needs, and other expected discharge requirements. It is advisable to check **McKesson's InterQual manual,** *Acute Pediatric Criteria,* which provides objective criteria to justify acute levels of care based upon severity of illness and intensity of services required.

Chapter 85
Diabetic Ketoacidosis (Case 43)

Meg A. Frizzola DO

Case: A 10-year-old girl presents to the emergency department with abdominal pain, headache, and "confused and slurred" speech for the past 12 hours. Her parents report she has lost approximately 10 pounds in the past month and has seemed to have very frequent urination and insatiable thirst, drinking several liters of water a day.

Differential Diagnosis

Diabetic ketoacidosis (DKA)	Hyperosmolar hyperglycemic nonketotic state (HHNK)

Speaking Intelligently

When I am presented with a patient with the constellation of symptoms described above, I strongly suspect DKA and work to both resuscitate the patient and achieve a diagnosis. Initial focus on the ABCs of airway, breathing, and circulation is appropriate, as well as obtaining an initial set of vital signs and attempting to place at least one large IV for eventual fluid resuscitation. Laboratory values are extremely important in diagnosis, so I immediately obtain a blood gas and a dextrostick as well as a urine specimen to determine the presence of glucose and/or ketones. Electrocardiogram (ECG) monitoring is important because of the electrolyte abnormalities. Patients with DKA can be assumed to have at least a 10% fluid deficit and will require volume resuscitation; however, cerebral edema is a real and serious complication, and judicious fluid use is warranted. It is best to start with 10 to 20 mL/kg of an isotonic solution, such as normal saline (0.9% sodium chloride). Although fluid resuscitation is crucial, insulin administration, typically in the form of a continuous infusion, is important to stop the ketosis and reverse the acidosis. Bicarbonate is generally not indicated to treat the acidosis. Finally, the level of obtundation/depressed consciousness is important to assess. Neuroimaging and appropriate management of cerebral edema with mannitol or 3% saline should be instituted if necessary (see Chapter 81, Raised Intracranial Pressure).

PATIENT CARE

Clinical Thinking
- Support airway, breathing, and circulation.
- Is there evidence of **neurologic impairment?** Do I have to immediately treat **cerebral edema?**
- Are there other contributing factors, such as infection, stress, or missed insulin dose, that led the patient to develop DKA?
- What is the **degree of dehydration** of this patient?

History
- Consider contributing conditions, such as infection, missed dose of insulin, pregnancy, or stress that led to the development of DKA.
- Consider family history of type 1 diabetes or other autoimmune disorders.
- Ensure low likelihood of ingestion or starvation before arriving at diagnosis of DKA.
- Often history of vomiting, headaches, polyuria, and polydipsia with significant weight loss over brief period of time.

Physical Examination
- Vital signs: Expect to see tachycardia, sometimes with hypotension, elevated respiratory rate, afebrile (usually). Hypertension may be a warning sign of cerebral edema.
- General appearance: ill-appearing, malaise, obtundation or confusion.
- Head, ears, eyes, nose, and throat (HEENT) exam will reveal dry mucous membranes, acetone (fruity) breath.
- Kussmaul respirations may be noted.
- Check pupils and fundi for signs of cerebral edema and increased intracranial pressure (ICP).
- May have vague, diffuse abdominal pain.

Tests for Consideration
- **Arterial blood gas levels:** Crucial to obtain pH and bicarbonate level to determine degree and etiology of acidosis $156
- **Electrolyte levels, blood urea nitrogen (BUN), and creatinine level:** Important to monitor sodium, potassium, bicarbonate, chloride, magnesium, phosphorus, BUN, and creatinine level $68
- **Complete blood count (CBC) with differential:** Important if suspect infection $53
- **Glucose level:** Elevated above 200 mg/dL $29
- **Hemoglobin A1C:** Useful for determining degree of control of diabetes $25
- **Urinalysis:** Check for presence of ketones and glucose $110
- **β-Human chorionic gonadotropin in adolescent female patients** $25
- **Osmolality:** Can be helpful in determining other sources of anion gap metabolic acidosis such as ethanol ingestion $25
- **Serum acetone** $25

IMAGING CONSIDERATIONS

→ **Head computed tomography (CT):** Will need emergently if evidence of significant cerebral edema. $750
→ **Chest radiograph:** If pneumonia is suspected as an infectious etiology for presence of DKA. Patients also can develop acute respiratory distress syndrome (ARDS) as a rare complication. $75

Clinical Entities   Medical Knowledge

Diabetic Ketoacidosis

Pφ   ***Diabetic ketoacidosis*** results from absolute or relative insulin deficiency along with the effects of counterregulatory hormones such as catecholamines, glucagon, cortisol, and growth hormone. In type 1 or juvenile diabetes low levels of insulin along with high levels of the counterregulatory hormones yield a catabolic state in the body, causing the liver and kidney to produce increased levels of glucose, impaired peripheral glucose use that leads to hyperglycemia and hyperosmolarity, and increased lipolysis and ketogenesis that leads to ketonemia and metabolic acidosis.

TP   The typical child with DKA will present with polyuria, polydipsia, weight loss, headache, confusion, muscle pain, abdominal pain, vomiting, and shortness of breath. On physical examination, patient will appear dehydrated with dry mucous membranes, sunken eyes, and poor skin turgor. They often have a fruity smell (acetone production). They may be tachycardic and tachypneic with abnormal breathing pattern (Kussmaul respirations) and may have significant diffuse abdominal pain.

Dx   Diagnosis can be made by performing the testing mentioned above. In particular, the patient must be hyperglycemic with blood glucose levels greater than 200 mg/dL with an anion gap metabolic acidosis (serum bicarbonate level less than 15 mEq/L) and ketosis with elevated serum ketones (β-hydroxybutyrate and acetoacetate) or ketonuria.

Tx   Goals of therapy are to correct acidosis and reverse ketosis, correct dehydration, and restore blood glucose to normal levels. Begin with fluid resuscitation; give 10 to 20 mL/kg fluid bolus with an isotonic crystalloid, normally 0.9% sodium chloride. After initial fluid bolus, begin IV fluid therapy with the goal of replacing the fluid deficit over the next 24 to 48 hours at an even rate, typically using 0.9% sodium chloride with a mix of up to 40 mEq/L total of potassium chloride and potassium phosphorus. Patients should not have potassium added until the serum potassium is less than 5.0 mmol/L. They are total body potassium depleted, but the acute acidosis shifts potassium out of the cells, giving high serum levels transiently. Always remember, cerebral edema is a potential complication, occurring in 1% of patients with DKA, so careful management of fluid status is critical. When blood glucose level approaches 300 mg/dL, dextrose must be added to the fluid solution. Insulin infusion rate is typically 0.1 unit/kg/hr. It is important to remember that blood glucose levels return to normal earlier than ketosis resolves and insulin therapy should never be discontinued until ketoacidosis is resolved. It is important to note that despite the degree of acidosis, sodium bicarbonate use is not recommended, because its use has been associated with higher incidence of cerebral edema. If cerebral edema is suspected, CT scan and appropriate treatment should be initiated. **See Nelson Essentials 171.**

Hyperosmolar Hyperglycemic Nonketotic State

Pφ | **Hyperosmolar hyperglycemic nonketotic state** develops secondary to decreased insulin activity, not insulin deficiency. This leads to hyperglycemia and hyperosmolarity without development of ketoacidosis. The hyperglycemia and hyperosmolarity result in an osmotic diuresis, causing severe dehydration, electrolyte disturbances, and altered mental status.

TP | HHNK most commonly develops in patients with type 2 diabetes who have a concurrent illness that causes them to have reduced fluid intake. Neurologic changes noted such as delirium, drowsiness, coma, seizures, visual changes, hemiparesis, and sensory deficits may have been present for weeks. The patients will complain of polyuria and polydipsia and will appear dehydrated. The patients are typically tachycardic and tachypneic and exhibit hypotension. Abdominal pain is usually absent.

Dx The diagnostic triad for HHNK is hyperglycemia (serum glucose >600 mg/dL), hyperosmolarity (>320 mOsm/kg), and mild metabolic acidosis. Ketosis is typically absent. Sodium levels may be low, normal, or elevated; total body potassium is low, regardless of the serum value; magnesium and phosphorus levels will be low. BUN and creatinine level are elevated, serum creatinine phosphokinase (CPK) level may be elevated (rhabdomyolysis may trigger or occur with HHNK). It is also important to look for other signs of infection as mentioned above; concurrent illness is often a trigger.

Tx The goals of therapy include restoring hemodynamic stability, correcting electrolyte disturbances, gradual correcting of hyperglycemia and hyperosmolarity, and treating underlying causes. Fluid resuscitation is as outlined for DKA. If the patient is hypotensive, a 20-mL/kg bolus of isotonic fluid should be given. Potassium replacement is important; once rehydration and insulin are started, serum potassium levels quickly fall. The typical insulin infusion is 0.1 unit/kg/hr. **See Nelson Essentials 171.**

ZEBRA ZONE

a. **Salicylate intoxication:** May present as a late metabolic acidosis in addition to respiratory alkalosis with stupor

b. **Starvation:** Can be a cause of ketonuria, but usually low or normal glucose

c. **Diabetes insipidus:** Inadequate antidiuretic hormone (ADH) in the central form or inability to respond to ADH (nephrogenic DI); presents with polyuria and polydipsia and dehydration.

Practice-Based Learning and Improvement: Evidence-Based Medicine

Title
Risk factors for cerebral edema in children with diabetic ketoacidosis

Authors
Glaser N, Barnett P, McCaslin I, et al

Reference
N Engl J Med 344:264-269, 2001

Problem

Investigation into risk factors associated with cerebral edema development in children with diabetic ketoacidosis

Comparison/control (quality of evidence)

Case-control study with cited references in peer-reviewed journal

Outcome/effect

Children with DKA who have low partial pressures of arterial carbon dioxide and high serum urea nitrogen concentrations at presentation and who are treated with bicarbonate are at increased risk for cerebral edema.

Historical significance/comments

Historically, patients with DKA who presented with severe acidosis were routinely given bicarbonate to help correct their acidosis. This article helped to change that management strategy, and now bicarbonate is rarely used in the treatment of DKA despite the degree of acidosis.

Interpersonal and Communication Skills

Be Alert for Issues of Adolescence

Many patients with DKA present during adolescence. Although this may be a consequence of metabolic changes occurring at this age, it often is a sign of changing attitudes consistent with adolescent development. Adolescents prefer not to be different. They wish to eat/drink the same as their peers. This is compounded by an adolescent's needs to be in control of his/her own body. Insulin administration and frequent blood glucose monitoring challenges that control. It is not unusual for teenagers with diabetes to stop using insulin or to skip doses in their desire to be "normal." It is important to explore these thoughts and feelings when confronted with adolescents recovering from DKA.

Professionalism

Explore Precipitating Factors

It is important for clinicians who care for patients with DKA to determine the underlying factors that have contributed to the need for hospital admission. Using the ecologic model[2] (formerly called the biopsychosocial model), which postulates that diseases occur within ecological contexts and are significantly influenced by social behaviors, the supervising physician should initiate a root cause analysis focused on ameliorating or eliminating the factors that precipitated the episode of DKA in his/her patient.

References

1. Characteristics of California children with single versus multiple diabetic ketoacidosis hospitalizations (1998-2000). *Diabetes Care* 28:2082-2084, 2005.
2. Brieger WR: Health behavior and the ecological model. Johns Hopkins Bloomberg School of Public Health. Available at http://ocw.jhsph.edu/courses/ SocialBehavioralFoundations/PDFs/Lecture2.pdf.

Chapter 86
Trauma (Case 44)

Paul M. Shore MD, MS

Case: A 6-year-old pedestrian child has been hit by a car traveling at moderate speed (30 mph)

Differential Diagnosis	
Chest injuries	Spinal cord injury
Abdominal injuries	Traumatic brain injury (TBI)

Speaking Intelligently

I approach the trauma patient with the assumption that immediately life-threatening injuries exist, and it is up to me and the trauma team to identify and treat them. I follow protocols outlined by the American College of Surgeons in their Advanced Trauma Life Support course. The patient is first approached with a primary survey looking at the ABCDEs, in which immediately life-threatening injuries to the airway, breathing, and circulation are recognized and treated aggressively. Next, a secondary survey is undertaken, and a more thorough examination is performed. Radiographic and laboratory examination may follow, and injuries not apparent on physical examination are identified. Finally, a disposition is determined as to where the patient will receive further definitive management (e.g., surgery) or stabilization (e.g., home, ward, or intensive care unit).

PATIENT CARE

Clinical Thinking
- **Primary Survey (A,B,C,D,Es)**
- *Airway:* The patient's airway may be obstructed by direct trauma, debris, or by neurologic impairment (e.g., coma or seizure). If the airway is patent, proceed to "breathing." If not, obtain a patent airway. Caution must also be taken to **maintain a stable cervical spine** during any airway procedures.
- *Breathing:* "Breathing" refers to the act of respiration, which may be impaired by direct trauma to the thorax or neurologic impairment. If the patient's breathing is adequate, proceed to "circulation." If not, identify and treat the problem immediately.
- *Circulation:* "Circulation" refers to the patient's blood volume and cardiac function. Patients should have two large-bore peripheral IVs placed immediately upon arrival, and isotonic crystalloid should be administered. Control any obvious source of external bleeding with externally applied pressure.
- *Disability:* Gross neurologic disability should be recognized during the primary survey. The patient's level of consciousness should be assessed using the Glasgow Coma Scale (GCS). If the GCS is ≤8 or deteriorating, the trachea should be intubated under the assumption that airway patency or respiratory drive will soon be lost. Examine the pupils: if anisocoria is present without eye trauma, the patient should be treated immediately for intracranial hypertension. A cervical collar should be placed on the patient to immobilize the neck.
- *Exposure:* The patient's clothing is removed to facilitate a complete physical examination.
- **Secondary Survey**
- Proceed to the secondary survey *only* if the complete primary survey has identified no immediately life-threatening injuries.

- The secondary survey should be a careful, systematic, head-to-toe evaluation of the patient with careful attention paid to all potential injuries.
- Always logroll the patient (keeping the neck stable) to examine the back.
- Radiographic examination of the patient should be done in the trauma room and should include plain films of the chest, cervical spine, and pelvis if injury to these areas is suspected. Clinical findings or mechanism of injury should guide the need for computed tomography (CT) scans of the head, neck, chest, abdomen, or pelvis following the initial stabilization. Blood can be drawn for a laboratory panel (see below) while IV access is obtained.
- All historical and physical examination findings should be recorded on a flow sheet designed specifically for acute trauma. The leader of the team should therefore call out each finding (including normal findings) as they are identified.
- **Occult Trauma**
  - Nonaccidental trauma (child abuse) patients often present with a history of trauma that may be inaccurate, conflicting, or entirely absent, and their arrival to medical attention may be delayed. They may present with symptoms that are nonspecific or subtle, such as vomiting, irritability, or "not acting right."
  - Near-drowning typically causes hypoxic-ischemic injury. However, because the events of a near-drowning are often unwitnessed (e.g., patient found at the bottom of a pool), a traumatic injury may have occurred.
- **Patterns of Injury**
  - Various mechanisms often produce patterns of injury that may increase the clinical suspicion of particular injuries. For example, automobile passengers restrained with a seat belt may have injuries to the liver, spleen, intestines, pelvis, or lower spine that are heralded by abdominal bruising that traces the seat belt.
- **Pediatric Considerations**
  - Compared with those of adults, the heads of children, particularly infants, are larger relative to their bodies. Children are therefore more likely to sustain cervical spine injuries.
  - The skeletons of children have much more cartilage than adults, making them more flexible. Organ injury, such as pulmonary or cardiac contusions, can therefore occur without overlying fractures to herald them. Spinal cord injuries can occur without bony fractures (known as spinal cord injury without radiographic abnormality, or **SCIWORA**). Fractures of long bones often involve cartilaginous growth plates.
  - Both adults and children can exsanguinate internally, into the chest, abdomen, retroperitoneum, pelvis, or thighs. Infants can also exsanguinate into the head (into the brain or, more commonly, into the subgaleal potential space).

History
- History of the **patient** should focus on age, relevant past medical history, allergies, and last meal.
- History of the **trauma** should focus on details of the mechanism may provide clues to the pattern and severity of injuries.
- History of **prehospital care** should focus on patient complaints and interventions by emergency medical services providers.

Physical Examination
- Vital signs: Tachycardia should be considered as a sign of hypovolemia and impending hypovolemic/hemorrhagic shock; tachypnea, particularly with desaturation, should be considered as a sign of hemothorax, pneumothorax, pulmonary contusion, or airway compromise. Hypopnea indicates central nervous system dysfunction.
- Head, ears, eyes, nose, and throat (HEENT): Carefully note fractures underlying scalp lacerations; pupillary and extraocular muscle examinations if the nasal septum is midline; if the oropharynx is normal or injured (e.g., missing teeth); if the jaw is tender or cannot open fully.
- Neck: Carefully note if the trachea is midline (it may deviate away from a tension pneumothorax). Ensure neck immobilization, but carefully remove immobilizer (while holding the neck stable) to examine the cervical spine for tender areas or step-offs during the secondary survey.
- Chest: Tachypnea, grunting, flaring, or retracting suggests lung injury. Lack of breath sounds suggests hemothorax or pneumothorax.
- Cardiovascular: Tachycardia, delayed capillary refill, or weak pulses mean impending hemorrhagic shock until proven otherwise. Muffled heart sounds suggest pericardial effusion.
- Abdomen: A tense abdomen suggests intraperitoneal bleeding. Gently press on the anterior iliac crests to assess pelvic stability.
- Genitourinary: Always perform a rectal examination before placing a Foley catheter; an unstable prostate or blood at the urethral orifice suggests urinary injuries. Priapism and lack of rectal tone strongly suggest spinal cord injury.
- Neurologic: Assess the level of consciousness using the Glasgow Coma Scale. Assess all extremities for sensory and motor deficits.
- Musculoskeletal: Inspect all extremities visually and by palpation, looking for fractures. For suspicious areas, assess the sensation and quality of pulse to identify a neurovascular injury. Logroll the patient, and palpate the entire spine to identify points of tenderness or step-off.

Tests for Consideration
- **Complete blood count (CBC):** To assess degree of blood loss $110
- **Electrolytes, blood urea nitrogen (BUN), creatinine, glucose levels:** To assess hydration status and renal function $115

- **Aspartate transaminase (AST), alanine transaminase (ALT), γ-glutamyltransferase (GGT), alkaline phosphatase levels:** If suspect liver trauma — $45
- **Amylase lipase levels:** If suspect pancreatic trauma — $56
- **Arterial or venous blood gas levels:** To assess acidosis or elevated PCO_2 in impending respiratory failure — $45
- **Prothrombin time (PT), partial thromboplastin time (PTT):** To identify coagulopathy — $75
- **Urinalysis:** To identify microscopic blood — $35

IMAGING CONSIDERATIONS

→ **Chest radiograph:** To identify pneumothorax, hemothorax, pulmonary contusion — $120
→ **Cervical spine radiograph of the cervical spine:** If suspect cervical spine trauma — $800
→ **Computed tomography (CT) scan of the cervical spine:** If suspect cervical spine trauma — $500
→ **Pelvic radiograph:** If suspect pelvic trauma — $150
→ **Head CT:** To identify acute bleeding herniation — $1000
→ **Abdomen/pelvis CT:** To evaluate extent of trauma when suspected — $1100

Clinical Entities — Medical Knowledge

Chest Injuries

Pφ Children have a significantly more flexible rib cage compared to that of adults. Therefore a significant injury can be present without rib fractures. The presence of rib fractures indicates an injury of significant force. Injuries include pulmonary contusion, pneumothorax, and hemothorax.

TP Pulmonary contusion presents with worsening hypoxemia. Crackles are often present on lung examination.
  Pneumothorax presents with tachypnea and hypoxemia. Breath sounds are absent on the affected side, with hyperresonance to percussion. If the pneumothorax continues to expand, a tension pneumothorax may result, with hemodynamic compromise due to impaired venous return. There may be tracheal shift and distended neck veins.
  With hemothorax breath sounds will be absent over the affected side, with dullness to percussion.

Dx   Pulmonary contusion is often noted as an infiltrate on chest radiograph as a radiolucent area and possibly a line representing the visceral pleura.

   Pneumothorax will be visible on chest radiograph.

   Hemothorax is identified on chest radiograph, but thoracentesis to remove the serosanguineous fluid is confirmatory.

Tx   Patients with pulmonary contusion may require intubation and ventilation with positive end-expiratory pressure (PEEP) to manage hypoxemia.

   Pneumothorax should be treated either with needle decompression followed by chest tube placement, or one can directly to chest tube placement, depending on the patient's respiratory status.

   Hemothorax should be treated by chest tube placement. **See Nelson Essentials 133 and 138.**

Spinal Cord Injury

Pφ   Until about 8 years of age children have anatomic differences in the spine that predisposes to different types of *spinal cord injury.* Their head is larger in proportion to the body and the neck muscles are weaker and less well developed. The orientation of the vertebral bodies is different, resulting in force being shifted to the ligaments and ligamentous injury being more common rather than fractures.

TP   Children may present with back pain or with focal neurologic deficits. High-level injuries can present with impaired respiratory effort or neurogenic shock.

   Children may have fractures with or without subluxation, subluxation alone, or SCIWORA, which is unique to pediatrics.

Dx   Magnetic resonance imaging (MRI) and plain films of the spine are helpful in making a diagnosis. SCIWORA presents as a significant injury with normal imaging and alignment of the cord.

Tx   Initial resuscitation with fluids is important. Transport with the spinal axis immobilized is challenging in infants and children, but important to prevent further injury. Corticosteroids are controversial but typically are administered in the period immediately following injury. **See Nelson Essentials 42.**

Traumatic Brain Injury

Pφ **Traumatic brain injury (TBI)** results from the impact of trauma to the brain. A mix of forces may be involved—direct contact as well as acceleration-deceleration type of injury from the brain moving in a fixed cavity. Because the child has a larger head to body ratio, these acceleration-deceleration forces are more significant, and children often suffer more diffuse brain injury. These forces inflict the primary injury. In addition, there may be injury to arteries, resulting in epidural hematoma or tears in bridging veins resulting in subdural hematoma.

TP Children may present with altered mental status and/or focal neurologic deficits. Pupillary exam may reveal anisocoria.

Dx Head CT will demonstrate fractures, subdural and epidural hematomas, mass lesions, parenchymal hemorrhage, and cerebral edema. The full extent of diffuse injury may not be apparent on the initial scan, and MRI may be indicated later for prognostic information.

Tx The goal of treatment is to minimize secondary injury because there is no specific treatment for the primary injury. See Chapter 81, Raised Intracranial Pressure. **See Nelson Essentials 184.**

Abdominal Injuries

Pφ Children are at increased risk for **abdominal injuries** because their smaller size results in a larger amount of force per unit area. An additional injury risk is related to the abdominal wall musculature and connective tissues being less well developed.

TP Abdominal tenderness or distention may be present. Bruising from a seat belt may be present over the abdomen.

Dx If there is suggestion of an abdominal injury (i.e., distention, free fluid on focused abdominal sonography for trauma [FAST] imaging) in a hemodynamically unstable patient, operative exploration is indicated. Otherwise, diagnostic imaging with CT scanning is indicated.

Tx Most solid organ injuries respond to nonoperative management, and surgery is usually not warranted. Serial hemoglobin levels are monitored, and transfusion may be indicated. However, if a patient is hemodynamically unstable, then operative intervention may be necessary. Evidence of bowel perforation also requires operative intervention. **See Nelson Essentials 42.**

ZEBRA ZONE

Consider Underlying Medical Conditions

Few diagnoses can masquerade as acute trauma. However, one must always ask if an underlying medical condition caused or predisposed the patient to the particular trauma. Occasionally a medical condition is detected incidentally on examination. For example, a pathologic fracture may occur in a child with an underlying bone disease. Other examples might include **seizures, encephalitis, osteosarcoma, toxic ingestions, obstructive hydrocephalus, or sinus cavernous hemangiomas.**

Practice-Based Learning and Improvement: Evidence-Based Medicine

Title
Outcomes and delivery of care in pediatric injury

Authors
Densmore JC, Lim HJ, Oldham KT, Guice KS

Reference
J Pediatr Surg 41(1):92-98, 2006

Problem
How to allocate resources effectively in designing pediatric trauma systems and delivering care. Is there a substantial benefit to being cared for in a children's hospital versus an adult hospital or a children's unit within an adult facility? Is that benefit substantial enough to risk overtriaging and overburdening the limited pool of pediatric surgeons?

Intervention
The database of pediatric inpatient admissions and selected pediatric injury cases was reviewed. Data were separated by age and injury severity score (ISS). Outcomes reviewed were in-hospital mortality, length of stay, and total charges.

Outcome/effect
In the youngest (0 to 10 years) and most severely injured (ISS >15) patients all outcomes—in-hospital mortality, length of stay, and total charges—were reduced significantly with care in a children's hospital (p <0.001).

Historical significance/comments
There has been much debate about whether care in a children's hospital is superior for the pediatric trauma patient. Much of the literature up to this point has been equivocal. This study looking at a large number of patients suggests that maybe pediatric trauma patients need to be triaged differently with the youngest and sickest being preferentially treated at a children's hospital.

Interpersonal and Communication Skills

Understand Children's Reaction to Pain, Discomfort, and Anxiety

Trauma is terrifying, particularly for small children who may be in pain, bewildered, and separated from their parents. Talking to the child in a soothing voice, using his/her first name, and focusing his/her attention away from the medical personnel and treatment may be an extremely effective form of anxiolysis.

Professionalism

Behavior in the Trauma Bay: Respectful and Considerate Interactions With Colleagues and Staff

The trauma bay is the epitome of "organized chaos" but represents an intricately choreographed dance when done properly. The trauma team consists of a command physician, one or more assistants, several nurses, often several physician extenders, generally several social support personnel, and, transiently, the emergency medical services personnel. Each member of the team should have an assigned role, such as "airway physician" or "nurse left." Each should remain in his/her assigned position, but should be aware of others and offer help when needed. Remain quiet unless you have something specific to say. The rule is that only the command physician's voice should be heard. The student or resident should have his/her role defined before the arrival of the patient, whether observer or command physician.

Systems-Based Practice

Regionalized Trauma Systems Reduce Mortality

Regionalization of trauma care has decreased preventable deaths from trauma by making resources and expertise available in one location to care for the trauma patient. For pediatric patients, it has been demonstrated that mortality decreases when a child is cared for in a specialized pediatric trauma center and not in an adult facility. After adjusting for injury severity and patient age, research has shown that the primary factors contributing to the reduced mortality are treatment at a tertiary center, reduced prehospital time, and direct transport from the scene to tertiary centers. Therefore the integration of trauma care services into a regionalized system reduces mortality. Overall, **tertiary trauma centers** and **reduced prehospital times** are the essential components of an efficient trauma care system.[1]

Reference

1. Sampalis JS, Denis R: Trauma care regionalization: A process-outcome evaluation. *J Trauma* 46(4):565-579, 1999.

Chapter 87
Status Asthmaticus (Case 45)

Venkat R. Shankar MD, MBA

Case: A 6-year-old child known to have asthma has been having increasing difficulty breathing for the past 24 hours. He developed a cold and a runny nose 2 days ago, and has been taking repeated "breathing treatments" overnight without any relief. Since this morning, he has been unable to speak in sentences and cannot walk to the bathroom.

Differential Diagnosis

Asthma	Congestive heart failure	Pneumonia

Speaking Intelligently

Status refers to a condition that persists despite appropriate therapy. Children in status asthmaticus typically appear very ill and distressed. The most critical aspect of management is to assess the degree of oxygenation using pulse oximetry and to provide supplemental oxygen. I also assess mental status as a marker of ventilation—the degree to which they are responsive. Lack of adequate responsiveness is often the harbinger of respiratory arrest. One of the first priorities is to administer inhaled beta-agonists in addition to supplemental oxygen. Establishing vascular access and administering intravenous methylprednisolone early are also key. I usually do not obtain an arterial blood gas determination—as the decision to assist with mechanical ventilation is usually evident based on clinical examination.

PATIENT CARE

Clinical Thinking

- Can I reverse the process with aggressive **bronchodilators** and **anti-inflammatory** therapy (i.e., corticosteroids)?
- Is the child dehydrated from poor oral intake and insensible fluid losses due to hyperpnea?
- Hypoxemia can be life threatening; however, one can withstand a significant degree of hypercapnia.

History

- **Previous history** of wheezing, "bronchitis," and seasonal cough is suggestive of asthma.
- Nocturnal or exercise-induced cough may also be suggestive of asthma.
- Fever may be present, although a high degree of fever could indicate pneumonia.
- Exposure to tobacco, animals, pollen, or other allergens may suggest an asthma trigger.
- A history of sudden choking may suggest foreign body aspiration, not asthma.
- Symptoms of poor feeding or growth or easy fatigue may suggest a cardiac etiology.

Physical Examination

- Vital signs: The child is tachypneic with increased work of breathing with intercostal, subcostal, and supraclavicular retractions. Tachycardia and bounding pulses are common. Decreased oxygen saturation on room air pulse oximeter may be present.
- **Pulsus paradoxus,** an exaggerated decrease in systolic blood pressure on inspiration (greater than 10 mm Hg), is suggestive of severe disease.
- In general, the child may appear distressed. The **inability to speak** in short sentences is a sign of severe status asthmaticus.
- On lung examination, air entry may be severely diminished, and wheezing may not be audible in severe cases. Prolonged expiratory phase is typical.
- A heart murmur or gallop and hepatomegaly may suggest congestive heart failure as an etiology rather than asthma.
- Evaluation of **mental status** is helpful in deciding the severity of asthma and need for assisted ventilation.

Tests for Consideration

- **Electrolytes:** To assess degree of dehydration and presence of acidosis. $115

- **Arterial blood gas (ABG) levels:** May help in cases that are borderline for intubation $45
- **Complete blood count (CBC):** May help differentiate an infectious process from asthma, or asthma with secondary pneumonia $110

IMAGING CONSIDERATIONS

→ **Chest radiographs:** May be useful in ruling out other causes, such as cardiac failure, and in identifying complications of asthma such as atelectasis, and pneumothorax, pneumonia, or pneumomediastinum $120

Clinical Entities	Medical Knowledge

Asthma

Pφ	***Asthma*** is caused by inflammation of the airways, resulting in bronchoconstriction. Mucus production and broncospasm are prominent features resulting in mucus plugging of the airways. The overall result is resistance to airflow, particularly on exhalation, resulting in air trapping lung hyperinflation. Asthma is thought to be immune-mediated and triggered by pollutants, allergens, infections, weather changes, and exercise.
TP	Patients present with difficulty breathing, chest tightness, tachypnea, and cough. On examination, diffuse expiratory wheezing, decreased aeration, and prolonged expiratory phase are typical findings, along with prominent accessory muscle use. In more severe cases with severe obstruction, wheezing may not be appreciated due to severely decreased air movement.
Dx	Diagnosis is based on history and clinical examination. Chest radiograph study may demonstrate hyperinflation due to air trapping from obstruction. Pulmonary function testing in an older child may be helpful, revealing a decrease in forced expiratory flow. Peak flow may be helpful in selected cases, when formal pulmonary testing is not available, but note that it is effort-dependent.

Tx   The mainstay of treatment is supplemental oxygen and inhaled beta-agonists such as albuterol, which may be administered intermittently or as a continuous inhalation in the setting of status. Beta-agonists cause smooth muscle relaxation and subsequent bronchodilation. Ipratropium bromide may also be useful for additional bronchodilation, particularly in the emergency department. Corticosteroids are important to decrease inflammation. Careful monitoring of response to each intervention—noting oxygen saturation, respiratory rate, quality of air movement, degree of alertness, and perceived work of breathing—helps to decide further management and to determine the appropriate setting for continued care (inpatient floor vs. the intensive care unit). Magnesium sulfate and terbutaline may be helpful adjuncts in severe cases. Bilevel positive airway pressure (BiPAP), a form of noninvasive ventilation, may help to decrease work of breathing. Heliox, a gas mixture of helium and oxygen, allows for more laminar gas flow in the airways, and may overcome airway resistance and improve delivery of inhaled medications to the more distal airways. Patients who require magnesium, terbutaline, heliox, and/or BIPAP require admission to the intensive care unit. **See Nelson Essentials 78.**

Congestive Heart Failure

Pφ   *Congestive heart failure* (CHF) results when the heart is unable to eject enough blood to sustain the body's metabolic needs and can be due to myriad causes related to inadequate contractility, problems with afterload (such as aortic stenosis), or problems with preload (volume overload such as in ventricular septal defect). Congenital heart disease or any myocardial dysfunction (such as cardiomyopathy or myocarditis) can lead to the end point of CHF. In left-sided heart failure, the congested pulmonary circulation can lead to pulmonary edema, which may mimic the signs and symptoms of asthma.

TP   *Congenital heart lesions* such as a large ventricular septal defect (VSD) typically present with congestive heart failure, if the diagnosis is not previously known, around 6 to 8 weeks of age as the pulmonary vascular resistance reaches nadir and left-to-right shunting increases. There will be a history of difficulty feeding, sweating with feeds, failure to thrive, and tachypnea with increased work of breathing. A harsh, systolic murmur and inspiratory crackles may be auscultated, and hepatomegaly may be detected on abdominal examination. *Myocarditis* may present with a viral prodrome and then tachypnea, crackles or wheezing on lung examination, and often a gallop cardiac rhythm. Patients will be ill-appearing and poorly perfused (cool extremities, diminished pulses, and/or delayed capillary refill).

Dx	Echocardiography will confirm the diagnosis. Chest radiography may be helpful in demonstrating cardiomegaly and pulmonary congestion.
Tx	Treatment of congestive heart failure includes supplemental oxygen to maintain optimal oxygenation, administration of diuretics (to remove excessfluid), and digoxin and other inotropic agents (to increase myocardial contractility). Use of vasodilators and afterload-reducing agents (angiotensin-converting enzyme [ACE] inhibitors) may be indicated to improve cardiac output by decreasing peripheral vascular resistance. Surgical intervention may be indicated for certain congenital heart lesions. (See Chapters 65, The Newborn With a Murmur, and 90, Myocarditis.) **See Nelson Essentials 145.**

Pneumonia

See Chapter 83, Acute Respiratory Failure.

ZEBRA ZONE

a. **Foreign body inhalation:** In younger infants and toddlers can produce sudden onset of cough and respiratory distress or complete occlusion of the airway with respiratory arrest. (See Chapter 44, Difficulty Breathing.)

b. **Vocal cord dysfunction:** This poorly understood disease typically occurs in adolescent girls and is characterized by sudden onset of breathing difficulty in a manner that can that masquerade as asthma.

Practice-Based Learning and Improvement

Title
Assessment and treatment of acute asthma in children

Authors
Chipps BE, Murphy KR

Reference
J Pediatr 147:288-294, 2005

Problem
Review of acute asthma and its management in children

Comparison/control (quality of evidence)
Review article with cited references in peer-reviewed journal

Historical significance/comments
Up-to-date review of both standard therapies and new opportunities in the treatment of asthma

Interpersonal and Communication Skills

Using Open-Ended and Closed-Ended Questions Appropriately

Although open-ended questions usually produce more information when taking a history, there are situations in which closed-ended questions (those that can be answered with a simple "yes" or "no") are also used effectively. Status asthmaticus can be a life-threatening condition. Medications need to be administered quickly, a history needs to be obtained, and the family may be frightened and require reassurance. Time is of the essence, and the patient in status asthmaticus is unlikely to be able to give more than a one- or two-word response. This is a situation in which a few closed-ended questions can help clarify the initial history so that therapy can be started promptly. Once initial therapy has been started and the patient is stable, a more extensive history and examination can be performed.

Professionalism

Advocacy: Patient Well-Being May Require Elimination of Environmental Tobacco Smoke

Children with asthma often have attacks triggered by pollutants such as cigarette smoke. It can be frustrating to care for a child with asthma whose family continues to expose the child to *environmental tobacco smoke (ETS)*. Educating the family and directing them to smoking cessation resources is part of the responsibility of the pediatric physician, because it significantly affects the child's well-being. It is important to be supportive and nonjudgmental, and to understand that behavior change is difficult and can take time. However, based on the clinical course and severity of the child's asthma, it may be necessary to involve child protective services when families are unable to eliminate ETS exposure.

Systems-Based Practice

Practice Cost-Effective Health Care Without Compromising Quality

There is little evidence to suggest that obtaining routine chest radiographs in all children who present with acute asthma changes the clinical management or outcomes. However, if there is suspicion of complication—pneumothorax, pneumomediastinum—appropriate imaging studies should be obtained. Similarly, there is no proven reason for obtaining routine arterial blood gas levels to diagnose or monitor the degree of airway obstruction or to assess the need for assisted ventilation. Although radiographs and blood gas determinations may at times be used to support decisions, actions in these matters should be based on best clinical judgment.

Chapter 88
The Chronic Child (Case 46)

Danna Tauber MD, MPH

Case: A 10-year-old girl with a diagnosis of spinal muscular atrophy type II presents to the emergency department (ED) with fatigue, weight loss, morning headache, and shortness of breath.

Differential Diagnosis

Congenital neuromuscular disorders	Static encephalopathy/hypoxic ischemic encephalopathy
Metabolic disorders	Bronchopulmonary dysplasia (BPD)/ chronic lung disease

Speaking Intelligently

When I evaluate a child in chronic respiratory failure, I first think about the underlying disease process that led to the child's current status. In a child who has progressive muscle weakness, the time course to respiratory failure can be protracted, and earlier interventions may help stave off impending respiratory failure. In cases of static encephalopathy, a child's airway may be compromised, with an acute presentation and necessary emergent interventions, or the course may be more chronic with recurrent aspiration pneumonias leading to lung damage and eventual respiratory failure. The time course can vary, and earlier interventions can be helpful. In all cases, careful discussion with the child's caretakers regarding treatment options is very important.

PATIENT CARE

Clinical Thinking
- Is the child in imminent danger of respiratory arrest?
- What is the nature of the respiratory failure: **airway obstruction** versus **parenchymal lung disease** versus **respiratory muscle weakness.**

History
- Underlying medical conditions
- Chronicity of respiratory illness
- Recent fever or evidence of respiratory infection
- History of swallowing difficulty or history of emesis or feeding intolerance
- History of **weight loss**

Physical Examination
- Vital signs including weight
- Assessment of airway: Is there audible breathing, stridor, suprasternal retractions?
- Auscultation of breath sounds
- Evaluation of work of breathing: thoracoabdominal asynchrony, intercostal muscle activity
- Assessment of muscular tone, control of secretions, mental status

Tests for Consideration
- **Arterial blood gas levels:** To check for compensated respiratory acidosis $45
- **Electrolyte levels:** To check serum bicarbonate $115
- **Pulmonary function testing:** To evaluate for obstruction or restrictive breathing pattern $255
- **Overnight polysomnogram:** To check for upper airway obstruction versus centrally mediated hypoventilation without airway compromise or a mixed pattern with elements of obstruction and hypoventilation $450

IMAGING CONSIDERATIONS

→ Chest radiograph	$75
→ Videofluoroscopic swallow study	$675
→ Laryngoscopy or bronchoscopy	$2200

Congenital Neuromuscular Disorders

Pφ   ***Congenital neuromuscular disorders*** result in progressive muscle weakness, which eventually include the muscles of respiration. Respiratory involvement can begin in infancy, early childhood or, late adolescence. The respiratory insufficiency may initially present with retained secretions leading to atelectasis and infections. As muscle weakness progresses, impaired ventilation during sleep becomes an issue. With progression of weakness, swallowing can also become impaired, and the patient can be at risk for aspiration of food or liquids into the lung. Eventually daytime ventilation becomes impaired with worsening hypercapnia and hypoxemia.

TP   Presentation depends on the age, the specific disease, and the extent of muscle degeneration. Infants with aggressive neuromuscular diseases can present with increased work of breathing or apnea. Older children with slowly progressive disease can present with recurrent respiratory infections.

Dx   Diagnosis is made on initial presentation of muscle weakness with muscle biopsy and in some cases genetic testing. Respiratory insufficiency or failure is diagnosed with clinical findings and arterial blood gas evaluation, which will demonstrate hypercarbia and some degree of hypoxemia, the extent of which is determined by the degree of respiratory insufficiency.

Tx   Early on, assisting the patient with airway secretion clearance can prevent atelectasis and infection. This includes manual chest physiotherapy, aerosol therapy, and cough assist devices. If the patient has evidence of nocturnal hypoventilation, then treatment with noninvasive mechanical ventilation (bilevel positive airway pressure [BiPAP]) can improve ventilation, quality of sleep, and even daytime level of functioning. Once ventilation has deteriorated permanently, the patient can transition to either noninvasive ventilation (sip ventilation [mouthpiece intermittent positive pressure ventilation] and BiPAP) or invasive ventilation via a tracheostomy tube. **See Nelson Essentials 182.**

Metabolic Disorders

Pφ *Metabolic disorders* include a large number of diseases with different etiologies. The final outcome is decreased energy production in the cells due to errors in metabolism. The impact on respiration comes from involvement of respiratory muscle cells and cells of the central nervous system.

TP There is not a typical presentation due to the large variety of disorders. Patients with the same disorder can present differently depending on which organ system is more involved. Feeding is frequently impacted, as is level of cognitive and muscle functioning. Impaired ventilation more or less follows the same progression as in the neuromuscular disorders.

Dx Diagnosis can be made on newborn genetic screening, muscle biopsy, and blood tests for specific metabolic markers.

Tx Treatment varies depending on the level of dysfunction. In patients with airway involvement, surgery to remove airway obstruction can be helpful as can placement of a tracheostomy tube. Airway clearance devices, noninvasive mechanical ventilation, and invasive mechanical ventilation can also be used depending on the level of impairment. **See Nelson Essentials 51.**

Static Encephalopathy/Hypoxic-Ischemic Encephalopathy

Pφ *Static encephalopathy* is irreversible, permanent brain damage that can result from multiple different causes. Examples include prolonged cardiac arrest, trauma, stroke, and infection. This can result in poor airway tone, swallowing dysfunction with aspiration, gastroesophageal reflux with or without aspiration, and impaired control of breathing.

TP Respiratory complications from static encephalopathy can present differently. Immediately after the injury the patient can require ventilatory support or stabilization of the airway. Years after the original injury, there can be partial or complete airway obstruction. Central or obstructive or mixed apnea may develop over time.

Dx Diagnosis of encephalopathy can be made with an electroencephalogram (EEG), magnetic resonance imaging (MRI), or computed tomography (CT) scan of the brain. For airway compromise, laryngoscopy and bronchoscopy can be helpful to determine the exact location and nature of the airway impingement. Overnight polysomnogram should be done to determine if there is obstructive or central apnea.

Tx   Treatment is individualized and may includes tracheostomy
      tube placement, gastrostomy tube placement, noninvasive
      mechanical ventilation, invasive mechanical ventilation, and
      airway clearance devices. **See Nelson Essentials 64.**

Bronchopulmonary Dysplasia/Chronic Lung Disease

Pφ   *Bronchopulmonary dysplasia (BPD)* results from either
      premature birth or term birth with the development of
      respiratory distress syndrome (RDS) and need for mechanical
      ventilation and supplemental oxygen therapy. BPD can vary
      in severity with the most severe cases requiring prolonged
      mechanical ventilation, including home ventilator support. The
      exact cause is likely multifactorial, including prematurity of the
      lung parenchyma, infection and inflammation, oxygen toxicity,
      and barotrauma from mechanical ventilation leading to lung
      injury and poor nutrition. Pathology findings include
      atelectasis, metaplasia, fibrosis, and overdistended alveoli.

TP   Initial presentation of BPD is at birth with respiratory distress
      syndrome and hypoxemia. Once the infant has been diagnosed
      with BPD and discharged from the neonatal intensive care unit
      (NICU), he/she can present with respiratory infections,
      including respiratory syncytial virus (RSV) bronchiolitis, which
      in these infants can be very severe and present with apnea or
      respiratory distress and hypoxemia. Other presentations include
      an infant with BPD having a "BPD spell," in which the infant
      has poor aeration and significant hypoxemia.

Dx   Diagnosis of BPD is made if the infant required supplemental
      oxygen and/or mechanical ventilation for the first 28 days of
      life and continues to require supplemental oxygen at 36 weeks
      postmenstrual age. Severe BPD is defined as requiring greater
      than 30% supplemental oxygen or positive pressure ventilation
      at 36 weeks postmenstrual age. There is retained CO_2 with a
      compensatory metabolic alkalosis.

Tx   Treatment includes diuretic therapy if there is evidence of
      pulmonary edema and bronchodilators and systemic
      corticosteroids for bronchospasm; intubation with mechanical
      ventilation for the severe cases with marked CO_2 retention and
      respiratory failure. **See Nelson Essentials 61.**

ZEBRA ZONE

The diagnoses primarily considered in this chapter may themselves be considered "Zebras." When taking care of the chronic child it is also important to remember that "common things are common." Always consider acute infections and other common reasons for a downturn in a patient's condition, no matter how esoteric or complex their underlying diagnosis.

Practice-Based Learning and Improvement: Evidence-Based Medicine

Title
Mechanical ventilation beyond the intensive care unit

Authors
Make BJ, Hill NS, Goldberg AI, et al

Reference
Chest 113(suppl):289S-344S, 1998

Problem
Management of patients requiring long-term mechanical ventilation

Comparison/control (quality of evidence)
Consensus statement of the American College of Chest Physicians

Outcome/effect
Provides guidelines for the management of chronically mechanically ventilated children

Historical significance/ comments
Good reference on approach to chronic long-term ventilator management

Interpersonal and Communication Skills

Encourage Patient (Family) to Participate in Decisions to the Extent Desired

The primary care physician or hospitalist can sometimes feel overwhelmed and "out of the loop" when involved in the care of a chronically ill child. These patients often have multiple subspecialty physicians who provide care. More importantly, the parents are usually very knowledgeable and savvy about the health-care system. Chronically ill children often have had numerous admissions and previous interventions with varying success. Their parents may want to participate in any major care decision and to share the historical perspective of what has and hasn't worked for their child's problems.

Care coordination with all of the stakeholders (the family, physicians, social workers, nurses, other therapists, and home care providers) is key to smoothly transitioning a child from the acute care setting back to the home setting. This will ensure a continuation in care in the home setting.

Professionalism

Social Justice: Allocation of Resources

The H1N1 pandemic, which began in 2008-2009, prompted examination of how, should the need arise, decisions about allocation of limited resources, such as ventilators, would be made.[1,2] Who should and would have priority? Should a child who has a chronic illness with little chance for long-term survival be taken off a ventilator and the ventilator given to an acutely ill child who has a good chance for survival and a healthy life? Who will make, enforce, and carry out decisions about allocation of ventilators, and what will be the physician's role in the process?

Systems-Based Practice

Health-Care Economics: Claims, Coding, and Billing

Obtaining adequate reimbursement for the additional services associated with providing a medical home to children with special needs is essential. It is critically important to work with insurance carriers, Medicaid and State Children's Health Insurance Program (SCHIP) officials, and managed care executives on a proactive basis to avoid the added financial risk that comes with caring for these children. According to the American Academy for Pediatrics' *Coding for Pediatrics*,[3] in order to increase their efficiency, physicians must:

- Code correctly
- Follow Current Procedural Terminology (CPT) guidelines
- Use the most specific International Classification of Diseases (ICD) code possible
- Use modifiers when appropriate
- Know their carriers
- Know their contracted fee schedule
- Check every explanation of benefits
- Develop a relationship with one person at every insurance carrier
- File appeals and follow up their status promptly
- Document all provided services

References

1. Kinlaw K, Levine R: Ethical guidelines in pandemic influenza, 2007. Available at: http://www.cdc.gov/od/science/phethics/panFlu_Ethic_Guidelines.pdf.
2. Centers for Disease Control and Prevention: Ethical considerations for decision making regarding allocation of mechanical ventilators during a severe influenza pandemic or other public health emergency. Available at: http://www.cdc.gov/od/science/integrity/phethics/docs/ethical-considerations-allocation-mechanical-ventilators-in-emergency-201011.pdf.
3. Bradly J, Salus T: *Coding for pediatrics: A manual for pediatric documentation and reimbursement*, 8th ed. Elk Grove Village, IL, 2003, American Academy for Pediatrics.

Chapter 89
Status Epilepticus (Case 47)

Matthew J. Kapklein MD, MPH

Case: A 6-year-old boy presents to your hospital's emergency department after collapsing at school and beginning to have tonic-clonic movements. On arrival to the emergency department 30 minutes later, he is noted to be unresponsive, with rhythmic, jerking movements of all extremities. He is tachycardic and hypertensive, and his respirations are irregular.

Differential Diagnosis

Brain problems affecting gross structure	Brain problems affecting function	Non–central nervous system problems affecting the brain
Intracranial hemorrhage (intraparenchymal or extraparenchymal)	Epilepsy	Toxin exposure
Tumor	Diffuse infections: meningitis, encephalitis, meningoencephalitis	Electrolyte disturbance or metabolic problems
Abscess	Atypical febrile seizure	
Hypoxia of any etiology		

Speaking Intelligently

Although many children are able to maintain adequate oxygen saturation during status epilepticus, I always assume they are hypoventilating. Management of airway, breathing, and circulation (ABCs) comes first. The decision of when to stabilize the airway will be determined by three patient factors: (1) current status, (2) anticipated response to interventions, (3) actual response. For example, a patient who fails to respond to intravenous phenytoin, phenobarbital, and lorazepam and is receiving an infusion of midazolam before traveling to the computed tomography (CT) scanner may well require endotracheal intubation simply because of the anticipated additional respiratory depressive effects of the infusion. If you intubate, remember that a paralytic agent will eliminate your ability to monitor the neurologic examination for a period of time, so I try to avoid them or use a short-acting paralytic. Stopping the seizures themselves is largely a matter of selecting supportive therapies (i.e., different classes of antiepileptic drugs) until control is obtained. I generally start with benzodiazepines and if control is not obtained will load with a medication like phenytoin (fosphenytoin) or phenobarbital. In addition, one needs to think of and look for specific treatable causes (e.g., hyponatremia, hypoglycemia, subdural hematoma). If you are considering the possibility of a treatable infection, it is a good idea to give antibiotics early, even if you are planning a lumbar puncture (which may be delayed by clinical instability, seizures, or the need for imaging). Status epilepticus is associated with increased insensible fluid losses (excessive motor activity, hyperthermia, tachycardia, metabolic demand), so generous hydration with hemodynamic support as needed is a must.

PATIENT CARE

Clinical Thinking
- Does this patient need a secure airway?
- The longer the patient seizes, the more dangerous it becomes to the brain. Use agents with the most rapid onset first. The rectal, intranasal, or intramuscular route may be your first choice if the patient does not yet have an IV or intraosseous (IO) line.
- Start by looking for specific diagnoses that are rapidly detectable and treatable, such as **hyponatremia, hypocalcemia, hypoglycemia, hypoxemia, dysrhythmia, meningitis, some toxins, bleeds, or tumors.**

History
• Does the child have an **underlying seizure disorder?**
• If **febrile,** is this a simple febrile seizure or a CNS infection? Fevers also lower seizure thresholds in children with epilepsy.
• **Trauma** can either be the causative agent of seizures or occur as a direct result (e.g., the child who collapses and hits her head).
• How was the child behaving before the seizure?
• Where was the child found? Did the child have access to medications or other **poisons?**

Physical Examination
• Vital signs: Most actively seizing children are tachycardic and hypertensive, with irregular and/or ineffective respirations.
• As always, start with the ABCs.
• Look for stigmata of an underlying neurodevelopmental disorder (e.g., microcephaly, contractures, dysmorphic features).
• Remember toxidromes: Some require specific therapies.
• Pupil examination can be helpful—unequal pupils may suggest an etiology requiring rapid surgical intervention.

Tests for Consideration
• **Bedside glucose:** Hypoglycemia may be a treatable cause $45
• **Electrolytes:** Hyponatremia, hypocalcemia, and hypomagnesemia are all treatable causes of seizures $115
• **Arterial blood gas levels:** Degree of acidemia may affect decision to intubate $45
• **Drug levels:** For those patients known to be on antiepileptic medications $60
• **Lumbar puncture:** Important but can wait until no longer seizing $135

IMAGING CONSIDERATIONS

→ **Head CT:** To rule out mass lesions $1000
→ **Electroencephalogram (EEG):** To determine type of underlying seizure disorder (after it stops) or see if your patient may still be seizing without your knowledge (i.e., nonconvulsive status epilepticus) $225
→ **Magnetic resonance imaging (MRI):** To delineate small structural abnormalities $1800

Brain Problems Affecting Gross Structure

Pφ   These disorders share the common feature of increased intracranial pressure.

Intracranial hemorrhage may be spontaneous or traumatic, and seizures may result from direct neuronal injury or irritation by blood.

Tumors and other masses may arise from anywhere inside the cranial vault. In certain positions these may obstruct CSF flow and cause an obstructive hydrocephalus.

Abscesses may form via direct extension from another site (sinusitis, mastoiditis, meningitis) or hematogenous spread.

TP   *Headache:* The classic presentation of a spontaneous subarachnoid hemorrhage is that of a sudden-onset "worst headache of life," whereas tumors and abscesses are usually slower growing and hence associated with a more chronic history.

Vomiting: Elevated intracranial pressure stimulates the brain's vomiting center. The classic presentations of brain tumors is vomiting in the morning, not associated with nausea.

Mental status changes: These may be subtle or nonexistent in focal lesions like tumors and abscesses.

Trauma: History or physical findings of trauma may be present, although in nonaccidental trauma (abuse) the history may be of an injury that is minor or nonexistent.

Dx   All require imaging to diagnose. CT is the usual first choice (fast), but you may need contrast to see abscesses or an MRI to see small lesions.

Tx   Treatment is aimed at reducing the size of the lesions, in addition to supportive care.

Intracranial hemorrhages may require surgical decompression if they are focal.

Tumors usually require surgical resection, although corticosteroids may be used to reduce vasogenic edema preoperatively.

Abscesses are treated with long-term antibiotics and, rarely, surgery. **See Nelson Essentials 184.**

Brain Problems Affecting Function

Pφ These problems are characterized by altered brain function in the presence of no or minimal changes in gross brain structure.

   Seizure disorders (epilepsy) are the most common cause of status epilepticus in children and are characterized by one or more foci of abnormal electrical activity in brain cells. An important subtype here is febrile seizures (see below).

   Diffuse infections (meningitis, encephalitis, meningoencephalitis) can be bacterial or viral. Although they may be associated with structural changes (e.g., cerebral edema), they also cause altered brain function through inflammation and altered cell membrane permeability.

TP **Seizure disorders** may occur in previously healthy children and in children with known neurologic problems (e.g., cerebral palsy, neurofibromatosis) at any age.

   CNS infections are typically characterized by a period of altered mental status (e.g., lethargy, confusion) before the onset of seizures and are often associated with fevers.

Dx **Seizure disorders,** although the most common, are also diagnoses of exclusion and are usually diagnosed by EEG.

   Infections are diagnosed by lumbar puncture or a combination of MRI and serologic studies.

Tx **Seizure disorders** are usually treated with prophylactic antiepileptics, the type determined by the child's age and EEG profile. Many families are given a dose of diazepam to keep at home, which may be administered rectally in the case of unremitting seizures.

   Infections are treated with appropriate antimicrobial therapy. **See Nelson Essentials 181.**

Non–Central Nervous System Problems Affecting the Brain

Pφ These problems are all characterized by profound CNS effects in the presence of a structurally normal brain, usually due to a systemic illness.

Toxins and *metabolic disturbances* can be present in the bloodstream, including medications (isoniazid, theophylline), environmental poisons (lead, carbon monoxide), electrolyte imbalances (hyponatremia), and inborn errors of metabolism.

Febrile seizures are an important subtype of seizures, listed here because fever itself (which lowers seizure threshold in everyone) is the "cause" of the seizure—these are usually brief and benign. Simple febrile seizures are defined as occurring in children **6 months to 5 years of age,** being **generalized,** lasting **less than 15 minutes,** and **not recurring** within 24 hours. Complex febrile seizures are febrile seizures lasting longer than 15 minutes (i.e., febrile status epilepticus), focal seizures, or recurrent seizures within 24 hours. Fever of any origin can be the cause, but it is typically a viral infection that, at its onset, causes an abrupt rise in temperature.

TP These problems are typically associated with systemic, as well as CNS, manifestations. Although many toxins are associated with solely CNS manifestations, it is important to look for clues in the history (e.g., ingestions, exposures), physical examination (e.g., pupillary changes, odors), or laboratory studies (e.g., anion or osmolar gaps, electrolyte disturbances). Many children with inborn errors of metabolism have other evidence of prolonged systemic disease, such as impaired weight gain or developmental delay.

Dx History and initial physical examination alone are usually sufficient to rule in febrile seizures, and many toxins as potential causes. It may be a challenge is to find the source of the fever.

Blood tests demonstrating electrolyte disturbances, abnormal metabolites, and characteristic toxin profiles can aid in diagnosis.

Tx As always, treatment is aimed at stopping seizures along with respiratory and hemodynamic support. Toxins and inborn errors of metabolism may have specific antidotes, electrolyte abnormalities require correction, and the source of fever may require treatment with antimicrobial agents. **See Nelson Essentials 185.**

ZEBRA ZONE

Not all that convulses is a seizure. Remember that *myoclonic jerks, dystonic reactions* to medications, *agitation* in spastic individuals, and uncontrolled *tics* can all mimic seizures.

Practice-Based Learning and Improvement: Diagnostic Assessment

Title
Practice parameter: Diagnostic assessment of the child with status epilepticus (an evidence-based review): Report of the Quality Standards Subcommittee of the American Academy of Neurology and the Practice Committee of the Child Neurology Society

Authors
Riviello JJ, Ashwal S, Hirtz D, et al

Reference
Neurology 67(9):1542-1550, 2006

Problem
Childhood status epilepticus

Intervention
Different modes of diagnostic testing

Comparison/control (quality of evidence)
Evidence-based review and practice guideline

Historical significance/comments
The current state of the art, endorsed by the American Academy of Neurology, American College of Emergency Medicine, American Academy of Pediatrics, and American Epilepsy Society

Interpersonal and Communication Skills

Communicate Effectively: Limit Hysteria, Calm Families, Focus on Real Priorities

Parents who have experienced it will say that there is no more frightening experience than the sight of one's own child convulsing. Parents may panic. Do not be surprised if some details of the history are forgotten in the initial interview, which often takes place by necessity at the time of resuscitation and stabilization. It may be wise to assign a team member whose sole role initially is to comfort and inform family members.

Such panic may spread to health-care personnel. A team leader speaking calmly but firmly as the initial evaluation and resuscitation proceeds will help reduce the level of tension. Convulsions may distract caregivers from more important issues, such as a compromised airway. Part of the provider's role is to focus attention on problems in the order of their priority.

Professionalism

Personal Biases Should Not Interfere With Best Professional Judgment

Many children with status epilepticus have profound neurological impairment at baseline, and health-care providers may be prone to feelings of "futility" or "resource waste" because these children often require ever-increasingly aggressive interventions. It is important to remember that in our society, parents have the right to determine what is in the best interest of their children unless they give compelling evidence that they are incapable of doing so. This includes decisions about life-sustaining treatment for neurologically impaired individuals. Families are entitled to our respectful treatment, regardless of whether we agree with their decisions.

Systems-Based Practice

The Role of the Hospital Formulary

The hospital formulary plays a vital role in containing rising drug costs and promoting patient safety. The broad definition of hospital formulary (HF) is the array of drugs and therapeutics available in a particular hospital. Agents included in the HF are at the discretion of the appropriate parties on the medical staff, who, in conjunction with the hospital pharmacy department, make decisions about what will and will not be included in the formulary. Formulary management processes generally include the determination of therapeutic protocols and guidelines as well as the power to place restrictions on the prescribing of certain medications within the hospital. Optimally, formulary management leads to best quality for patients through the selection of medications that maximize value relative to costs. Physician involvement is integral to the process.

Chapter 90
Myocarditis (Case 48)

Aaron D. Kessel MD

Case: A 4-year-old child with respiratory distress, tachypnea, and tachycardia

Differential Diagnosis

Pneumonia	Bronchiolitis/dehydration/viral illness	Myocarditis/dilated cardiomyopathy
Pericarditis	Pneumothorax	Asthma

Speaking Intelligently

When evaluating a patient in respiratory distress, I first consider the ABCs: airway, breathing, and circulation. When I suspect a cardiac etiology, I obtain a chest radiograph and an electrocardiogram (ECG). I feel it is prudent to consult a cardiologist quickly, because the management of a cardiac illness can be complicated and beyond the scope of many practitioners. It is important to closely monitor the hemodynamic status because patients with myocarditis may have a rapidly changing course and immediate adjustments in medical care are required. Transfer to a tertiary care facility with intensive care specialists and cardiologists should occur immediately after stabilization.

PATIENT CARE

Clinical Thinking
- Address the **ABCs** before further intervention.
- There are many possible causes of tachypnea and tachycardia. Consider the most likely for age and history first.

History
- How long has the patient had the current symptoms?
- Has the child had fever, symptoms of a **viral illness,** or any sick contacts?
- Does the patient have any other **medical problems?** Has the patient suffered from a similar episode in the past?
- Has the child had other symptoms during the same time period?
- Do these symptoms affect daily activities? Has the patient had a normal energy level since the symptoms began?
- Has the patient been gaining weight appropriately?

Physical Examination
- Vital signs: Note tachypnea and/or tachycardia. The patient may have decreased oxygen saturation secondary to pulmonary edema. If critically ill, these may be associated with hypotension. The patient may also have a fever.
- There may be respiratory distress with tachypnea, retractions, and nasal flaring. Note **crackles** and decreased breath sounds at the lung bases.
- Cardiac examination may reveal:
  - Tachycardia (regular or irregular rhythm)
  - An S_3/S_4 gallop from volume overload and cardiac wall impairment
  - A **friction rub**
  - A new-onset systolic **murmur** from mitral or tricuspid insufficiency
  - Abdominal examination may reveal **hepatomegaly** secondary to congestive heart failure.
- Extremity examination may reveal **pallor,** increased time of capillary refill, **poor pulses, cool extremities,** and edema.

Tests for Consideration
- **Complete blood count (CBC):** White blood cells (WBCs) when infection is suspected; hemoglobin to assess oxygen-carrying capacity — $110
- **Electrolyte levels:** To examine metabolic and renal function. Sodium may be decreased and blood urea nitrogen (BUN) increased with fluid overload in congestive heart failure (CHF) — $115
- **Liver function tests:** May be elevated with hepatic congestion in right-sided heart failure — $65
- **Arterial blood gas (ABG), including lactate,** demonstrate ventilatory status and acid-base status. Elevated lactate level is a sign of anaerobic metabolism and may indicate poor perfusion. — $45
- **Cardiac enzyme levels:** Troponin I/T and creatine kinase, myocardial (CK-MB): Elevation reveals cardiac ischemia. — $75
- **Blood culture** — $55
- **Viral culture** — $55

- **Viral titers:** Adenovirus, echovirus, cytomegalovirus (CMV), Epstein-Barr virus (EBV), human immunodeficiency virus (HIV) $50-$250 per test
- Nonspecific indicators of systemic inflammation:
  - **C-Reactive protein:** $65
  - **Erythrocyte sedimentation rate** $65

IMAGING CONSIDERATIONS

→ **Chest radiograph:** To evaluate lung fields, pulmonary vasculature, and heart size. $75
→ **ECG:** Often shows sinus tachycardia, low voltages, and inverted T waves. May demonstrate arrhythmias, including ventricular tachycardia (VT), supraventricular tachycardia (SVT), premature atrial complexes (PACs) and premature ventricular contractions (PVCs). $150
→ **Echocardiogram:** To evaluate left ventricular function and size, and atrioventricular (AV) valve function. $325

Clinical Entities   Medical Knowledge

Myocarditis/Dilated Cardiomyopathy

Pφ   ***Myocarditis*** is a viral infection (usually adenovirus or echovirus) of the cardiac muscle. Various cells within the immune system (most notably T cells) invade the muscle to eradicate the viral pathogens and damage myocytes in the process, which are replaced by fibrotic and necrotic tissue. As a result, ventricular size enlarges, and the diseased myocardium is unable to adequately eject blood because of impaired contractility. ***Dilated cardiomyopathy*** occurs when the heart has decreased function secondary to dilation and decreased contractility. It may occur as a primary insult or secondary to myocarditis.

TP   Presentation usually consists of tachycardia, tachypnea, and decreased oxygen saturation. Patients may also have hepatomegaly, cool extremities, poor capillary refill, and peripheral edema. In the advanced stages of the disease they may present with severe respiratory distress and hypotension. These symptoms may be preceded by a viral prodrome of myalgias, arthralgias, and fever.

Dx   Chest radiograph reveals cardiomegaly. Confirmatory tests include echocardiography, which displays decreased cardiac function, and electrocardiography, which may show arrhythmias. Viral culture/titers and polymerase chain reaction (PCR) testing for adenovirus, coxsackievirus, CMV, EBV, or HIV may yield an etiology. PCR has been found to be more sensitive than viral cultures or acute and convalescent titers.

    Magnetic resonance imaging may be used to monitor disease progression. Myocardial biopsy is considered the diagnostic gold standard; however, biopsy results are positive in only 20% to 50% of cases.

Tx   The treatment goal is to maintain adequate cardiac output by improving the heart rate, blood pressure, and tissue perfusion. This is accomplished with afterload reducing agents (milrinone), inotropes (dopamine, dobutamine), and diuretics (furosemide, thiazides). In the acute stage an antiarrhythmic agent may be needed to control unstable cardiac rhythms. Controversial therapy aimed at decreasing the inflammation includes corticosteroids, immunosuppressive agents (azathioprine, tacrolimus, cyclophosphamide), and intravenous immunoglobulin (IVIG). IVIG has proven to be the most effective of these medications. Long-term agents to improve myocardial function include digoxin to increase contractility, as well as angiotensin-converting enzyme (ACE) inhibitors and spironolactone to restore the renin-angiotensin axis and reduce afterload. **See Nelson Essentials 145.**

Bronchiolitis/Dehydration/Viral Illness

Pφ   A *viral illness* may mimic myocarditis. Patients may be dehydrated secondary to vomiting and diarrhea, leading to tachycardia. They may have increased respiratory secretions causing tachypnea and decreased oxygen saturation. Fever may produce both tachypnea and tachycardia.

TP   Patients may present with fever, respiratory distress, tachycardia, vomiting, and diarrhea. They may also have a rash, a sore throat, and other signs of a viral infection. They often have sick contacts with similar symptoms.

Dx   Diagnosis can be made with the clinical findings and history given above. Confirmatory testing may be done to look for etiologies such as respiratory syncytial virus, influenza virus, or adenovirus. A chest radiograph may reveal bilateral increased interstitial markings without focal findings.

| Tx | Treatment usually consists of symptomatic care. (See Chapter 44, Difficulty Breathing.) **See Nelson Essentials 109.** |

Pneumonia

See Chapter 44, Difficulty Breathing, and Chapter 83, Acute Respiratory Failure.

Pneumothorax

Pφ	A *pneumothorax* occurs from abnormal accumulation of air between the parietal and visceral pleura of the lungs. A complicated pneumothorax (or a tension pneumothorax) occurs when there is a constant air leak into the pleural space and may become a life-threatening emergency.
TP	Patients with a simple pneumothorax may not have any symptoms. Those with a complicated or larger pneumothorax present with respiratory distress and chest pain.
Dx	Diagnosis is made by physical examination, which may show decreased breath sounds on the affected side in addition to chest radiograph, which will demonstrate air in the pleural space.
Tx	Treatment is removal of the air from the pleural space. If the pneumothorax is large, or if the patient is symptomatic, a chest tube is inserted to evacuate the air. In the case of a tension pneumothorax, immediate decompression may be indicated by insertion of a needle in the second interspace in the midclavicula line. See Chapter 95, Chest Pain. **See Nelson Essentials 138.**

Asthma

See Chapter 31, Cough, Chapter 44, Difficulty Breathing, and Chapter 87, Status Asthmaticus.

Pericarditis

| Pφ | *Pericarditis* is pericardial inflammation with polymorphonuclear infiltration of the pericardial tissue that surrounds the heart. The pericardium may have a fibrous reaction with exudates and adhesions. |

TP	The typical patient has chest pain that is worse with lying supine, swallowing, or moving. Patients may complain of dyspnea if pericarditis progresses to cardiac tamponade. They may also have tachypnea, tachycardia, and fever.
Dx	A friction rub, best heard at the left lower sternal border, may be appreciated. Electrocardiography may show diffuse ST-segment elevation. Chest radiograph may have cardiomegaly due to effusion. In addition, echocardiography and CT scan may reveal effusions. With pericardial tamponade, hypotension, pulsus paradoxus, tachycardia, and distant heart sounds may be present.
Tx	Treatment includes aspirin and nonsteroidal antiinflammatory medications for pain. Drainage of effusion is undertaken if tamponade is present. **See Nelson Essentials 148.**

ZEBRA ZONE

Myocarditis is usually the zebra. Kudos to those who diagnose it acutely.

Practice-Based Learning and Improvement: Evidence-Based Medicine

Title
Pediatric myocarditis: Presenting clinical characteristics

Authors
Durani Y, Egan M, Baffa J, et al

Reference
Am J Emerg Med 27:942-947, 2009

Problem
Myocarditis is often misdiagnosed at initial presentation

Comparison/control (quality of evidence)
Review of presenting signs and symptoms of pediatric myocarditis

Outcome/effect
Demonstrates that viral infection is the most common presenting diagnosis of myocarditis

Historical significance/comments
Demonstrates the common signs and symptoms that distinguish myocarditis from other disease states at presentation

Interpersonal and Communication Skills

Identify and Engage Appropriate Resources and Communicate Directly

Because of the severity of this illness it is important to transfer the patient to a tertiary care center that is equipped to treat critically ill children. This includes a pediatric intensive care unit and a cardiology team. Prompt person-to-person communication with these professionals will assist in obtaining the diagnosis and treatment rapidly, allow for the receiving team to ask specific questions, and avoid confusion and delays in deciphering information once the patient arrives in a new setting.

Professionalism

Being Aware of the Limits of Our Expertise

It is incumbent upon us as medical professionals to know what we know, to know what we don't know, and to be comfortable asking for help from others when we suspect we have reached the limits of our expertise. The diagnosis of myocarditis presents such a challenge. As soon as a diagnosis of myocarditis is suspected, a primary care physician should arrange transfer to an appropriate facility where tertiary care can be provided. Failure to recognize the need for help early in this process may result in an avoidable deterioration in a patient's clinical status.

Systems-Based Practice

Informed Consent and Patient Bill of Rights

The child with myocarditis often requires procedures such as central venous access or cardiac catheterization for diagnosis and treatment. Given the severity of illness of these patients, these procedures have a higher incidence of complication and even mortality. When obtaining informed consent for procedures, it is of paramount importance to communicate these risks honestly. Minimizing the known risks with the good intention of "not alarming" a parent is ultimately not helpful. If a patient or parent agrees to the procedure, but these risks have not been outlined or understood, then informed consent has not been truly obtained. See Chapter 104, Informed Consent, for a more detailed discussion of this matter.

Professor's Pearls
Section VI: The Pediatric Intensive Care Unit
Lewis P. Singer MD, FCCM

Consider the following clinical problems and questions posed. Then refer to a discussion of these issues by Lewis P. Singer MD, FCCM, Professor of Clinical Pediatrics, Department of Pediatrics, Albert Einstein College of Medicine, Bronx, New York.

1. **Case:** A 3-week-old infant was transferred to the pediatric critical care unit because of a gradual onset of tachypnea and difficulty feeding. The infant has good symmetric breath sounds, no cardiac murmur, a soft abdomen with the liver palpated 3 cm below the costal margin, and warm hands and feet. What further information do you need to help you make a diagnosis? What would be the next step in management?

2. **Case:** A 13-year-old boy is admitted to the hospital with weakness 2 weeks after receiving an influenza vaccine. He initially had difficulty walking and is now unable to stand without support. He has a history of asthma. On examination, there is marked weakness of his lower extremities with absent ankle and knee deep tendon reflexes (DTRs). What is his likely diagnosis? At what point would you place this patient in an intensive care unit for closer monitoring and support?

3. **Case:** A previously healthy 4-year-old child is admitted to the intensive care unit after presenting to the emergency department with a seizure. The child developed a high fever, cough, and poor urine output over the previous day. The chest radiograph demonstrated right lower lobe consolidation. The child does not appear dehydrated. What are the possible diagnoses? What complication should you be concerned about?

4. **Case:** A previously healthy 6-week-old male infant is admitted with diarrhea and assessed to be 10% dehydrated. The baby's birth weight was 3.4 kg. His weight 1 week ago during a well child visit was 4.2 kg. Despite adequate fluid resuscitation, the child remains acidotic and has an ashen color but has begun to make urine. Why is the child still acidotic?

5. **Case:** A previously healthy 19-year-old presents to the emergency department with a chief complaint of light-headedness and concern for the way she is breathing. Her vital signs are temperature of 39° C (102.2° F), heart rate of 154 beats per minute, respiratory rate of 40 breaths per minute, and a blood pressure of 80/30 mm Hg. Her skin is erythematous. What are the most likely diagnoses? What should be her initial management?

6. **Case:** A 3-week-old infant is admitted to the intensive care unit for management of abdominal distention and respiratory compromise. The baby was born at home, has been poorly feeding over the last few days, and did not pass meconium until the third

day of life. What is the baby's most likely diagnosis? What is the most concerning complication? What should be the best management for this young infant?

7. **Case:** A 16-year-old is admitted to the hospital with a history of a sore throat on treatment with penicillin. She now has neck pain, cervical swelling and tenderness, and continued high fever, and she has developed tachypnea. Chest radiograph demonstrates bilateral "cannonball" infiltrates. What is her diagnosis? Which imaging study might confirm the diagnosis? How should this patient be managed?

8. **Case:** A 3-month-old infant who was born prematurely at 25 weeks' gestation comes to your office for a checkup. The baby has bronchopulmonary dysplasia and is taking both hydrochlorothiazide and aldactone. The family is planning a trip to Disney World. Is it safe for this child to fly on a commercial jet? What are the issues involved?

Discussion by Lewis P. Singer MD, FCCM, Professor of Clinical Pediatrics, Department of Pediatrics, Albert Einstein College of Medicine, Bronx, New York.

1. **Discussion:** Evaluation of any patient should be done in a systematic manner, including the evaluation of vital signs, which in this patient makes the diagnosis. The vital signs revealed a temperature of 37° C (98.6° F), a respiratory rate of 72 breaths per minute, a heart rate of 300 beats per minute, and a blood pressure of 66/36 mm Hg. The heart rate is consistent with a supraventricular tachycardia (SVT). An electrocardiogram (EKG) should be performed and a pediatric cardiologist consulted. Though vagal maneuvers can be tried, intravenous adenosine is usually diagnostic and therapeutic. Long-term management will likely include propranolol. Digoxin is usually not prescribed because digoxin promotes conduction through the bundle of Kent in patients with Wolff-Parkinson-White syndrome (WPW) with the risk for inducing ventricular tachycardia and subsequent ventricular fibrillation. WPW may present with SVT and not be diagnosed until multiple EKGs are performed over an extended period of time.

2. **Discussion:** This patient likely has a postvaccination ascending paralysis—Guillain-Barré syndrome. Because of potential respiratory compromise, this is a medical emergency. Difficulty with speaking or swallowing indicates bulbar palsy. Bradycardia, hypotension, or hypertension may develop. Approximately 30% of patients with Guillain-Barré syndrome will require respiratory support. Monitoring the forced vital capacity (FVC) is very helpful in determining which patients will require respiratory support. When the FVC falls below 20 mL/kg or the child develops evidence of bulbar palsy, the child should be placed in the intensive care unit. As the FVC approaches 10 mL/kg, the child should be electively intubated.

3. **Discussion:** Fever, cough, and pulmonary infiltrate in a child, associated with oliguria and no signs of dehydration, could be a classic presentation for atypical hemolytic uremic syndrome (HUS) associated with invasive pneumococcal disease. The complications of seizures and renal failure are both due to microangiopathic hemolysis. In a recent paper from the United Kingdom there was an increasing incidence of this pneumococcal-associated syndrome. Early mortality was eight times higher than with diarrhea-associated HUS. The pneumococcal vaccine did not cover most pneumococcal strains isolated.

4. **Discussion:** Though there are many causes for acidosis, oximetry may be diagnostic. Methemoglobinemia is sometimes induced during infantile diarrhea. This usually occurs in infants under 3 months of age. The level of methemoglobinemia is very variable but has been reported as high as 57%. Young infants are highly susceptible due to their high levels of fetal hemoglobin, which is much more easily oxidized to methemoglobin than adult hemoglobin, and because their red blood cells have lower activity of NADH methemoglobin reductase. Treatment with intravenous methylene blue or vitamin C along with intravenous hydration should be considered.

5. **Discussion:** In a patient who is not immunosuppressed, septic shock is unusual, but toxic shock syndrome can occur in any patient with a staphylococcal or streptococcal infection. This is characterized by the typical signs and symptoms of septic shock with marked fever, tachycardia, tachypnea, and hypotension. A patient may present with light-headedness and progress to depressed mental function. This patient was having difficulty breathing, which was an early sign of impending respiratory failure. Other associated abnormalities are erythroderma; conjunctival injection; pharyngeal inflammation; and renal, hepatic, and myocardial dysfunction. Hydrops of the gallbladder and thrombocytopenia are not uncommon. One to 3 weeks after onset of the illness, the patient generally develops desquamation of the digits, palms, and soles.

6. **Discussion:** Hirschsprung disease would be at the top of the differential diagnosis in a baby who did not pass meconium until the third day of life. Babies who have untreated Hirschsprung disease are at risk for toxic megacolon with subsequent perforation, peritonitis, and septic shock. Bowel decompression with a colostomy is potentially lifesaving. Another diagnosis to consider is a midgut volvulus in a patient with malrotation.

7. **Discussion:** This patient has Lemierre disease, a rare complication of pharyngeal infection in which Fusobacterium species cause a suppurative thrombophlebitis. Computed tomography (CT) scan with contrast of the neck would confirm the diagnosis of septic

thrombophlebitis of the jugular and surrounding veins throwing septic emboli to the lungs, causing the radiographic "cannonball lesions." Blood cultures may be positive. High-dose penicillin and metronidazole is therapeutic.

8. **Discussion:** A child with bronchopulmonary dysplasia who requires diuretic therapy has at least moderate chronic respiratory failure with a metabolic alkalosis from a combination of diuretic therapy and chronic CO_2 retention. Let's assume the baby's normal Po_2 is 65 mm Hg in room air at sea level. Commercial airliners are pressured to an atmospheric pressure comparable to 8000 feet above sea level, 572 mm Hg compared with 760 mm Hg at sea level. People with normal pulmonary physiology will have an arterial Po_2 of approximately 70 mm Hg during a flight. Assuming that our patient's alveolar-arterial gradient (23 mm Hg) remains the same at 8000 feet as it is at sea level, using the alveolar gas equation, we can predict that the baby's Po_2 will be below 50 mm Hg. This child may fly to Disney World but definitely needs supplemental oxygen during the flight to prevent cyanosis.

Section VII
THE EMERGENCY DEPARTMENT

Section Editor

Magdy W. Attia MD

Section Contents

Chapter 91
Focused Evaluation of the Emergent Pediatric Patient: An Introduction for the Student

R. Jason Adams MD and Magdy W. Attia MD

The pediatric emergency department is a relatively new subspecialty. With the unfortunate inaccessibility of primary care and the readily available medical information of the Internet stirring the anxiety of parents, concerns and chief complaints of short duration may present to the emergency department (ED) rather than to the primary care physician. There has been an exponential increase in ED visits throughout the country, resulting in increased utilization of resources and increased wait times for care. Patients with a wide variety of chief complaints and diagnoses are evaluated and treated routinely. The ability to perform a rapid but focused evaluation, while considering the possibility of a serious underlying disease state, is an essential skill required to efficiently triage the child with severe illness or trauma who needs immediate treatment.

Medical Knowledge and Patient Care

When first assessing a child in the ED, the physician should immediately determine whether the patient is ill-appearing or toxic. In the case of an unresponsive patient in shock, resuscitative measures to stabilize the airway, breathing, and circulation (ABCs) should be promptly initiated. For trauma cases, a rapid assessment using the primary survey should be carried out to identify and treat life-threatening injuries.

The history will be focused on:

- **Chief complaint:** The chief complaint will steer the physician in the direction of an organ system. Further questioning in a non-leading manner typically refines the chief complaint(s) and could redirect the physician to other organ systems that could be involved.
- **Onset of symptoms:** Insidious versus sudden. For instance, sudden onset of abdominal pain is more concerning than pain developing over weeks.

- ***Duration of symptoms:*** The ED physician can be challenged by a convoluted or protracted history of the present illness, but must remain focused on recent changes in symptoms in order to address the emergent needs.
- ***Associated symptoms:*** Symptoms such as pain, rash, respiratory symptoms, nausea and vomiting, though nonspecific, could be diagnostic clues and should be elicited in the review of systems.
- ***Past medical history:*** This is an integral part of the history. For example, patients with a chronic underlying medical condition such as chronic lung disease with episodic acute illness may require a more thorough evaluation than a child who is perfectly healthy with the same complaints of a fever and cough. Similarly, the child with previous intra-abdominal surgery who presents with abdominal pain may be more worrisome and may present a greater diagnostic challenge than a patient without a history of prior surgery.

The information obtained in the history will focus your attention to expected findings on physical examination. Unlike the examination performed during a well child visit encounter, the examination in the ED is derived primarily from the chief complaint and the history of present illness. The challenge to the clinician's medical knowledge is to identify the relevant components of the focused physical examination in this setting. Important aspects of the physical examination include:

- Vital signs: Temperature, heart rate, respiratory rate, and blood pressure. Obtaining, documenting, and interpreting vital signs of the patient in the emergency department are imperative.
- General: Unresponsiveness, irritability or lethargy, hydration status, toxic appearance, and response to interventions, including examination, All yield clues to the seriousness of the illness. Similarly, in trauma cases, the primary survey will identify life-threatening injuries such as hemorrhage, tension pneumothorax, and cardiac tamponade.
- Head, ears, eyes, nose, and throat (HEENT): Anterior fontanelle, if open—bulging may be a sign of meningitis; tympanic membranes—bulging, erythema, presence of pus, immobility; eyes—injection, erythema, discharge, extraocular movements, fundoscopic examination when indicated; mouth—gum swelling/tenderness; throat—vesicles/ulcers, tonsillar injection/exudates; sinus tenderness.
- Neck: Neck stiffness/decreased range of motion, especially flexion; Brudzinski sign is involuntary hip/knee flexion with active flexion of neck. In the case of trauma, cervical spine (C-spine) tenderness. The clinician should follow the C-spine clearance protocol.
- Lymph: Lymphadenopathy of cervical, axillary, or inguinal areas.

- Chest: Crackles/rales/rhonchi—especially if focal; cough—observe for type and quality; presence of retractions or differential air exchange.
- Heart: Heart rate; abnormal sounds, especially murmurs, gallops, rubs, or distant heart sounds.
- Abdomen: Tenderness, rebound, guarding; liver/spleen size; masses; costovertebral angle (CVA) tenderness.
- Extremities: Joint erythema/swelling/tenderness/warmth; range of motion; Kernig sign is pain with flexion of hip and extension of knee.
- Neurologic findings: Motor tone, strength, reflexes, sensory examination, and gait.
- Skin: Rash, petechiae, purpura; erythema/induration/fluctuance.

Practice-Based Learning and Improvement

The Emergency Department: A Rich Setting for Practice-Based Learning and Improvement

For students and trainees in particular, the emergency department is a perfect opportunity to fulfill the competency of Practice-Based Learning and Improvement. When challenged by a case, identify your personal areas of weakness and/or inexperience. Search the literature and discuss the case with your mentors. Assimilate what you have learned, and apply it to your practice.

Interpersonal and Communication Skills

Multitasking in the Emergency Department Can Distract Even the Best Communicators

The emergency department is a busy place where physicians are called upon to see multiple patients at the same time. Effective communication with the patient and his/her family is essential to ensure a complete understanding of the problem. The family should be continuously kept up to date on the patient's status, and should be notified of any changes. Understandably, physicians are called upon to see other patients. In such instances, be sure to assign a nurse or other liaison to keep patients and their caregivers updated and informed.

Professionalism

Communication and Collaboration: Be Prepared for Your Consultants

Before discussing a patient with a consultant, a physician should have already acquired detailed information about all aspects of the case, including the following: history of present illness or mechanism of injury; vital signs; physical examination findings; past medical history, including medications and allergies. A social history, including mention of the caregivers who have brought the child to the emergency department, is also relevant.

Systems-Based Practice

Bill for What Is Documented; Avoid Accusations of Fraud

"If it's not documented, it's not done." Although many practitioners know this to be a false statement, it is of critical importance when physician billing is concerned. Physician services are billed based upon the level of complexity of the patient encounter. A focused encounter is often (but not always) just that: a focused physical examination and a focused problem set. A physician's documentation must accurately reflect the complexity of an encounter (according to the established codes), and billing must be consistent with such documentation. Physicians should not subject themselves to accusations of fraud by billing at levels that are not consistent with what has been documented.

Chapter 92
Dehydration (Case 49)

Cara B. Doughty MD, MEd *and*
Deborah Hsu MD, MEd

Case: A 3-month-old male infant with persistent low-grade fever, nonbilious/nonbloody vomiting, and copious diarrhea

Differential Diagnosis

Gastroenteritis: viral or bacterial	Pyloric stenosis
Milk-protein allergy	Intussusception

Speaking Intelligently

When faced with a dehydrated child, my management is primarily determined by the child's degree of dehydration. With **mild to moderate dehydration,** slow oral rehydration is generally effective, except in patients with ongoing active emesis. In cases of **moderate to severe dehydration,** I proceed directly to intravenous hydration and administer isotonic saline at 20 mL/kg. I reevaluate the patient after each bolus of fluid, assessing the response. I observe vital signs and urine output closely, and, so that I can best determine disposition, I note whether or not the child can tolerate oral fluids. In some situations an anti-emetic may be indicated, but one must be careful not to mask another diagnosis when suppressing vomiting by pharmacologic means. If the child is moderately dehydrated or otherwise ill-appearing, it is generally wise to check serum electrolytes.

PATIENT CARE

Clinical Thinking
- Monitor and support **airway, breathing, and circulation.**
- What diagnostic tests, if any, would be useful to help you make an accurate diagnosis or formulate a treatment plan?

- In determining disposition, consider clinical criteria, availability of home care and close follow-up, ability to return if condition worsens, and parental understanding of and willingness to follow the care plan.

History

- Consider underlying **chronic medical conditions.**
- Fever in an otherwise healthy child with these symptoms is most commonly a viral gastroenteritis.
- History of other **sick contacts** and recent **medications** may yield clues to the diagnosis.
- A history of recent **travel,** unusual **food intake,** or exposure to reptiles, along with bloody diarrhea, may increase concern for bacterial gastroenteritis.
- Determine amount of **oral intake,** frequency and amount of **vomiting** and **diarrhea,** and **urine output.**

Physical Examination

- Vital signs: **Tachycardia** can be an early sign of dehydration, or related to fever and anxiety. Hypotension is a late and ominous finding.
- Realize that the normal range for heart rate, blood pressure, and respiratory rate varies with age.
- Change in weight from baseline, if known, helps to assess degree of dehydration.
- Clinical assessment includes pulse, blood pressure, skin turgor, decreased tearing, dry mucous membranes, a sunken fontanelle in infants, decreased urine output, and systemic signs such as lethargy.
- Complete examination with particular focus on heart, chest, abdominal, genitourinary examination, and neurologic examination.

Tests for Consideration

- **Electrolytes:** Bicarbonate to assess acidosis, sodium to identify hypernatremia or hyponatremia, hypokalemia secondary to potassium losses in emesis or stool. $29
- **Urinalysis:** If concern for urinary tract infection; specific gravity can assist in assessing degree of dehydration in older infants and children. $38
- **Complete blood count (CBC):** If concern for bleeding, infection, hemolytic uremic syndrome (HUS) $53
- **Specific stool studies in select cases** *Clostridium difficile* **toxin)**
  - **Stool occult blood** $170
  - **Stool white blood cells** $80
  - **Bacterial culture** $170
  - **Rapid rotavirus antigen** $170
  - **Stool ova and parasites, usually obtained on 3 consecutive days** $202 each
  - *Clostridium difficile* **toxin** $169

IMAGING CONSIDERATIONS

→ **Abdominal obstruction series:** If concern for bowel obstruction, ileus, intussusception $219
→ **Abdominal ultrasound:** If concern for intussusception, pyloric stenosis, appendicitis $846
→ **Abdominal/pelvic computed tomography (CT):** If concern for intraabdominal or pelvic mass, or appendicitis $1691

Clinical Entities   Medical Knowledge

Gastroenteritis

Pφ **Viral gastroenteritis:** Viruses causing gastroenteritis include rotaviruses, caliciviruses, astroviruses, adenoviruses types 40 and 41, and some picornaviruses. Viruses infect and destroy enterocytes, resulting in transudation of fluid into the intestinal lumen. They are predominantly transmitted via the fecal-oral route, with peak incidence in children 3 to 24 months of age. Cases and hospitalizations typically peak during the winter months, with up to 7% to 10 % of all pediatric hospitalizations resulting from acute gastroenteritis.

Bacterial gastroenteritis: Bacterial sources of gastroenteritis include but are not limited to *Salmonella, Campylobacter, Shigella,* enterohemorrhagic and enterotoxigenic *Escherichia coli, Clostridium perfringens* and *C. botulinum, Staphylococcus aureus,* group A streptococcus, *Yersinia enterocolitica,* and *Listeria monocytogenes.* Most of these bacteria are the cause of foodborne-disease outbreaks resulting from multiple factors but most commonly improper food storage and poor hygiene practices of food handlers, with direct person-to-person spread being a common cause. Young children and immunocompromised patients are at highest risk for developing serious consequences.

TP Infectious gastroenteritis typically presents with fever, vomiting, diarrhea, abdominal cramping, myalgias, and varying degrees of dehydration. Although no one clinical feature distinguishes viral from bacterial gastroenteritis, watery nonbloody stools without mucus are more likely viral. Symptoms may change as the disease develops and may differ within a family.

Dx   Diagnosis is primarily clinical. It is most important to assess for signs of dehydration and evidence for competing diagnoses that would require a different approach. In a straightforward case without severe dehydration, no diagnostic tests are needed unless a bacterial etiology is suspected, in which case stool cultures may be indicated.

Tx   Treatment of both viral and bacterial gastroenteritis is supportive and primarily depends on the patient's degree of dehydration and ability to maintain hydration.

Antibiotic therapy should be administered in select cases to those in whom a pathogen has been isolated with ongoing symptoms after identification of the pathogen (such as *Shigella* and *Clostridium difficile*) or in patients who develop bacteremia, sepsis, or other extraintestinal infections such as osteomyelitis or meningitis.[1,2] **See Nelson Essentials 112.**

Milk-protein allergy

Pφ   Cow or milk is a common cause of food allergy, affecting about 2.5% of children in the first 2 years of life. These allergies may be IgE mediated, causing gastrointestinal (GI) anaphylaxis, or non–IgE mediated, which causes dietary protein–induced proctitis/colitis, enteropathy, or enterocolitis. Most infants with *milk-protein allergy* develop tolerance with resolution of symptoms by 3 years of age.

TP   Patients with IgE-mediated allergy causing GI anaphylaxis typically present with acute-onset nausea, vomiting, abdominal pain/cramping, and/or diarrhea within minutes to 6 hours after ingestion.

Patients with non–IgE mediated allergies have more subacute or chronic symptoms.

Infants with protein-induced enterocolitis are often ill-appearing and present with chronic GI symptoms of vomiting, diarrhea, and malabsorption resulting in failure to thrive (FTT), and/or melena. However, patients with dietary protein–induced **proctitis/colitis,** present with microscopic gross blood in the stool. Although the blood loss may cause mild anemia, these patients are unlikely to be ill-appearing or have FTT as seen in patients with dietary protein–induced **enterocolitis.** Symptoms typically resolve with removal of the causative agent.[3]

Dx   Dietary trials and skin tests are used for diagnosis.

Tx   Treatment includes removal of the causative agent and supportive care with intravenous fluid hydration and electrolyte imbalance correction an needed. (See Chapter 34, Diarrhea.) **See Nelson Essentials 129.**

Pyloric Stenosis

Pφ   In infantile hypertrophic *pyloric stenosis* the pylorus is
elongated and thickened, leading to near-to-complete
obstruction of the gastric outlet. The etiology is unclear, but
most likely multifactorial, ranging from genetic predisposition
to environmental factors. Administration of macrolides
(specifically oral erythromycin) is associated with increased
risk for developing pyloric stenosis.

TP   Patients typically present between 3 and 6 weeks of age with
nonbilious projectile emesis immediately after feeds. It occurs
in 2 to 3.5 live births, with a male predominance. The so-called
"hungry vomiter" is hungry soon after vomiting and demands to
be refed quickly. In the past, infants have been described as
being emaciated and dehydrated at presentation with
electrolyte abnormalities revealing a hypochloremic metabolic
alkalosis; now with earlier diagnoses, infants with pyloric
stenosis are typically well nourished with no or very minimal
electrolyte abnormalities.

Dx   The classic teaching is a palpable "olive" on physical
examination (unlikely to be palpable unless the patient is
completely relaxed). Pyloric ultrasound is the imaging study of
choice for diagnosis. Before the advent of ultrasonography,
upper gastrointestinal contrast study was used to confirm
diagnosis with the "string sign" demonstrated by the slow
passage of barium through the narrowed pyloric channel. In
addition, electrolyte levels should be obtained for these infants
to screen for the electrolyte abnormalities mentioned above.

Tx   In the emergency department, ensure adequate hydration for
these patients. Patients with normal electrolyte levels and mild
dehydration may be managed with maintenance intravenous
fluids (IVF). If the patient is moderately to severely dehydrated,
IVF resuscitation with isotonic solution should be administered.
Patients should not undergo surgical correction, the definitive
treatment for this condition, until after any metabolic alkalosis
and volume depletion have been corrected have been corrected
because metabolic alkalosis has been associated with an
increased risk for postoperative apnea in these infants.[4] **See
Nelson Essentials 128.**

Intussusception

See Chapter 94, Abdominal Pain.

ZEBRA ZONE

a. **Hemolytic uremic syndrome (HUS):** This disorder consists of microangiopathic hemolytic anemia, thrombocytopenia, and acute renal injury. The majority of children with HUS have Shiga toxin–associated HUS caused mostly by strains of Shiga toxin–producing *E. coli.*

b. **Short bowel syndrome:** Consider if the patient was a former premature infant who had necrotizing enterocolitis and extensive intestinal resection.

c. **Intracranial mass:** Consider if the patient has prolonged vomiting and little or no diarrhea along with other signs of increased intracranial pressure, such as headache on morning waking.

d. **Appendicitis:** In older children, appendicitis is a common cause of dehydration; children often present with abdominal pain, vomiting, inability to tolerate oral intake, and subsequent development of dehydration.

Practice-Based Learning and Improvement: Evidence-Based Medicine

Title
Usefulness of the serum electrolyte panel in the management of pediatric dehydration treated with intravenously administered fluids

Authors
Wathen JE, MacKenzie T, Bothner JP

Reference
Pediatrics 114:1227-1234, 2004

Problem
Evaluate the utility of routinely ordering the serum electrolyte panel in the treatment of dehydrated patients receiving intravenous fluids

Intervention
Prospective study of pediatric patients ages 2 months to 9 years receiving IVFs in a pediatric emergency department. Attending physicians documented whether they would have ordered electrolytes before knowing laboratory results. Outcomes included whether electrolyte results changed clinical management, and correlation of disposition with electrolyte results.

Comparison/control (quality of evidence)
Prospective study of 182 patients. No control group.

Outcome/effect
The authors defined significant electrolyte abnormalities as bicarbonate <16 mEq/L, glucose <60 mg/dL, blood urea nitrogen (BUN) >17 mg/dL, K <3.5 mEq/L, or Na >150 mEq/L. Eighty-eight patients (48%) had one or more abnormalities found, but in only 19 patients (10.4%), the electrolytes changed clinical management (IV glucose, potassium supplementation, longer observation).

Historical significance/comments
Serum electrolytes may not be necessary in the management of every infant and child presenting to the emergency department with dehydration.

Interpersonal and Communication Skills

Acknowledge the Caregiver's Burden

Caregivers may be tired and sleep deprived from having had to care for a child requiring frequent diaper changes or multiple changes of clothing after bouts of emesis. When appropriate, give positive reinforcement to the caregiver who has spent time trying to keep the child well hydrated. An expression of empathy for what the caregivers have had to endure with their child's illness often goes a long way in reinforcing the caregivers' positive behaviors and in reassuring everyone concerned that the child will be well as long as adequate fluid intake can be maintained.

Professionalism

Anticipate and Respond to Parental Expectations

Parents are often aware that children with vomiting and diarrhea get admitted to the hospital to receive intravenous fluid. You will at times encounter parents who will expect that this will be done for their child. When you determine that a child is a candidate for oral rehydration, be sensitive to the possibility that the expectations of the parents may be quite different from your own. Your anticipation, understanding, and compassion will help avoid a situation that is potentially confrontational.

Systems-Based Practice

The Emergency Medical Treatment and Active Labor Act and Its Provisions

Although most hospital emergency departments are equipped to deal with a severely dehydrated child in shock, such a case often is not routine unless the hospital is a pediatric hospital. Hence, institutions often seek to transfer such patients to a pediatric facility as soon as possible. Before transferring such a patient, however, hospitals and physicians have an ethical and legal responsibility to stabilize and treat such patients. The legal burden comes from the **Emergency Medical Treatment and Active Labor Act (EMTALA).** EMTALA was initially designed to prevent hospitals from "dumping" patients without means to pay onto other hospitals. EMTALA imposes three requirements on institutions that provide emergency medical services (i.e., the institution has an emergency department [ED]):

- The hospital must provide an appropriate medical screening examination to anyone coming to the ED seeking medical care.
- For anyone who comes to the hospital and is determined to have an emergency medical condition, the hospital must treat and stabilize the emergency medical condition.
- A hospital must not transfer an individual with an emergency medical condition who has not been stabilized unless several conditions are met, which includes arranging and implementing an appropriate transfer.

References

1. Wong CS, Jelacic S, Habeeb RL, et al: The risk of the hemolytic-uremic syndrome after antibiotic treatment of *Escherichia coli* 0157:H7 infection. *N Engl J Med* 342:1930, 2000.
2. Harper MB, Fleisher GR: Infectious disease emergencies. In Fleisher GR, Ludwig S, editors: *Textbook of pediatric emergency medicine*, Philadelphia, 2010, Wolters Kluwer/Lippincott Williams and Wilkins.
3. duToit G, Meyer R, Shah N, et al: Identifying and managing cow's milk protein allergy. *Arch Dis Child Educ Pract Ed* 95:134-144, 2010.
4. Steven IM, Allen TH, Sweeney DB: Congenital hypertrophic pyloric stenosis: The anesthetist's view. *Anaesth Intensive Care* 1:544, 1973.

Chapter 93
Lumps and Bumps (Case 50)

Maria Stephan MD

Case: An 8-month-old who presents with a neck lump

Differential Diagnosis

Lesions Occurring Anywhere on the Body	Lesions Occurring in Specific Anatomic Locations

Cutaneous:
  Abscess
  Nevus
  Warts
  Molluscum contagiosum
  Insect bites
  Sebaceous cysts
  Hemangioma
  Pyogenic granuloma
	Head and neck:
	Cutaneous:
	  Neck sinus
	  Periauricular skin tag and sinus
	Deep:
	  Thyroglossal duct cyst
	  Branchial cleft cyst
	  Cystic hygroma
	  Lymphadenopathy
	  Tumor/neoplasm

Subcutaneous:
  Hemangioma
  Lipoma
	Trunk:
	  Epigastric hernia
	  Supernumerary nipple

Deep:
  Foreign body
  Hematoma
  Benign or malignant tumor
	Upper extremity:
	  Granuloma annulare
	  Ganglion cyst

	Lower extremity:
	  Ganglion cyst, Baker cyst
	  Erythema nodosum
	  Pseudorheumatoid nodule
	  Hidradenitis suppurativa (groin)

Speaking Intelligently

Many conditions can be diagnosed on visual inspection. Clues from the history can make the process of distinguishing between entities easier. A good history is paramount. On initial inspection, I ask about the following: known duration, change in size, presence of pain or inflammation, how many there are, and where they started.

Have there been exposures to any potentially inciting agents such as drugs, insects, foods, chemicals or trauma? Are there any systemic manifestations such as fever, weight loss, arthralgias, or arthritis? The location of the lesions is often suggestive of the cause. For example, in the head and neck region, swollen nodes are often in response to focal infectious processes occurring in areas that drain to the region of the nodes. Timing, duration, and age of the patient are also informing: congenital anatomic defects of the neck, for example, are often inapparent at birth, but may develop into significant cystic masses over time.

PATIENT CARE

Clinical Thinking
- What are the patient's **vital signs?** Is there any indication of systemic involvement or patient distress?
- If the lesions are on the body, look for signs of **infection, inflammation,** or **redness** with surrounding cellulitis.
- Does the lesion feel hard or cystic?
- Is the lesion the same color as skin or is it pigmented?

History
- See Speaking Intelligently.

Physical Examination
- Essentially all lesions originating in the skin of children are benign.
- Most inflammatory conditions present as red papules or nodules.
- Vascular tumors are usually bright red or purple with sharply demarcated borders.
- Determine how deep in the skin this lesion occurs and its size. If it is a cutaneous lesion, the skin does not move over the surface and puckers when the adjacent skin and tissue are compressed and elevated.
- If the bump is palpated over the underlying fascia, it is in the subcutaneous tissue and is essentially benign. However, if the lesion is fixed to the underlying fascia, or the examiner cannot be sure, then the possibility of malignancy should be considered.
- Examine the lesion for **signs of infection**—tenderness on palpation, redness or cellulitis of the surrounding skin; note if the central area is fluctuant, as in an abscess.
- The location of a lesion will often define its etiology.

Tests for Consideration
- **Complete blood count (CBC)** An elevated white blood cell count can strengthen your diagnosis of an infectious process. A low platelet count is consistent with the diagnosis of petechiae. **$35**

- **Erythrocyte sedimentation rate (ESR):** If considering an underlying systemic inflammatory process, either ESR or CRP (or both) is often elevated $25
- **C-reactive protein** $25
- **Blood culture:** Cultures identify specific bacterial etiologies and may allow narrowing of your antibiotic therapy $100
- **Throat culture** $20
- **Test for mononucleosis and streptococci:** When appropriate to evaluate cervical lymphadenopathy $45
- **Purified protein derivative (PPD):** When tuberculosis is in the differential diagnosis $10
- **Aspiration of the node for culture and sensitivity:** May be required to define the process as specific and guide appropriate antibiotic therapy .... $100-$1000

IMAGING CONSIDERATIONS

→ **Ultrasound of lesions:** For questions of cystic versus solid $325
→ **Neck computed tomography (CT) with contrast:** Can be helpful in determining anatomic relationship of mass or abscess to important structures $1200

Clinical Entities	Medical Knowledge

Warts

Pφ	**Warts** are viral-induced intraepidermal tumors caused by human papillomavirus. Spontaneous resolution occurs in 9 to 24 months. They may be characterized on the basis of their appearance (flat, plantar, venereal).
TP	Most are skin colored, sharply demarcated papules that have a firm and rough surface. They are often asymptomatic, although on pressure-bearing surfaces they may be painful.
Dx	Diagnosis is made by visual inspection.
Tx	Cryotherapy—using a cotton swab dipped in liquid nitrogen, applied to the center of the wart for 20 to 30 seconds. Other topical therapies exist but require several weeks of therapy. These include salicylic acid paint (10%); salicylic acid plaster (40%); cantharidin applications; and podophyllin (25%) used for venereal warts. Most of these treatments are applied by specialty physicians. **See Nelson Essentials 98.**

Molluscum Contagiosum

Pφ	*Molluscum contagiosum* is a white or whitish-yellow papule with central umbilication caused by a poxvirus.
TP	The papules tend to be clustered, occurring anywhere on the skin surface. They may be in the genital area of adults as a sexually transmitted disease.
Dx	Diagnosis is made by visual inspection, as described above. In addition, Wright stain of the contents reveals epidermal cytoplasmic viral inclusions.
Tx	Sharp dermal curettage is the treatment of choice. Spontaneous resolution occurs in 2 to 3 years. **See Nelson Essentials 98.**

Abscess/Furuncle

Pφ	A *furuncle* is a deep lesion of bacterial folliculitis usually caused by staphylococcus or streptococcus.
TP	A painful, erythematous, indurated nodule may be single or occur in crops. It is often associated with a surrounding red flare. As the lesion matures, a central pustule develops and ruptures with drainage of contents.
Dx	Diagnosis is made by visual inspection.
Tx	First-line therapy for early nonfluctuant lesions is an oral antistaphyloccocal drug that also covers methicillin-resistant staphylococcus. (clindamycin or trimethoprim/sulfamethoxazole plus rifampin). **See Nelson Essentials 98.**

Nevus

Pφ	A *nevus* is a benign hamartoma of melanocytes. Nevi are extremely common. A congenital nevus has an increased risk for malignant transformation into malignant melanoma, although this transformation is rare during childhood. Dysplastic nevi develop in the second decade of life, have haphazard coloration, and are larger than 7 mm with poorly demarcated borders. Their morphologic appearance is intermediate between malignant melanoma and benign nevi.
TP	A benign nevus is an evenly pigmented brown lesion.
Dx	Referral to dermatology may be indicated with biopsy for histologic study in certain cases.
Tx	Refer to a specialist for treatment. A nevus may require surgical excision. **See Nelson Essentials 193.**

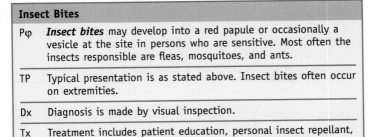

Insect Bites

Pφ   *Insect bites* may develop into a red papule or occasionally a vesicle at the site in persons who are sensitive. Most often the insects responsible are fleas, mosquitoes, and ants.

TP   Typical presentation is as stated above. Insect bites often occur on extremities.

Dx   Diagnosis is made by visual inspection.

Tx   Treatment includes patient education, personal insect repellant, and, for mild disease, corticosteroid creams. **See Nelson Essentials 195.**

Sebaceous Cysts

Pφ   *Sebaceous cysts* are formed from hair follicles that become blocked by a keratin plug or inflammation in a superficial scar over the surface. As epithelium continues to turn over, desquamated stratum corneum remains trapped in the follicle and keratin distends the follicle, forming the cyst.

TP   They may occur anywhere on the body where hair is located. The borders are smooth and well demarcated. They are concerning if located on the face, for cosmetic reasons, or if irritated by pressure, in which case they become inflamed.

Dx   Diagnosis is made by visual inspection and palpation.

Tx   Treatment is generally unnecessary. However, excision may be required for cosmetic or symptomatic lesions. When infected, cysts should be drained, irrigated, and allowed to heal by secondary intention. **See Nelson Essentials 188.**

Hemangioma

Pφ   *Hemangioma,* if capillary (strawberry birthmark), is a benign tumor of dilated blood vessels. It is the most common tumor of infancy.

TP   Generally, hemangiomas grow from birth to 6 months of age. Growth can happen very quickly. Involution of the lesion begins at 6 to 18 months, but lesions can last up to 5 years. Over time, the color changes from strawberry red to a more violaceous hue.

Dx   Diagnosis is made by visual inspection.

Tx   Treatment includes parental counseling. However, if the
      hemangioma occurs in an area causing organ compromise (e.g.,
      airway obstruction, compromised vision), other therapies may
      be required. These include excision, radiation, embolization,
      and laser therapy. **See Nelson Essentials 194.**

Lipoma

Pφ   *Lipoma* is a very common hamartoma of fatty tissue.

TP   Lipomas may occur anywhere on the body. The tumor has a
      characteristic soft appropriate texture with discrete borders.
      Lipomas are sometimes sensitive to pressure. Paraspinal lipomas
      may protrude deeply between the transverse spinous processes
      and encroach on spinal nerve foramina.

Dx   Diagnosis is made by clinical examination. Magnetic resonance
      imaging may be if the lesion is noted to be midline over the
      spine and needs to be differentiated from other conditions.

Tx   Excision is required if diagnosis is in doubt or if symptomatic.
      See Nelson Essentials 126.

Pyogenic Granuloma

Pφ   *Pyogenic granuloma* is a common skin growth. It is felt to be
      the site of skin trauma.

TP   It is a small, bright red, glistening bump. It looks like a
      hemangioma, but with a thin white border where it meets the
      skin. Left untreated, pyogenic granulomas grow slowly and
      bleed easily when abraded by minor trauma.
          Frequently granulomata may be noted in the umbilicus after
      sloughing of the umbilical cord.

Dx   Diagnosis is made by inspection.

Tx   Treatment includes silver nitrate, electrocautery, or excision.
      See Nelson Essentials 194.

Thyroglossal Duct Cyst

Pφ   *Thyroglossal duct cysts* develop along the line of descent of
      the thyroid gland in the neck, anywhere from the base of the
      tongue to the sternal notch.

TP	They are usually midline, near the hyoid bone, in children 2 to 10 years of age. They are soft and smooth and may move when the child swallows. With infection, they become red and tender and may drain.
Dx	Diagnosis is usually made by inspection and palpation. Ultrasound and contrast neck CT may be useful.
Tx	If the cyst is infected, antibiotics (covering mouth and skin flora) are indicated. Surgical excision is the treatment of choice. **See Nelson Essentials 50.**

Cystic Hygromas

Pφ	*Cystic hygromas* are cystic lymphatic malformations occurring in the posterior triangle of the neck.
TP	They are soft, mobile, and nontender. They vary in size, occur in the neck, and are often present at birth. Respiratory compromise can occur with large lesions.
Dx	Diagnosis is made by ultrasound or contrast neck CT.
Tx	Surgical excision is the treatment of choice. **See Nelson Essentials 50.**

Branchial Cleft Anomalies

Pφ	*Branchial cleft anomalies* are lesions occurring from defects in the development of the second branchial arch resulting in firm masses along the anterior border of the sternocleidomastoid muscle.
TP	Branchial cleft sinuses are painless and present with drainage at the junction of the middle and lower thirds of the sternocleidomastoid muscle. Cysts will be fluctuant, mobile, and nontender if the tract is blocked; or warm, red, and painful if infected.
Dx	Diagnosis is made by ultrasound or contrast neck CT.
Tx	Antibiotics are indicated if infected. Surgical excision is the treatment of choice. **See Nelson Essentials 50.**

Lymphadenopathy/Lymphadenitis

Pφ Cervical **lymphadenopathy** is the most common reason for neck masses in children. Etiologies for lymphadenopathy include bacterial or viral infections from local, regional, or systemic disease. Supraclavicular lymphadenopathy is considered pathologic, and a biopsy of a supraclavicular mass should be performed.

    Lymphadenitis occurs when acute infection is present in the lymph node. Bacteria are the most common causes and include methicillin-resistant *Staphylococcus aureus* and group A beta-hemolytic streptococci, as well as anaerobes such as *Peptostreptococcus*. If located in the inguinal area, consider sexually transmitted diseases as a possible etiology.

TP Usually one or more nodes are warm, red, tender, and enlarged. Often the cervical nodes are affected in children.

Dx Diagnosis is usually made by inspection and palpation. Ultrasound, contrast neck CT, needle aspiration, and PPD may be helpful for correct diagnosis.

Tx Antibiotics are indicated for infection. Incision and drainage may be required. **See Nelson Essentials 99.**

Ganglion Cysts

Pφ **Ganglion cysts** arise from tendon sheaths or the synovium of a joint.

TP Ganglion cysts are tense cystic masses that may present over the wrist, palm, or dorsum of the hand or fingers. Pain is a frequent complaint. In the lower extremities, ganglion cysts characteristically involve the ankle and feet.

Dx Diagnosis is made by inspection and palpation.

Tx Spontaneous resolution and recurrence occur. Surgical excision may be indicated. **See Nelson Essentials 203.**

Erythema Nodosum

Pφ **Erythema nodosum** is a vascular hypersensitivity reaction that occurs in the subcutaneous fat. No obvious cause is found in 50% of cases. Infections, especially streptococcal disease, histoplasmosis, tuberculosis, and *Yersinia* are known causes. Medications, such as oral contraceptives, estrogens, and sulfas; and chronic inflammatory diseases, such as sarcoidosis and inflammatory bowel disease, are also associated with erythema nodosum.

TP	Red, dusky, or violaceous tender nodules usually present on the shins but can be located in other areas.
Dx	Diagnosis is made by visual inspection. Sometimes it may be difficult to distinguish from other inflammatory processes. However, erythema nodosum lacks systemic toxicity and the lesions are nondraining lesions, thereby making it easier to differentiate from other diseases. If in doubt, a biopsy may be helpful.
Tx	Treatment includes identification and elimination of the cause, use of nonsteroidal antiinflammatory drugs, and elevation. **See Nelson Essentials 97.**

ZEBRA ZONE

a. Neuromas, fibromas, and neurofibromas: These arise from neural cells and can be benign or malignant varieties. They are also associated with systemic syndromes, such as neurofibromatosis.

b. Bony exostoses: These are typically benign growth from a bone. They can be damaging if in a critical area such as the spine.

Practice-Based Learning and Improvement

Title
Lumps and bumps in children

Author
Putnam TC

Reference
Pediatr Rev 13:371-378, 1992

Problem
Extensive review of superficial masses in children

Comparison/control (quality of evidence)
Review article with cited references in peer-reviewed journal

Historical significance/comments
Excellent overview of diagnosis and management of these lesions

Interpersonal and Communication Skills

Strive for Accuracy in Terminology

The primary care physician must often discuss cutaneous and subcutaneous lesions with a specialist (e.g., dermatologist, general surgeon). Knowledge of common dermatology vocabulary and its correct usage is paramount when describing lesions accurately to other health-care professionals. The clinician must use nouns descriptive of the patient's lesion (e.g., papule, nodule, mass, blister). Accuracy in this terminology is as important as discussing specific lung or cardiac findings. Incorrect description or misuse of such terminology may lead to misdiagnosis and/or an unnecessary workup.

Professionalism

Advocate by Being Careful and Comprehensive: Avoid Shortcuts

Physicians are often under time pressures when seeing patients. It is tempting therefore, when the chief complaint is a localized skin finding, to "speed up" the visit by a quick inspection, without examining the skin completely, which may be indicated. The physician who takes shortcuts and does not undress the patient fully may make an incorrect diagnosis and, by so doing, harm the patient.

Systems-Based Practice

Payment for "Cosmetic" Procedures

Surgical excision is medically justifiable for many of the reasons discussed in this chapter. Some lesions, however, are removed for cosmetic reasons only. Medicare, Medicaid, and most commercial insurance companies will not cover the cost of services they consider to be purely cosmetic. As the physician, it is your responsibility to medically justify such procedures to the insurance carrier, when you are able to do so honestly. When you are unable to do so, be sure that patients are aware that the burden of payment for such procedures may be their own responsibility.

Chapter 94
Abdominal Pain (Case 51)

John M. Howard DO,
Ruth D. Mayforth MD, PhD, and
Reza J. Daugherty MD

Case: A 5-year-old boy with a 2-day history of abdominal pain presents to the emergency department.

Differential Diagnosis

Appendicitis	Intussusception	Malrotation with midgut volvulus	
Gastroenteritis	Mesenteric adenitis	Constipation	Urinary tract infection Pyelonephritis

Speaking Intelligently

Obtaining an accurate description of pain is crucial: ***onset, quality, location, duration, and associated symptoms***. I use the information and physical examination to formulate and narrow my differential diagnosis and to determine the level of urgency. Patients with a possible surgical diagnosis are a top priority, as are patients who will require hydration and/or antibiotics. Knowledge of the differential diagnosis based on age is also essential, because there are unique diagnoses within each of the pediatric age-groups.

PATIENT CARE

Clinical Thinking
- A careful history and physical examination remain the cornerstones of assessment of the acute abdomen. When the patient is too young to provide a history, it is obtained from parents or adult caregivers.
- An important first step is to reassure the patient and family that the examination will be performed gently. Distracting the patient during the physical examination will often be helpful.
- If the patient has systemic manifestations of his/her illness, then resuscitative management should be initiated even while the diagnosis is in the process of being determined.

- Assess hydration status and provide IV fluids.
- Determine if surgical consultation is required.
- The use of CT to evaluate patients with abdominal pain has become quite prevalent in adults. This may not, however, be the best practice in pediatrics, as radiation may pose a long-term risk of cancer.
- Inquire about previous episodes of abdominal pain. Was a diagnosis obtained?

History

- Determine the location, onset, duration, severity, and type of pain. Is it constant or episodic? Has the pain shifted in location?
- Fever, anorexia, and behavioral changes, including lethargy, should be noted.
- Ask about emesis, diarrhea, constipation, passage of flatus, or blood in the stools.
- Note any previous abdominal surgery.
- In adolescent girls, note menstrual and sexual history.
- Has there been a previous consideration of *functional* abdominal pain? (A careful history and physical examination that is unrevealing, with judicious laboratory testing, may support this diagnosis; but it is still surely a **diagnosis of exclusion.**)

Physical Examination

- A complete examination is performed looking for signs and symptoms of inflammation and hypovolemia (e.g., prolonged capillary refill). The examination should also include attention to nonabdominal conditions that can present as abdominal pain (e.g., streptococcal pharyngitis, lower lobe pneumonia.)
- A detailed abdominal examination includes identifying the point of maximal tenderness. When palpating, the examination should begin away from the point of maximal tenderness and work toward tender areas. Focal peritoneal findings (tenderness to palpation and percussion, guarding, and rebound) may be present. Generalized peritonitis may present with more diffuse abdominal pain; in generalized peritonitis diffuse guarding would be expected. In advanced peritonitis the abdomen may appear "rigid."

Tests for Consideration

- **Complete blood count (CBC):** A leukocytosis, especially with a left shift, suggests an inflammatory process — $40
- **Urinalysis:** To rule out urinary tract infection, nephrolithiasis, or pyelonephritis — $50
- **Stool studies (culture, ova, and parasites):** If persistent diarrhea, gastroenteritis presentation — $120

IMAGING CONSIDERATIONS

→ **Obstruction series:** Look for evidence of obstruction (distended bowel loops, air fluids levels) or perforation (abdominal free air). Radiodense items such as kidney stones, gallstones, or an appendicolith (rare) may be visible. $200

→ **Ultrasonography:** No radiation or oral contrast is needed. False negatives do occur. Evaluates for intussusception, kidney stones, gallstones, appendicitis, and possible ovarian pathology $350

→ **Computed tomography (CT):** CT is used rarely and judiciously in small children. Substantial radiation dose and long delay in order to fill GI tract with contrast $800

→ **Barium swallow study:** Upper gastrointestinal tract to identify the ligament of Treitz if concern for malrotation $500

→ **Air-contrast enema:** If concern for intussusception—this may be both diagnostic and therapeutic $350

Clinical Entities	Medical Knowledge

Appendicitis

Pφ	The appendiceal lumen is initially obstructed (presumably by stool), leading to inflammation in the appendiceal wall; this leads to edema and bacterial overgrowth, resulting in erosion of the mucosal surface. This allows bacterial translocation, inflammation, ischemia, and ultimately perforation of the appendix with release of fecal contents and bacteria, leading to peritonitis.
TP	Classically, periumbilical abdominal pain precedes vomiting and is associated with low-grade fevers and anorexia. As the inflamed appendix makes contact with the peritoneum, the pain "migrates" from the periumbilical area and pinpoint tenderness is noted at the McBurney's point in the right lower quadrant (RLQ). If the appendix lies in an atypical orientation, the area of referred pain may be offset from the RLQ.

Dx   The diagnosis is based on clinical suspicion and supported by
     examination findings, laboratory test results, and imaging. An
     elevated white blood cell (WBC) count and absolute neutrophil
     count support this diagnosis. An elevated C-reactive protein
     level may also be an early marker for acute *appendicitis,* but
     sensitivities and specificities are not superior to WBC alone.[1]
     Urinalysis may demonstrate pyuria, hematuria, and/or
     bacteriuria. Abdominal pain films are not specific for acute
     appendicitis. An appendicolith is present in 10% of studies.
     CT studies with contrast or an ultrasound are preferred imaging
     studies. Ionizing radiation exposure with ultrasound, however,
     is operator-dependent and patient body habitus.

Tx   Intravenous fluids are administered for dehydration and third
     space losses. Antibiotic prophylaxis is indicated in early
     appendicitis, for wound infections or intra-abdominal abscess.[2]
     Finally, can be performed depending on the surgeon's
     preference. In children, perforated appendicitis with intra-
     abdominal fluid and a suspected appendiceal phlegmon or
     abscess is often treated with hospitalization and IV antibiotics;
     "interval appendectomy" is usually performed 6 to 8 weeks later
     when the child has recovered from the acute illness. **See
     Nelson Essentials 129.**

Intussusception

Pφ   Intussusception is an obstruction caused by bowel telescoping
     in on itself. The intussusceptum tunnels into the
     intussuscipiens, pulling mesentery and vasculature into the
     distal lumen. Venous and lymphatic congestion develops,
     causing intestinal edema, and possibly ischemia from obstructed
     arterial flow.

TP   Typical patients are 3 to 24 months old, but can be up to 6
     years and present with episodes of sudden-onset severe, colicky
     abdominal pain with irritability and drawing up of the knees.
     The patients are often lethargic between episodes. Patients
     often present following a viral prodrome. The classic triad of
     colicky pain, vomiting, and bloody mucous stool (current jelly
     stool) is relatively uncommon.[3]

Dx   A sausage-shaped mass in the RUQ may be palpable. Stool for
     occult blood may be positive. An obstruction series may be
     normal or may reveal a mass effect, usually in the RUQ with
     distended proximal bowel loops. The preferred study is an
     abdominal ultrasound, which may demonstrate a "bull's-eye" or
     "coiled spring" representing the intussusception.

Tx   A contrast enema is diagnostic and is therapeutic in 80% to 90% of cases. Air reduction is preferred because of a higher success rate and fewer complications. If used, contrast must be refluxed into the terminal ileum to ensure complete reduction. There is a 10% risk for recurrence after successful reduction by contrast enema. When an enema fails or if peritonitis is present, surgery is indicated. Surgery may consist of simple manual reduction or may require resection of an identified lead point or necrotic bowel. Some centers administer prophylactic antibiotics before contrast enema in the rare event of perforation during reduction. **See Nelson Essentials 129.**

Malrotation With Midgut Volvulus

Pφ   Malrotation results from the improper rotation of the intestines during embryogenesis. Improper fixation of the mesentery of the bowel to the posterior abdominal wall causes it to twist and obstruct, causing a volvulus.

TP   *Malrotation with volvulus* may occur in any infant or child. Presentation is usually bilious emesis and abdominal pain. The pain is severe and constant and can be associated with gross blood from the rectum—an indication of significant ischemia and possible necrosis of the bowel. Older children (>1 year) constitute 25% of these cases. On examination, the abdomen may be distended and diffusely tender.

Dx   Suspect malrotation in all children with sudden onset of bilious vomiting, severe abdominal pain, and hemodynamic instability. Clinically unstable patients should proceed directly to surgery for exploratory laparotomy. Stable patients are evaluated with plain radiographs, upper gastrointestinal (GI) contrast study, barium enema, or ultrasound. Plain films may be normal or may demonstrate a gasless abdomen or mild intestinal dilation. Especially concerning is the malpositioning of an orogastric or nasogastric tube in the duodenum or a "double bubble" sign consistent with duodenal obstruction. An upper GI study is the gold standard for visualization of the duodenum and the position of the ligament of Treitz. In malrotation, the ligament of Treitz may appear on the right side of the abdomen, or the duodenum may have a "corkscrew" appearance. Ultrasound may illustrate an abnormal position of the superior mesenteric vein or a dilated duodenum as a result of obstruction by Ladd bands.[4]

Tx   Fluid resuscitation should be administered. A nasogastric or orogastric tube is placed to decompress the stomach. Broad-spectrum antibiotics are initiated to cover for bowel flora. Surgical correction is urgently required and is life-saving. **See Nelson Essentials 129.**

Gastroenteritis

Pφ   Gastroenteritis is caused by a number of common pathogens, including both viruses and bacteria.

TP   The typical patient presents with vomiting followed by diarrhea. However, there may be only vomiting or only diarrhea. Stools may contain blood, more commonly with bacterial enteritis. Patients may have abdominal pain and signs of dehydration.

Dx   A history of sick contacts, travel, antibiotic use, and possible seafood ingestion should be obtained. The degree of dehydration should be assessed and serum electrolytes should be checked in severely dehydrated patients. Stools can be sent for analysis for fecal leukocytes, culture, and ova and parasites.

Tx   Mild to moderate dehydration is managed with oral rehydration with commercially available pediatric oral electrolyte solutions, which can often be done at home. For severe dehydration, significant emesis or high stool output may prevent adequate oral rehydration, making intravenous rehydration necessary. Antibiotics may be indicated for patients with diarrhea caused by *Clostridum difficlle, Shigella,* or *Salmonella.* See Chapter 34, Diarrhea, and Chapter 92, Dehydration. **See Nelson Essentials 112.**

Mesenteric Lymphadenitis

Pφ   Mesenteric lymphadenitis is inflammation of the mesenteric (usually ileocolic) lymph nodes, and may be due to either bacterial or viral pathogens. It may occur with streptococcal pharyngitis, and in children is more commonly associated with a primary enteric pathogen.

TP   The presentation is variable and may include fever, RLQ pain, anorexia, nausea, vomiting, and occasionally diarrhea. The site of tenderness may shift when the patient changes position (in contrast to appendicitis, where it usually remains in the same location). The patient may have pharyngitis.

Dx	Leukocytosis is common. A throat culture for *Streptococcus* should be obtained if pharyngitis is present. The diagnosis is generally one of exclusion. Ultrasonography with graded compression or CT may be useful in the diagnosis and in excluding appendicitis.
Tx	The disease is generally self-limited; hospital admission may be indicated for rehydration and for serial examinations to rule out an early appendicitis that may be missed on diagnostic imaging.

Constipation

See Chapter 35, Constipation.

Urinary Tract Infection/Pyelonephritis

See Chapter 41, Dysuria.

ZEBRA ZONE

a. **Trauma:** Although trauma cases are usually easily identified, it is important to check for a history of recent trauma in presentations of abdominal pain.

b. **Incarcerated hernia:** Much less common in a 5 year old than in infants.

c. **Presentations of nonabdominal pathology:** Note that there are entities in which the pathology is **not** primarily intra-abdominal, yet the child may present with a chief complaint of abdominal pain. Such entities include diabetic ketoacidosis, hemolytic-uremic syndrome, Henoch Schönlein purpura, pneumonia, and streptococcal pharyngitis.

Practice-Based Learning and Improvement: Evidence-Based Surgery

Title
Early analgesia for children with acute abdominal pain

Authors
Green R, Bulloch B, Kabani A, et al

Reference
Pediatrics 116(4):978-983, 2005

Problem
Use of analgesia in children with acute abdominal pain

Intervention
Intravenous morphine versus normal saline placebo

Comparison/control (quality of evidence)
Randomized, double-blind, placebo-controlled trial of early analgesia with either intravenous morphine or normal saline in children 5 to 16 years of age

Outcome/effect
Morphine did not increase the rate of missed appendicitis. It was found to be effective in treating acute abdominal pain and did not affect emergency physicians' or surgeons' confidence in the diagnosis of acute appendicitis.

Historical significance/comments
Physicians had withheld analgesia during early evaluation of abdominal pain for acute appendicitis. It was thought that analgesia may mask subtle findings on the examination that could interfere with surgical evaluation and ultimately delay the diagnosis of acute appendicitis. This paper refuted those claims and supported physicians' decisions to treat abdominal pain with satisfactory levels of analgesia. (Whereas early analgesia has proved safe and beneficial in the pediatric population, the same schema may not apply in all *adult* cases, in whom other diagnoses [e.g., bowel obstruction] are frequent considerations, and severity of the condition could be masked.)

Interpersonal and Communication Skills

Seek Out Unexpressed Concerns

Abdominal pain is a common pediatric complaint, and sometimes despite a complete evaluation, no etiology is found. Once the results of the evaluation have been reviewed with the family, the family may continue to worry. Ask family members if they have other issues or concerns. They may be secretly worried that their child has cancer or another underlying problem that has not yet been discovered. At times, such concerns have been stimulated by the family's knowledge of some other child who presented similarly and was ultimately discovered to have a serious problem. Knowing this upfront may allow you to dispel unfounded concerns. You may actually be able to demonstrate that this "secret worry" has already been considered and eliminated as a potential cause. Seeking out such unexpressed concerns is a skill applicable to numerous clinical situations.

Professionalism

Improve Quality of Care by Ensuring Appropriate Follow-Up

Arranging for proper follow-up is essential to improving quality of care. A patient may have a surgical problem causing abdominal pain, yet have an unremarkable abdominal examination and a negative initial diagnostic workup. Computed tomography, for example, if performed too early in the course of appendicitis, may be falsely negative. It is important to advise the family that appropriate follow-up should be arranged if symptoms persist, change, or worsen. In some cases, a preplanned follow-up examination the following day by either the pediatrician or a pediatric surgeon is advisable. If there is a concern that the parents may delay in seeking medical attention if the child's condition should worsen, admission for observation may at times be an appropriate course of action.

Systems-Based Practice

Careful Documentation Spawns Good Practice and May Avoid Malpractice

Abdominal pain is a very common complaint, but only rarely a serious medical concern. However, despite the best care, a vague abdominal complaint can turn into catastrophe. It is important for physicians to develop a formal and proactive approach to lowering the risk for lawsuits in everyday practice. Plaintiff's allegations tend to concentrate on failure to document an adequate examination and failure to provide proper follow-up care. Be mindful of the areas of greatest risk in your field of medicine and understand the common pitfalls of these clinical conditions. Develop good habits in documenting care. Good documentation leads to better care; at some point in your career, it may also offer protection from legal action.

References

1. Stefanutti G, Ghirardo V, Gamba P: Inflammatory markers for acute appendicitis in children: Are they helpful? *J Pediatr Surg* 42(5):773-776, 2007.
2. Andersen B, Kallehave F, Andersen H: Antibiotics versus placebo for prevention of postoperative infection after appendicectomy. *Cochrane Database Syst Rev* (3):CD001439, 2005.
3. Heldrich FJ: Lethargy as a presenting symptom in patients with intussusception. *Clin Pediatr (Phila)* 25(7):363-365, 1986.
4. Dufour D, Delaet MH, Dassonville M, et al: Midgut malrotation, the reliability of sonographic diagnosis. *Pediatr Radiol* 22(1):21-23, 1992.

Chapter 95
Chest Pain (Case 52)

Steven M. Selbst MD

Case: A 7-year-old boy was hanging drywall when he felt a sharp pain in his left shoulder. The pain has persisted and he has shortness of breath with exertion.

Differential Diagnosis

Musculoskeletal Causes	Respiratory Causes	Gastrointestinal Disease
Muscle strain	Asthma	Gastroesophageal reflux
Costochondritis	Pneumonla	Esophagitis
Trauma (contusion)	Pleural effusion	Retained foreign body
Trauma (fracture)	Pneumothorax	

Nonorganic Causes	Cardiac Causes—problems with perfusion/cardiac output
Anxiety	Rhythm disturbances
Stress	Ischemia

Speaking Intelligently

When I evaluate a child with chest pain, I recognize that the etiology of chest pain in children is usually not related to the heart. Still, each patient must be taken seriously, because occasionally a child with chest pain is found to have a serious medical problem. My first step is to ascertain that the child is hemodynamically stable before I proceed with a detailed evaluation. I connect the child to a monitor and evaluate cardiac rate, rhythm, and oxygen saturation. It is crucial to be sure the patient does not need cardiovascular or respiratory support immediately. If there are signs of poor perfusion, I start an intravenous line and give a bolus of normal saline, 20 mL/kg over the next hour. Although many children with chest pain (especially chronic pain) do not need laboratory or diagnostic studies, a chest radiograph and an electrocardiogram can be helpful in determining if the chest pain and other associated signs and symptoms are related to cardiac or pulmonary pathology.

PATIENT CARE

Clinical Thinking
- Support airway and breathing.
- Support circulation.

History

- History of **trauma** is concerning. A minor chest wall injury or muscle strain should improve over time.
- The **description** of pain is sometimes helpful. "Burning pain," worse with lying down, is associated with esophagitis.
- **Nausea, vomiting,** and anorexia are often related to gastrointestinal (GI) disorders, but these are very nonspecific.
- **Dizziness** with standing suggests dehydration but could also be related to cardiac insufficiency.
- **Shortness of breath** and **pain worse with exertion** are very concerning. These symptoms make a respiratory or cardiac cause seem more likely.
- **Onset** of pain is important. Acute pain (<48 hours) is more likely to have an organic cause. Chronic pain (>6 months) is more likely to be psychogenic or idiopathic. In an older child with sudden onset of pain, consider an arrhythmia, pneumothorax, or musculoskeletal injury. In a young child with sudden onset of pain, consider a foreign body (coin) in the esophagus or chest injury.
- Ask about **family history.**
- **Severity** and **frequency** of chest pain is sometimes revealing.
- Determine if the pain is **induced by exercise** or exertion.
- Consider recent use of **cocaine.**
- Inquire about recent significant **stress** (e.g., move, death of loved one, serious illness).
- Determine if there are **associated complaints.**
- **Past medical history** is sometimes revealing.

Physical Examination

- If the child is in significant **distress,** emergency care and stabilization are required. Consider pneumothorax or arrhythmia.
- **Vital signs** give crucial information. Orthostatic changes suggest depleted intravascular volume (dehydration) but could relate to cardiac insufficiency (pump failure).
- **Fever** is notable and serves as a "branch point" in narrowing the differential diagnosis.
- An abnormal **cardiac examination** (heart murmur, rub, arrhythmia) clearly points to a cardiac condition. Absence of such findings does not rule out cardiac disease.
- If the child appears **chronically ill,** chest pain may be part of a serious illness such as malignancy (Hodgkin lymphoma) or systemic lupus erythematosus.
- If skin **bruising** is present, chest pain may be related to unrecognized trauma.
- If the **abdominal examination** is abnormal, chest pain may be related to a GI disorder with pain referred to the chest.
- If **arthritis** is present, consider a collagen vascular disease, which may manifest as pleural effusion and chest pain.
- If the child is unusually **anxious,** consider pain related to stress.

- If the **chest examination** reveals rubs, decreased breath sounds, or wheezing, this may suggest pneumonia or asthma with overuse of chest wall muscles. If subcutaneous emphysema is palpable on chest or neck, consider a pneumothorax or pneumomediastinum.
- **Tenderness** of the chest wall or costochondral junctions suggests musculoskeletal pain or costochondritis. However, this finding may be nonspecific.

Tests for Consideration
- **Electrocardiogram (ECG)** $150
- **Exercise stress test** $290
- **Pulmonary function tests** $26
- **Drug screen:** If cocaine use is suspected $235

IMAGING CONSIDERATIONS

→ **Chest radiograph** $75
→ **Echocardiogram** $325

Clinical Entities   Medical Knowledge

Musculoskeletal Causes

Pφ	Musculoskeletal pain is due to **strain** of chest wall muscles in rough play, wrestling, carrying heavy books, or exercising. **Costochondritis** is a subset that involves the costochondral junctions where the ribs attach to the sternum. Pain may be bilateral and is exacerbated by physical activity or breathing. This pain may last for weeks. Also, direct **trauma** to the chest may result in a mild contusion or a **rib fracture**.
TP	The child presents with pain associated with movement of chest wall muscles or upper extremities. Pain is often sharp and may radiate to the back.
Dx	Diagnosis is made by reproducing pain on physical examination, by palpation or moving upper extremities and chest wall muscles. Eliciting tenderness over the costochondral junctions is usually sufficient to make the diagnosis of costochondritis. Diagnostic studies are not needed unless there was significant trauma and rib fracture is suspected.
Tx	Treatment consists of rest and analgesics, such as acetaminophen or nonsteroidal anti-inflammatory agents. **See Nelson Essentials 141.**

Respiratory Causes

Pφ	Respiratory conditions cause chest pain in a variety of ways. *Asthma* and *pneumonia* may lead to chest pain by causing overuse of chest wall muscles with increased work of breathing. Exercise may induce chest pain related to asthma. Occasionally a *pleural effusion* associated with pneumonia irritates the diaphragm and causes pain. *Pneumothorax* leads to sudden sharp chest pain and respiratory distress when an unrecognized subpleural bleb ruptures. This can occur with cough, sneezing, sudden movement, or minimal trauma.
TP	The child presents with tachypnea, and often there is use of accessory muscles (retractions). There may be decreased breath sounds with asthma, pneumonia, or pneumothorax. Those with pneumonia usually have fever. There may be palpable subcutaneous air with pneumomediastinum or pneumothorax.
Dx	Diagnosis is made by physical examination. A chest radiograph often confirms the condition when atelectasis, infiltrate, or pneumothorax is noted. A treadmill test may diagnose exercise-induced asthma.
Tx	Treatment for asthma consists of bronchodilators and corticosteroids. Pneumonia is treated with antibiotics. Pneumothorax is sometimes treated with needle aspiration and placement of a chest tube, although a small pneumothorax can be managed with cautious observation in the hospital. **See Nelson Essentials 141.**

Gastrointestinal Disease

Pφ	*Gastroesophageal reflux* causes burning pain of the esophagus (esophagitis), which may be secondary to an infection such as candida, herpes, or CMV. Pain may also develop in a young child when a *coin lodges* in the esophagus, resulting in obstruction and surrounding irritation.
TP	Patients with esophagitis complain of burning midsternal chest pain, which worsens when the patient eats spicy foods or reclines. The child with a coin in the esophagus will have sudden midsternal chest pain and associated dysphagia and drooling.
Dx	Diagnosis of esophagitis is made by taking a careful history. A trial of antacids is both diagnostic and therapeutic. A chest radiograph will confirm a coin lodged in the esophagus.

Tx   Treatment of reflux consists of antacids. A coin in the esophagus of a symptomatic patient must be removed promptly, usually by endoscopy in the operating room or with a balloon catheter in the radiology suite under fluoroscopic guidance. **See Nelson Essentials 141.**

Cardiac Causes—Problems with Perfusion/Cardiac Output

Pφ   *Supraventricular tachycardia (SVT)* or *ventricular tachycardia* causes sudden palpitations and possibly chest discomfort. Hypertrophic cardiomyopathy is an inherited disorder and may cause *ischemia,* especially when the patient exercises. Myocarditis is usually caused by a viral infection (coxsackievirus) and also may lead to ischemic pain.

TP   Children with arrhythmias usually feel palpitations and present acutely with chest discomfort. Some present with syncope.

Dx   An ECG may reveal an arrhythmia or evidence of structural heart disease such as hypertrophic cardiomyopathy or long QT syndrome. Signs of ischemia may be noted. An EKG shows nonspecific changes with myocarditis, such as arrhythmia or ST-segment changes. A Holter monitor is useful to detect arrhythmias not noted on EKG. A chest radiograph reveals cardiomegaly with myocarditis. An echocardiogram detects cardiac conditions such as hypertrophic cardiomyopathy. It also reveals poor cardiac muscle function with myocarditis (see Chapter 90, Myocarditis).

Tx   All of these conditions require urgent cardiology consultation. Treat those symptomatic with SVT with intravenous adenosine or with synchronized cardioversion, and admit the patient to the hospital for further monitoring. Myocarditis requires supportive care and hospital admission. **See Nelson Essentials 141.**

Nonorganic Causes

Pφ   Although it is known that *anxiety* and *stress* affect somatic sensation, the specific mechanisms by which they cause chest pain remain unclear.

TP   The child with stress-related pain or conversion disorder is usually older than age 12 and may appear anxious or unconcerned. There may be hyperventilation or a normal examination.

Dx   Diagnosis is made by taking a careful history. There is often a recent major stressful event such as separation from friends, divorce in the family, or school failure that correlates temporally with the chest pain.

Tx   Psychological counseling is generally helpful. **See Nelson Essentials 141.**

ZEBRA ZONE

a. **Pulmonary embolism:** Consider PE in teenage girls who use oral contraceptives, following abortions, and in teens with recent leg trauma. Chest pain is often accompanied by tachypnea and respiratory distress.

b. **Pill esophagitis:** Pain is more likely if patient takes pills with little water and lies down soon afterward. Many drugs produce an acidic solution or gel as they dissolve.

c. **Myocardial infarction:** Consider MI in patients with known underlying heart disease such as anomalous coronary arteries or past history of Kawasaki disease and in patients with longstanding diabetes mellitus. Also consider MI in teenagers who abuse cocaine.

d. **Pericarditis:** An uncommon infection of the pericardium characterized by fever, respiratory distress, and sharp stabbing mild sternal pain that is relieved when the patient sits up and leans forward. A friction rub, distant heart sounds, neck vein distention, and pulsus paradoxus are classic features.

e. **Tumor:** Chest pain may be the presenting finding of a malignancy involving the chest such as Hodgkin or non-Hodgkin lymphoma.

f. **"Texidor's twinge" or "stitch in the side":** Characterized by brief, sharp, unilateral pain that improves with straightening up or taking shallow breaths. Cause is uncertain.

Practice-Based Learning and Improvement: Evidence-Based Medicine

Title
Pediatric chest pain: A prospective study

Authors
Selbst SM, Ruddy RM, Clark BJ, Santulli T

Reference
Pediatrics 82:319-323, 1988

Problem
Review of etiology of chest pain in children presenting to an urban pediatric emergency department

Comparison/control (quality of evidence)
Prospective study with a large sample size of more than 400 children with chest pain over a 1-year study period; limited by its setting in the emergency department, so more likely to include those with acute chest pain

Outcome/effect
Most children with chest pain have a benign outcome. Cardiac disease is rarely found in children with chest pain.

Historical significance/comments
A cautious approach to children with chest pain is needed. Not all children with chest pain require extensive laboratory testing.

Interpersonal and Communication Skills

Elicit Patient's and Family's Concerns

It is important to relieve the anxiety and concerns of the patient and family when possible. Often families are frightened about chest pain because of media reports of sudden death in young athletes. Most children with chest pain can be reassured after a complete history and physical examination. However, when there are concerning features in the history and/or examination, inform the parents of the need to consult a cardiologist, and, when necessary, admit the patient to the hospital for supportive care and observation.

Professionalism

Be Mindful that Hindsight is 20–20

In many conditions, including chest pain, symptoms and signs change over time, making it easier for the physician who sees the patient after days, weeks, or even months have passed to "put the pieces together" and make a correct diagnosis. Due to these factors, it is important to remain nonjudgmental of physicians who may have seen a child earlier in the course of the illness and may have failed to make the correct diagnosis.

Systems-Based Practice

Medical Liability: Avoid Unnecessary Testing, but Document Your Reasoning

A careful history and physical examination often point to the cause of chest pain. For many conditions (musculoskeletal chest pain, psychogenic pain, or gastroesophageal reflux), expensive diagnostic studies are not helpful and are unnecessary. Diagnostic tests should be used when diagnostic uncertainty exists and/or to confirm findings in the history and physical examination. For those patients with acute pain or worrisome findings on history or physical examination, additional studies such as a chest radiograph and electrocardiogram may be required. Further testing may be guided by findings on the initial studies with help from a consultant. If no further studies are to be pursued, be sure to document your findings and the rationale as to why further testing is not indicated.

Chapter 96
Physical Abuse (Case 53)

Sara L. Beers MD

Case: A 15-month-old boy was brought in by emergency medical services after becoming unresponsive in the bathtub while in the care of his mother's boyfriend, who stated that the child may have fallen off the couch earlier in the afternoon.

Differential Diagnosis

Abusive head trauma	Abusive abdominal trauma
Abusive fractures	Abusive burns

Speaking Intelligently

Nonaccidental trauma or physical abuse should always be considered when there is no history or only a minor history of trauma with significant findings. Cervical spine (C-spine) precautions should be implemented immediately. The child's airway, breathing, and circulation should be assessed and supported. The child needs to be completely undressed, while simultaneously being placed on cardiopulmonary monitors. A quick secondary survey needs to be performed. This includes log-rolling the child while holding C-spine precautions to assess the child's back and buttocks. A Glasgow Coma Scale (GCS) score should be assigned. If the GCS score is altered, the child needs to have a stat computed tomography (CT) scan of the head. One should strongly consider obtaining an abdominal CT at the same time when nonaccidental trauma is on the differential. Intravenous access should be obtained with bedside testing for glucose, hemoglobin, and venous blood gas levels. Additional blood should be obtained for complete blood count (CBC), prothrombin time (PT), partial thromboplastin time (PTT), international normalized ratio (INR), aspartate aminotransferase (AST), alanine aminotransferase (ALT), amylase, lipase, and a type and crossmatch. Obtaining blood should not delay going to the CT scanner.

PATIENT CARE

Clinical Thinking
- Support airway, breathing, and circulation.
- The **differential is broad** when initially evaluating a child with abuse because rarely is that given in the history.
- Things to consider include **ingestion, infection, seizure,** and **hypoglycemia.**

History
Obtain and document a thorough history of the explanation of the injury and/or the day's events from the caregiver. This information may later become important to the investigators and/or prosecutors. The following are aspects of a history that may be particularly concerning for abuse:
- No explanation or vague explanation with a significant injury.
- An important detail of the explanation changes significantly.
- An explanation that is inconsistent with the pattern, age, or severity of the injury or injuries.
- An explanation that is inconsistent with the child's physical and/or developmental capabilities.
- Different witnesses provide markedly different explanations for the injury or injuries.
- Delay in seeking care.

Physical Examination
- Always **completely undress** the child because some injuries resulting from physical abuse may be missed otherwise (e.g., burns to the bottoms of the feet).
- A complete neurologic assessment, including reflexes, cranial nerves, sensorium, gross motor, and fine motor abilities, should be performed.
- Take note of any tenderness or swelling, especially when palpating the child's extremities, head, and ribs because there may be new or healing fractures.
- Look closely in the child's mouth for caries (which may indicate neglect) and at the frenulum (which often is torn in cases of forced feeding).
- A thorough examination of the child's skin is very important, looking for bruises, lacerations, burns, or bites. (Remember to look at the child's ears because this is often a site of bruising from the ears being pulled.)
- If the child is stable, the height, weight, and fronto-occipital (FOC) circumference should be carefully measured and plotted on a growth chart.
- Always perform a thorough genitourinary (GU) examination on children with suspected physical abuse to check for signs of sexual abuse.

Tests for Consideration

• CBC with differential	$53
• Diffuse intravascular coagulation (DIC) panel (PT, PTT, fibrinogen, D-dimer)	$75
• Liver enzymes (AST, ALT)	$75
• Pancreatic enzymes (amylase, lipase)	$45
• Urinalysis	$38

IMAGING CONSIDERATIONS

→ **Head computed tomography (CT):** Abnormal neurologic examination, scalp/head swelling or bruising on physical examination, or a child less than 2 years old with other injuries of concern for physical abuse. — $750

→ **Head magnetic resonance imaging (MRI):** Not as readily available as CT. Often obtained after a CT. Better characterization of cerebral edema, more sensitive for subtle intracranial injuries, better dating of intracranial injuries. — $1800

→ **Abdominal CT:** If concern for abdominal trauma (IV contrast). — $950

→ **Skeletal survey:** Recommended for all children under the age of 2 years with injuries concerning for physical abuse. Consider repeating in 2 weeks. — $225

→ **Radionuclide bone scan:** Better for acute rib fractures and subtle nondisplaced long-bone fractures. — $560

Clinical Entities — Medical Knowledge

Abusive Head Trauma

Pψ *Abusive head trauma* has the highest morbidity and mortality of all abusive injuries. Intracranial bleeds are often subdural (tearing of bridging veins) but can also be subarachnoid, epidural, or intraparenchymal. The bleed may be an acute bleed or multiple bleeds of varying ages. As the bleeding and/or swelling of the brain continues, the intracranial pressure rises (see Chapter 81, Raised Intracranial Pressure). Skull fractures that are especially concerning for abuse are multiple, complex, diastatic, or occipital in location. There may or may not be external signs of trauma with scalp swelling or bruising. **Retinal hemorrhages** may also be seen in infants with abusive head injuries.

TP	Infants with intracranial injuries and/or skull fractures often have nonspecific symptoms. The more severe the head injury, the more likely the infant is to have symptoms that range on a continuum from decreased responsiveness, irritability, lethargy, and limpness to coma and death.
Dx	Diagnosis is suspected with presentation and confirmed with head imaging (initially a head CT). **See Nelson Essentials 22.**
Tx	With epidural and subdural bleeding a neurosurgical intervention to drain the clot is almost always necessary. Because these events develop quickly, the risk for impending herniation is very high. Immediate medical management includes the following: respiratory and hemodynamic support, head of bed elevation with the neck midline, osmotherapy with 3% saline or mannitol, and adequate sedation and pain control. Hyperthermia should be avoided, and any seizure activity should be aggressively treated. If hypertension, bradycardia, and other signs of herniation are present, then hyperventilation is appropriate.

Abusive Abdominal Trauma

Pψ	*Abusive abdominal trauma* is caused by crushing, sudden compression, and/or shearing mechanisms. It is the second most fatal form of child abuse. With severe blows to the flank, the child may sustain renal trauma. Severe blows to the abdomen may result in liver, spleen, or pancreatic contusions or lacerations. Intestinal contusions or perforations may also occur.
TP	A typical presentation is peritonitis with abdominal distention, pain, and vomiting. There may or may not be external signs of trauma. With significant intraabdominal bleeding, the child may present in hypovolemic shock.
Dx	The diagnosis is suspected with clinical presentation; however, confirmatory imaging is almost always needed. This may be done with a bedside ultrasound (FAST) to quickly look for free fluid. An abdominal CT with IV contrast is more sensitive. A CBC, AST, ALT, amylase, and lipase, are also be obtained.
Tx	Treatment depends on the extent of the injury. Consult a pediatric surgeon as soon as possible. Some intraabdominal injuries may be managed medically with serial imaging and supportive care. Other injuries will require immediate repair in the operating room. **See Nelson Essentials 22.**

Abusive Burns

Pψ	The pathophysiology involves injury to the epidermis with first-degree burns and to the underlying dermis with second-degree (partial thickness) and third-degree (full thickness) burns.
TP	The typical presentation of *abusive burns* will include uniform depth of the burn with distinct borders compared with accidental burns, which will often have splash marks, varying depths, and indistinct borders. A common pattern of abusive immersion burn involves simultaneous scald burns of the buttocks, perineum, and both feet.
Dx	Diagnosis of burns is made clinically. The "rule of nines" can be used to determine total body surface area. Diagnosis of abusive versus accidental burns involves careful consideration of the caregiver's history and the pattern of the burn.
Tx	Initial treatment is support of the ABCs: airway, breathing, and circulation. Remove all of the child's clothing. Fluid resuscitation is often necessary with crystalloid (normal saline or Ringer's lactate solution). The burns are covered with cool, saline-soaked gauze. Pain control is paramount. Second- and third-degree burns will require debridement. Extensive burns, circumferential burns, and burns of the hands and feet may require inpatient treatment. **See Nelson Essentials 22.**

Abusive Fractures

Pψ	Fractures are seen in 5% to 18% of abused children. Long-bone fractures, including spiral/oblique fractures and metaphyseal fractures, should be evaluated closely for nonaccidental causes. Rib fractures (usually posterior or lateral) may occur from a squeezing mechanism.
TP	Clinical presentations of *abusive fractures* are variable. The caregiver may seek care when he/she notices swelling or tenderness in a specific area or with decreased use of an extremity. Older or healing fractures may not be detected on examination.
Dx	The diagnosis with an imaging study. Fractures may be diagnosed with a skeletal survey when nonaccidental trauma or abuse is suspected. Skeletal surveys are mandatory in all cases of suspected abuse in children under 2 years old. A bone scan may identify acute rib fractures and subtle nondisplaced long-bone fractures.

Tx   Treatment depends on the type and age of the fracture. Rib
      fractures heal well without intervention. Long-bone fractures
      usually require splinting or casting. Significant angulation or
      displacement of fractures may require sedation and reduction.
      See Nelson Essentials 22.

ZEBRA ZONE

a. **Idiopathic thrombocytopenic purpura (ITP):** Low platelets can
   cause significant bruising with very minor trauma.

b. **Osteogenesis imperfecta:** "Brittle bone disease" may present
   with multiple fractures at different stages of healing without
   abusive trauma.

c. **Hemorrhagic disease of the newborn:** Similar to ITP with
   presentation of bruising and bleeding in the absence of trauma.

d. **Glutaric aciduria type 1:** Inborn error of metabolism associated
   with spontaneous intracranial hemorrhage.

Practice-Based Learning and Improvement

Title	
The battered child	
Authors	
Kempe CH, Silverman FN, Steele BF, et al	
Reference	
JAMA 181(1):17-24, 1962	
Problem	
Incidence of child abuse unknown and unrecognized	
Intervention	
Survey of district attorneys who reported a large number of children who were severely beaten	
Comparison/control (quality of evidence)	
Survey with descriptive statistics	
Outcome/effect	
Incidence of child abuse cases identified	
Historical significance/comments	
This important study contributed to the fact that mandatory reporting laws were enacted in all 50 states.	

Interpersonal and Communication Skills

The Documentation of Abuse Is an Important Communication

In cases of child abuse it is essential to ensure that medical record documentation is thorough and accurate. This may include quotes from the child or family members, if appropriate. Complete documentation of the timeline of events is important. Be sure to document all caregivers who may have had contact with the child during the possible times the injury is estimated to have occurred. This is obviously important for the patient as well as for any future legal actions that may result.

Professionalism

Altruism and Advocacy: The Duty to Report Abuse

Child abuse presents in many different ways, and sometimes a clinician may have concerns about abuses that are not shared by his/her physician colleagues. It is important to pay attention to and to respect another physician's concerns about possible abuse and not attempt to dissuade them from contacting the local social services department that investigates potential abuse cases. Every physician's responsibility is to protect the children for whom he/she cares; if a physician is concerned about the possibility of abuse, the physician is obligated to report it.

Systems-Based Practice

Health Law: The Obligation Is to Report, Not to Prove

Cases of alleged abuse are not often clear-cut and require further evaluation based upon initial suspicion. Health-care workers who suspect abuse of a child are required to report such suspicion to their local child protective service agency. All 50 states have statutes that mandate the reporting of suspected child abuse and neglect, and the health-care worker is not required to prove abuse before reporting it. Most insurance companies will pay for hospital admission for the protection of children in cases of suspected abuse, but they are not federally required to do so.

Chapter 97
Pediatric Poisonings
(Case 54)

Jannet Lee-Jayaram MD *and*
Christopher J. Haines DO, FAAP, FACEP

Case: A 13-month-old boy is brought into the emergency department (ED) because he is "not acting right." He vomits and then starts to have a generalized tonic-clonic seizure. Eventually, his family brings in an empty jar that smells strongly of the medicinal odor that was noted on the child on arrival.

Differential Diagnosis

Camphor	Salicylates	Hydrocarbons

Speaking Intelligently

When I suspect a patient has ingested a toxic substance, I start with the ABCDEs (see Clinical Thinking). Simultaneously, I obtain a focused history and perform a physical examination while trying to fit the information into a particular toxidrome. A toxidrome is a pattern of signs and symptoms that are consistent with a specific toxic exposure. I consider the potential manifestations of the toxidrome and what problems may progress to become urgent/emergent. My decision to observe in the emergency department (ED), discharge home, or admit to the hospital is based on recognition of the specific ingestion and the patient's clinical status. If ingestion is suspected, I often consult with the poison control center. The number **1-800-222-1222** is used throughout the United States to speak with a poison control center.

PATIENT CARE

Clinical Thinking
- **A**irway: If the airway is patent, should the airway be secured now before there is progressive loss of airway maintenance?

- *B*reathing: How is the breathing, and does it need support?
- *C*irculation: Do the vital signs seem to imply impending hemodynamic instability? Have I secured vascular access? Do I need to administer volume or vasopressor support?
- *D*isability: What is the patient's mental status, and do I expect further deterioration?
- *D*econtamination: Is there continued exposure to toxic substance from the skin or the clothes? Have I been careful to wear **personal protective equipment?** What, if any, method of decontamination should be used? What was the time of the exposure/ingestion? Will decontamination be successful and safe?
- *D*extrose: Have I checked a bedside serum glucose level?
- *E*xposure: Have I exposed the body to look for other signs of injury or clues to a diagnosis? Have I checked a temperature?
- *E*lectrocardiogram (ECG): Is the patient on a monitor, and have I ordered an ECG to identify arrhythmias and specific toxidromes?
- Does this patient have a recognizable **toxidrome?** Does this particular ingestion have an **antidote?** Are there recommended support measures? Is the substance something that can and should be removed with hemodialysis?
- Is the patient a teenager with intentional ingestion with multiple substances?
- Is the patient pregnant?

History
- What medications are kept in the home (over-the-counter medications, prescription medications, cultural remedies)?
- Knowing medical conditions of others in the home provides clues to what medications are in the home.
- Ask for the bottle of the ingested substance to **estimate the dose** in mg/kg.
- Find out the **exact time** of ingestion to correlate expected symptoms and the current patient status.
- Separate the teenager from the caregiver to promote open communication and honesty and facilitate patient-doctor communication.

Physical Examination
- Initial assessments starts with the **ABCDEs** as above.
- **Tachycardia** does not necessarily reflect intravascular volume depletion, which can occur if the ingestion causes excessive vomiting. Tachycardia may be due to the anticholinergic properties or impending hemodynamic collapse or may be a sign of autonomic stimulation. Bradycardia may represent direct cardiac effects or generalized autonomic depression.
- **Tachypnea** with respiratory alkalosis classically presents in early aspirin toxicity. Tachypnea may be present if a substance was

aspirated. Bradypnea can occur with generalized autonomic depression.

- **Hypotension** is a late sign of shock in children.
- **Hyperthermia** can be seen in aspirin toxicity and may lead the clinician to incorrectly diagnose the patient with an infection.
- An age-appropriate **mental status** examination can be performed quickly. Caregivers are the best resource to identify if the child is at baseline activity and level of consciousness. Children may be appropriately somnolent if it is past their usual bedtime.
- **Pupillary size, bowel sounds, mucosal moisture,** and **skin moisture** are clues to whether a cholinergic or anticholinergic toxidrome is present. Diaphoresis may indicate a sympathomimetic ingestion.
- **Odors** can be helpful in identifying specific ingestions. Characteristic odors may include but are not limited to the menthol camphor odor, minty oil of wintergreen (methylsalicylate) odor, and bitter almond odor associated with cyanide.
- **Depressed affect** may be noted in the teenager who intentionally ingested multiple substances to commit suicide or ask for help.

Tests for Consideration

- **Arterial blood gas levels:** Metabolic acidosis, respiratory alkalosis ... $156
- **Electrolytes:** Anion gap and calculated serum osmolarity ... $68
- **EKG:** Prolonged corrected QT interval (QTc), widened QRS, terminal R wave in aVR ... $150
- **Bedside blood glucose level:** If hypoglycemia is present, initiate immediate treatment. ... $12
- **Acetaminophen level:** Early toxicity is clinically silent. ... $53
- **Salicylate level:** Follow decreasing levels, dialysis indications ... $53
- **Other specific drug levels as warranted** ... $53
- **Urine drug screen:** Rarely helpful immediately, varies by institution ... $235

IMAGING CONSIDERATIONS

→ **Chest radiograph:** Indicated with hydrocarbon ingestions for aspiration pneumonitis ... $75
→ **Abdominal radiograph:** May identify iron or aspirin bezoars ... $45

Camphor

Pφ	*Camphor* is a common ingredient in many topical liniments, with a distinct pungent odor. It is an aromatic terpene ketone that easily crosses the blood-brain barrier.
TP	Camphor ingestion manifests as gastrointestinal (GI) distress and central nervous system (CNS) hyperactivity or depression. There is usually a distinct odor. There may be vomiting or abdominal pain. CNS hyperactivity manifests early on and may include delirium and seizures, which can be followed by CNS depression, coma, and central hypoventilation. Seizures may be paroxysmal and refractory to typical treatment.
Dx	Diagnosis is made by history and clinical findings.
Tx	Treatment is supportive. Seizures are treated with benzodiazepines and barbiturates. If intubation and muscle relaxation become necessary, continuous electroencephalogram (EEG) monitoring is indicated to monitor seizure status. Asymptomatic patients may be discharged home after a 6- to 8-hour period of observation. **See Nelson Essentials 45.**

Salicylates

Pφ	*Salicylates* are found in aspirin but many nonaspirin exposures, such as Pepto-Bismol and Ben-Gay, occur in pediatrics. They are in high concentration most notably as methylsalicylate or oil of wintergreen. Salicylates directly stimulate the central respiratory system, increase pulmonary vascular permeability, increase glucose consumption, enhance insulin secretion, inhibit glycogenolysis, and uncouple oxidative phosphorylation. The kidney responds with diuresis and large urinary losses of bicarbonate, potassium, and sodium, leading to metabolic acidosis.
TP	Classically, the patient presents with tachypnea causing respiratory alkalosis. However, pediatric patients may present already in severe metabolic acidosis. The oil of wintergreen odor, hyperthermia, tachycardia, and tachypnea may be present. Lethargy, seizures, and coma may develop. Vomiting may contribute to dehydration. Noncardiogenic pulmonary edema is an ominous sign. Cardiovascular deterioration may be rapid.

Dx   Diagnosis can be made by history and clinical findings. Salicylate levels, blood gas levels, and serum electrolyte levels aid in the diagnosis and management. A nomogram exists but is not helpful in prognosis.

Tx   Treatment is supportive. Intravenous fluids should be administered to expand intravascular volume and maintain high urine output. Urine alkalinization of the urine with intravenous sodium bicarbonate will enhance urinary excretion of salicylate. Definitive treatment is elimination by hemodialysis. Institution of therapy is guided by the severity of the clinical presentation and not the serum salicylate level. **See Nelson Essentials 45.**

Hydrocarbons

Pφ   *Hydrocarbons* are liquid at room temperature and are found in fuels (lamp oil and lighter fluid), solvents, and household cleaners (pine oil and furniture polish). Their major toxicity is related to their low viscosity, leading to aspiration and severe pneumonitis. Some hydrocarbons may cause CNS depression, GI irritation, and cardiotoxicity.

TP   A small amount of liquid can cause significant pneumonitis (<2 mL). This occurs during initial ingestion or after vomiting. The patient may present with respiratory distress, including coughing, choking, gagging, tachypnea, and hypoxia.

Dx   Diagnosis is made with history and clinical findings. A chest radiograph is obtained in those with respiratory symptoms at presentation. Although findings consistent with pneumonitis may not be demonstrated on the initial film.

Tx   Treatment is supportive. Routine antibiotics and corticosteroids are not indicated. Gastric decontamination is not indicated, and every effort is made to prevent vomiting, which increase risk for aspiration. Patients who remain asymptomatic and have a normal chest radiograph at 4 to 6 hours may be discharged home. The patient who is symptomatic or who has an abnormal chest radiograph should be admitted for further management. **See Nelson Essentials 45.**

ZEBRA ZONE

a. **Gamma hydroxybutyrate (GHB) overdose:** GHB is a dose-related central nervous system depressant that interacts with dopamine, serotonin, γ-aminobutyric acid (GABA), and opioid systems. It is a date-rape drug, notorious for its amnestic and hypotonic effect. It is voluntarily used for its euphoric and aphrodisiac effects at clubs, raves, and parties. Because of the steep dose-response curve, it can rapidly lead to respiratory depression, bradycardia, and coma.

Practice-Based Learning and Improvement: Evidence-Based Pediatrics

Title
Position paper: Gastric lavage

Authors
American Academy of Clinical Toxicology, European Association of Poisons Centres and Clinical Toxicologists

Reference
J Toxicol Clin Toxicol 42(7):933-943, 2004

Problem
Routine use of gastric lavage in poisoned patients

Intervention
Large-bore orogastric tube lavage

Comparison/control (quality of evidence)
Literature review of animal, volunteer, and clinical studies of gastric lavage and position statement by toxicologists

Outcome/effect
Animal studies demonstrated no substantial drug recovery after 60 minutes. Volunteer studies provided insufficient support because of high variability of marker recovery, and one implied increased propulsion of material further into small intestine. Clinical studies demonstrated no clinical benefit, and there was association with higher prevalence of intensive care unit (ICU) admissions and aspiration pneumonitis.

Historical significance/comments
Gastric lavage, once regularly practiced in EDs for theoretic benefit, should not be employed routinely, if ever. Risks and complications far outweigh any theoretic benefit that may come from substance recovery.

Interpersonal and Communication Skills

Avoid Blame but Seize the Opportunity for Discussions of Safety

Pediatric poisonings may cause caregivers to feel guilty about their role in the ingestion. Caregivers may become defensive as they are questioned about how long the child was unsupervised, how the medications were accessed, or what substances are kept in the house. The clinician should be sensitive to the viewpoint of the caregiver and not assign blame, but all visits for real or possible ingestions should provide the perfect opportunity to review safety, injury prevention, and poison-proofing of the home.

Professionalism

Respect for Others: The Complexities of "Confidentiality" in the Pediatric Patient

In pediatrics the level of confidentiality between the patient and physician changes over time. Young adolescents must be introduced to the idea that their relationship with their physician is confidential and be guided to take control of their health-care needs as they progress to the age of majority. **Confidentiality must be broken if doing so serves the best interests of the patient who is still a minor.** An example of when confidentiality should be broken is if the adolescent says that he or she plans to commit suicide by taking an overdose. Even in instances in which it is not *essential* to break confidentiality, the clinician should encourage and facilitate open discussion between the family and patient, while still supporting the adolescent's emerging autonomy.

Systems-Based Practice

Utilize Poison Centers and Poison Help Hotlines

With the ever increasing pharmacologic therapies available to both adults and children, the possible toxicity from an agent alone or in combination has become very complex. In addition to requiring the help of other specialists in the management of the acutely poisoned child, **early contact with toxicologists will help guide your management, decision making, and identification of the substance ingested.** America's poison centers are open 24 hours a day, 7 days a week. The Poison Help hotline, 1-800-222-1222, serves as a key medical information resource and helps reduce costly emergency department visits.

Chapter 98
Petechial Rash (Case 55)

Sabina B. Singh MD

Case: A 4-year-old child presents with fever and a red rash that began today (petechial).

Differential Diagnosis

Meningococcemia	Trauma	Enteroviral infection
Rocky Mountain spotted fever (RMSF)	Henoch-Schönlein purpura (HSP)	Thrombocytopenia

Speaking Intelligently

Petechial and purpuric rashes are amongst the most feared rashes in medicine. Petechiae are pinpoint (<3 mm) flat round lesions under the skin caused by intradermal hemorrhage. They are nonblanching. Purpura are larger in size and form when the petechiae coalesce.

Patients who are ill appearing and have abnormal vital signs need emergent medical care.

Infection with *Neisseria meningitidis* or *Rickettsia* is the primary concern in these patients, because these infections can be rapidly fatal. Early recognition of these disease processes is paramount, and early treatment will improve outcomes. In addition to examining the skin rash, all other systems should be examined. Ill-appearing patients need aggressive treatment with initial emphasis on the airway, breathing, and circulation (ABCs). First the airway should be assessed for patency, the breathing assisted (oxygen supplementation to intubation), followed by IV access. While inserting the IV, blood should be drawn for a complete blood count (CBC), blood culture, chemistry, prothrombin time (PT), and partial thromboplastin time (PTT), and an initial fluid bolus of normal saline, 20 mL/kg, should be given. Broad-spectrum antibiotics should be given early and not withheld for the lumbar puncture. Patients refractory to fluid resuscitation may require vasopressor support. Parents should be kept informed.

Patients with suspected meningococcemia should be placed on respiratory isolation.

PATIENT CARE

Clinical Thinking
- Assess for **airway, breathing,** and **circulation.** Address deficiencies before progressing in the evaluation.
- Laboratory studies should be rapidly evaluated and interpreted.
- Aggressive **fluid resuscitation** with crystalloid fluids (20 mL/kg).
- Use of **vasopressors** in fluid refractory shock.
- Early **broad-spectrum antibiotic** administration.
- **Respiratory isolation** and **personal protective equipment.**

History
- History of onset, progression, site, and severity of the rash itself.
- **Fever** suggests a potential infectious cause of the petechial rash.
- History of **bleeding diathesis** in family or patient, such as easy bruising, gingival bleeding, heavy menstrual cycles, or history of blood transfusion.
- History of prior injuries, scars, or bruising.
- History of **recent trauma** and illness.
- Recent **medication use,** which may precipitate platelet dysfunction.

Physical Examination
- Vital signs: Changes associated with sepsis are hyperpyrexia, hypopyrexia, tachypnea, tachycardia, and hypotension.
- Airway, breathing, and circulation are the primary concern in ill patients.
- Head: Evidence of trauma.
- Head, ears, eyes, nose, and throat (HEENT): Oral petechiae, rhinorrhea.
- Skin: Petechial/purpuric rash, including location, size, characteristics, and progression (Figure 98-1).
- Neurologic: Evaluate mental status, **signs of meningeal irritation (Kernig sign and Brudzinski sign),** and focal neurologic deficits.
- Examination should be directed toward assessment of all organ systems and adequate end-organ perfusion, including mental status, neurologic deficits, and urine output.

Tests for Consideration
- **CBC** — $53
- **Blood culture** — $100
- **Chemistry panel** — $29
- **Inflammatory markers (erythrocyte sedimentation rate[ESR], C-reactive protein [CRP]** — $25 each
- **PT/PTT, bleeding time** — $75
- **Fibrinogen** — $55
- **Cerebrospinal fluid (CSF):** Cell counts, chemistries, and culture — $175

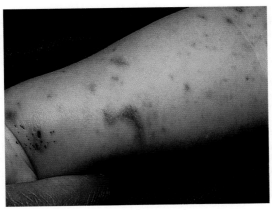

Figure 98-1   Petechial rash.

IMAGING CONSIDERATIONS

→ **Head CT:** If evidence of focal neurologic deficit $750

Clinical Entities	Medical Knowledge

Meningococcemia

Pφ *N. meningitidis* is the causative agent of ***meningococcemia.*** It is a rapidly progressing disease transmitted through respiratory secretions. Humans are the only known host. *N. meningitidis* invades endothelial cells of small blood vessels and causes damage by liberating endotoxin. Consequently, endothelial permeability increases, resulting in shock and multiorgan failure and disseminated intravascular coagulation (DIC).

TP Meningococcal disease is a continuum. Patients may present following a viral prodrome with fever, headache, myalgias, and arthralgias, or they may present in shock. Clinical deterioration may be precipitous. Classic skin findings are a petechial/purpuric rash. Extracutaneous manifestations include changes in mental status, neck stiffness, irritability, seizure, and unstable vital signs.

Dx   History and physical examination often alert the physician to the diagnosis. A high white blood cell count and pleocytosis on the CSF are supporting evidence. Confirmation is provided when the blood or CSF culture is positive for *Neisseria*. Skin scrapings and punch biopsies can also identify infection with *N. meningitidis*.

Tx   Treatment is aggressive resuscitation and early initiation of broad-spectrum parenteral antibiotics (penicillin or cephalosporins). In penicillin-allergic patients chloramphenicol is the drug of choice. Droplet isolation must be instituted in cases of presumed infection. Furthermore, intimate patient contacts and health-care workers who may have been in contact with the patient must receive prophylaxis with antibiotics. **See Nelson Essentials 100.**

Rocky Mountain Spotted Fever

Pφ   ***Rocky Mountain spotted fever*** is a tickborne disease due to *Rickettsia rickettsii* infection. Bacteria are introduced into the bloodstream by infected ticks after a blood meal of greater than 6 hours. *Rickettsia* enter the bloodstream and target vascular endothelial cells, leading to increased vascular permeability, leading to multisystem organ dysfunction. Infection is characterized by fever, myalgias, headache, and petechial rash. It is the most common fatal tickborne disease, and therefore it is imperative to maintain a high index of suspicion for RMSF. In the United States, RMSF is more common in the Southeast states.

TP   Typically patients will have a history of tick attachment. Fever is nearly ubiquitous. A rash is present in 85% to 90% of patients. It typically begins as blanching maculopapular lesions, which can progress to petechial or purpuric. Lesions start around the wrists and ankles with involvement of the palms and sole; the rash then spreads in a centripetal manner to the rest of the body. Central nervous system changes include confusion and lethargy. Pulmonary involvement may lead to acute respiratory distress syndrome. Gastrointestinal (GI) manifestations may include GI bleeding and focal hepatocellular necrosis. Renal failure may also occur.

Dx	Diagnosis can be suggested by history and physical examination. Results of laboratory studies should be evaluated. Nonspecific signs of RMSF include hyponatremia, anemia, thrombocytopenia, and elevated liver function test results. Cerebrospinal fluid evaluation should be completed to rule out other infectious causes. Serologic assays to detect IgG levels are done for definitive diagnosis.
Tx	Treatment consists of early recognition of the disease. If the tick is still present, it should be removed. Provide aggressive fluid resuscitation as needed. Tetracycline or chloramphenicol is the antibiotic of choice, even in children under 9 years of age. Antibiotic prophylaxis is not indicated. **See Nelson Essentials 122.**

Enteroviral Infection

Pφ	Enteroviruses are a group of single-stranded RNA virus belonging to the Picornaviridae family. The enteroviral group consists of coxsackievirus, echovirus, and poliovirus. Transmission occurs via the fecal-oral route. These viruses enter the human host through the gastrointestinal or respiratory tract. Replication causes minor viremia on the third day of infection, followed by a second major viremic episode on days 3 to 7.
TP	*Enteroviral infection* can cause a constellation of symptoms, but most cases include fever, viral prodrome, and gastrointestinal symptoms. Exanthematous rashes may occur as maculopapular, blanching rash mimicking rubella and usually have a benign 3- to 5-day course. It may occur following cessation of fever. Cardiac involvement, central nervous system involvement, oral lesions, and musculoskeletal pain may also be presenting signs.
Dx	Diagnosis is based on clinical judgment in conjunction with seasonal outbreak patterns and other historical features. Definitive diagnosis made by recovering the organism from throat, blood, urine, and stool cultures. Physicians should use ancillary studies to eliminate bacterial causes of illness. Blood: CBC, chemistries, inflammatory markers. Cerebrospinal fluid: Cell count, chemistries, culture, and enteroviral polymerase chain reaction (PCR) testing.
Tx	Treatment is supportive. Antibiotics can be given prophylactically to those patients with severe illness while awaiting culture and PCR results. **See Nelson Essentials 122.**

Trauma	
Pφ	Traumatic petechiae are commonly associated with increased intrathoracic pressure. Common causes are prolonged vomiting, whooping cough, strangulation, and crush injury to the chest and abdomen. Petechiae are usually located above the nipple lines secondary to reflux of blood through the valveless veins of the head and neck.
TP	Patients are **well appearing,** with petechiae limited to the face, neck, and upper trunk (usually above the nipple line).
Dx	Diagnosis may be based on a **well-appearing** patient with adequate history of vomiting or coughing before development of lesions . More ominous causes of petechiae must be ruled out.
Tx	Treatment is supportive care. **See Nelson Essentials 42.**

Henoch-Schönlein Purpura	
Pφ	**Henoch-Schönlein** purpura is an inflammatory disorder characterized by generalized small vessel vasculitis. It has a multifactorial etiology. All organ systems may be affected. HSP is characterized by petechial/purpuric rash, migratory polyarthritis, renal involvement, and gastrointestinal involvement.
TP	Patients are commonly well appearing and afebrile. There is usually a history of prodromal illness, followed by rash, abdominal pain, edema, vomiting, and arthritis. A petechial rash that can progress to purpura is commonly seen localized to lower extremities.
Dx	Evaluation should include a CBC, ESR, urinalysis, and a chemistry panel. Additional serologic studies may be added in cases of unknown etiology.
Tx	Treatment is supportive care. Minor complaints may be treated symptomatically. Corticosteroid therapy should be initiated for intestinal complications. **See Nelson Essentials 87.**

Thrombocytopenia

Pφ Thrombocytopenia is defined as a decreased platelet count. Etiologies can be divided into increased destruction, decreased production, or sequestration. Multiple etiologies exist; a partial list includes:
- **Decreased production**
  - □ Malignancies
  - □ Bone marrow suppression
- **Increased destruction**
  - □ **Idiopathic thrombocytopenic purpura (ITP)** is a clinical syndrome secondary to decreased circulating platelets, which manifests clinically as easy bruising. Platelets become coated with autoantibodies, resulting in phagocytosis and a quantitative platelet deficit.
  - □ Thrombocytopenic purpura
  - □ Disseminated intravascular coagulation
- **Sequestration**
  - □ Splenic sequestration
  - □ Arteriovenous malformation

TP Petechiae and purpura may be present along with self-limited small vessel bleeding. Spontaneous bleeding is a feared outcome but usually does not occur with platelet counts greater than 10,000/μL

Dx CBC with peripheral smear should be done, as well as coagulation studies. Bone marrow biopsy should be considered, to rule out causes of thrombocytopenia such as malignancy.

Tx The goal is to keep platelets at an acceptable level. Most patients do not require treatment. Corticosteroids are the mainstay of treatment; however, they change bone marrow morphology. Therefore a bone marrow aspiration should be done before instituting therapy. Intravenous immunoglobulin as well as intravenous RhoGAM are secondary options. **See Nelson Essentials 151.**

ZEBRA ZONE

a. **Nonaccidental trauma (child abuse):** Must always be considered. Careful history taking is imperative. In these cases the physical findings are not consistent with the history given. Caregiver reliability must also be assessed.

b. **Infectious endocarditis:** Is infection of the endocardial surface of heart. Infected clots form and can break up and spread throughout the body. Classic signs that are a result of hematogenous spread consist of petechiae, splinter hemorrhages (dark red linear nailbed lesions), Osler nodes (tender subcutaneous nodules), Janeway lesions (nontender maculae on palms and soles), and Roth spots (retinal hemorrhages with small, clear centers).

Practice-Based Learning and Improvement: Evidence-Based Medicine

Title
Goal-directed management of pediatric shock in the emergency department

Authors
Carcillo JA, Han K, Lin J, Orr R

Reference
Clin Pediatr Emerg Med 8(3):165-175, 2007

Problem
Pediatric septic shock

Intervention
Multiple goal-directed therapies in the management of pediatric sepsis

Comparison/control (quality of evidence)
Review article with cited references in peer-reviewed journal

Outcome/effect
Early goal-directed management of pediatric shock improve outcomes.

Historical significance/comments
Early recognition of sepsis is imperative during the initial assessment of patients. Management has evolved to a set of time-sensitive goal-driven therapies that when addressed have improved patient outcomes.

Interpersonal and Communication Skills

Implement "Repeat-Backs" While Avoiding Condescension

The parents and family members of patients with idiopathic thrombocytopenic purpura (ITP) should be advised about the possibility of an intracranial bleed with minor trauma when the platelet levels are low. It is important to take the time to explain the risks clearly, in lay language, and with the goal of achieving complete understanding by the family. One approach to doing this is to have family members repeat back instructions and warnings. This technique is applicable at all levels of family literacy. When using this technique for clear communication, physicians should be vigilant to avoid condescension in their words or demeanor.

Professionalism

Commitment to Professional Responsibility: Rid the Workplace of Sexual Harassment

It is 2 AM. You have just watched your female PGY1 resident successfully complete a lumbar puncture on a young child with a petechial/purpuric rash who is suspected of having meningococcemia. The tap was obtained on the first stick, and a prompt diagnosis was made. You witness your (male) chief resident congratulating the PGY1, putting his arm affectionately around her. The affection is obviously unwanted. **Sexual harassment** has become a national concern and one that is increasingly recognized in the field of medicine. Studies show that female students encounter an unacceptable amount of sexual harassment in medical training from fellow students, patients, faculty, and doctors with whom they work. This behavior affects learning opportunities. Medical educators need to address issues of gender, sexual harassment, and the setting and maintaining of proper boundaries in order to prevent a hostile learning environment from developing.[1]

Systems-Based Practice

Patient Identification and Patient Safety

You have just completed a lumbar puncture. How focused are you on labeling your tubes? Misidentification of patients is a major source of error: in the laboratory, with medication, in radiologic procedures, in transfusion, and in surgical procedures. Accurate patient identification should be accomplished by matching two identifiers of the patient to two identifiers linked to the procedure. Acceptable identifiers include the patient's name, birth date, address, telephone number, or medical record number. In pediatrics, patients often cannot articulate many of these, so the wristband serves as this source of identification. The procedure-linked identifiers should match at least two patient identifiers. In high-risk environments, it is best that two independent providers confirm this identification. Incorrectly identifying the patient's medical record can also serve as a source of error. This can lead to ordering medications on the wrong patient, interpreting laboratory results incorrectly, or transmitting false information in the record that is acted upon by others.

Reference

1. Mann BD: Surgery: A Competency-Based Companion, Philadelphia, 2009, Saunders, p 276.

Chapter 99
Animal Bite (Case 56)

Arezoo Zomorrodi MD
and John M. Loiselle MD

Case: A 1-year-old boy is brought to the emergency department for two puncture marks on his cheek.

Differential Diagnosis

Dog bite	Cat bite
Bat bite	Human bite

Speaking Intelligently

When I evaluate a bite wound, I first search for and address limb- or life-threatening injuries. I establish the severity of the injury by determining the depth of the wound and involvement of underlying soft tissue, muscle, or bone. I ensure proper blood flow to and neurologic function of the injured area. As I thoroughly examine the wound, I consider the need for wound irrigation, primary closure, antimicrobial prophylaxis, and proper pain control. Among the key priorities for animal bite wound care is the restoration of normal function and prevention of infection. Animal bites that penetrate the skin are considered dirty wounds. Wounds in highly vascular areas such as the face and scalp are at lower risk of bacterial infection.[1] Primary closure of a wound is associated with higher infection rates, although carefully selected wounds can be repaired with little risk of infection.[2,3] Thorough irrigation with a high volume of saline delivered under high pressure is the most effective means of cleaning the wound and minimizing the risk for infection,[4] and I therefore irrigate all bite wounds meticulously. I choose prophylactic antibiotics to cover the expected bacteria in the mouth of the biting animal. Animal wounds that become infected contain predictable pathogens.[5,6] A 3- to 5-day course of prophylactic antibiotics is recommended for wounds considered to be at high risk for infection.[7] Amoxicillin-clavulanate is the most commonly chosen antibiotic for animal bite prophylaxis.[7,8] These recommendations are based on consensus opinion, because there are no definitive studies that demonstrate a reduction in infection rate as the result of prophylactic antibiotics.[9]

PATIENT CARE

Clinical Thinking
- Perform the **primary survey,** concentrating on immediate threats to the patient's airway, breathing, and circulation (ABCs).
- Assess injuries to the neck or chest and any uncontrolled hemorrhage.
- Control active bleeding by applying direct pressure to the wound.
- Perform the **secondary survey** with meticulous assessment of all wounds, the extent of each injury, and involvement of any underlying structures.
- Although the cosmetic aspect of injuries may be most obvious, attend to potential life- and limb-threatening injuries first.
- **Tetanus toxoid booster** administration is based on the child's immunization status.
- Dogs, cats, and bats are among animals that can transmit **rabies.** The need for rabies postexposure prophylaxis depends on the animal's immunization status and health, local epidemiology, and the ability to quarantine the animal for observation.

History
- Elapsed time since the bite
- Wound care before arrival
- Species of biting animal
- General health of biting animal

- Immunization status and availability of the animal for observation or testing
- Underlying medical conditions and immune status of the patient
- Immunization status of the patient
- Allergies to medications
- Response to previous wounds, including scarring or keloid formation
- Recent oral intake if procedural sedation is anticipated

Physical Examination
- Assess vital signs. Tachycardia may occur on the basis of anxiety, pain, or blood loss. Hypotension may be a sign of uncompensated hemorrhagic shock.
- Make note of the normal range for heart rate, blood pressure, and respiratory rate for the patient's age.
- Initial assessment should focus on the ABCs.
- The patient must be undressed completely to accurately document the extent of injuries.
- Assess for signs of airway involvement because the face is a common location of injuries. Penetrating wounds to the neck may involve the trachea. Vascular injuries in the neck can produce an expanding hematoma.
- Evaluate perfusion of involved structures.
- Test function of injured sites.
- Perform neurovascular examination of areas distal to the site of injury.

Tests for Consideration
- **Complete blood count (CBC):** Laboratory evaluation is generally unnecessary except in the rare instance of major hemorrhage, in which case serial hemoglobin levels should be performed. $35

IMAGING CONSIDERATIONS

→ Medical imaging may be necessary, depending on the potential for injury to underlying structures.

→ **Computed tomography (CT) scan of the head:** If there is penetrating injury of the scalp and there is concern for skull fracture or intracranial air. $750

→ **Plain radiographs:** If there is a concern for underlying fractures. $75

Clinical Entities	Medical Knowledge

Dog Bites

Pφ **Dog bites** account for 80% to 90% of mammalian bites. In 1994 an estimated 4.7 million dog bites occurred in the United States. Dogs belong to the victim's family in 15% to 30% of cases. Dogs typically produce lacerations or crush injuries. They are capable of generating tremendous force with their jaws. The hand is commonly bitten.

Dog bites are at risk for transmitting infections with common organisms, including *Staphylococcus aureus,* viridans streptococci, *Pasteurella multocida* and *Eilkenella* species. Dogs can carry and transmit rabies.

TP Patient identifies dog bite.

Dx Radiographs should be obtained to evaluate for underlying fractures. Dog bites to the scalp in young infants can penetrate the calvarium. A CT of the head should be considered in infants less than 1 year of age with penetrating wounds to the scalp to rule out a depressed skull fracture or presence of intracranial air.

Tx Proper wound irrigation should be performed. A 3- to 5-day course of prophylactic antibiotics is recommended for high-risk wounds. The decision to provide postexposure rabies prophylaxis following a dog bite depends on the dog's immunization history, the local epidemiology of rabies, the general health of the dog, and the ability to quarantine and observe the dog. All dog bites are considered tetanus prone, and tetanus toxoid booster administration should be based on the child's immunization status. **See Nelson Essentials 122.**

Cat Bites

Pφ **Cat bites** account for 5% to 10% of mammalian bites. Cats are likely to inflict puncture wounds due to the nature of their needle-sharp teeth. Cats are at risk for transmitting rabies and tetanus. Bacterial infection of cat wounds occurs at a higher rate than other animal bites because of the nature of the inflicted wounds and the difficulty in cleaning them. Puncture wounds inoculate bacteria deep within the wound. Punctures cannot be adequately disinfected, and attempts to irrigate the site may force bacteria deeper into the wound. Coring out a puncture wound is not helpful and adds to the area of damage. *Pasteurella* is the predominant bacteria infecting cat bite wounds. These polymicrobial infections also commonly include staphylococcal and streptococcal species.

TP	These wounds are often inflicted in the victim's hand or arm when the cat is fighting, anxious, or presented with an unfamiliar or unwanted handler. The inflicted wounds initially appear minor, and medical care is often delayed. Most patients only seek care once infectious symptoms appear.
Dx	Diagnosis is made by the history and characteristics above. Medical imaging is rarely required and should be obtained if there is concern for underlying fracture.
Tx	Cat bites generally do not require sutures. Because of the high risk for infection, primary closure is frequently contraindicated. Most clinicians recommend antibiotic prophylaxis for full-thickness bites because of the high risk for infection and the difficulty in irrigating the wound. Postexposure rabies prophylaxis depends on the cat's immunization status, the local epidemiology of rabies, the general health of the cat, and the ability to quarantine and observe the cat. Tetanus toxoid booster should be administered based on the immunization status of the patient. **See Nelson Essentials 122.**

Human Bites

Pφ	Humans inflict 2% to 3% of bite wounds that come to medical attention. **Human bites** are considered tetanus prone and at risk for other bacterial infection. *Eikenella corrodens* is present in 30% to 50% of all infected human bites and is resistant to cephalosporins and antistaphylococcal penicillins.[10]
TP	Human bites often produce hematomas or crush wounds but can also penetrate the skin. Toddlers often inflict injuries during altercations or in the course of exploratory behavior. A clenched fist used to strike an opponent in the mouth is another common means of sustaining a human bite wound. Adult bites may be encountered in cases of child abuse.
Dx	The distance between the impressions left by the canine teeth of the biter can be used to determine the age of the assailant. DNA from the biter can also be recovered from a fresh bite wound.
Tx	Perform aggressive local wound irrigation. Ensure adequate tetanus immunization. Initiate a 3- to 5-day course of prophylactic antibiotics for high-risk wounds. **See Nelson Essentials 122.**

Bat Bites	
Pφ	Bats rarely if ever inflict cosmetically significant wounds. Most bites are undetectable. Bats are at high risk for carrying rabies, and transmission can occur without a visible bite.
TP	A child is considered to have a significant exposure if found in a room with a live bat or handling a dead bat.
Dx	Diagnosis is usually made based on the history, and medical imaging is rarely required.
Tx	Clean wound thoroughly with soap and water. Do not suture bat bites. Initiate rabies postexposure prophylaxis. The complete series of immunization can be discontinued if the bat is available for testing and the results are negative. Administer tetanus toxoid booster based on patient's immunization status. **See Nelson Essentials 122.**

Practice-Based Learning and Improvement: Evidence-Based Medicine

Title
A comparative double-blind study of amoxicillin/clavulanate versus placebo in the prevention of infection after animal bites

Authors
Brakenbury PH, Muwanga C

Reference
Arch Emerg Med 6;251-256, 1989

Problem
Evaluate the utility of prophylactic antibiotics for prevention of animal bite–associated wound infections.

Intervention
Prospective, randomized, double-blind placebo-controlled study of patients age 6 years and above with full-thickness animal bites. Patients were randomized to either treatment with amoxicillin-clavulanate or placebo for 5 days.

Comparison/control (quality of evidence)
Prospective, randomized, double-blind, placebo-controlled study

Outcome/effect
Infection occurred in 7 out of 29 (24%) children in the treatment group and 5 out of 25 (20%) children in the placebo group. Wound infection was reduced significantly by antibiotic prophylaxis in wounds more than 9 hours old ($p = .023$). Antibiotics did not

significantly decrease infection rates in hand bites as compared with general bites.

Historical significance/comments

This study evaluated mainly dog bites, and the results cannot be extrapolated to other mammalian bites. The total number of hand bites in the study was small. The infection rate was higher than in comparative studies.

Interpersonal and Communication Skills

The Importance of Person-to-Person Communication

An unprovoked animal bite can be a sign of a public health risk that must be communicated to the appropriate health department. The animal may be dangerous to others. Certain animals such as skunks, bats, coyotes, and foxes (among others) may have contracted rabies, which means postexposure prophylaxis decisions will need to be made regarding your patient. Because of the seriousness of these events and the importance of prompt receipt of information, person-to-person direct communication should occur whenever possible. This allows you as the health-care professional to discuss the details of the incident with the public health officer and for you both to discuss and clarify the issues. Although it may be easier to leave a voice mail, send an e-mail, or text page, you have no assurance that your message has been received. Although it may be stating the obvious, the importance of person-to-person communication applies to many matters of communication in medicine.

Professionalism

Involving Consultants: Balancing Parental Expectation and Actual Need

Injuries inflicted by an animal bite can be psychologically traumatic for the child and the parent. Parents may harbor feelings of guilt that they were unable to protect their child. They are often concerned about disfiguring scars as a result of the bite, especially when these occur on the face. It is common for parents to request a plastic surgeon for the repair. The emergency physician must be realistic about his or her skill in laceration repair and consult a more skilled practitioner when necessary. However, most minor lacerations do not require specialized plastic closure, and, after acknowledging the parental concerns, the physician should explain to the parents that the type of repair and anticipated outcome will not differ regardless of who performs the closure.

Systems-Based Practice

Reporting to the Centers for Disease Control and Prevention

State health departments should be the primary contact for physicians during consultation about possible human rabies cases. After consultation with the appropriate physicians, it may be deemed necessary to send human samples for rabies testing to the Rabies Laboratory at the Centers for Disease Control and Prevention (CDC). Any questions regarding likelihood of a case, sampling techniques, and shipping can be answered by calling the Rabies Section at the CDC at (404)-639-1050.

Physicians must complete the associated form detailing the clinical history of the patient and provide the name and phone number of the physician who should be contacted with the test results in addition to state health department authorities. This form must accompany any samples sent to the Rabies Laboratory at the CDC.

References

1. Rutherford WH, Spence RAJ: Infection in wounds sutures in the accident and emergency department. *Ann Emerg Med* 9:350-352, 1980.
2. Chen E, Hornig S, Shepherd SM, Hollander JE: Primary closure of mammalian bites. *Acad Emerg Med* 7:157-161, 2000.
3. Maimaris C, Quinton DN: Dog-bite lacerations: A controlled trial of primary wound closure. *Arch Emerg Med* 5:156-161, 1988.
4. Speigl JD, Szabo RM: A protocol for the treatment of severe infections of the hand. *J Hand Surg* 13A:254-259, 1988.
5. Dire DJ: Cat bite wounds: Risk factors for infection. *Ann Emerg Med* 20:973-979, 1991.
6. Talan DA, Citron DM, Abrahamian FM, et al: Bacteriologic analysis of infected dog and cat bites. *N Engl J Med* 340(2):85-91, 1999.
7. American Academy of Pediatrics: Bite wounds. In Pickering L, editor: *2006 Red book: Report of the Committee on Infectious Diseases*, ed 27, Elk Grove Village, IL, 2006, American Academy of Pediatrics, pp 191-195.
8. Smith MR, Walker A, Brenchley J: Barking up the wrong tree? A survey of dog bite wound management. *Emerg Med J* 30:253-255, 2003.
9. Medeiros I, Saconato H: Antibiotic prophylaxis for mammalian bites. *Cochrane Database Syst Rev Cochrane Library* (4), 2004.

Professor's Pearls
Section VII: The Emergency Department
Magdy W. Attia MD

Consider the following clinical problems and questions posed. Then refer to a discussion of these issues by Magdy W. Attia, MD, Academic Chief, Division of Pediatric Emergency Medicine, Department of Pediatrics, Nemours, Wilmington, Delaware.

1. You are evaluating a 3-week-old in the emergency department (ED) because of inconsolable crying. The newborn has had no fever and if anything appears to be pacified by more feeding. His young mother believes he has "belly pain" because he is drawing his legs up. He was a product of 34 weeks of gestation. His mother reported that labor and delivery were uncomplicated. The newborn has regained his birth weight and is thriving well. His vital signs are rectal temperature, 37.5° C (99.5° F); heart rate (HR), 160 beats per minute; respiratory rate (RR), 44 breaths per minute. Examination reveals a crying, difficult-to-console newborn, but good color, strong muscle tone, and lustrous cry. What is the differential diagnosis?

2. You are presented with a 2-year-old with sudden onset of fever and rash. The child has had chills and appeared ill. The family reports no known sick contacts. You can confirm that all her immunizations are up to date as you review her electronic medical record. Her presenting vital signs were temperature, 39° C (102.2° F); HR, 150 beats per minute; RR, 24 breaths per minute; blood pressure (BP), 76/44 mm Hg. She is lethargic and has a diffuse nonblanching rash. Her neck is supple. Her extremities are warm. The remainder of her examination is nonrevealing. The supervising physician ordered a blood count, for which results are typically received in 2 hours, and the physician is waiting for the results before proceeding to the next step in the management! What is your interpretation of this presentation? What is the significance of the vital signs? Would you approach this patient differently?

3. A 7-year-old child presents to the ED with a 4-day history of sore throat and fever. His mother noticed a lump in left side of his neck. What are the seven elements a clinician must comment on when describing a lump?

4. A 10-month-old has a 3-day history of fever and numerous bouts of vomiting and diarrhea. The stools are very watery and voluminous. The infant is becoming progressively more lethargic. How do you assess the hydration status of this patient? What are the appropriate interventions?

Discussion by Magdy W. Attia, Academic Chief, Division of Pediatric Emergency Medicine, Department of Pediatrics, Nemours, Wilmington, Delaware.

1. The list of differential diagnosis of the fussy infant or newborn is quite long. A thorough examination coupled with accurate assessment of the history and vital signs is crucial. The list is best generated if approached as a head-to-toe examination. In our case, there is no fever, which can lower the possibility of an infectious etiology, although it does not eliminate it completely. The examiner has to assess the head for any nonaccidental injury, and the anterior and posterior fontanel should be palpated for bulging as an indication of increased intracranial pressure. The eyes should be assessed for corneal abrasions and the ears for foreign bodies and infections. The nasal passages should be assessed for patency, and buccal mucosa and throat examination should be thorough to identify any potentially painful lesions. The neck should be assessed for the presence of masses or cysts. The chest should be examined for possible rib factures elicited by crepitus and tenderness. The lung fields should be auscultated for air exchange and any adventitious sounds. The heart should be evaluated for rate and murmurs, and the femoral pulses should be palpated. Assess the abdomen for tenderness and masses. Newborn neuroexamination is focused on muscle tone. The extremities were warm and without tenderness or deformities. No hair tourniquet was found. Although you think that this was a thorough examination, there is one part of the exam that was not addressed. Which one is it?

   In this case the examiner did not inspect the diaper area. On the return visit the newborn was found to have fullness in his left hemiscrotum, and the left testicle was firm and tender. A Doppler ultrasound confirmed the presence of testicular torsion.

   The head-to-toe examination of the fussy infant should include careful inspection of the perineum and palpation of the scrotal sac for torsion and hernias.

2. Fever and petechiae is a serious presentation and, once encountered, should be addressed aggressively and in a timely manner. This patient is likely suffering from meningococcemia and has developed septic shock based on her tachycardia and low normal blood pressure. The mainstay of the management is rapid sampling of blood for culture and a complete blood count, which may provide some prognostic values, but should *not* delay initiation of antibiotic therapy. Simultaneously, this patient should be aggressively resuscitated for her hypotension with a rapid infusion of crystalloid fluid such as normal saline or lactated Ringer's. Vasopressors and ventilatory support should be

immediately considered if there is a suboptimal response to fluid resuscitation. Lumbar puncture should be performed if the patient is stable and can tolerate the procedure. Performance of a lumbar puncture should *not* delay therapy as outlined earlier.

3. When describing a mass, the clinician must comment on location, size, consistency (soft, firm, hard, cystic), tenderness, mobility, and the appearance of the skin overlying the lesion and if there are any palpable sinus tracks. Gathering these characteristics by physical examination assists the clinician in generating a sound list of differential diagnosis.

    In our case the lump was in the submandibular area; measured 3 cm in diameter; was firm, tender, and mobile; and there was an overlying erythema. Clearly this presentation is consistent with cervical adenitis.

4. Assessment of the hydration status is an important clinical skill. The most objective method is to compare recent weights using the same scale and without clothing. This is, however, not always possible. The earliest, most sensitive way to assess intravascular volume depletion is the heart rate. An elevated heart rate at rest in this scenario is indicative of volume depletion. Assessment of urine output is helpful but can be difficult because of the associated diarrhea. Some diapers can absorb a fair amount of urine before it is noticeable by the caregiver. The remainder of physical findings can be subjective, including sunken fontanel (if open), sunken eyes, dry mucous membranes, poor skin turgor, and cool extremities. Findings in mental status such as listlessness, lethargy, or unresponsiveness are an indication of severe dehydration.

    The novice clinician may forgo some historical information that is helpful in this evaluation—for instance, how many times the child vomited and had diarrhea and also the type of diarrhea. Another important element of the history is the amount of intake in the period preceding evaluation.

    In this case, the infant had 3 days of symptoms and is exhibiting change in mental status. She is severely dehydrated. Rapid infusion of crystalloid such as normal saline or lactated Ringer's solution is required. Peripheral venous access can be difficult to establish in these cases. The clinical team must avoid delayed access and search for alternative means to access the vascular space. An intraosseous line can be established rapidly and used for infusion until a more secure access is obtained.

Section VIII
THE COMPETENCIES: CHALLENGES AND PERSPECTIVES

Section Contents

Chapter 100
Giving Bad News

Sharon Calaman MD

Medical Knowledge and Patient Care

How we deliver bad news impacts more than just the patient; it affects the entire family. Bad news has been described as "any information that produces a negative alteration to a person's expectations about their present and future."[1] Bad news may not always seem obvious, but even "simple" problems such as a cleft lip or a birthmark may impact a family's expectations. Bad news has many forms in pediatrics—ranging from birthmarks that may need surgical removal, genetic disorders that affect the family in the future, chronic disease that has an impact on a young child and family for life, to the impending death of a child.

How bad news is delivered is critical. Years later people remember how and the circumstances under which the news was delivered. The level of physician control, the time it takes to get to the point, the caring about the parents' feelings, the confidence the physician has, the amount of information given, the amount that the physician shows his or her own feelings, and how much the physician allows parents to talk and express their own feelings have been looked at in various settings.[2-4] The common thread in these studies, whether looking at delivering news that a child is dying to something as seemingly simple as a cleft palate, is that parents expect to be given time to talk and be heard during delivery of bad news. When asked by questionnaire years later, parents remember not being asked how they felt. They want the physician to show caring and confidence, but also to allow the parents some time to show their feelings and to talk.[1-4]

Parents have also expressed a strong desire to be put in touch with other parents in similar situations, yet in one study only 19% were referred.[2] This is important to consider when breaking bad news—making the offer to put the parent in touch with other parents or support groups.

Physicians need to be careful about making judgments as to the value of bad news. In looking at the delivery of bad news to families with children born with cleft palate, a treatable disorder without long-term consequences, the parental experience is greatly affected by the manner in which the news is delivered. The experience of being in the delivery room with a child being born disfigured was devastating for some families when they were not prepared—some families reported delays in full disclosure, which was difficult and unnecessarily stressful. Families expressed that they wished to be given basic information right at the time of delivery and more detailed information within the next 48 hours. One mother said, "A lot of the medical staff said, 'If you have to have a problem, this is a good problem to have. Other problems are much worse.' My response was that this was in fact the biggest problem right now in my life."[3] One has to be careful about letting one's opinion affect the delivery of information.

Parents of children with Down syndrome were questioned as to their experience when the bad news was delivered and what they wished would have happened. They expressed that it was important for both parents to hear the news together privately and then to be able to spend some time alone preferably with their child to process the diagnosis. They wished for follow-up 24 to 48 hours later with more information.[2] Parents of children with developmental delay felt that they could have been given more information at the early encounters.[2] Parents recalling their experiences receiving bad news also remember the circumstances—being given the news in the middle of rounds, where they felt rushed and felt that the doctor was protecting himself or herself from his or her own emotions by not facing them, as opposed to other physicians who took the time to sit down.[5]

Complete and honest information is important to families as well. One must be prepared to address questions that come up with different forms of bad news. In looking at end-of-life care, parents commented on conflicts between physicians and wished that they could at least meet with all parties involved rather than not understanding all the issues at stake.[4] Information needs to be simple and nonconflicting.[6]

One key issue in pediatrics is whether or not the child should be part of the discussion. Disclosure to the child should be encouraged when the family is ready. The emphasis needs to be on supporting the family and helping them with their decisions, not forcing them to make a decision that they are uncomfortable with.[7] In a study looking at parents of children who died from malignancy, parents were asked by questionnaire whether or not they had disclosed to the child that the child was going to die. Thirty-four percent had, and none of those parents had regrets about having talked to their children. Sixty-seven percent had not, and of those 27% had regrets that they had not spoken with their children.[8]

In the intensive care unit setting in particular, diagnoses are often discovered and children often die. The team needs to be aware of the impact of body language. Moreover, the language used and body language can give the family the sense that you have given up on them when their child is dying, at a time when they may need your presence more than ever. In a study exploring a family's desire to meet with physicians even after their child's death, it was found that parents did want to meet and to have a chance to clear the air and settle unresolved questions. They felt the lack of that meeting showed lack of physician interest.[9] In contrast, positive recollections of physicians' breaking bad news were described in the setting where the doctor stayed involved even when the child was no longer on that physician's service.[5]

If the news is about an incurable diagnosis, thought needs to be given to addressing end-of-life issues such as comfort care, withdrawing support, and do not resuscitate (DNR) orders. Care needs to be taken to give clear information. A team approach is best so that there are no conflicting messages and the appropriate support can be present, such as child life and social work. In some institutions specific palliative care teams exist to help medical teams and patients deal with these issues.

Interpersonal and Communication Skills

Share Information and Check for Understanding

Delivering bad news in a compassionate and empathetic way is a skill physicians should master. Many parents are overwhelmed or shocked by bad news, so what is discussed may not be fully comprehended. Therefore it is essential to summarize the salient points before the end of the meeting and to ask the parents what they have heard.

There are several simple things that can be done to ensure that the parents are as comfortable as possible before hearing the news. The meeting should occur in a private area with ample seating and with tissues and a wastebasket available. Paper and pens should also be available in case you are asked to write something down or the parent wishes to take notes. Make sure the meeting begins by introductions of everyone present and that you understand the relationships of everyone in the room. Once the discussion begins, adhere to the following basic principles:

- Body language is important—be aware of your posture, of how you hold your arms.
- Use easy-to-understand language—don't hide behind medical jargon.

- Be honest—expect to have to repeat yourself.
- Make contact information and written information available if possible.
- Involve people who may be essential for long-term follow-up—the primary pediatrician, the appropriate subspecialists.
- Use empathetic listening skills—expect to listen as much as talk.
- Arrange a follow-up discussion to allow for further questions as the information is processed.
- Don't be afraid to show empathy and emotion.

Professionalism

Resolve Team Conflicts First

Often the team will have conflicts about prognosis and treatment options. These need to be resolved, often with a team meeting of the multidisciplinary medical team, before speaking with the family. Information given to the family must be clear, accurate, and consistent.

Systems-Based Practice

Financial Implications of End-of-Life Care

Discussing end-of-life care with your patients or their families has significant financial implications. In *Improving Care for the End of Life: A Sourcebook for Health Care Managers and Clinicians,* the authors state the following:

> The Medicare hospice financing structure is very different from its other reimbursement programs. Most hospice payments are based on an all-inclusive per diem rate, except for physician services, which are mostly paid in the conventional manner (Part B physician billing). The Medicare hospice benefit is available only to individuals who are eligible for Medicare Part A, whose physicians certify that the prognosis is "less than six months," who understand the nature and purpose of palliative care, and who understand that by selecting hospice, they waive their right to certain other Medicare services. For qualified patients, the benefit includes most costs for prescription drugs, durable medical equipment, and care provided through an interdisciplinary team that assesses the needs of each patient and family and develops and implements an appropriate care plan. Hospice patients are distinctly less likely to have surgery, hospitalization, resuscitation, or other "high-tech" interventions (though these services are not explicitly precluded by the Medicare regulations).[10]

References

1. Fallowfield L, Jenkins V: Communicating sad, bad, and difficult news in medicine. *Lancet* 363:312-319, 2004.
2. Sharp MC, Strauss RP, Lorch SC: Communicating medical bad news: Parents' experiences and preferences. *J Pediatr* 121:539-546, 1992.
3. Strauss RP, Lorch C, Kachalia B: Physicians and the communication of "bad news": Parent experiences of being informed of their child's cleft lip and/or palate. *Pediatrics* 96:82-90, 1995.
4. Meyer EC, Ritholz MD, Burns JP, Truog RD: Improving the quality of end-of-life care in the pediatric intensive care unit: Parents' priorities and recommendations. *Pediatrics* 117:649-657, 2006.
5. Davies R, Davis B, Sibert J: Parents' stories of sensitive and insensitive care by paediatricians in the time leading up to and including diagnostic disclosure of a life limiting condition in their child. *Child Care Health Dev* 29:77-82, 2003.
6. Barnett MM: Effect of breaking bad news on patients' perceptions of doctors. *J R Soc Med* 95:343-347, 2002.
7. Hilden JM, Watterson J, Chrastek J: Tell the Children. *J Clin Oncol* 18:3193-3195, 2000.
8. Kreicbergs U, Valdimarsdottir U, Onelov E, et al: Talking about death with children who have severe malignant disease. *N Engl J Med* 351:1175-1186, 2004.
9. Meert KL, Eggly S, Pollack M, et al and the NICHHD Collaborative Pediatric Critical Care Research Network: Parents' perspectives regarding a physician-parent conference after their child's death in the pediatric intensive care unit. *J Pediatr* 151:50-55, 2007.
10. Lynn J, Schuster JL, Kabcenell A: "Medicare Reimbursement," *Improving Care for the End of Life: A Sourcebook for Health Care Managers and Clinicians*, New York, 2000, Oxford University Press.

Chapter 101
Difficult Encounters

Cynthia DeLago MD, MPH

Speaking Intelligently

The primary goal of any patient/caregiver encounter is to develop a partnership that ultimately results in the best medical decisions for the patient. How well you communicate with patients and caregivers determines how successful you will be at achieving your goal. Good interpersonal relations and communication skills will help you deliver medical and systems-based information and provide good patient care. These skills will help you negotiate medical treatment. Because "difficult encounters" are so tenuous, they require a high degree of professionalism; a misstep can sabotage everything. When an unpredictable event occurs, such as the sudden death of a child, you do not have much time to accrue the medical knowledge or learn the systems-based practices; therefore it is important to learn about these beforehand. Medical knowledge about child abuse is especially important because this knowledge will help you recognize child abuse and neglect in the first place. During more slowly evolving situations, it is important to know the most current information about the disease or situation.

Medical Knowledge and Patient Care

What defines a "difficult encounter"? For me, it is every time I have to deliver bad news or exchange emotionally charged information with a child's caregiver or family or with an adolescent patient. Examples of these types of encounters are:

- Informing parents/caregivers their child has died
- Informing parents their child has a serious or terminal disease
- Telling parents I suspect someone abused their child and I have to take protective action
- Confronting a substance-impaired caregiver and taking protective action
- Informing parents of a medical error
- Telling a teenager bad news, such as a positive human immunodeficiency virus (HIV) test

A more insidious type of difficult encounter occurs with parents of children with terminal, chronic, or fabricated disease (Munchausen syndrome by proxy). Over time the doctor-patient relationship may become strained because the parent becomes increasingly dissatisfied and demanding, despite tremendous effort by the doctor. In this case, almost every encounter with the parent is difficult.[1] Decision making in palliative care of a dying child may lead to difficult discussions about how much or how little treatment should be given.[2]

When a child dies suddenly, it is important to understand that sudden death is more common than anticipated death in this age-group. Unexpected child death may spark secondary reactions, such as posttraumatic stress disorder in parents, families, and health-care workers. Doctors should inform family members of this and encourage them to seek help if they develop symptoms. The same is true for involved members of the health-care team.

When a child is diagnosed with a terminal or chronic disease, caregivers need accurate, consistent information about the illness, treatment options, and prognosis. Caregivers/parents, and at times the child, need to be involved in the decision-making process. Their opinions need to be respected. Physicians caring for terminally ill children should be knowledgeable about palliative care and pain management. It is important to develop a care plan including directives about life-sustaining measures.[2] The goal is to keep the child comfortable and prevent unnecessary procedures and therapies.

Medical knowledge of risk factors, signs, symptoms, and physical examination findings about physical/sexual abuse and child neglect is the key to recognition. Heightened awareness leads to timely reporting to child protection agencies and law enforcement and can potentially save the child's life or prevent future mental and physical disability in the child and his or her siblings.[3]

Practice-Based Learning and Improvement

Learn by Reviewing: What Precipitated the Encounter? How Was It Handled?

By now you should realize that some "difficult encounters" are unavoidable but can be greatly diffused by having effective communication skills, relevant medical knowledge, and awareness of systems-based practices and by demonstrating professionalism. By striving to provide excellent patient care, you will make good decisions, even if you cannot always make everyone happy.

Some difficult encounters can be prevented or dealt with more effectively by applying practice-based learning and improvement principles. Examples of these types of encounters include those involving medical errors, parent anger and frustration regarding office practices, or parental mental health issues. After such an encounter, all involved should evaluate what precipitated the encounter and how it was handled. Resources such as books, journal articles, and Web-based materials pertaining to the situation can help identify ways to change office policies or to discuss the difficult situations with the child's parent. References 1 to 6 are particularly helpful resources for handling various "difficult encounters." Mental health professionals can offer advice about improving therapeutic relationships with difficult caregivers.[1] Other subspecialists can help improve disease management in your office, including developing guidelines for appropriate referrals to them.

Interpersonal and Communication Skills

Communicate Effectively With Families

During your medical school career, you should learn skills to communicate effectively with caregivers, patients, and their families. Maintaining good eye contact and positioning your body to be at the same level as the person with whom you are speaking help create a setting that will allow equal exchange of thoughts and ideas. During "difficult encounters" it is important to:

- Reflect on your own emotions and thoughts before you begin the conversation with the parent or adolescent. For example, in cases of child abuse, your first reaction is to be angry at anyone who would hurt a child. The person who brought the child to your office may not be the perpetrator. If you approach the caregiver as an angry person, you will not communicate effectively. Therefore you must acknowledge your anger and then refocus on the goal of providing good patient care. This will allow you to regain your composure and direct the conversation to arrive at the best outcome for the child.
- Be honest with the caregiver or adolescent, and get to the point. Evasive answers heighten anxiety and interfere with the interpersonal relationship you are trying to develop.[7]
- Be caring. When delivering bad news, parents want doctors to show they care. They appreciate it when doctors give them time to talk and express their emotions.[7]
- Be patient and available. When first presented with bad news, patients and parents cannot comprehend everything you are telling them. You must give them time to process the information. They may ask you to repeat what you said several times, and they will have questions. Often they think of questions or require further clarification hours to days later. Answer their phone calls, and be physically available.
- Define the caregiver's unresolved issues. In chronic disease management situations, parents who become increasingly dissatisfied and demanding over time may have unresolved issues. They may be grieving the loss of their child's potential, and this interferes with their child's care. Setting aside consultative time to discuss this may bring resolution.[1]
- Have the most current medical knowledge and know the systems involved with ensuring the delivery of this child's medical care before speaking with the family. Take the time to consult with subspecialists and learn about the disease and treatment beforehand so the patient or caregiver hears the same information from all doctors involved. Explain what happens next, and facilitate this by arranging subspecialist appointments, helping parents navigate health insurance issues, and providing resource information.

Professionalism

Listen and Recognize Your Own Response to Emotionally Charged Encounters

Difficult encounters are uncomfortable and may occur often. Examples include situations related to a child's terminal illness and death, medical errors or misadventures, or caregivers with mental health problems. Staying calm, being clear and confident, letting families speak and listening to what they have to say, taking sufficient time, allowing silence for families to process information, and saying "sorry" are essential elements. Emotional outbursts directed at you as the physician should not be taken personally: platitudes, excuses, and justifications have no place in the conversation. Showing emotion about tragic situations is natural; families and patients appreciate genuine expressions of sadness and concern.[7,8] It is important to remain available to the patient and family after the conversation; give them a way to contact you directly, and check back with them unprompted. Be sure to contact parents/caregivers without delay if you learn about new or relevant information pertaining to their child.

Systems-Based Practice

The Hospital and Medical Ethics

The hospital ethics committee is an advisory group usually appointed by the hospital executive medical board to act as patient advocate on bioethical issues and to develop and recommend hospital and clinical policies and guidelines that define ethical principles for conduct within the hospital. It will also provide advisory consultation and review in cases in which ethical dilemmas are perceived by the patient/patient's family, surrogate, or the physician/medical team. Committee members consist of doctors, nurses, social workers, an attorney, a chaplain, a medical ethics professional, and preferably a member of the community.

Examples of ethical and medical-legal issues usually addressed by the hospital ethics committee include:

- Withholding or withdrawing life-sustaining treatment
- Recommended procedures for determining brain death
- Guidelines for do not resuscitate (DNR) orders
- Refusal of blood transfusions
- Management of patient/family complaints
- Research involving human subjects
- Disagreement between care providers or between providers and patients/families regarding the ethical aspects of a patient's care

References

1. Stein MT, Jellinek MS, Wells RD: The difficult parent: A reflective pediatrician's response. *Pediatrics* 114:1492-1495, 2004.
2. Institute of Medicine, Committee on Palliative and End-of-Life Care for Children and Their Families, Board on Health Sciences Policy: Communication, goal setting and care planning. In Behrman RE, Field MJ, editors: *When children die: Improving palliative and end-of-life care for children and their families*, Washington, DC, 2003, National Academies Press. Available at http://www.nap. edu/openbook.php?isbn=0309084377.
3. Office on Child Abuse and Neglect (HHS); Goldman J, Salus MK, Wolcott D, Kennedy KY: *A coordinated response to child abuse and neglect: The foundation for practice*. Child Welfare Information Gateway, 2003. Available at http://www. childwelfare.gov/pubs/usermanuals/foundation/foundation.cfm.
4. Truog RD, Christ G, Browning DM, Meyer EC: Sudden traumatic death in children: "We did everything, but your child didn't survive." *JAMA* 295(22):2646-2654, 2006.
5. Fraser JJ Jr, McAbee GN; Committee on Medical Liability: Dealing with the parent whose judgment is impaired by alcohol or drugs: Legal and ethical considerations. *Pediatrics* 114(3):869-873, 2004.
6. Cahill L, Sherman P: Child abuse and domestic violence. *Pediatr Rev* 27:339-345, 2006.
7. Strauss RP, Sharp MC, Lorch SC, Kachalia B: Physicians and the communication of "Bad News": Parent experiences of being informed of their child's cleft lip and/or palate. *Pediatrics* 96:82-89, 1995.
8. Meyer EC, Ritholz MD, Burns JP, Truong RD: Improving the quality of end-of-life care in the pediatric intensive care unit: Parents' priorities and recommendations. *Pediatrics* 117:649-657, 2006.

Chapter 102
Teamwork and Communication

Sara L. P. Ross MD

Medical Knowledge and Patient Care

Background

It is estimated that a doctor performs 160,000 to 300,000 interviews during a lifetime career, making the medical interview the most commonly performed procedure in clinical medicine.[1] Multiple evidence-based studies have shown that the interpersonal and communication skills of doctors correlate with improved health outcomes, improved quality of health care provided, and enhanced patient satisfaction. Improved communication enriches the overall health of patients by increasing the efficiency and cost-effectiveness of health-care delivery and enhances the satisfaction of both patients and practitioners. More than a decade ago, Kaplan, Greenfield, and Ware[2] presented data from four clinical trials conducted in varied practice settings among chronically ill patients. The trials demonstrated improved patient health from physiologic, functional, and subjective standpoints related to specific aspects of physician-patient communication.[2] A cross-sectional observational study of 7204 adults revealed that physicians' comprehensive knowledge of patients and patients' trust in their physician were the variables most strongly associated with therapy compliance, and trust was the variable most strongly associated with patients' satisfaction with their physician.[3]

In addition, poor communication and lack of caring or collaboration in health-care delivery is often associated with the development of mistrust by the patient and the decision to litigate with filing of malpractice claims.[4] As early as 1997, the *Journal of the American Medical Association*[5] published a study of 124 primary care physician, general surgeon, and orthopedic surgeon offices in Oregon and Canada assessing the differences in communication behaviors of "no-claims" and "claims" physicians. No difference was noted between the physicians in the surgical practices, but among the primary care physicians, "no-claims" primary care physicians used more statements of orientation (educating patients on what to expect), laughed and used more humor, and tended to use more facilitation (soliciting patients' opinions, verifying understanding, encouraging patient feedback). "No-claims" physicians spent more time in routine visits than "claims" primary care physicians, and the length of the visit was an independent predictor of the claims status.[5] The first study revealing a clear relationship between communication and malpractice in surgeons was reported in 2002. It was found that a surgeon's tone of voice in routine visits is associated with malpractice claims history.[6]

To address the importance of training in effective communication, in 1999 the Accreditation Council for Graduate Medical Education (ACGME)[7] endorsed six general competencies that postgraduate residents should demonstrate, one of which was interpersonal skills and communication. Starting in 2004, all national and international medical graduates applying for postgraduate training in the United States were required to demonstrate competence in clinical, interpersonal, and communication skills on the U.S. Medical Licensing Examination (USMLE) clinical skills examination.[8]

Communication With Patients/Family

At the beginning of a patient encounter, the clinician should always introduce himself/herself to the patient/family. The truth is that patients/family want to know, and be reminded, who the members of the medical team are. Numerous doctors, nurses, and technicians may come in contact with a critically ill patient every day, and it is unrealistic to expect that patients/families remember names and faces during this extremely stressful experience.

When a patient's/family's first language is something other than English, a "nonfamily" interpreter should be used whenever possible. An interpreter allows for better clarity and simplicity in exchange of medical information and permits families to focus on key elements of medical decision making that require their consent or involvement.

When establishing a relationship with a patient/family, it is always important to elucidate the primary medical concerns and reason for seeking medical attention. Although this seems obvious, the "chief complaint" often does not correlate with the ultimate reason for admission. A further adjunct to this is to ask patients/families what they hope to "get" out of the hospital visit. One may find the medical team goals to be very different from the patient/family goals.

During a patient's hospitalization, the family is often the first to notice changes in patient status, from new complaints of pain, to changes in level of consciousness, or technical differences like a persistently elevated heart rate. It is important to be receptive to new or ongoing concerns from patients/families because their comments may herald important changes in the patient's condition.

Families pay close attention to medical rounds and desire to, and should, be included. It has been shown that parent involvement on medical rounds is perceived to improve communication and lead to better care and increased satisfaction for both families and members of the medical team.[9] In addition, if a parent/guardian is unable to be present during medical rounds, he/she should be contacted frequently during hospitalization by a member of the medical team to discuss the patient's condition.

Communication about the Patient

For any given patient, there may be dozens of students, house staff, attending physicians, consultants, nurses, respiratory therapists, nurse practitioners, and physician assistants that make up the medical team. Teamwork and ongoing communication among these groups are essential to the well-being of each patient. Discussion of patient status and goals is not isolated to morning rounds or sign-out. It is imperative that patient reassessment and communication between nurses, house staff, and attendings occur on an ongoing basis throughout the day and night. It is important to be aware of the roles of each member of the medical team and ancillary staff to avoid duplicating or overlooking aspects of the care plan.

Often patient acuity warrants immediate involvement of multiple subspecialty services, and delay and inefficiency may have deleterious or even life-threatening effects. If there is uncertainty about the need for consultation, it is always safer to seek the involvement of subspecialty services early, rather than during or after an emergency situation has arisen. When asking for consultation, one should approach consultants with specific questions and not hesitate to discuss any points of confusion with more senior members of the medical team. Most importantly, students and house staff must be readily available to all members of the medical team, especially the bedside nursing staff.

There will undoubtedly be times when members of the medical team disagree about the approach for a patient. Multidisciplinary discussion is welcomed and necessary to the delivery of superior care. However, patients/families should be shielded from disputes among members of the medical team. A unified approach to patient care is both reassuring to patients/family and embodies the team approach that is necessary for the delivery of effective care to critically ill patients.

With regard to the form of communication, one must develop both verbal and written communication skills. Daily notes should reflect key events over the past 24 hours; have a clear, concise plan; and be readable. Another written form of communication being used more frequently is a "daily patient care goal" document. This is a daily summary of the medical plan outlined on rounds for each patient that remains at the bedside for access by all members of the medical team. This has been shown to streamline communication among team members[10] and, by doing so, may reduce medical errors.

Finally, with the restrictions placed on house staff work hours, more house staff are required to complete the medical team. This affords additional opportunities for transfer of information and potential for failure of communication. It is imperative that a comprehensive discussion of daily patient events and care plans be carried out among colleagues changing shifts to provide seamless, exemplary care to patients. The use of structured templates for transferring of information has proven to be an effective method of higher-quality communication.

Interpersonal and Communication Skills

Workplace Communication: Listen and Consider What Others Have to Say about Relevant Issues

Patients are cared for by a variety of health-care practitioners who are part of a health-care team. These patients issues are often complicated, and their medical condition may change precipitously. It is important to listen to information provided by all members of the health-care team, in addition to the patient's family. Family, patients, and bedside nurses are usually the first to notice a change in patient condition. Respiratory therapists may be the first to alert you to a change in respiratory status.

Professionalism

Be Available—in Person or by Pager

Multidisciplinary discussion of patient care is encouraged and necessary. Disagreements regarding management will occur and should be addressed exclusive of the patient/family so that the patient/family can be approached with a cohesive plan of care.

Systems-Based Practice

Teamwork, Transition of Care, and the Joint Commission National Patient Safety Goals

Transition of care between teams is a critical time and has been shown to be a source of medical error. In order to minimize error The Joint Commission has adopted medication reconciliation as one of its National Patient Safety Goals. Medication reconciliation is the process by which the new care team reviews all medicines the patient is currently taking or was taking at one time and confirms that they are being administered as desired. This process is designed to reduce the number of adverse drug events (ADEs) in hospitalized patients. ADEs are known to lead to increased morbidity and mortality, extra costs, and longer lengths of stay.

References

1. Rider EA, Keefer CH: Communication skills competencies: Definitions and a teaching toolbox. *Med Educ* 40:624-629, 2006.
2. Kaplan SH, Greenfield S, Ware JE: Assessing the effects of physician-patient interactions on the outcomes of chronic disease. *Med Care* 27(3 suppl):S110-S127, 1989.
3. Safran DG, Taira DA, Rogers WH, et al: Linking primary care performance to outcomes of care. *J Fam Pract* 47(3):213-220, 1998.
4. Beckman HB, Markakis KM, Suchman AL, Frankel RM: The doctor-patient relationship and malpractice: Lessons from plaintiff depositions. *Arch Intern Med* 154(12):1365-1370, 1994.
5. Levinson W, Roter DL, Mullooly JP, et al: Physician-patient communication: The relationship with malpractice claims among primary care physicians and surgeons. *JAMA* 277(7):553-559, 1997.
6. Ambady N, Laplante D, Nguyen T, et al: Surgeons' tone of voice: A clue to malpractice history. *Surgery* 132(1):5-9, 2002.
7. Accreditation Council for Graduate Medical Education (ACGME): *General competencies: ACGME outcome project*, Chicago, IL, 2001, ACGME. Available at http://www.acgme.org/outcome/comp/compFull.asp
8. Klass D, De Champlain A, Fletcher E, et al: Development of a performance-based test of clinical skills for the United States Licensing Examination. *Federal Bull* 85:177-185, 1998.
9. Jarvis JD, Woo M, Moynihan A, et al: Parents on rounds: Joint decision making in rounds in the PICU result in positive outcomes and increased satisfaction. *Pediatr Crit Care Med* 6:626(abstract), 2005.
10. Pronovost P, Berenhotz S, Dorman T, et al: Improving communication in the ICU using daily goals. *J Crit Care* 18(2):71-75, 2003.

Chapter 103
Patient Safety

Todd Sweberg MD

Medical Knowledge and Patient Care

Background: The Institute of Medicine Report

In 1999 the Institute of Medicine released a report estimating that up to 98,000 people die each year in U.S. hospitals because of inadequate patient safety. Inpatient areas, especially critical care units, are particularly vulnerable to error. A complex interaction of attending physicians, residents, fellows, nurse practitioners, physician assistants, nurses, and pharmacists are responsible for the continuous and high-risk care dedicated to these patients; often there are multiple subspecialty services participating in patient care as well. Communication between team members may be fragmented and incomplete, leading to mistakes. In addition, the severity of disease leaves patients particularly vulnerable to morbidity and mortality resulting from medical error.

The Pediatric Experience

In the pediatric intensive care population, up to 8% of patients experience complications of care, and 4.6% of patients may experience iatrogenic illness, including infection, adverse drug reactions, and improper procedures.[1,2] Iatrogenic illness results in the need for further treatment, increasing risk to the patient from exposure to medications or procedures and causing increased expenditures. Studies show that preventable medical errors are more frequent in younger patients, in those with prolonged intensive care unit (ICU) stays, and in those with more severe illnesses. Although most mistakes are minor (78%), up to 3% may be serious events.[3] In light of this increasing burden of evidence, much focus has been placed on system-wide improvements in patient safety. A large contribution to the change in culture has been driven by The Joint Commission, which provides national accreditation to hospitals meeting certain standards. Approximately half of The Joint Commission's standards are safety related, covering topics including medication use, infection control, surgical safety, sedation and restraint use, staffing, fire safety, medical equipment safety, and emergency management. These national standards are designed in an attempt to ensure consistent application of care and thus reduce the risk for adverse events. One component of this system is The Joint Commission's Sentinel Event Policy. Under this program, events that result in unexpected death or serious injury are evaluated by the hospital using a root cause analysis. This analysis is expected to result in changes to organizational systems and processes limiting the risk for similar events occurring in the future. These events and the interventions undertaken as a result may be reported to The Joint Commission and shared with health organizations throughout the country.

Pay-for-Performance as Incentive to Safer Care

In addition to The Joint Commission, private groups have emerged as a driving force in patient safety. One example is The Leapfrog Group. This group consists of several large corporations that are significant purchasers of health care. They produce a voluntary quality and safety survey that hospitals may choose to participate in. The results, emphasizing quality of care and safety, are published and publicly available. Meeting these types of standards may allow hospitals to negotiate preferred rates of reimbursements with insurers, adding a monetary incentive to the delivery of safe care. Some of the measures that The Leapfrog Groups tracks and reports include the use of computerized order entry, adherence to national quality practices, and the staffing of intensive care units with physicians specifically trained in intensive care medicine, all initiatives that have been shown to play a role in improving the quality of care and reducing medical errors.

This pay-for-performance model has gained popularity with both private and public insurers, and recent legislation requires the Centers for Medicare and Medicaid Services (CMS) to initiate this type of approach for Medicare.[4] In order to ensure adherence to the quality and safety measures outlined in pay-for-performance programs, many hospitals and physicians have implemented care bundles. Based on disease or type of procedure, these bundles outline a consistent approach to care, incorporating the most recent safety and quality data.

"Bundles" for Consistency of Quality

Bundles have been incorporated into care in a variety of ways. Most intensive care units employ ventilator bundles, which outline specific care procedures that should be used on all mechanically ventilated patients. This usually includes the elevation of the head of the bed (>30 degrees), closed suctioning systems, and daily extubation readiness tests, designed to help avoid ventilator-associated pneumonias. Similar bundles are used to avoid central venous catheter infections. Central line bundles dictate hand washing, full barrier protection, and antiseptic skin preparation before insertion. Further requirements include sterile technique when accessing the line and daily review of the need for central venous access.

Computerized Order Entry

Another approach that has gained momentum is the use of computerized order entry. The potential benefits include reduced transcription errors, as well as prompts that warn against potential overdose, allergy, or adverse drug interactions. These systems have been shown to reduce the rate of medical errors.[5] A newer application of computerized order entry has been the use of bar coding to ensure that the right patient is receiving the ordered medication. In these systems, a nurse must scan a bar code on the patient's identification band, as well as on the medication, before administering the medication.

Standardized Drip Concentrations

A further area in which medication ordering has been modulated in an effort to improve patient safety has been the use of standardized drip concentrations. Historically, each time a vasoactive drip was ordered, a concentration was calculated based on the child's weight, and the medication was then mixed to the appropriate concentration by the pharmacist or at the bedside by the nurse. This introduced potential for error in calculation and in mixing of the medication each time. By using a standardized concentration of premixed medications, the possibility of mixing error is greatly reduced and the only calculation needed is the appropriate administration rate of the drip. These standard concentrations have been used in conjunction with smart pumps to further reduce error. By entering the concentration of the medication, the patient's weight, and the desired dose, the pump calculates the appropriate rate of administration. The adoption of fixed medication concentration and smart pump technology has been shown to reduce medication errors by up to 70%.[6]

Interpersonal and Communication Skills

Workplace Communication: Provide Person-to-Person Communication When Possible

Communication among providers is another area in which systematic approaches may improve patient safety. Because the acute and rapidly changing environment present in the ICU, the discussion of plans is frequently fragmented. Nurses may miss rounds on their patients while performing other vital duties. Residents with less experience in critical care medicine may not fully understand the daily plan. The implementation of a daily goals worksheet may improve complete communication of daily goals to the entire medical care team.[7] These daily worksheets generally provide a checklist of goals for the day. They often contain prompts to stimulate discussion regarding the continued need for central lines and Foley catheters (which are prone to infection during prolonged use). Completed at the time of rounding on the patient and left at the bedside, they provide a record for all health-care providers to refer to throughout the day regarding the aims of care for the patient.

Professionalism

Reducing the Authority Gradient Facilitates "Stopping the Line" for Patient Safety

The term "authority gradient" refers to the balance of decision-making power or the steepness of command hierarchy in a given situation. Members of a crew or organization with a domineering, overbearing, or dictatorial team leader experience a *steep* authority gradient. Expressing concerns, questioning, or even simply clarifying instructions in such an environment would require considerable determination on the part of a team member who perceives his/her input as devalued or frankly unwelcome. Although most teams require some degree of authority gradient (otherwise roles are blurred and decisions cannot be made in a timely fashion), *it is important to create an environment in which all members of the team would be comfortable speaking up to "stop the line" when there is a concern for patient safety.*[8]

Systems-Based Practice

The Joint Commission: Reporting of Sentinel Events

A sentinel event is an unexpected occurrence involving death or serious physical or psychologic injury, or the risk thereof. Serious injury specifically includes loss of limb or function. Such events are called "sentinel" because they signal the need for immediate investigation and response. The Joint Commission has issued criteria for reporting an occurrence as a sentinel event. Failure to comply with the reporting requirement will place the facility on accreditation-watch status. If a recipient of care is affected by one or more of the items listed below, then the incident must be reported to The Joint Commission:

- An event resulting in an unanticipated death or major permanent loss of function, not related to the natural course of the patient's illness or underlying condition
- Suicide during continuous care
- Infant abduction or discharge to the wrong family
- Rape
- Hemolytic transfusion reaction involving the administration of blood or blood products having major blood group incompatibilities
- Surgery on the wrong patient or body part

References

1. Stambouly JJ, Pollack MM: Iatrogenic illness in pediatric critical care. *Crit Care Med* 18(11):1248-1251, 1990.
2. Stambouly JJ, McLaughlin LL, Mandel FS, Boxer RA: Complications of care in a pediatric intensive care unit: A prospective study. *Intensive Care Med* 22(10):1098-1104, 1996.
3. Larsen GY, Donaldson AE, Parker HB, Grant MJC: Preventable harm occurring to critically ill children. *Pediatr Crit Care Med* 8(4):331-336, 2007.
4. Rosenthal MB, Dudley RA: Pay-for-performance: Will the latest payment trend improve care? *JAMA* 297(7):740-744, 2007.
5. King WJ, Paice N, Rangrej J, et al: The effect of computerized physician order entry on medication errors and adverse drug events in pediatric inpatients. *Pediatrics* 112(3, pt 1):506-509, 2003.
6. Larsen GY, Parker HB, Cash J, et al: Standard drug concentrations and smart-pump technology reduce continuous-medication-infusion errors in pediatric patients. *Pediatrics* 116(1):e21-e25, 2005.
7. Pronovost P, Berenholtz S, Dorman T, et al: Improving communication in the ICU using daily goals. *J Crit Care* 18(2):71-75, 2003.
8. AHRQ Patient Safety Network: http://psnet.ahrq.gov/popup_glossary.aspx?name =authoritygradient.

Chapter 104
Informed Consent

James S. Killinger MD *and*
Marilyn C. Morris MD, MPH

Medical Knowledge and Patient Care

Informed consent has been at the forefront of medical ethics since the middle of the twentieth century. In the United States the courts have been essential to the creation of a framework of consent to treatment. Legal decisions dating back to the early twentieth century have clarified the autonomy of the competent individual to make personal health-care decisions. Although children are not seen as competent in most legal aspects, the principles that govern consent to treatment in competent adults are important to the understanding of the application of this concept to minor children.

Legal Decisions

Early in the twentieth century, a landmark case decided in the Court of Appeals of New York helped to solidify the role of individuals in making medical decisions for themselves.[1] Mary Schloendorff had consented to have an examination of a uterine fibroid performed under anesthesia but specifically did not consent to its removal while a patient at New York Hospital. While she was under anesthesia, the surgeon removed her tumor without her consent.[1] In the opinion following the legal action brought by Mrs. Schloendorff, future U.S. Supreme Court Justice Benjamin Cordozo wrote that "[e]very human being of adult years and sound mind has the right to determine what shall be done with his own body; and a surgeon who performs an operation without his patient's consent commits an assault, for which he is liable in damages, except in cases of emergency where the patient is unconscious, and where it is necessary to operate before consent can be obtained."[2]

The term *informed consent* was used for the first time in a legal brief filed in *Salgo v Leland Stanford Jr University Board of Trustees* in 1957.[3] Martin Salgo suffered permanent paralysis as a result of translumbar aortography, and he sued his physicians for failing to warn him about the risk for paralysis.[3] The court found that the treating physicians had a duty to disclose "any facts which are necessary to form the basis of an intelligent consent by the patient to proposed treatment. Likewise the physician may not minimize the known dangers of a procedure or operation in order to induce his patient's consent."[4] In this decision, the duty of the physician to explain the risks and benefits, as well as alternative therapies, is highlighted and proves to be an essential component of true informed consent.

These court decisions and the many that followed set the framework for the concept of informed consent in terms of consent to treatment. The principles of autonomy and competence are introduced in *Schloendorff*, and the process of clearly explaining the risks, benefits, and alternatives for each intervention is outlined in *Salgo*.

Autonomy

According to Faden and Beauchamp,[3] autonomous actions are truly autonomous only if the subject acts (a) intentionally, (b) with understanding, and (c) without controlling influences. Whether an action is done intentionally is an objective determination. It is the other two conditions that truly determine the autonomous action and thus are so vital to the principle of informed consent. Patients have a wide variability in their understanding of information of diagnoses, procedures, risks, or prognoses.[3] It is the responsibility of the health-care provider to determine what is relevant and to communicate this in a way that the subject is able to comprehend.

In addition, practitioners must not coerce patients to consent; "the concept of informed consent presupposes that patients have moral and legal rights to refuse any medical intervention."[5] It is the obligation of the person obtaining the informed consent to do so with the understanding that the patient has the right to refuse the intervention. Often the patient's refusal may be due to fear, lack of understanding, or denial of the necessity of an intervention. Reassurance, clear explanation of the relevant information, and compassion are important in discussing any intervention with a patient. This takes time and effort on the part of the physician but often will lead to a more favorable situation. It may also mean that the subject fully understands the intervention, the need for the intervention, and the consequences of not giving permission for the intervention and still does not wish to go through with the intervention.

Competence

Without compelling evidence to the contrary, U.S. law assumes that adults are competent and able to make decisions for themselves. When the adult patient is temporarily incompetent (the intubated patient in the intensive care unit in need of lifesaving coronary revascularization therapy), a living will, power of attorney, or legal statute will dictate a surrogate decision maker for the patient. In the case of the previously competent patient who is no longer competent, it is critical to take into account their past wishes, and the decision maker (e.g., spouse, adult child, court-appointed guardian) should make decisions through the concept of substituted judgment, meaning that they should make decisions in accordance with what the now incompetent patient would want.

The doctrine of informed consent has only limited direct applications in pediatrics, because in most scenarios minor children are incompetent and dependent upon adults for medical decision making.[5] As a result, the American Academy of Pediatrics Committee on Bioethics released a policy statement in 1995 suggesting that parents or other surrogates provide informed permission for diagnosis and treatment of children with the assent of the child whenever appropriate."[5] With this in mind, parents or other surrogates will use the best-interests standard, which weighs quality-of life-considerations against potential burdens of therapy, or the rational-parent standard, which requires the surrogate to demonstrate the ability to prioritize options for the child using the parent or guardian's own value system.

Pediatrics differs dramatically from adult medicine in the area of withholding consent for "indicated" therapy. Although a competent adult may refuse therapy, the same is not generally true for parents and children. For example, a competent adult may refuse treatment for leukemia, but if a parent wishes to refuse proven therapy for a child with leukemia, the medical team may take legal action on behalf of the minor patient. The thought is that to do so enables the minor's future autonomy. However, the court sometimes sides with the family, particularly if the patient is an adolescent and wants to forgo therapy.

Mature Minors

There are circumstances—which vary from state to state—in which a minor child has the legal capacity to make independent medical decisions. One circumstance is in the legally emancipated minor. In many states this category of patients includes those minors who marry, enter military service, live outside their parents' home and are no longer financially dependent on their parents, and those who are parents or are pregnant.[5] In another circumstance, states may give decision-making authority to minors who seek treatment for certain medical conditions (sexually transmitted diseases, pregnancy, and drug and alcohol abuse).[6]

Assent

Assent of the minor patient is dependent upon the developmental stage of the patient. It is the responsibility of the physician to understand age-appropriate development when engaging a patient in a discussion regarding assent to an intervention. The American Academy of Pediatrics Committee on Bioethics, in their policy statement on informed consent, has included the following guidelines with respect to assent[5]:

Assent should include at least the following elements:

1. Helping the patient achieve a developmentally appropriate awareness of the nature of his or her condition.
2. Telling the patient what he or she can expect with tests or treatment(s).
3. Making a clinical assessment of the patient's understanding of the situation and the factors influencing how he or she is responding (including whether there is inappropriate pressure to accept testing or therapy).
4. Soliciting an expression of the patient's willingness to accept the proposed care. Regarding the final point, no one should solicit a patient's views without intending to weigh them seriously. In situations in which the patient will have to receive medical care despite his or her objection, the patient should be told that fact and should not be deceived.

Clarity

Informed consent is not a parent's signature on a form. Informed consent, informed permission, and informed assent all are predicated on the clear sharing of information and values among the physician, parent, and, at times, the patient.[5] Discussions in this area revolve around three main issues when it comes to medical therapeutics: risks, benefits, and alternatives to a particular intervention. In order for the physician to discuss any potential intervention, he or she must know the risks, benefits, and alternatives before any discussion with the family is to occur.

Being prepared for the discussion with the family allows for more clarity and instills more confidence in the medical team. For example, the team caring for a patient decides that a patient needs a blood transfusion, and two of the major risks of this intervention are infection and allergic reaction. The person obtaining consent should be able to communicate to the family how likely it is that each of those two events will occur. Secondly, the family should understand the benefits of a blood transfusion in the particular clinical situation. Lastly, what are the alternatives? Any person obtaining consent in this situation should be able to anticipate these concerns and have the information available for the family when they ask.

Treatment without Consent

Consent for medical treatment may be implied (or assumed) in emergency situations.[3] The idea here is that delaying care in order to obtain informed consent could cause serious or permanent harm. However, short of an urgent circumstance, implied consent does not apply, and informed consent should be obtained.

Interpersonal and Communication Skills

- Be patient when discussing what may seem to be simple interventions with families. Even the most sophisticated parents are in a very high stress environment when their child is ill and will often need time to fully understand the intervention.
- Open discussions—Sit down when discussing interventions with families.
- Share information—Be clear in explaining the intervention, and do so in language that the patient and family will understand; use a foreign language interpreter when appropriate.

Professionalism

- Allow for enough time to discuss interventions with families.
- Know the limits—It is important to have a complete understanding of the intervention that informed consent is needed for. Know the data on the risks and alternatives for interventions.
- Respect others—Be accountable to children and their families, working cooperatively with them. Be available if the family has questions after agreeing to the intervention, and be considerate and empathetic when discussing complicated interventions, without condescension. Be sure that the team taking care of a patient understands the reason for any intervention. Families will often ask several other people on the team their opinions before agreeing to any intervention. Mixed messages are very difficult for families in high-stress environments like the pediatric intensive care unit.

References

1. Osman H: History and development of the the doctrine of informed consent. *Int Electr J Health Educ* 4:41-47, 2001.
2. *Schloendorff v Society of New York Hospital,* 211 NY 125 (1914).
3. Faden RR, Beauchamp TL: *A history and theory of informed consent*, New York, 1986, Oxford University Press.
4. *Salgo v Leland Stanford etc Bd Trustees,* 154 Cal App 2d 560 (1957).
5. Committee on Pediatric Emergency Medicine: Consent for emergency medical services for children and adolescents. *Pediatrics* 111(3):703-706, 2003.
6. Sigman GS, O'Connor C: Exploration for physicians of the mature minor doctrine. *J Pediatr* 119(4):520-525, 1991.
7. Beauchamp TL, Childress JF: *Principles of biomedical ethics*, ed 5, New York, 2001, Oxford Univeristy Press.

Chapter 105
Ethics in the Neonatal Intensive Care Unit: The Limits of Viability

Helen M. Towers MD

Medical Knowledge and Patient Care

The limits of viability encompass three different groups of infants in the neonatal intensive care unit (NICU). Some infants are born with evidence of congenital anomalies that are incompatible with life. These infants are generally identified in the antenatal period by ultrasound or chromosome analysis or by physical examination very shortly after delivery. In these unfortunate cases, there may be no medical interventions available to correct the underlying problem. No ethical dilemma regarding the provision of care exists, and the infants are offered comfort care. The families are generally provided with social support, and palliative support services as available. Other infants reach the limit of medical viability by virtue of congenital or acquired illnesses that lead to death despite extensive resuscitation efforts. These cases also generally do not generate ethical dilemmas, because all available resources have been used. The third group of infants consists of infants born at the gestational limit of viability, which is generally accepted as that time period between 22 and 25 completed weeks of gestation. Infants with birth weight less than 700 g make up approximately 5% of NICU admissions but account for almost one third of the deaths in the NICU. Because of the uncertainty of outcome at this gestational age, the decisions regarding the provision of medical care to these infants are laden with medical, social, and bioethical implications and remain some of the most difficult decisions that neonatal practitioners and the families of these tiny infants face together. The following areas are helpful in gathering the information required to make an informed and ethical decision in these situations.

Gestational Age

In vitro fertilization is clearly associated with an accurate date of conception. The accuracy of gestational dating in spontaneous pregnancies is greatest in the first trimester, approaching ±5 days, and has been greatly enhanced by early prenatal care and ultrasound evaluation. Gestational age based on a composite of menstrual history, early pregnancy examination, laboratory data, and ultrasound examination has been seen to predict survival better than estimated fetal weight. Fetal weight estimates may vary as much as 15% to 20%. Postnatal examination generally underestimates gestational age in infants less than 28 weeks.

Birth Weight[2]

Most infants with birth weight above 800 grams who receive optimal neonatal intensive care survive. There are few survivors with birth weight less than 400 grams. In the past two decades improvements in neonatal care have led to greater numbers of infants with birth weights ranging from 450 to 700 grams surviving at least the first day of life, but the success rate has reached a plateau in the last 10 years. Interestingly, one report suggests that if the infant survives until the fourth day of life, the likelihood of survival to discharge approaches 80% for this group of extremely low-birth-weight (ELBW) infants and was greater than 50% for those infants weighing less than 600 grams. Therefore most tiny infants who die in the NICU do so within the first 72 hours of life. This observation may counteract arguments that scarce health-care dollars invested in NICU care are spent on infants who do not survive.

Medical Outcomes

The two questions most commonly proposed to physicians during antenatal counseling at the gestational limit of viability are generally "Will my baby survive?" and "Will my baby survive neurologically intact?" The outcome figures from national and local sources should be used when counseling because these outcome data may differ significantly. Reported data suggest highest survival levels of approximately 25% for infants born at 23 completed weeks, 60% at 24 completed weeks, and 70% at 25 weeks. Data from individual units may vary considerably, and the prediction for intact survival for any individual infant is impossible. Reported outcomes on infants born under 26 weeks completed gestation reveal a high prevalence of neurologic and developmental disabilities, including cerebral palsy, deafness, blindness, and mental retardation. One study of surviving infants less than 26 weeks gestation reported 46% of infants had moderate or severe disability at 6 years of age, and 34% had mild disability. Surviving male infants were seen to have an increased risk for disability.

Condition at Birth[3,4,7]

Because of the nonuniformity in application of resuscitation measures to infants at the threshold of viability, there are insufficient data indicating that the condition at birth is predictive of outcome. Scores of illness severity have been developed to attempt to predict survival or nonsurvival of infants admitted to intensive care units. These scores include the APACHE, PRISM, and SNAP scoring systems and are based on physiologic parameters that include respiratory support, heart rate, blood pressure, oxygenation status, and other measures. The predictive power for nonsurvival using these score systems is rarely greater than 50%. Clinical experience and intuition of the health-care providers are also inaccurate predictors of nonsurvival.

Parental Wishes[5]

Parents are the surrogate decision makers for their children and retain the right to jointly make decisions with the physician regarding the initiation or noninitiation of intensive care at the threshold of gestational viability. For those cases in which uncertainty prevails it is not uncommon to initiate intensive care, with the caveat that as more information becomes available or the infant fails to respond to therapeutic interventions, intensive measures may not be escalated or might subsequently be withdrawn and comfort care provided. Frequent reevaluation of the medical situation is required, and frequent communication between the parents and health-care team is of paramount importance so that the course of action chosen is medically appropriate and consistent with the family's own personal values and goals.

Comfort Care

In those situations in which the decision is made to withhold resuscitation, discontinue resuscitation, or forego other life-supporting treatments, an active plan of comfort care is initiated. This includes careful handling, maintaining warmth, avoidance of invasive procedures, and unobtrusive monitoring. Support for the parents by social services, chaplain support, or other bereavement support should be offered. An awareness and respect for cultural and religious diversity is particularly important at these times. Parents can and should be asked to share their preferences for end-of-life care.

Ethics Committees

There are occasions when complex and difficult decisions may need to be negotiated between families, physicians, and nursing staff. Multidisciplinary ethics committees have played an important role in assisting all parties in voicing their concerns and will generally provide an objective recommendation after due consultation and consideration. Any member of the family or health-care team is at liberty to request their counsel.

Bereavement Counseling

Referral for counseling after the demise of an infant is helpful and should be extended to the family. Developmentally appropriate sibling support can be offered to help explain the loss to other family members. Many institutions hold annual memorial services to which families return year after year.

In summary, the decision-making process surrounding the delivery of an infant at the gestational threshold will likely never be absolutely applicable to every case, precisely because it is filled with the complexities of the individual family and their circumstances. As medical advances continue, the ethical questions regarding how we apply these technologies to fragile and vulnerable infants at the threshold of biologic viability will remain, and it is important that they continue to be asked.

Interpersonal and Communication Skills

Encourage Partnership Between the Physician and the Family

Meetings with the health-care team before delivery, even surrounded by the stresses of impending preterm delivery, can provide opportunities for families to ask questions, weigh options, and learn about the risks inherent in early delivery. A clear delineation of the current situation and potential options needs to be presented in an unbiased but sympathetic manner to parents and updated regularly as information becomes available. The decision to either continue care or withdraw support when the outcome is unknown or uncertain should not be a unilateral decision made by either party, but ideally should be a consensus partnership between the physician and the family taking in all the particulars of the individual situation.[6]

Professionalism

Place the Family's Values Ahead of One's Own

Personal biases and values of the physician or other health-care providers may conflict with parental choices. It is important to be conscious of the potential for difference in opinion and to respect parental autonomy, as long as the decisions remain medically appropriate.

Systems-Based Practice

Medical Ethics: American Medical Association Standards of Conduct

As a member of the medical profession, a physician must recognize responsibility to patients first and foremost, as well as to society, to other health professionals, and to oneself. The following principles of medical ethics adopted by the American Medical Association are not laws, but standards of conduct that define the essentials of honorable behavior for the physician[8]:

I.   A physician shall be dedicated to providing competent medical care, with compassion and respect for human dignity and rights.

II. A physician shall uphold the standards of professionalism, be honest in all professional interactions, and strive to report physicians deficient in character or competence, or engaging in fraud or deception, to appropriate entities.

III. A physician shall respect the law and also recognize a responsibility to seek changes in those requirements that are contrary to the best interests of the patient.

IV. A physician shall respect the rights of patients, colleagues, and other health professionals, and shall safeguard patient confidences and privacy within the constraints of the law.

V. A physician shall continue to study, apply, and advance scientific knowledge, maintain a commitment to medical education, make relevant information available to patients, colleagues, and the public, obtain consultation, and use the talents of other health professionals when indicated.

VI. A physician shall, in the provision of appropriate patient care, except in emergencies, be free to choose whom to serve, with whom to associate, and the environment in which to provide medical care.

VII. A physician shall recognize a responsibility to participate in activities contributing to the improvement of the community and the betterment of public health.

VIII. A physician shall, while caring for a patient, regard responsibility to the patient as paramount.

IX. A physician shall support access to medical care for all people.

References

1. Lantos JD, Meadow WL: *Neonatal bioethics: The moral challenges of medical innovation*, Baltimore, 2006, Johns Hopkins University Press.
2. Tyson JE, Nehal PA, Langer J, et al: Intensive care for extreme prematurity—moving beyond gestational age. *N Engl J Med* 358(16):1672-1681, 2008.
3. Janvier A, Barrington KJ: The ethics of neonatal resuscitation at the margins of viability: Informed consent and outcomes. *J Pediatr* 147(5):579-585, 2005.
4. Peerzada JM, Richardson DK, Burns JP: Delivery room decision making at the threshold of viability. *J Pediatr* 145(4):492-498, 2004.
5. Meadow W, Frain L, Ren Y, et al: Serial assessment of mortality in the neonatal intensive care unit by algorithm and intuition: Certainty, uncertainty and informed consent. *Pediatrics* 109:878-886, 2002.
6. AAP policy statement: Perinatal care at the threshold of viability. *Pediatrics* 110(5):1024-1027, 2002.
7. Marlow N, Wolke D, Bracewell MA, et al for the EPICure Study Group: Neurologic and developmental disability at six years of age after extremely preterm birth. *N Engl J Med* 352(1):9-18, 2005.
8. http://www.ama-assn.org/ama/pub/physician-resources/medical-ethics/code-medical-ethics/principles-medical-ethics.shtml

Chapter 106
The Challenge of Immunization Refusal

Stephen C. Eppes MD

Medical Knowledge and Patient Care

Background and Scope of the Problem

Recent surveys have demonstrated that 85% of U.S. pediatricians encountered immunization refusal during the preceding 12 months,[1] only 77% of 3-year-olds had received all recommended vaccines,[2] and 25% of parents believe a theory that the total number of vaccines and number administered simultaneously harm the immune system.[3] This is difficult for physicians because prevention is an important aspect of pediatric care, and immunization is a cornerstone of prevention. If parents disagree with the physician about immunization, trust, which is so important in a productive physician-patient relationship, is undermined. Some physicians may fear legal repercussions from failing to immunize, or worry about resurgence of disease. Frustration, disappointment, and even anger may result when physicians are unable to provide this critical aspect of well child care.

Approach to Vaccination Refusal

Some physicians dismiss families who decline vaccination. Because children need access to health care for reasons other than immunization, the American Academy of Pediatrics (AAP) discourages dismissal unless a substantial level of distrust or philosophical differences has developed.[4]

The first step in dealing with vaccine refusal is to explore with the family their basis of **concern or reservation about vaccines.** Their vaccine fears may be based on relatively weak conceptual grounds, which may be overcome with education. Some families have more deep-seated belief systems, often rooted in dubious information and recommendations. **The clinician must understand the belief system in order to confront it.** To simply dismiss the family's concerns will cause some to seek another health-care provider who will acquiesce to their requests or demands. The physician should be honest about what is known (and not known) about risks and benefits of immunization.[4] The family should be counseled about disease prevalence, both in the United States and globally, because of increased international travel. Counseling should include estimates of potential morbidity and mortality should the child become infected.

Most modern-day parents have never seen the diseases that currently available vaccines prevent. The U.S. vaccination program may be a victim of its own success. **Some parents now wonder why their children must receive shots to prevent diseases that they perceive do not even exist.** Parents may be aware of vaccine preservatives, adjuvants, other additives, or residual substances from the production process. Gelatin and egg proteins may be present in quantities sufficient to cause severe hypersensitivity reactions, but these are quite rare. Minute amounts of other substances, including thimerosal, formaldehyde, aluminum, antibiotics, and yeast proteins have never been shown to be harmful in either experimental animals or humans.[5]

Parents are often influenced by misinformation. Sources of misleading information include well-meaning friends and family members, books devoted to the hazards of vaccines, and even some antivaccination health-care practitioners. The Internet is a major vehicle for dissemination of antivaccination material that may sound official. Many sources refer to dubious scientific studies, whereas others emphasize heart-wrenching personal testimonies about children who were allegedly harmed by vaccines, and others decry health-care conspiracies.

To address parental concerns, physicians should understand the considerable effort and **multiple steps are required to develop safe, effective vaccines and put them into routine use.** This complex process initially involves animal and human safety testing followed by large-scale testing for efficacy, immunogenicity, and safety in the target population, followed by Food and Drug Administration (FDA) approval and licensure. The Advisory Committee on Immunization Practices (ACIP) advises the Centers for Disease Control and Prevention (CDC), and the candidate vaccine is recommended for addition to the immunization schedule. Next, independent professional organizations (e.g., the AAP) release their recommendations with modifications as appropriate. Finally, public and private insurance companies approve vaccine coverage and put it into action in the community.

Vaccine safety is of paramount importance for the ACIP, professional organizations, practitioners, and parents. However, **"safe" does not imply "risk free."** All vaccines have potential adverse reactions that are usually discovered before licensure. Minor side effects such as injection site pain may be fairly frequent with some vaccines. Major adverse events must be very uncommon for a vaccine to ever achieve licensure. Sometimes rare but important side effects are captured only by postmarketing surveillance. Physicians should know and remind parents that reports of adverse events associated with vaccinations are continuously reviewed by the FDA.

For parents (and sometimes children), immunizations are a memorable event such that, *if a child develops a condition in temporal relationship to receipt of a vaccine(s), they may assume a causal relationship,* when the timing may be a chance coincidence. There are several well-publicized "associations" that lack credible evidence.

- *Measles, mumps, and rubella (MMR) vaccine and autism:* MMR is administered shortly after the first birthday, when certain developmental abnormalities, including autism, are likely to be identified. Multiple published studies from the United States and Europe have failed to identify a causal relationship of MMR and autism spectrum disorders.[6]
- *Thimerosal and autism:* Thimerosal (an organic mercury compound) was a common vaccine preservative, and concern arose for potential neurotoxicity. However, based on scientific evidence, the toxicity of trace amounts of thimerosal in vaccines appears to be nil. There is no credible epidemiologic link to autism or other neurologic conditions. However, as a precautionary measure, thimerosal is no longer used in routinely recommended childhood vaccines (except for certain influenza vaccines). The incidence of autism has continued to rise despite reduction or elimination of thimerosal (see Chapter 26, Autism).[6]

In addition to the lack of credible scientific evidence for a link between MMR and/or thimerosal and autism, the U.S. Court of Federal Claims in the Omnibus Autism Proceeding has concluded that there is no association (and therefore no basis for medicolegal liability).

Interpersonal and Communication Skills

Counsel and Advocate for Vaccination Using a Nonjudgmental Approach

A nonjudgmental approach with a well-organized dialogue will be the most successful. The physician's understanding of the family's concerns and the manner in which the conversation is begun may have significant impact. Emphasizing benefits, as opposed to risks, may work better for some families. On the other hand, some parents may be more comfortable choosing the risks they would be willing to accept for their children, rather than having risks forced upon them. Parents like these will be unlikely to respond to a discussion of mandatory requirements and legal ramifications. The main focus should be the welfare of the child, even though the physician and parents may not always agree on what is in the child's best interest. As the physician-patient relationship develops over time, with open communication and mutual respect, parents may be willing to reconsider their previous objection to immunization.

Professionalism

Social Justice: The Obligation to Limit Vaccine-Preventable Disease

Parental permission must be obtained before children receive immunizations, and parents are free to decline immunization, unless their decision places the child at substantial risk for serious harm.[4] The physician who understands disease epidemiology, risks for infection, and likely outcome of an infection has a critical role in protecting the child and is responsible for presenting information to help the family reconsider their position.[7]

Families who refuse to vaccinate their children because of perceived risks, philosophical objections, inconvenience, or cost are often referred to as "free riders."[1,4] They indirectly benefit from vaccines because of the immunity of others that results in low levels of infection within the population (i.e., herd protection). Some questioning parents may respond to this argument of "social justice" when they realize that immunization can be viewed as a civic responsibility that promotes a safe environment for medically fragile/vulnerable individuals such as the very young, immunocompromised, and cancer patients.

Practice-Based Learning and Improvement

Stay Informed of Advances in Vaccinology

There have been major advances in vaccinology with several newly approved vaccines over the last few years, resulting in considerable information for the physician to comprehend and put into clinical practice. There are vaccines currently in clinical development at least some of which will ultimately become FDA approved and incorporated into the vaccine schedule. To keep up with new vaccine information and changing immunization schedules requires taking an active role in continued learning. There are online opportunities for learning about immunization on several excellent websites:

- American Academy of Pediatrics http://www.aap.org
- American Academy of Family Physicians http://www.familydoctor.org
- AAP Childhood Immunization Support Program http://www.cispimmunize.org
- Immunization Action Coalition http://www.immunize.org
- National Network for Immunization Information http://www.immunizationinfo.org

Systems-Based Practice

Cost-Effectiveness of Publicly Funded Vaccination Programs

The cost-effectiveness of currently recommended childhood vaccines has been established, in both quality-adjusted life years for individuals and net cost savings to society. That said, physicians should be sensitive to the possibility that the cost of office visits, vaccines, and vaccine administration may be the reason some parents hesitate about immunization. Offices and clinics should work with these families accordingly to help get their vaccines paid for in either the private or public (Vaccines for Children [VFC]) sector. Physicians who immunize qualified children should be familiar with the VFC program in their state. VFC is a government-sponsored program that provides all vaccines on the current schedule free of charge to children with public insurance (i.e., Medicaid) and to children who lack insurance. It is a carefully structured program that tracks recipients' records and requires participating offices to maintain separate storage and recording of the vaccine stock. An accurate office record-keeping system is required to satisfy requirements and audits of the VFC program.

If physicians are concerned about liability associated with failing to vaccinate, they should carefully document the discussion of risks and benefits and the family's refusal in the medical record. The use of a waiver is a helpful strategy: If parents have to sign a document acknowledging the risks and benefits have been explained and that they are declining to have their child vaccinated, it may help persuade them to reconsider. If they do sign, the waiver is an important piece of documentation and should be kept in the child's medical record.

References

1. Lyren A, Leonard E: Vaccine refusal: Issues for the primary care physician. *Clin Pediatr* 45:399-404, 2006.
2. Centers for Disease Control and Prevention: The National Immunization Survey. Available at http://www.cdc.gov/nis/.
3. Offit PA, Quarles J, Gerber MA, et al: Addressing parents' concerns: Do multiple vaccines overwhelm or weaken the infant's immune system? *Pediatrics* 109:124-129, 2002.
4. American Academy of Pediatrics, Committee on Bioethics: Responding to parental refusals of immunization of children. *Pediatrics* 115:1428-1431, 2005.
5. Offit PA, Jew RK: Addressing parents' concerns: Do vaccines contain harmful preservatives, adjuvants, additives, or residuals? *Pediatrics* 112:1394-1401, 2003.
6. National Network for Immunization Information: Available at http://www.immunizationinfo.org/iom_reports_detail.cfv?id=42.
7. Levi BH: Addressing parents' concerns about childhood immunizations: A tutorial for primary care providers. *Pediatrics* 120:18-26, 2007.

Chapter 107
Building Rapport With the Pediatric Patient: A Retrospective Perspective

Deena K. Roemer

The extraordinary progress in medicine has largely been due to tremendous advances in science and technology over the past few decades. However, before surgical robots and lasers in the operating room, and before millimeter-size incisions became the norm, the practice of medicine relied more heavily on the time-tested commodity of skillful rapport. Although mastering medical knowledge and clinical skills has been a major focus until this stage of your medical education, consider that your capacity to build rapport can effectively bring the art to the science, and this is what can make a good physician great.

Having spent the better part of my teenage years and well into my twenties dealing with a chronic illness, I now realize that disappointments in my physician relationships during my early years as a patient remained with me for 15 years. As I approach my thirtieth birthday and yet another bout with ulcerative colitis, I welcome the opportunity to share some thoughts, hoping to transform my previous disappointments into a reflection that may be useful to the next generation of caring physicians.

Establishing rapport is essential to the healing relationship. Though some physicians may have more innate skill than others, the best ways to develop rapport can be taught. Its mastery may, at times, seem as difficult as decoding the Rosetta stone. You speak one language, "Doctor," while the patient speaks "Kid," and far too often the intended message is lost in translation. Medical jargon can sound sterile to a sick child and can be the fast track to disengagement and feelings of defeat. On the other hand, good communication skills will make life easier for both doctor and patient from the initial encounter through the phases of diagnosis and disease management. There is tremendous power in doctor-patient collaboration when you have successfully recruited the patient to be an active participant in his or her care.

The key to "how to" lies in focusing on one's *interactions* with the patient as much as one focuses on the desired treatment outcomes. By concentrating effort on the *specific practice* of interpersonal skills and communication, the real physician partnership based on rapport can be created.

HOW TO MAKE A GOOD FIRST AND CARING IMPRESSION

Most articles that highlight the value of building rapport focus on making a good first impression and stress the importance of introducing yourself, making eye contact, smiling, and addressing the patient by name. All are true. My perspective as a patient is that in a high-anxiety setting like a hospital, rapport requires more than a handshake: it requires offering up your humanity. How can you let your humanity shine through?

1. **Acknowledge the child's hardship.** Diagnoses and doctor's orders are often met with resistance. Ordering a child to complete a battery of medical tests or ingest daily medication is easy. Getting the child to comply is a different story. Tests and treatments may come with unpleasant prep activities and side effects. Thus it may be perceived that the child is being asked to choose an unknown pain or discomfort over the pain and discomfort that is already familiar. It is a good idea to acknowledge the anticipated hardship and validate the child's fears, anxiety, and discomfort. Be honest and forthright. Downplaying anticipated side effects may diminish your future credibility. Honest information can be delivered with carefully chosen and sensitive words.

2. **Break out the drawing board.** Medical knowledge is a string of complex concepts, and for pediatric patients and parents, it is useful to SIMPLIFY and DIAGRAM. Spend time on explanations, and use age-appropriate language. Use visuals such as drawings or models to help explain an illness within the context of the body at large. If age appropriate, consider drawing a diagram, and have the child color it. Analogies are your friend and are great for helping children visualize and process content. If a child has a basic understanding of what is going on in his/her body, the child may be more likely to help you fight it.

3. **Much like a teacher, be suggestion oriented.** Providing helpful information that may not be found elsewhere (i.e., an insider's tip) can make you invaluable. There are many day-to-day challenges a child with a chronic illness must face. Offer suggestions for daily coping as often as possible. Even if your patient does not follow every suggestion, it will show your recognition of the child's daily struggle and your active attempts to seek ways to ease it.

4. **Seek out the psychologic and social issues.** The physical effects of a chronic illness are usually visible. The emotional and psychologic impact may be less transparent, yet equally painful. Research shows that psychologic issues motivate 65% of primary care visits.[1] Parents are more likely to disclose psychologic issues when a pediatrician shows interest, asks direct questions, and listens attentively.[2] While treating the body, do not forget the mind: when an emotional issue or social barrier to successful treatment is uncovered, take the time to point your patient in the direction of help.

5. **Engage, empower, and encourage the child's input from day one!** You will give patients many important instructions over the course of their treatment; but once they leave your office, the sphere of your influence is limited unless they have been specifically empowered to take the initiative with their illness. Encourage the patient to learn about the illness (perhaps consider a reading assignment), to ask questions, and to keep a record of how he or she is feeling. If there is a protracted treatment plan, ask for feedback at each stage. Set goals, and as small successes become evident, be sure the patient is directly associating those successes with his or her own efforts.

6. **Make yourself accessible.** Be accessible beyond the time spent in the examination room. A doctor's office is an intimidating place, and parents and children are likely to feel overwhelmed just by the setting alone. Within the realm of reasonable expectations and your own personal boundary preservation, let your patient and the family know how to contact you, and respond as promptly as possible to their communications. Evidence-based studies show that good communication and focus on the relationship between patient and physician correlate directly with improved quality of care, including symptom improvement,[3-7] increased patient adherence to treatment plans,[8] better management of chronic conditions,[9-11] increased patient and physician satisfaction,[12,13] and reduced risk of medical errors.[14]

The above thoughts are merely the personal reflections of a single patient, who (despite whatever implicit criticisms may be manifest) is ultimately grateful for her medical care and to those practitioners who have rendered it. Nonetheless, the sentiments and recommendations found herein seem to be corroborated fully by a review of the extant literature on this important subject.

References

1. Kahn RS, Wise PH, Finkelstein JA, et al: The scope of unmet maternal health needs in pediatric settings. *Pediatrics* 103:576-581, 1999.
2. Wissow LS: Pediatrician interview style and mothers' disclosure of psychosocial issues. *Pediatrics* 93:289-295, 1994.
3. Mumford E, Schlesinger HJ, Glass GV: The effects of psychological intervention on recovery from surgery and heart attacks: An analysis of the literature. *Am J Public Health* 72:141-151, 1982.
4. Uhlmann R, Inui TS, Peconaro RE, et al: Relationship of patient request fulfillment to compliance, glycemic control and other health care outcomes in insulin-dependent diabetes. *J Gen Intern Med* 3:458-463, 1988.
5. Brody DS, Miller SM, Lerman CE, et al: Patient perception of involvement in medical care: Relationship to illness attitudes and outcomes. *J Gen Intern Med* 4:506-511, 1989.
6. Stewart MA: Effective physician patient communication and health outcomes: A review. *Can Med Assoc J* 152:1423-1433, 1995.
7. Stewart M, Brown JB, Donner A, et al: The impact of patient-centered care on outcomes. *J Fam Pract* 49:796-804, 2000.

8. DiMatteo MR: The role of effective communication with children and their families in fostering adherence to pediatric regimens. *Patient Educ Couns* 55:339-344, 2004.

9. Heisler M, Bouknight RR, Hayward RA, et al: The relative importance of physician communication, participatory decision making and patient understanding in diabetes self management. *J Gen Intern Med* 17:243-252, 2002.

10. Gascon JJ, Sanchez-Ortuno M, Lior B, et al: Why hypertensive patients do not comply with treatment: Results from a qualitative study. *Fam Pract* 21:125-130, 2004.

11. Cabana MD, Slish KK, Evans D, et al: Impact of physician asthma care education on patient outcomes. *Pediatrics* 117:2149-2157, 2006.

12. Flocke SA, Miller WL, Crabtree BF: Relationships between physician practice style; patient satisfaction, and attributes of primary care. *J Fam Pract* 51:835-840, 2002.

13. Daghio MM, Ciardullo AV, Cadioli T: GPs' satisfaction with the doctor-patient encounter: Findings from a community based survey. *Fam Pract* 20:283-288, 2003.

14. Woolf SH, Kuzel AJ, Dovey SM, et al: A string of mistakes: The importance of cascade analysis in describing, counting, and preventing medical errors. *Ann Fam Med* 2:317-326, 2004.

Chapter 108
The Core Competencies in a Disaster Zone: The Haitian Experience

Glenn R. Stryjewski MD, MPH

As a physician educator in the United States, I believe in the values set forth by the Accreditation Council for Graduate Medical Education (ACGME) in their outcomes project. The six core competencies capture the many facets of what defines excellent physicians and the quality of care they deliver. The question in Haiti, however, was whether these competencies maintain their relevance amidst a disaster. If so, then are the competencies different in Haiti than in the well developed health care environment of the United States?

MEDICAL KNOWLEDGE

"You Know What You Know"

The truth of this aphorism became apparent upon first patient contact and served as a source of discomfort for me throughout my time in Haiti. It exposed my dependence on others as a safety net for my own knowledge gaps. I am a pediatric critical care physician by trade. In some ways my training provided me with much of the requisite knowledge to care for the injured children of Haiti. However, the bits of knowledge I did not possess, I rarely had the opportunity to ask about or search for in the medical literature. I was surrounded by wonderful and intelligent practitioners, but certainly I did not have the usual array of subspecialists from whom I so frequently draw knowledge. Their absence was magnified by the presentation of unique diseases such as tetanus, something we are rarely called upon to treat in the highly immunized community in which I practice. However, my discomfort with my knowledge base made me fail back upon my years of study and practice and doctoring processes I had learned. I was forced to make diagnoses and treatment decisions about which I was unsure. But the solid foundations of medical knowledge from medical school and residency carried the day. I was compelled to reinvigorate my history-taking skills; my physical examination skills were revitalized; and, once again, clinical judgment reigned over sophisticated testing. My eyes, ears, nose, and hands, combined with the knowledge of anatomy and physiology I had acquired over time, helped me do what I was trained to do. My discomfort waned as my inner physician once again resurfaced.

PATIENT CARE

What Is Quality Care?

We apply a certain standard of care that we feel is adequate and appropriate to deliver within our local health care environment. Most of us feel that we deliver a high standard of care every day. So what is quality care when there is no standard to compare it with? We lacked needed supplies, so we improvised where possible. Substitutions that we would never have made at home suddenly seemed justifiable. Was this delivering poor-quality patient care? Honestly, this took some time to get used to. Initially, this felt awful, as if we were doing a disservice to the very people we were trying to help. Perhaps we should just go home. How could we even consider using amoxicillin alone to treat a massive cellulitis on an injured leg? How could we provide deep sedation without a pulse-ox monitor? How could we care for a premature newborn without any ability to keep the baby warm? It was impossible to provide care at the level we would have provided in Philadelphia. What we did in Haiti, however, was raise the standard of available patient care the best we could. Ultimately, we met the community standard and exceeded it by far. We created a pediatric intensive care unit (PICU) and neonatal intensive care unit (NICU). As far as we could tell, these were the only functioning PICU and NICU in the country! Despite unfortunate imbalance in health care standards worldwide, patient care is as much what we do as how we do it. Care was delivered with compassion, concern, and empathy. We tried our best to offset the shortcomings in our provision of care with compassion in our demeanor and with vigilance in our follow-up and daily concern.

PRACTICE-BASED LEARNING AND IMPROVEMENT

Integrate Evidence With Values
In the United States, I am a strong proponent of the principles of evidence-based medicine (EBM). EBM teaches us to integrate the best available evidence from the scientific literature **with the situation, beliefs, and values of our individual patient.** Many of us are oblivious to the latter part of this definition and associate EBM only with reading and quoting from the latest journal articles. So how does one practice EBM when the ability to access the medical literature does not exist? In Haiti, the best level of evidence became our own personal experiences. Practice-based learning was supplanted by trial and error. Medline was replaced by the best advice of our colleagues. Good communication and professionalism compensated for the absence of search engines, and we remained steadfastly guided by the beliefs and values of our patients.

INTERPERSONAL AND COMMUNICATION SKILLS

Bonding Through Nonverbal Communication
Even in the United States it can be difficult to care for a patient who speaks a language unfamiliar to others. In general, we teach that the use of an interpreter is of paramount importance unless you are fully fluent in a given language. In Haiti, where Creole is the predominant language, very few of the U.S. physicians had any familiarity with the language and interpreters were scarce. We were also faced with many orphans, so parents were not available to assist in communication with a young child. We communicated in any way we could and this bonded us: We made drawings, gestures, and noises that were quite amusing. Although not the most efficient method of communicating, the doctor-patient relationship was enhanced. In pediatrics, laughter is a powerful tool. We became closer to our patients because of it. It provided a therapy to the children, which in some instances was better than anything else we could provide.

PROFESSIONALISM

Let the Welfare of the Patient Reign Above All Else
The professionalism of the staff in Haiti exceeded my expectations. Though in retrospect I might have anticipated how highly the concept

of teamwork might be valued among a group of those self-selected for self-sacrifice, I was constantly amazed at our group's responses to the professionalism challenges we faced. Despite the lack of resources, there was rarely disagreement over their use. Doctors, nurses, respiratory therapists, physical therapists, pharmacists and lay people all led and all followed. Unanimous decisions were the rule. In the few instances when treatment decisions were not unanimous, compassionate, well-thought conversations took place. It was obvious that the welfare of the patient reigned above all else. This sacred value of patient care reminded me of why I chose medicine, how I felt when I was new to it, and why it is both career and passion to so many of us.

SYSTEMS-BASED PRACTICE

Systems, What Systems?

Insurance companies, third-party payers, billing, oversight, and regulatory authorities did not exist. There was never a need to call to justify a prescription or write a letter of medical necessity. No need to prepare for a visit from The Joint Commission. At first this was liberating. But I was surprised that my experiences in Haiti taught me something about the value of these systems. Although frustrating at times, we all need to be stewards of the financial resources that enable us to deliver good care. Insurance companies that pay for physician and hospital services frustrate us at times when they question our decisions to save themselves money. Interestingly, the limitations posed by the financial realities in Haiti made us want to take responsibility for the finances of the decisions we made; and the absence of someone else's oversight made us realize that a good system needs checks and balances. Similarly, The Joint Commission is responsible for many of the system processes that we must have in place in our health care system. Again, I learned in Haiti that there is value to having a group empowered to think about how health care can be delivered better to keep patients safe. I would have been comforted to think that a group such as The Joint Commission was monitoring the care we delivered in order to maximize its quality. Even with the shortcomings and frustrations of our systems, one learns to appreciate "systems" when systems do not exist.

Credits

Text

Principles of professionalism in text and Table 4-1: From American Board of Pediatrics (2003). Appendix F: professionalism. In: Program director's guide to the ABP: resident evaluation, tracking & certification. Chapel Hill, NC: American Board of Pediatrics.

Definition of professionalism in text in chapter 4: From ACGME Competency definitions: Used with permission of Accreditation Council for Graduate Medical Education (c) ACGME 2011. Please see the ACGME website: www.acgme.org for the most current version.

Definition of interpersonal and communication skills in chapter 5: From ACGME Competency definitions: Used with permission of Accreditation Council for Graduate Medical Education (c) ACGME 2011. Please see the ACGME website: www.acgme.org for the most current version.

Definition of practice-based learning and improvement competency in Table 6-1: From ACGME Competency definitions: Used with permission of Accreditation Council for Graduate Medical Education (c) ACGME 2011. Please see the ACGME website: www.acgme.org for the most current version.

Tables 24-1 and 24-2: From Tanner JM: Growth at Adolescence, 2nd ed. Oxford, England, Blackwell Scientific Publications, 1962, with permission from Wiley.

Systems-Based Practice competency, Chapter 43: Used with permission of the American Academy of Pediatrics, content from http://www.aap.org/visit/coml.htm, copyright American Academy of Pediatrics, 2011.

Section I Appendix 1

ACGME Competency definitions: From ACGME Competency definitions: Used with permission of Accreditation Council for Graduate Medical Education (c) ACGME 2011. Please see the ACGME website: www.acgme.org for the most current version.

Figures

Figures 13-1 through 13-8: Developed by the National Center for Health Statistics in collaboration with the National Center for Chronic Disease Prevention and Health Promotion, 2000.

Figure 13-9: The Recommended Immunization Schedules for Persons Aged 0 through 18 Years are approved by the Advisory Committee on

Immunization Practices (http://www.cdc.gov/vaccines/recs/acip), the American Academy of Pediatrics (http://www.aap.org), and the American Academy of Family Physicians (http://www.aafp.org). From the Centers for Disease Control and Prevention. Available at http://www.cdc.gov/vaccines/recs/schedules/child-schedule.htm#hcp. Centers for Disease Control and Prevention. Recommended immunization schedules for persons aged 0–18 years—United States, 2011. MMWR 2011;60(5).

Figures 16-1 through 16-4, 38-2A and B, 38-3, 38-4 (modified), 38-5 (modified), 99-1: From Zitelli B, Davis HW: Atlas of Pediatric Physical Diagnosis, 5th edition. Copyright 2007, Elsevier.

Figures 17-1, 17-2 (modified), 17-3 (modified), 38-2C, 73-1, 75-1, 83-1: From Kliegman RM, Behrman RE, Jenson HB, Stanton BF: Nelson Textbook of Pediatrics, 18th edition. Copyright 2007, Elsevier.

Figures 24-1 and 24-2: Courtesy of J. M. Tanner, MD, Institute of Child Health, Department for Growth and Development, University of London, London, England.

Figure 38-1: Modified from Drake R, Vogl WA, Mitchell A: Gray's Anatomy for Students, 2nd edition. Copyright 2010, Elsevier.

Figure 39-1: From Wagner EH. Chronic disease management: What will it take to improve care for chronic illness? Effective Clinical Practice. 1998;1:2-4, American College of Physicians.

Figure 60-1: Reproduced with permission from Bhutani, VK, Johnson, L, Sivieri, EM: Predictive ability of a predischarge hour-specific bilirubin for subsequent significant hyperbilirubinemia in healthy term and near-term newborns. Pediatrics, 103: 6-14, Fig. 2, Copyright © 1999 by the AAP.

Figure 60-2: Reproduced with permission from AAP Clinical Practice Guideline. Subcommittee on Hyperbilirubinemia: Management of hyperbilirubinemia in the newborn infant 35 or more weeks of gestation. Pediatrics, 114: 297-316, Fig. 3, Copyright © 2004 by the AAP.

Figure 64-1: From Brenner BM: Brenner and Rector's The Kidney, 8th edition. Copyright 2008, Elsevier.

Figure 66-1: From Osborn L, DeWitt T, First L, Zenel J: Pediatrics. Copyright 2005, Elsevier.

Index

The letter *t* indicates a table, *b* indicates a box, and *f* indicates a figure.